Steves' Review of Nuclear Medicine Technology

Preparation for Certification Examinations

FOURTH EDITION

Norman E. Bolus, MPH, CNMT
Assistant Professor and Director
Nuclear Medicine Technology Program
University of Alabama at Birmingham
School of Health Professions
Birmingham, Alabama

Amy Byrd Brady, BS, CNMT
Teacher, Clinical Coordinator
Nuclear Medicine Technology Program
University of Alabama at Birmingham
School of Health Professions
Birmingham, Alabama

Published by
SOCIETY OF NUCLEAR MEDICINE
1850 Samuel Morse Drive, Reston, VA 20190–5316

Society of Nuclear Medicine, Inc.
1850 Samuel Morse Drive, Reston, VA 20190–5316

Made in the United States of America.

Library of Congress Cataloging-in-Publication Data

Bolus, Norman E., 1965–
Steves' review of nuclear medicine technology : preparation for certification examinations / Norman E. Bolus, Amy Byrd Brady. — 4th ed.
p. ; cm.
Review of nuclear medicine technology
Rev. ed. of: Review of nuclear medicine technology / Ann M. Steves, Patricia C. Wells. 3rd ed. c2004.
Includes bibliographical references.
ISBN 978-0-932004-87-1
1. Nuclear medicine--Examinations--Study guides. I. Brady, Amy Byrd, 1978– II. Steves, Ann M., 1947– Review of nuclear medicine technology. III. Society of Nuclear Medicine (1953–) IV. Title. V. Title: Review of nuclear medicine technology.
[DNLM: 1. Nuclear Medicine--Examination Questions. 2. Radionuclide Imaging—Examination Questions. 3. Technology, Radiologic--Examination Questions. WN 18.2]
R896.S74 2011
616.07'575—dc22

2011007810

Contents

Preface to the Fourth Edition

The *Review of Nuclear Medicine Technology* is now called the ***Steves' Review of Nuclear Medicine Technology*** in honor of Ann M. Steves, MS, CNMT, FSNMT, who has not only helped many nuclear medicine technology students successfully prepare for national certification examinations but has personally helped us prepare for such examinations. We are honored to have been two of the many students of Ann M. Steves, who has contributed so much to previous editions of the *Review Book* and to the field of nuclear medicine as a whole through her many years of service to the field. Ann Steves has been enjoying her retirement since July 2007.

Also, this edition will honor the late Professor Emeritus, Michael A. Thompson, who worked with Ann Steves at the University of Alabama at Birmingham (UAB) School of Health Professions in the Nuclear Medicine Technology Program and was also an instructor to both of us. As an honor to him, a portion of each book sold will go to a Memorial Scholarship Fund in Michael Thompson's name for students in this program.

The fourth edition updates the review book information to bring it in line with the fourth edition of the *Society of Nuclear Medicine (SNM) Curriculum Guide*. This new edition includes computed tomography (CT) and positron emission tomography (PET) instrumentation as integral parts of our field. Other added content from previous editions includes a radiation physics primer, a general introduction to pharmacology, a general counting statistics primer, an introduction to health informatics and research methods, an advanced nuclear cardiology primer, an advanced PET specialty exam primer, and a magnetic resonance imaging (MRI) primer. An effort has been made to update tables, images, and practice exams from previous editions along with the most current NRC regulations.

We thank the many contributors, reviewers, copyeditors, production staff, and all who took the time to review, suggest, comment, and correct parts of this review guide. We also thank our students who helped check many of the question sets and who helped find some of the images that are used in the review book.

It is our sincere hope that this *Review of Nuclear Medicine Technology* continues to be a guide to successfully prepare students for national board exams and as a reference for basic information in our field.

Norman E. Bolus
Amy Byrd Brady
February 2011

Preface to the Third Edition

The *Review of Nuclear Medicine Technology* has been helping nuclear medicine technology students prepare for national certification examinations for 12 years. A companion book of questions with annotated answers, *Preparation for Examinations in Nuclear Medicine Technology,* was published a year after the second edition of the *Review.* This current work combines both books. Chapters of new information covering patient care, instrumentation, and nuclear oncology have been added to the review portion of the book. Previous chapters have been updated and expanded to include topics such as electrocardiography, interventional drugs, and new therapeutic agents. Likewise, the review questions with their answers have been revised and rearranged into five practice examinations. Each practice examination includes 100 questions encompassing the areas of radiopharmacy, instrumentation, clinical procedures, and radiation protection.

The third edition has been in preparation for 2 years. Nuclear medicine has always been a dynamic field, but these 2 years have seen significant changes in nuclear medicine practice. As someone once said, "When you aim for perfection, you find it's a moving target." Although every effort has been made to include the most current information in this book, it is, like nuclear medicine, a work in progress.

One of the strengths of the review and preparation books has been the contributors who share their knowledge and expertise by volunteering to prepare a chapter or write review questions. I acknowledge all the individuals who contributed to this edition as well as to the previous ones. They enrich the work, and our profession is fortunate to have such dedicated members. Thanks are also due to those who worked behind the scenes to make this book a reality, including the Publications and Academic Affairs Committees of the Society of Nuclear Medicine Technologist Section and the publications staff in the Society of Nuclear Medicine office. Very special thanks and appreciation go to Nancy Knight who edited the book.

To all those who have been waiting for the third edition of the *Review,* I hope that it meets your expectations. Authors thrive on criticism. Recommendations for the next edition are welcomed and encouraged.

Ann Steves
stevesa@uab.edu

Note: Authors associated with nuclear medicine technology programs compiled their chapters from instructional materials presented to students in their respective programs. Material included in this book is not intended as a comprehensive review for any national certification examination.

Preface to the Second Edition

There are numerous changes and additions to this new edition. Many of them resulted from the comments and suggestions of individuals who used the first edition. Others occurred because of the innovations and alterations that have occurred in our profession. First, problem sets have been added to Chapter 1, Radiation Protection, and Chapter 3, Radiopharmacy. Solutions to problems are shown in detail in Appendix A. Second, NRC regulations have been updated throughout the text. Also, additional material has been added concerning pharmacologic stress testing, myocardial imaging protocols, and new radiopharmaceuticals such as [^{99m}Tc]sestamibi, [^{99m}Tc]bicisate, [^{89}Sr]chloride, [^{131}I]MIBG, Octreoscan, and OncoScint, among other topics.

Book publication is a detailed and laborious process. It is not possible without the hard work and cooperation of many talented and dedicated individuals.

I acknowledge all those who participated in making the first edition a success. To all those who purchased this book and took the time to contact me with their constructive criticism, I extend my thanks. I appreciated the compliments, but particularly valued the recommendations for the second edition.

I also acknowledge all those who worked to make the second edition a reality. I am particularly grateful to the contributors to the first edition who deemed this endeavor important enough to have a second go at it, and to Tim Baker who agreed to write a chapter after being accepted into medical school. Sheila Cooley and Maria Tyson performed most capably and efficiently as typists. Many other individuals, illustrators, photographers, and other production staff also deserve my thanks and appreciation for their efforts.

Finally, I thank the Publications Committee of the Technologist Section for their support of this project and the publications staff of the Society of Nuclear Medicine for their sage advice and assistance.

A.M.S.
1996

Preface to the First Edition

For some time now, candidates have been seeking a study guide to assist them in preparing for nuclear medicine technology certification examinations. This book was written with that objective in mind. It is intended as a summary of basic nuclear medicine technology practice, and it covers the material usually included on national certification examinations. The book is not designed to provide in-depth instructional content but rather to review the familiar concepts and principles and to emphasize their relation to clinical practice.

Certain topics are not included in this text. First, nuclear medicine technology certification examinations do not address all content areas included in an organized curriculum. Second, some subjects are better covered in other texts, for example, basic nursing care and computers.

The movement to replace the centimeter-gram-second (CGS) system with the meter-kilogram-second (MKS) system, also known as the Système International d'Unité (SI) units, in scientific work has not been completed. Therefore, CGS units as well as MKS (or SI) units are used throughout the text wherever possible. Since CGS units are cited in NRC and DOT regulations, only CGS units are quoted when referring to these regulations. Factors to convert from one system of units to another appear in Appendix F.

A publication of this kind is not possible without the hard work and cooperation of many individuals. Most obvious, of course, are the writers. Since "a picture is worth a thousand words," the colleagues who contributed the nuclear medicine images that appear in this book saved the authors much writing by illustrating their points. Certain individuals gave their permission to reprint previously published images; others such as Bob Bowen, Jackie Bridges, and the technical staff at Baptist Memorial Hospital East, Brad Pounds and Debora Reimers, scoured their patient files to find suitable images. Other colleagues also unselfishly gave their time to review this work and make helpful suggestions. Thanks to the typists and graphic artists who worked behind the scenes to make the book attractive and appealing. Special recognition goes to Lisa Morgan who accepted the challenge and formatted the entire text using a desktop publishing package.

The confidence and support demonstrated by the Publications Committee and the leadership of the Technologist Section during the time it took to complete this project are sincerely appreciated. I am especially grateful to the directors of the Nuclear Medicine Technology Certification Board for their important contribution to this book. Lastly, to the publications staff of the Society of Nuclear Medicine who offered both technical and moral support, go my appreciation and thanks.

A.M.S.
1992

Contributors to the First through Fourth Editions

Timothy Baker, MD
Supervisor, Nuclear Medicine
Walker Baptist Medical Center
Jasper, AL

Norman E. Bolus, MPH, CNMT
Assistant Professor and Director
Nuclear Medicine Technology Program
University of Alabama at Birmingham
School of Health Professions
Birmingham, AL

Crystal Botkin, MPH, CNMT, PET
Clinical Coordinator
Nuclear Medicine Technology Program
Medical Imaging and Radiation Therapeutics
Doisy College of Health Sciences
Saint Louis University
St. Louis, MO

Helen Drew, CNMT
Chief Technologist, In-Patient Services
Nuclear Medicine and Non-Imaging
Division of Nuclear Medicine
Johns Hopkins Hospital
Baltimore, MD

Remo George, MS, CNMT
Assistant Professor
Nuclear Medicine Technology Program
School of Health Professions
University of Alabama at Birmingham
Birmingham, AL

Robert Gladding, CNMT
Director
PET Operations
Miicro, Inc.
Chicago, IL

Amy Byrd Brady, BS, CNMT
Teacher, Clinical Coordinator
Nuclear Medicine Technology Program
University of Alabama at Birmingham
School of Health Professions
Birmingham, AL

William Hubble, MA, CNMT RT(R)(N)(CT), FSNMTS
Academic Chair/NMT Program Director
Associate Professor
Doisy College of Health Sciences
Department of Medical Imaging and Radiation Therapeutics
Saint Louis University
St. Louis, MO

Chalonda Jones-Thomas, MAEd, RT(R)(MR)(CT)(ARRT)
Assistant Professor, CT/MRI Clinical Coordinator
Nuclear Medicine Technology Program
School of Health Professions
University of Alabama at Birmingham
Birmingham, AL

Anthony Knight, MBA, CNMT, RT (N), NCT
Director
Nuclear Medicine Technology Program
University of Iowa Hospitals and Clinics
Iowa City, IA

Vivian Loveless, PharmD, BCNP, FAPhA
Associate Professor
University of Tennessee College of Pharmacy
Memphis, TN

Kathleen Murphy, MS, CNMT, NCT, FSNMTS
Professor and Director
Nuclear Medicine Technology Program
Gateway Community College
North Haven, CT

Liliana Navarrete, MS
Assistant Professor
Nuclear Medicine Technology Program
School of Health Professions
University of Alabama at Birmingham
Birmingham, AL

Pamela Paustian, MS, RHIA
Assistant Professor
Health Sciences Program
University of Alabama at Birmingham
Birmingham, AL

Melanie Stepherson, CNMT
Staff Technologist
Department of Nuclear Medicine
Mariner's Hospital
Islamorada, FL

Ann Steves, MS, CNMT, CPhT, FSNMTS
Associate Professor and Director
Nuclear Medicine Technology Program
School of Health Professions
University of Alabama at Birmingham
Birmingham, AL

Kathy Thomas, MHA, CNMT, FSNMTS
Senior Nuclear Medicine Technologist
City of Hope Medical Center
Duarte, CA

Patricia Wells, MAE, CNMT
Director
Nuclear Medicine Technology Program
Schools of Nursing, Medical Imaging, and Therapeutic Sciences
Muhlenberg Regional Medical Center
Plainfield, NJ

Dusty M. York, MAEd, ARRT(N)(CT), CNMT, PET
Assistant Professor and Clinical Coordinator
Nuclear Medicine Technology Program
Chattanooga State Community College
Chattanooga, TN

Note: Author titles and credentials were current at the time of his or her contribution to each edition.

Contributors to the Practice Examinations First through Fourth Editions

Norman E. Bolus, MPH, CNMT
Assistant Professor and Director
Nuclear Medicine Technology Program
University of Alabama at Birmingham
School of Health Professions
Birmingham, AL

Remo George, MS, CNMT
Assistant Professor
Nuclear Medicine Technology Program
School of Health Professions
University of Alabama at Birmingham
Birmingham, AL

Amy Byrd Brady, BS, CNMT
Teacher, Clinical Coordinator
Nuclear Medicine Technology Program
University of Alabama at Birmingham
School of Health Professions
Birmingham, AL

Elaine Markon, MS, RT(N), CNMT
Assistant Program Director
Nuclear Medicine Institute
The University of Findlay
Findlay, OH

Ann Steves, MS, CNMT, CPhT, FSNMTS
Associate Professor and Director
Nuclear Medicine Technology Program
School of Health Related Professions
University of Alabama at Birmingham
Birmingham, AL

Patricia Wells, MAE, CNMT
Director
Nuclear Medicine Technology Program
Schools of Nursing, Medical Imaging, and Therapeutic Sciences
Muhlenberg Regional Medical Center
Plainfield, NJ

Note: Author titles and credentials were current at the time of his or her contribution to each edition.

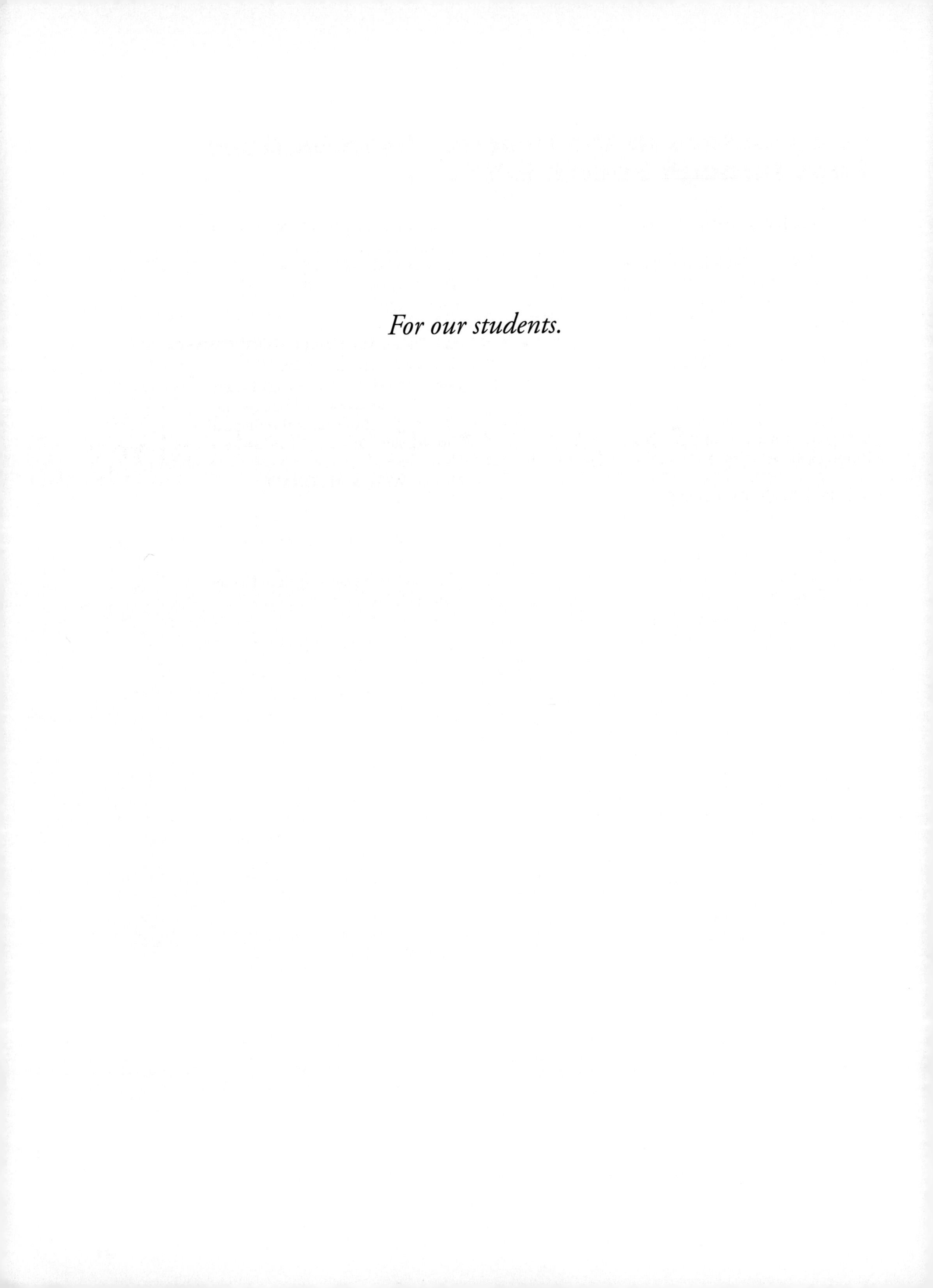

For our students.

PART I

Review of Nuclear Medicine Technology

CHAPTER 1 **Radiation Protection and Federal Regulations**

Patricia Wells, Ann Steves, Remo George, and Norman Bolus

Nearly all activities a nuclear medicine technologist engages in include elements of radiation protection. Prevention of unnecessary radiation exposure to oneself, co-workers, patients, and the general public is a routine part of competent clinical practice. This chapter reviews the principles of radiation protection and the implementation of these principles in the nuclear medicine department. It also reviews the federal agencies and regulations that control the use and handling of radioactive materials as related to nuclear medicine.

Regulatory Agencies

Various federal, state, and local government agencies have authority to regulate the use of radioactive materials. Jurisdiction over certain aspects of regulation is shared by more than one agency. Technologists need to be familiar with regulations at all levels that affect the practice of nuclear medicine technology. However, because the national certification examinations test knowledge of only federal regulations, this chapter discusses the three major federal agencies that control the use of radioactive materials in nuclear medicine practice.

Nuclear Regulatory Commission and State Agencies

The U.S. Nuclear Regulatory Commission (NRC) is responsible for regulation of the purchase, receipt, use, and disposal of radioactive materials. Table 1.1 is a list of reactor by-products and accelerator-produced radionuclides commonly used in nuclear medicine. By agreement with the NRC, some states, known as agreement states, accept responsibility for the regulation of all radioactive materials. If a licensee has its license in an agreement state then the licensee answers only to the state and does not have to answer directly to the NRC. The regulations established by agreement states must be at least as strict as those of the NRC. Federal facilities within the agreement states are regulated by the NRC. Such facilities include Veterans Affairs hospitals and military installations.

Authorization to use radioactive materials in humans is granted by the NRC or state agencies in the form of a facility license. There are several categories of licenses (see Table 1.2): each specifies which radioactive material is authorized for what purposes and who the authorized

Table 1.1 Reactor By-Products and Accelerator-Produced Radionuclides Commonly Used in Nuclear Medicine

Common reactor-produced by-products[a]	
^{99}Mo/^{99m}Tc	^{131}I
^{125}I	^{133}Xe
^{51}Cr	^{89}Sr
^{153}Sm	^{32}P
Common accelerator-produced radionuclides	
^{123}I	^{67}Ga
^{201}Tl	^{111}In
All positron emitters (except ^{82}Rb)	

[a]Some radioisotopes may be produced via an accelerator as well, but extraction techniques make them very costly.

Table 1.2 License Types (Program Codes) for Medical Facilities, Practices, and Laboratories

License title	NUREG-1556 Vol.
The code used depends upon whether licensee is a medical facility, private practice, mobile service, or laboratory	
Medical institution board	9 and 11
Medical institution—written directive required	9
Medical institution—written directive not required	9
Medical private practice—written directive required	9
Medical private practice—written directive not required	9
Mobile medicine service—written directive not required	9
Mobile medical service—written directive required	9
Medical therapy—other emerging technology	9
In vitro testing laboratories[a]	9
Additional license types (program codes) associated with medical use: the code used depends upon the medical device used[b]	
Eye applicators strontium-90	9
High-dose rate remote afterloader	9
Teletherapy	9
Gamma stereotactic radiosurgery	9
Pacemaker by-product and/or SNM—medical institution	17
Pacemaker by-product and/or SNM—individual	17
Source material shielding	17

[a]Not medical use but may be used for medical facilities and practices when it is the only by-product material used.
[b]Does not include research on human subjects. Licensing of individuals as nuclear medicine technologists is controlled only by state agencies. Not all states require licensing.

users are. Authorized users are responsible for supervising individuals working with radioactive materials, determining radiation safety procedures, and establishing dosage activity ranges.

Department of Transportation

The U.S. Department of Transportation (DOT) controls the packaging and interstate movement of hazardous materials, including radioactivity. Transportation of radioactive materials is permitted if adequate safeguards to contain both the material and the radiation it emits are in place. The type of packaging used to ship radioactive materials is classified as Type A or Type B. Type A is adequate for normal transport. Type B packaging is more accident resistant and is used for very large quantities of radioactive material. Most radiopharmaceuticals used in routine nuclear medicine practice are transported in Type A packaging.

Type A packages are labeled according to one of three categories based on the measured dose rate, in milliroentgens per hour (mR/hr), at the package surface and at 1 meter (m) from the surface. The dose rate measured at 1 m from the surface is called the transport index (TI), and it must appear on the label. The label must also specify the radionuclide and the amount of radioactivity contained in the package (Fig. 1.1).

DOT I (white):
- At contact not more than 0.5 mR/hr
- At 3 feet (1 m), no detected radioactivity (NDR)

DOT II (yellow):
- At contact not more then 50 mR/hr
- At 3 feet (1 meter) not more than 1 mR/hr

DOT III (yellow):
- At contact not more than 200 mR/hr
- At 3 feet (1 meter) not more than 10 mR/hr

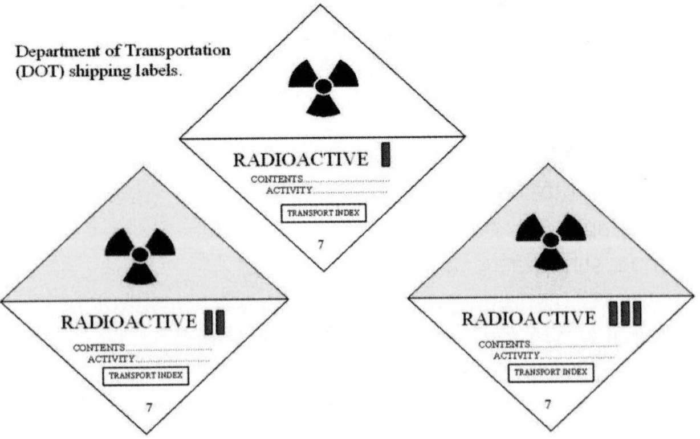

Figure 1.1 DOT I, II, and III shipping labels with limits for each label. (Courtesy of University of Alabama at Birmingham NMT Program Picture Library.)

Food and Drug Administration

The U.S. Food and Drug Administration (FDA) regulates and monitors the manufacture, distribution, safety, and effectiveness of radiopharmaceuticals. Only approved radiopharmaceuticals, those that have a new drug authorization (NDA), can be distributed for sale in the United States. All radiopharmaceuticals must be submitted for review by the FDA before an NDA is issued. A drug that is under investigation by the FDA for future approval is called an investigational new drug (IND) and may be used only in patients under very controlled conditions, which are specified by the FDA. A facility can use an IND only if it has been approved to join the study and the radionuclide is listed on that facility's license. Patients receiving INDs must give informed, written consent before dosage administration. The FDA also classifies devices according to risk. Only the highest-risk devices, such as mechanical heart valves and implantable infusion pumps, as well as some radiation therapy devices and equipment, require FDA approval before marketing. To receive FDA approval for these devices, the manufacturer must demonstrate that its devices provide a reasonable assurance of safety and effectiveness.

Federal Regulations

Selected federal regulations of the NRC, DOT, and FDA pertinent to nuclear medicine technologist certification are listed in Appendix A at the end of this book.

Practical Methods for Reducing Radiation Exposure

Three factors are involved in reducing external radiation exposure: time, distance, and shielding.

Time

Minimizing the amount of time spent in a radiation area (or radiation field) will limit the total radiation received. Practical applications of the time factor include working efficiently when handling radioactive materials and practicing new procedures with nonradioactive materials until the desired speed and accuracy are attained. The following equation is used to calculate the total radiation dose on the basis of the length of exposure, and the radiation dose rate (the dose per unit time) is used:

$$\text{total dose} = (\text{dose rate})(\text{time}).$$

Example 1. A technologist is standing next to a source that produces 0.5 mR/hr. What radiation dose will she receive if she remains there for 1.5 hr?

$$X = (0.5\ \text{mR/hr})(1.5\ \text{hr}) = 0.75\ \text{mR}.$$

Example 2. What will the radiation dose be to a technologist who handles a radioactive source for 5 min, if the source is producing 30 mR/hr?

$$X = \left(\frac{30 \text{ mR/hr}}{60 \text{ min/hr}}\right)(5 \text{ min}) = 2.5 \text{ mR}$$

(or $X = 30$ mR/hr $\times$ 1 hr/60 min $\times$ 5 min = 2.5 mR).

Distance

Increasing the distance from a radiation source will decrease the amount of radiation received. The radiation dose rate (the dose per unit time) from a small-volume radiation source varies inversely with the square of the distance from the source. This relationship is called the inverse square law. By doubling the distance, the radiation dose rate is reduced to one-fourth of the original. If the distance is halved, the dose rate is increased to four times the original. Table 1.3 outlines the steps taken to ascertain the new radiation dose resulting from a given change in distance.

The formula for the inverse square law is expressed as

$$(I_1)(D_1)^2 = (I_2)(D_2)^2$$

where I_1 is the dose rate (intensity) at distance D_1 from the source and I_2 is the dose rate (intensity) at distance D_2 from the source.

Example 1. If 10 mR/hr are measured at 3 m, what is the dose rate at 0.5 m?

$$(10 \text{ mR/hr})(3 \text{ m})^2 = (I_2)(0.5 \text{ m})^2$$

$$I_2 = \left(\frac{(20 \text{ mR/hr})(9 \text{ m}^2)}{0.25 \text{ m}^2}\right) = 360 \text{ mR/hr.}$$

Example 2. If 50 mR/hr are measured at 3 in. from a source, at what distance will 0.5 mR/hr be measured?

$$(50 \text{ mR/hr})(3 \text{ in.})^2 = (0.5 \text{ mR/hr})(D_2)^2$$

$$(D_2)^2 = \frac{(50 \text{ mR/hr})(9 \text{ in.}^2)}{0.5 \text{ mR/hr}}$$

$$(D_2)^2 = 900 \text{ in.}^2$$

$D_2 = 30$ in. (square root derived on both sides)

Practical applications of the distance factor include using tongs to handle vials of radioactive materials, storing radioactive materials away from high-occupancy areas, and using restraint devices to hold patients in position.

Table 1.3 Application of Inverse Square Law

Distance factor	Distance factor squared	Inverse square
2	$2^2 = 4$	$\frac{1}{4}$
3	$3^2 = 9$	$\frac{1}{9}$
4	$4^2 = 16$	$\frac{1}{16}$
$\frac{1}{2}$	$(\frac{1}{2})^2 = \frac{1}{4}$	4

Shielding

Shielding involves the use of a material, usually lead, leaded glass, or tungsten, to absorb the radiation transmitted from a source. The type of radiation determines the type of shielding to be used. Alpha particles, which are not currently used clinically (but may be used as radiotherapeutics in the near future), can be completely stopped by a sheet of paper. Complete absorption of beta particles can be achieved with only a few millimeters (mm) of plastic. Therefore, a plastic syringe provides adequate shielding of beta emissions.

Lead vial and syringe shields should not be used to shield a beta emitter, such as phosphorus-32 or strontium-89, because bremsstrahlung will be produced. Bremsstrahlung is radiation that results from the deceleration of the beta particles as they approach the nuclei of the lead atoms in the shield. As the beta particles slow down, they lose energy, which is released in the form of X rays. The amount of bremsstrahlung increases with the density of the material through which the beta particles pass. Consequently, a low-density material, such as plastic or Lucite, is recommended to absorb beta particles and to reduce the amount of bremsstrahlung produced in the shielding material.

For X and gamma rays, lead, leaded glass, or tungsten shielding is used to reduce, rather than completely absorb, the radiation emitted from a source. The ability of a material to absorb or attenuate X and gamma rays is expressed as the half-value layer (HVL). The HVL is defined as the thickness of a material required to reduce the radiation intensity to half its original value (Fig. 1.2). The effect of adding HVLs is seen in Table 1.4, which can be used to determine the decrease in exposure rate. A specific HVL is related to the photon energies of the X or gamma radiation as well as the type of shielding material (Table 1.5). This equation can also be used to calculate the exposure rate after shielding is added or the amount of shielding needed to decrease exposure to a desired level,

$$I = I_0 e^{-(0.693)(x/\text{HVL})},$$

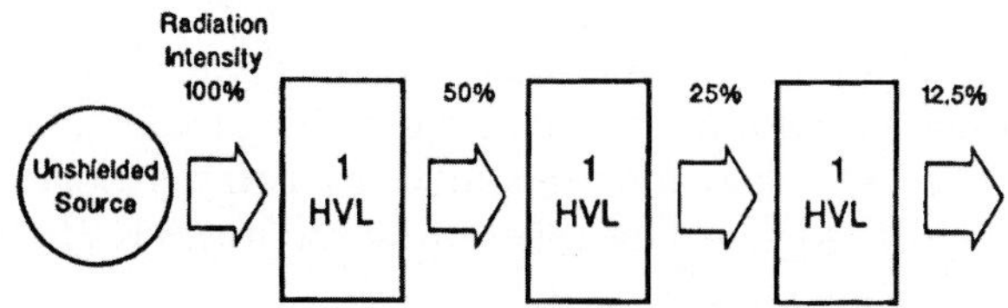

Figure 1.2 One half-value layer (HVL) of shielding material reduces radiation intensity to one-half of the original intensity. An additional HVL will halve radiation intensity again and so on.

Table 1.4 Effect of HVL

Number of HVLs	Percentage of original exposure rate (%)	Fraction of original exposure rate
1	50	0.50
2	25	0.25
3	12.5	0.125
4	6.3	0.063
5	3.1	0.031
6	1.6	0.016
7	0.8	0.008
8	0.4	0.004
9	0.2	0.002
10	0.1	0.001

Table 1.5 HVL of Lead for Selected Radionuclides

Radionuclide	Primary photon energy (keV)	HVL of lead (mm)
^{125}I	27.5	0.04
^{99m}Tc	140	0.27
^{51}Cr	320	2.0
^{131}I	364	3.0
^{18}F	511	4.1
^{137}Cs	662	6.5

where x is the thickness of shielding used, and HVL is the half-value layer for a specific shielding material and radionuclide. e is for the exponential in this equation. (For a review of the application of this equation, refer to *Practical Mathematics in Nuclear Medicine Technology.*) Some prefer the following equation instead of the previous one,

$$I = I_0 (0.5)^{x/\text{HVL}},$$

where x is the thickness of shielding used, and HVL is the half-value layer for a specific shielding material and radionuclide.

Positron emitters produce high-energy photons of 511 kiloelectron volts (keV), so heavy shielding is required. A number of 511-keV syringe shields and unit dose shields are now available. Remote injection systems should be used to decrease the radiation dose to the technologist during administration of positron-emitting tracers.

Example 1. If a source is producing an exposure rate of 45 mR/hr, what will the exposure rate be after 5 HVLs of shielding are placed over it?

From Table 1.4, 5 HVLs reduce the exposure rate to 3.1% of the original:

$$(45 \text{ mR/hr})(0.031) = 1.4 \text{ mR/hr}.$$

Example 2. The exposure rate from a source of iodine-131 (^{131}I) is 60 mR/hr. What will the exposure rate be if 12 mm of lead are used to shield it and 1 HVL = 3 mm?

$$\frac{12 \text{ mm}}{3 \text{ mm}} = 4 \text{ HVL}.$$

From Table 1.4, 4 HVL will decrease the exposure rate to 6.3% of the original:

$$(60 \text{ mR/hr})(0.063) = 3.8 \text{ mR/hr}.$$

Vial and syringe shields (which can reduce exposure by more than 90%), lead bricks (which can effectively attenuate and reduce exposure by 100%), and leaded-glass L-blocks (which vary in thickness and density) are all shielding devices that effectively reduce personnel radiation exposure.

Internal Exposure

Internal radiation exposure can result when radionuclides are inhaled, ingested, or absorbed through the skin. The following steps are recommended practices to minimize the possibility of internal contamination while working in the nuclear medicine department.

1. Refrain from eating, drinking, or smoking in areas where radionuclides are used.
2. Use automatic pipettes to measure or transfer radioactive solutions.
3. Wear protective clothing, such as lab coats and gloves, when handling radionuclides or objects that may be radioactive.
4. Monitor hands, clothing, and shoes after working with radionuclides.
5. Clean up radioactive spills promptly.
6. When working with ^{131}I solutions, keep vials tightly capped and open them only in a fume hood.
7. When performing lung ventilation studies with radioactive gases, ensure that gas trapping and room ventilation systems are working efficiently.

Personnel Monitoring

External radiation exposure levels received by nuclear medicine personnel can be documented with various dosimeter devices. The following types of dosimeters are most commonly used to measure personnel exposure.

Film Badges

The film badge consists of a plastic holder in which a strip of photographic film is held between a set of filters. After development, the amount of darkening (density) on the film is proportional to the amount of radiation absorbed. The three or four filters are each made of a different material (lead, copper, aluminum, plastic) so that the energy range and penetration of the radiation striking the badge can be assessed. The film badge holder also has an opening where the film can be exposed to beta particles and low-energy photons. Film badges are effective in measuring radiation exposures of 0.1 millisieverts (mSv) (10 mrem) to several sieverts (several hundred rem).

Film badges should be worn between the waist and the shoulder at the site of the highest exposure rate to the body. Because the latent image on the film tends to fade over time, it is recommended that film badges be processed monthly. The film in these badges is adversely affected by heat and moisture.

Thermoluminescent Dosimeters

A thermoluminescent dosimeter (TLD) uses special material, typically lithium fluoride crystals, that emits a quantity of light proportional to the amount of radiation absorbed by the crystals. The light is released and measured when the crystals are heated to an extremely high temperature. Filters may also be used in TLDs to distinguish nonpenetrating from penetrating radiation.

Although this type of dosimeter is more expensive than a film dosimeter, it is not readily affected by environmental conditions such as humidity and temperature. It does not fog with age as film does, so it can be used for 2 or 3 months if needed.

Because of the small size of the crystals, it is possible to use TLDs in the form of rings to monitor hand exposure. Ring badges should be worn on the forefinger of the dominant hand with the crystal facing the palm of the hand.

Optically Stimulated Luminescence Dosimeters

An optically stimulated luminescence dosimeter (OSL) uses a thin slice of aluminum oxide to detect radiation exposure. It is inserted into a light-proof envelope and placed in a cover that contains various filters. A laser is used to read the badge when it is returned to the supplier. Like a TLD, the OSL is resistant to heat, moisture, and aging. It is also more sensitive than a film badge and can be used to monitor a person over a longer period of time, up to 3 months.

Pocket Ionization Chambers

Pocket ionization chambers are useful supplementary monitoring devices. Immediate radiation exposure measurements are provided through a scale in the dosimeter itself or through a separate reading device. The amount of ionization is directly related to the amount of radiation exposure. Pocket dosimeters are expensive compared with film badges and TLDs and require careful handling to prevent inaccurate readings.

Nuclear Regulatory Commission Regulations

As of March 2010, NRC regulations are based on a risk-informed, performance-based approach. "Performance based" means the NRC will not, for the most part, specify exactly what methods must be used or how frequently radiation safety procedures must be performed. Instead, the licensee must develop policies and procedures that ensure that NRC requirements are met. The risk-informed approach has been adopted because scientific data have not demonstrated any health risk from radiation doses at or below the occupational limits set by the NRC. However, the NRC does require licensees to adopt practices that minimize radiation exposure to workers and to the general public as much as reasonably possible.

Radiation Exposure Dose Limits

Radiation exposure dose limits are expressed as dose equivalents. General exposure is measured with the total effective dose equivalent (TEDE), which is defined as the sum of the deep dose equivalent (DDE) and the committed effective dose equivalent (CEDE). The DDE refers to exposure to the internal organs from external sources, whereas the CEDE refers to exposure to the internal organs from internal sources. Because instances of internal exposure are rare in nuclear medicine technologists, the TEDE is essentially equivalent to the DDE. The shallow dose equivalent (SDE) is used to calculate the exposure to the skin or any appendage. The exposure limits do not include medical exposures received by individuals for their own healthcare.

The dose to the embryo/fetus of an occupationally exposed female can be calculated only after the woman has voluntarily provided a written declaration of pregnancy. After she declares her pregnancy, she becomes a "declared pregnant worker" and fetal monitoring for exposure is then required.

Table 1.6 lists the TEDE limits for occupationally exposed workers, the general public, and the embryo/fetus.

ALARA

To increase awareness of radiation protection techniques and to reduce occupational radiation exposure, the NRC subscribes to a philosophy called "as low as reasonably achievable" (ALARA). Individuals who practice the ALARA concept attempt to keep their radiation exposure as low as possible within the reasonable constraints of cost and patient needs.

Radiation Protection Programs

The NRC requires licensees to develop, document, and implement radiation protection programs that are appro-

Table 1.6 U.S. NRC Radiation Exposure Limits

Exposure	Millisieverts (rem)
Occupational exposures	
Whole-body TEDE[a]	50 (5)/year
Lens of eye (LDE)[b]	150 (15)/year
Any organ or tissue TEDE	500 (50)/year
Skin or any extremity (SDE)[c]	500 (50)/year
Member of general public TEDE	1 (0.1)/year
Embryo/fetus of occupationally exposed worker	5 (0.5) for entire pregnancy

[a]Total effective dose equivalent.
[b]Eye (lens) dose equivalent.
[c]Shallow dose equivalent.

priate for the amounts and types of radioactive materials being used at the facility. The licensee is also required to use procedures and engineering to help keep radiation exposure to workers and members of the general public ALARA.

Bioassays

A bioassay is any measurement of radioactivity that has been internalized by an individual (Fig. 1.3). This may be done as external counting or counting biological samples such as urine, blood, or other bodily fluids. Monitoring of thyroid uptake in personnel who handle volatile radionuclides is required if there is a possibility that inhaled activity exceeds NRC limits. In nuclear medicine departments, the most likely situation in which this may occur is with high therapeutic dosages of [^{131}I]sodium iodide.

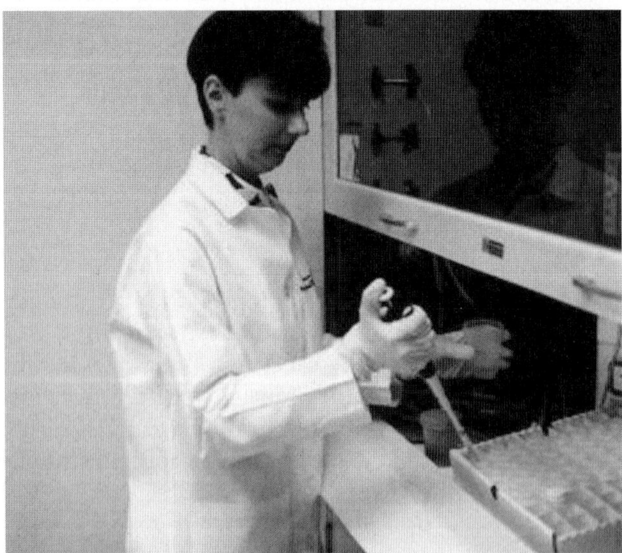

Figure 1.3 Typical bioassay of urine and/or blood samples. (Courtesy of University of Alabama at Birmingham NMT Program Picture Library.)

Radiation Areas

For purposes of radiation control, the NRC defines restricted and unrestricted areas. An unrestricted area is one in which access is not limited by or under the direct control of the licensee. Radiation levels in an unrestricted area must be such that anyone who is in the area will receive less than 0.02 mSv (2 mrem) in any 1 hr. If this radiation limit is exceeded, then the area is considered restricted and access to that area must be controlled. For example, in a nuclear medicine department, reception and waiting areas are unrestricted, whereas imaging rooms are restricted.

The NRC requires that restricted areas be posted with specific signs depending on the radiation level present (Fig. 1.4). Such signs display the conventional magenta radiation symbol on a yellow background with one of the following phrases.

- *Caution: radioactive materials*
  - These words are used to indicate any area in which certain quantities of radioactive materials are used or stored.
  - Found on entrances to work areas and nuclear medicine labs.
  - Indicate the potential presence of radiation sources and/or contamination.
  - Ingestion of food or drink is strictly prohibited in these areas.
  - No smoking or application of cosmetics is allowed in these areas.
  - Table 1.7 lists the radionuclides commonly used in the nuclear medicine department, with the amounts that require posting.
- *Caution: radiation area*
  - These words are used to denote areas in which an individual could receive more than 0.05 mSv (5 mrem) in 1 hour at 30 centimeters (cm) from the radiation source.
  - Commonly seen at entrances to nuclear medicine labs.
- *Caution: high radiation area*
  - These words are used to designate areas in which an individual could receive more than 1 mSv (100 mrem) in 1 hr at 30 cm from the radiation source.
  - Commonly seen in areas where radiation therapy is performed.
- *Grave danger: very high radiation area*
  - These words are used to designate an area in which an individual could receive an absorbed dose of more than 5 Grays, Gy (500 rad), in 1 hr at 1 m from the radiation source.
  - Not commonly seen in the hospital setting.

Table 1.7 Quantities of Selected Radionuclides Requiring Posting with "Caution: Radioactive Materials" Sign (U.S. NRC)

Radionuclide	Quantities exceeding
^{99m}Tc, ^{201}Tl, ^{67}Ga, ^{133}Xe, ^{51}Cr	10 mCi
^{111}In, ^{123}I, ^{153}Sm, ^{99}Mo, ^{57}Co	1 mCi
^{89}Sr, ^{32}P, ^{137}Cs	100 μCi
^{131}I, ^{125}I	10 μCi

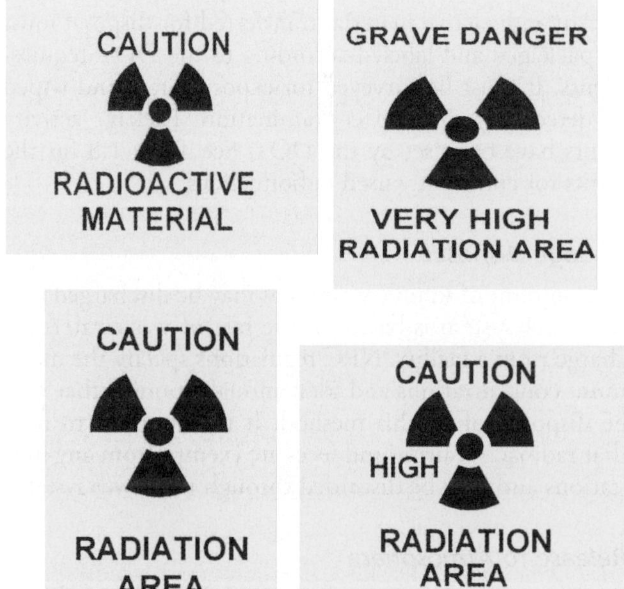

Figure 1.4 Radioactive caution signs. (Courtesy of University of Alabama at Birmingham NMT Program Picture Library.)

Receipt of Radioactive Materials

The NRC requires that all shipments of radioactive materials displaying a radioactive label (White I, Yellow II, or Yellow III; Figs. 1.1 and 1.2) be checked for contamination using a wipe test. They should be visually inspected for damage or to see if they are wet. A survey meter must be used to determine the exposure rate at 1 m and at the surface of the package. All surfaces must be checked when performing wipes or surveys. Packages must be monitored within 3 hr of receipt during regular working hours or, if they are delivered after hours, within 3 hr of the time the department reopens.

The procedure for monitoring and opening radioactive shipments includes the following stepped instructions:

1. Visually inspect the package for signs of damage or moisture.
2. If there are signs of damage or moisture, measure exposure rates at the package surface and at a distance of 1 m from the surface. If the exposure rate exceeds 200 mR/hr at the surface or 10 mR/hr at 1 m from the surface, the NRC and the carrier delivering the shipment must be notified immediately. Notification is usually accomplished through the institution's radiation safety officer (RSO).
3. Wipe the external surface of the package, assay the wipe, and decontaminate the exterior surface as required. If removable contamination exceeds 22 disintegrations per minute (dpm)/cm^2 (or 6600 dpm for a wiped surface area of 300 cm^2—which is approximately the size of an 8 × 11 in. standard piece of paper), notify the NRC and the carrier through the RSO.
4. After opening the package, verify that the contents match the packing slip and check the integrity of the radionuclide container.
5. Monitor the packaging material for contamination and remove the radiation labels before discarding the packaging material. If the materials are contaminated, dispose of them as radioactive waste.

The NRC requires wipe test readings to be recorded in disintegrations per minute. The efficiency of the well counter must be known to convert counts per minute (cpm) to disintegrations per minute using the following equation:

$$\text{efficiency} = \frac{\text{net cpm}}{\text{dpm}}.$$

Storage of Radioactive Materials

To comply with the principles of ALARA, radioactive materials that are being stored for later use must be shielded to minimize radiation levels in the work area. Vial shields and lead bricks usually provide sufficient protection. Vial shields and syringe shields must be labeled to identify the radiopharmaceutical and must be labeled with the radiation symbol. Storage areas must be posted with the appropriate radiation signs. If access to these areas cannot be limited, then these areas must be locked when nuclear medicine personnel are not present.

Certain radioactive materials may have additional storage requirements. Volatility of liquid radioactive sodium iodide can be minimized if the solution is kept refrigerated. Dosages of liquid [^{131}I]sodium iodide should be prepared under a fume hood.

Radioactive Waste Disposal

Radioactive materials must be disposed of carefully to limit exposure to occupationally exposed workers and members of the general public (Fig. 1.5).

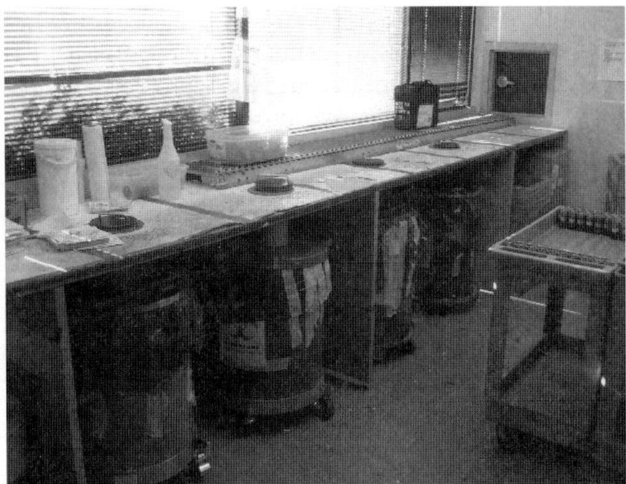

Figure 1.5 Typical radioactive waste storage area and separation of different radionuclides. (Courtesy of Cardinal Health Pharmacy, Birmingham, AL.)

Decay in Storage

Radioactive materials with a half-life of less than 120 days can be retained in a shielded storage area until they have decayed to a level of activity that equals background. (Commonly referred to as a "rule of thumb," one would decay the radioactive product for at least 10 half-lives before considering to discard it in regular or biological hazard trash.) When waste is placed in storage, it should be labeled with the date and the identity of the longest-lived radionuclide in the container.

For convenience, radioactive waste is separated according to half-life. Technetium-99m (^{99m}Tc) waste typically is segregated from other longer-lived waste such as thallium-201 and gallium-67, which have half-lives of approximately 3.0 and 3.3 days, respectively. Shorter-lived waste can then be disposed of more frequently than longer-lived waste to save storage space.

After the waste has been allowed to decay to background levels, it can be disposed of as regular garbage, after all radioactive labels have been defaced or removed. The labels may be left intact if the decayed materials are in containers that will be treated as biomedical waste. If the waste contains potentially biohazardous materials (used needles, syringes, etc.), it should be discarded with other biomedical waste.

Transfer to Authorized Recipient

Unused unit dosages and used dosage receptacles are usually returned to the commercial radiopharmacy that provided them. Long-lived radioactive waste, such as expired sealed sources, can be disposed of by transferring the material to an authorized commercial waste handler. Such companies either bury the material at an approved site or incinerate the waste.

Table 1.8 Package Limits for Shipment of Radioactive Waste Returned to Commercial Pharmacies

Radionuclide	Activity in MBq (mCi)
^{133}Xe	2000 (54.1)
^{201}Tl	1000 (27.0)
^{99m}Tc	800 (21.6)
^{67}Ga, ^{123}I	600 (16.2)
^{111}In	200 (5.4)
^{131}I, ^{89}Sr	50 (1.4)

Any radioactive material transferred for disposal must be packaged and labeled according to the DOT requirements. It must be surveyed for exposure rate and wiped to detect any external contamination. Package activity limits have been set by the DOT. See Table 1.8 for the limits for commonly used radionuclides.

Sewage Disposal

The amount of soluble waste that may be discharged into the sewer system is based on the rate of wastewater discharge from a facility. NRC regulations specify the maximum concentrations and total annual amounts that may be disposed of by this method. It is important to note that radioactive urine and feces are exempt from any limitations and may be discarded through the sewer system.

Release to Atmosphere

Radioactive gases may be discharged directly into the atmosphere in limited quantities. Maximum airborne concentrations are specified in the NRC regulations. The quantities of xenon-133 released by most nuclear medicine departments will not exceed these levels.

Regardless of the method of waste disposal used, records of the disposal must be maintained to document compliance with regulations.

Minimizing Contamination

The NRC requires licensees to use facility design and operational procedures to minimize contamination. This includes using nonporous materials where radioactive materials are prepared or stored, minimizing the number of areas where material is stored, and performing surveys with a frequency that will identify contamination. Plastic-backed absorbent pads should be used in preparation and administration areas to facilitate cleanup if spills occur.

Surveys for Contamination

Personnel must use a survey meter to check for contamination of their hands and feet before leaving the facility and should do the same before leaving for a meal. Personnel should survey their hands frequently.

Routine surveys of the nuclear medicine facility are required if workers are likely to receive more than 10% of the allowable limit for internal or external exposure or if members of the general public are likely to receive an exposure of more than 0.1 rem in an unrestricted area (Fig. 1.6). Frequent surveys should be performed for an adequate period of time that will permit the licensee to determine whether either of these criteria apply. If they do not, then surveys can be performed less frequently, such as weekly or even monthly. The use of long-term dosimeters placed in areas of highest exposure can also be used to determine whether frequent surveys are necessary.

Surveys should be performed more frequently, at least temporarily, when new personnel are hired, new procedures are instituted, or contamination is occurring. Surveys must be performed at the end of the day whenever therapeutic radionuclides are administered. Areas where the dosage was prepared and administered must be surveyed.

A properly calibrated survey meter must be used when performing surveys. The instrument must be sufficiently sensitive. When a trigger level is reached during surveys, the RSO must be notified. The trigger level must be set at no less than 0.05 mSv/hr (5 mrem/hr) for restricted areas and 2 μSv/hr (0.2 mrem/hr) for unrestricted areas.

Wipe Test for Removable Contamination

Routine wipe tests are performed using the same criteria as those required for surveys. Once the licensee has established that the criteria do not apply, then infrequent wipe tests can be performed on a monthly or even quarterly basis. Wipe test frequency should be increased whenever survey frequency is increased.

Wipe tests must be analyzed using an appropriate instrument, such as a well counter or an uncollimated gamma camera. The RSO must be notified if a trigger level of 22 dpm per cm^2 of removable contamination for beta- and gamma-emitting radionuclides is reached in either a restricted or unrestricted area.

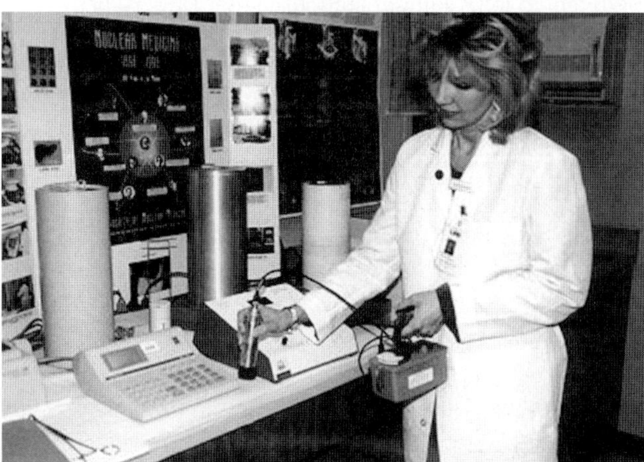

Figure 1.6 Typical survey of countertop work area. (Courtesy of University of Alabama at Birmingham NMT Program Picture Library.)

NRC regulations state that area survey and wipe records must be retained for 3 years. The record must include the date the survey was performed, the results, the instrument used, and the name of the individual who performed the survey.

Spill Procedures

Minor radioactive spills involving a small area or a relatively low radiation dose rate occasionally occur. The procedure for handling minor contamination is as follows:

1. Notify all persons in the immediate vicinity that a spill has occurred.
2. Contain the spill by placing absorbent material over liquids. Limit movement in the area until the extent of the spill is known and the area is isolated.
3. If clothing is contaminated, remove it before leaving the spill site. If skin is contaminated, wash it as soon as possible with warm water and soap. The use of abrasive cleansers and brushes to clean the skin should be avoided, because these can increase absorption, as can hot water.
4. Wear appropriate protective clothing, such as disposable gloves and shoe covers.
5. Place all materials used to clean the spill into plastic bags and dispose of them as radioactive waste.
6. Use a survey meter and wipe tests to determine whether all removable contamination has been removed.
7. Use absorbent paper and/or shielding to cover the area of the spill if activity remains after decontamination. Label the paper or shield with "Caution: Radioactive Material."
8. Report the spill to the RSO.

Major spills involving widespread areas of contamination or a high radiation dose rate are managed differently. The following procedure should be used:

1. Clear the immediate area. Notify all personnel not involved with the spill to leave the area.
2. Use absorbent paper to prevent the spread of contamination, but do not attempt to clean the spill.
3. Limit movement of contaminated personnel to prevent spread of contamination. Remove contaminated clothing before leaving the area.
4. Evacuate and close all doors to the area. Lock the doors or secure area to prevent entry.
5. Notify the RSO immediately. Cleanup and decontamination of major spills should be conducted under the supervision of the RSO.

6. Decontaminate personnel as described previously. The treatment of serious injuries always takes precedence over decontamination.

See Table 1.9 for a list of selected radionuclides and the amount of radioactivity that the NRC considers a major spill.

Radiopharmaceutical Preparation and Administration

An individual prescription, referred to as a written directive, is required for each individual patient who receives a therapeutic dosage of radionuclide. The authorized user also must establish a dosage range or a target dosage with percentage variation limits for each radiopharmaceutical for each type of diagnostic examination. For example, the authorized user may designate the dosage range for a bone scan as 555–925 MBq (15–25 mCi) [^{99m}Tc]oxidronate. The dosage must fall within this range, so nothing less than 555 MBq (15 mCi) or more than 925 MBq (25 mCi) could be administered to a patient. As an alternative, the target dosage can be set as 740 MBq (20 mCi) ±20%. In this case the acceptable range would be 592–888 MBq (16–24 mCi). Dosages above or below these limits may not be used. A dosage that falls outside the established range can be used only with written approval by the authorized user for the individual patient.

The authorized user should establish a standard method for determining pediatric dosages. Any dosage prepared from a bulk solution must be calibrated in a dose calibrator before administration to the patient. When a unit dosage supplied by a central radiopharmacy is used, a decay computation can be applied to determine the activity before administration. If the dosage has been manipulated (i.e., some radiopharmaceutical has been removed), then the dosage must again be calibrated in a dose calibrator before it can be administered.

Dosage records, which must be retained for 3 years, must include the patient's name and identification number (if one is used), radiopharmaceutical, prescribed dosage, actual dosage, time and date of determination, and name of the person calibrating the dosage.

Dosage Misadministration: A Medical Event

The NRC refers to a radiopharmaceutical misadministration as a medical event and clearly defines this term using two factors: error and excess exposure. The errors are as follows: the wrong radiopharmaceutical is administered, the dosage is administered to the wrong person, the dosage is administered by the wrong route, or the dosage differs from the prescribed dosage by more than 20% or falls outside the prescribed range. Excess exposure is defined as exceeding the following limits: 50 mSv (5 rem) effective dose equivalent, 500 mSv (50 rem) to any organ or tissue, or 500 mSv (50 rem) SDE to skin. *A medical event has occurred only when both an error and excess exposure have occurred.*

Other medical events defined in Title 10 Code of Federal Regulations (CFR) Part 35 include events in which a dose to an embryo or fetus exceeds 50 mSv (5 rem) from administration of by-product material to the mother without the approval of the authorized user, or if, as determined by a physician, there has been an unintended permanent functional damage to an organ or a physiological system of a patient or patient's lactating infant, following dose from the radiopharmaceutical administration. Written directives involving therapeutic amounts of ionizing radiation can lead to reportable events including the fetal exposures mentioned here. Generally, for most

Table 1.9 Major Spill Activities (U.S. NRC)

Activity (mCi)	Radionuclides
1	^{131}I, ^{32}P, ^{89}Sr
10	^{67}Ga, ^{111}In, ^{123}I
100	^{99m}Tc, ^{201}Tl

Table 1.10 Various Radiation Exposure/Event Cases and When the NRC Requires a Report to Be Given

Radiation exposure/event	Report to NRC within
Theft or loss of licensed material in quantities greater than 1.00 mCi—^{131}I 10.00 mCi—^{90}Y, ^{89}Sr, ^{32}P 100.00 mCi—^{153}Sm	Immediately
Fires or explosions causing excessive exposures	4 hr
Accidental administration of spreadable contamination	24 hr
>5.0 rem to fetus without authorized user physician approval	24 hr
>5.0 rem to nursing child causing organ or system damage	24 hr
Medical events	24 hr
Leaking sealed source	5 days
>0.1 rem to public	30 days
>5.0 rem to worker	30 days
>0.5 rem to minor	30 days
>0.05 rem/month, or >0.5 rem fetal dose	30 days
>20 mR/hr in unrestricted area	30 days
Theft or loss of licensed material in quantities greater than: 0.01 mCi—^{131}I 0.10 mCi—^{137}Cs, ^{32}P, ^{89}Sr, ^{90}Y 1.00 mCi—^{57}Co, ^{111}In, ^{123}I, ^{153}Sm 10.00 mCi—^{99m}Tc, ^{201}Tl, ^{67}Ga, ^{133}Xe, ^{18}F	30 days

diagnostic nuclear medicine studies, the NRC-defined medical events are not reportable (see 10CFR35).

The NRC must be notified of a medical event by telephone no later than the next calendar day. No patient identifiers must be used when communicating to the NRC to protect patient privacy. The technologist should notify the authorized user and RSO as soon as a medical event occurs so that these individuals can inform the NRC, the referring physician, and the patient (Table 1.10).

Release of Patients after Administration of Therapeutic Radiopharmaceuticals

A person who has received a therapeutic dosage of radiopharmaceutical can be released if it is determined that no individual in contact with the patient will receive more than 5 mSv (0.5 rem). If any person is likely to receive more than 1 mSv (0.1 rem) from the patient, then the patient must be given written instructions on how to minimize exposure to others.

References and Further Reading

Bixler A, Springer G, Lovas, R, 1999. Practical aspects of radiation safety for using fluorine-18. *J Nucl Med Technol.* 27:14–16.

Cherry SR, Sorenson JA, Phelps ME, 2003. *Physics in Nuclear Medicine.* 3rd ed. Philadelphia, PA: Saunders; 427–441.

Early PJ, Sodee DB,1995. *Principles and Practice of Nuclear Medicine.* 2nd ed. St. Louis, MO: Mosby; 323–325.

Federal Register Notice, 2002. Washington, DC: U.S. Government Printing Office; April 24.

Moore MM, 2004. Radiation safety in nuclear medicine. In: Christian PE, Bernier DR, Langan JK, eds. *Nuclear Medicine and PET: Technology and Techniques.* 5th ed. St. Louis, MO: Mosby; 184–210.

Powsner RA, Powsner ER, 1998. *Essentials of Nuclear Medicine Physics.* Malden, MA: Blackwell Science; 182–187.

Saha BS, 2003. *Physics and Radiobiology of Nuclear Medicine.* 2nd ed. New York, NY: Springer-Verlag.

Siegel JA, 2004. *Guide for Diagnostic Nuclear Medicine and Radiopharmaceutical Therapy.* Reston, VA: Society of Nuclear Medicine; 3–6, 9–13, 25–66, 81–105.

U.S. Nuclear Regulatory Commission, 2008. *Program-Specific Guidance about Medical Use Licenses.* NUREG-1556, Volume 9. Washington, DC: Nuclear Regulatory Commission.

U.S. Nuclear Regulatory Commission, 2009. *Federal Regulations.* Title 10, Chapter 1, Energy, Part 20. Washington, DC: U.S. Government Printing Office; January 1.

U.S. Pharmacopoeia Convention, 2000. *United State Pharmacopoeia 24* and *The National Formulary 19.* Rockville, MD: U.S. Pharmacopoeial.

Wells P, 1999. *Practical Mathematics in Nuclear Medicine Technology.* Reston, VA: Society of Nuclear Medicine; 81–82, 140–146, 154–158.

CHAPTER 2 **Patient Care**

Ann Steves, Chalonda Jones-Thomas, and Amy Byrd Brady

Basic patient care skills are integral to nuclear medicine technology practice. The patient typically is under the care of the technologist while in the nuclear medicine facility and may need care not directly related to the nuclear medicine examination. Certain skills (for example, administering an intravenous injection, performing cardiopulmonary resuscitation, or monitoring blood pressure) may be required as part of a nuclear medicine procedure.

Receiving the Patient

Patients should be acknowledged immediately upon entering the nuclear medicine facility. The technologist should keep in mind that the relationship with a patient begins as soon as the technologist introduces him- or herself. Greeting the patient establishes a rapport and sets the tone of the interaction between technologist and patient. At this time, the technologist can ascertain the identity of the patient by using two forms of identification and make a quick assessment of the patient's condition. Hospital patients are identified by checking the wristband against the patient identifying information (patient's name, medical record, or Social Security number) on the order for the nuclear medicine examination. The identity of outpatients can be verified by requesting unique information from the patient, such as Social Security number or birth date. Please note that a patient's information should always be kept confidential.

Next, the physician's order for the examination should be reviewed. Orders for hospitalized patients may be found in the medical record or in the hospital information system. Orders for outpatients may be called in from the referring physician's office or brought by the patient on the day of the examination. The clinical indication for the test should correlate with the patient's history. The technologist also should determine whether the patient has complied with the required preparations for the examination and whether there are any contraindications for completing the test. Gathering additional pertinent medical history from the patient or the medical record may assist the technologist in the completion of the examination or the physician in the interpretation of results.

The initial interaction between patient and technologist provides some clues about how best to explain the nuclear medicine procedure. Because no examination is ever routine to a patient, a technologist should address not only the technical requirements of the procedure but also questions and concerns the patient may express. Procedure explanations should be geared to the patient's level of understanding and present the most important information first.

Patient Transfer

Skillful application of the principles of body mechanics and transfer techniques helps ensure safety and comfort for both the patient and technologist. Proper body mechanics include using a strong base of support by spreading feet and flexing knees, lifting with large leg muscles, and avoiding twisting at the waist. Transfer methods must be chosen and adapted to the situation, on the basis of the ability, size, and strength of the individuals involved. The technologist should assess the strength, balance, mobility, understanding, and motivation of patients who are being moved. Some general guidelines include the following:

1. Assess the patient's ability to assist;
2. provide only the assistance necessary;
3. explain the move to the patient and let the patient see the destination;
4. pay attention to intravenous lines, catheters, chest tubes, oxygen tubing, etc.;
5. lock the imaging bed in place;
6. move the patient toward his or her strong side and assist on the weak side; and
7. obtain assistance from others when necessary.

Wheelchair-to-Bed Transfers

If the patient has generalized or one-sided weakness, using a transfer belt around the patient's waist may provide additional security during this transfer:

1. Lower the imaging bed to wheelchair level and lock bed in place;
2. place the wheelchair at a 45° angle to the bed, making sure that the patient's strongest side is closest to the bed;
3. lock wheelchair in place and raise footrests;
4. move patient to the edge of wheelchair seat;
5. if the patient needs assistance to stand, flex knees and brace patient's knees with your own;
6. place your arms under the patient's axillae or grasp transfer belt;
7. if the patient is able to help, ask the patient to push down on the armrests and lift up on the count of three (place the patient's hands on your shoulders if the patient cannot assist by pushing on the armrests);

8. pivot toward the patient's strong side so that the patient's back is toward the imaging bed;
9. flex knees to seat the patient onto the imaging bed; and
10. assist the patient into the supine position.

Stretcher-to-Bed Transfers

The patient who is unable to stand should be transported to nuclear medicine on a stretcher. Stretcher-to-bed transfers are best accomplished with two or three people when the patient is not able to assist with the transfer. The maneuvers described here will need to be performed several times to complete a transfer from the stretcher to the imaging bed or vice versa:

1. Lower the side rails and the head of the stretcher to the flat, horizontal position;
2. place the stretcher next to the imaging bed with patient's strongest side facing the bed;
3. adjust the height of the imaging bed to match that of the stretcher as closely as possible and then lock the bed and stretcher into place;
4. with the patient supine and the mover(s) on the far side of the imaging bed facing the stretcher, the single mover should place one arm under the patient's shoulder and the other under the pelvis, and ask the patient to push with feet and elbows while guiding the patient onto the bed (but if two movers are present, one can support the head and shoulders while the other lifts the pelvis and knees—both movers use a lift-and-pull motion); and
5. if the patient is unable to assist with the transfer, a lift or "draw" sheet may be necessary, and two or more movers may be needed in this situation: the patient's arms are crossed over the chest, and the movers grasp the edge of the sheet and, on the count of three, lift and pull the patient on to the imaging bed in several motions until the patient is completely on the imaging bed.

Contrast Media

Contrast media (also known as contrast agents) are pharmaceutical compounds used in imaging. Contrast media are used to distinguish adjacent tissues on an image. This is accomplished by enhancing the visual contrast, thus enhancing density differences within the area of interest, improving the visibility of adjacent anatomical structures, and outlining abnormalities. Contrast agents are usually administered orally or intravenously resulting in temporary density differences between tissues. Contrast media can also be administered intrathecally (into the subarachnoid space) or intra-articularly (into the joint space).

Types of Contrast Media

Contrast media are usually classified as negative or positive contrast agents. The classification is dependent on the contrast media's ability to absorb the X-ray beam. Negative contrast media are radiolucent, therefore X-ray photons are easily transmittable. Negative contrast media decreases the attenuation of the X-ray beam, which results in an increase in density (darkness) on the image. Examples of negative contrast media are gases such as air, oxygen, or carbon dioxide.

Positive contrast media, on the other hand, have an increased attenuation of the X-ray beam and produce a decrease density (darkness) on the image. Positive contrast agents are referred to as radiopaque because these types of contrast media are opaque to the X-ray photons. Positive contrast agents appear light or bright on the image. Positive contrast agents have a high atomic number. Examples of positive contrast media include the insoluble salt–barium sulfates and the variety of organic iodine compounds.

Barium Sulfates Contrast Agents

Barium sulfate ($BaSO_4$), often referred to as *barium,* has an atomic number of 56 and is often administered orally. Barium sulfate is an inert powder composed of crystals and is used for visualization of the gastrointestinal system. The powder is mixed with water before ingestion by the patient. Barium never dissolves in water, and the particles are suspended within water and may settle when the mixture sits for a period of time. Because barium sulfate never dissolves in water it is important to know the contraindications when administering. Barium sulfate is contraindicated if there is any chance that the mixture could go into the peritoneal cavity. Therefore, barium sulfate should not be used on patients with a perforated viscus or immediately before, during, or after surgery. In either case, water-soluble iodinated contrast media should be used instead of barium sulfate. Examples of water-soluble iodinated contrast media commonly used include Gastroview, Gastrografin, or Oral Hypaque, all of which can be readily absorbed by the body. A minor drawback to using water-soluble iodinated contrast agents as an oral agent is the bitter taste. Patients should be warned about the taste to increase the patient's cooperation. If the patient has a history of iodine sensitivity, water-soluble iodinated contrast media should not be used.

In some occasions positive and negative contrast media are used to obtain an optimal image. This is known as double contrast. Double-contrast techniques are widely used when evaluating certain diseases and conditions, for instance, when imaging the lumen of the colon or mucosa of the stomach to detect polyps, diverticulea, and ulcers. These are demonstrated better with the double-contrast technique.

Iodinated Contrast Agents

Iodinated contrast media may be injected directly into the patient's bloodstream. They are usually used to penetrate or perfuse blood vessels, organs, and vascular lesions. Ionic contrast media has a relative high atomic number of 53, making it radiopaque or positive. Although there are various brands of iodinated intravascular (IV) contrast agents in the marketplace, and each brand has distinctive properties, they all have one thing in common: all contain iodine. The more iodine contained in a contrast media's solution, the more X-ray photons will be attenuated during a procedure. Since different anatomical and pathological structures are perfused by IV contrast media at various rates and various extents, the contrast agent aids in delineating tissues and pathology on images. Tissues perfused by positive IV contrast media appear brighter on images. This increase in the brightness is often referred to as enhancement. It is important to understand that contrast media are a medication. Unlike most medications, contrast media are not used for their therapeutic qualities but for their distribution and elimination from the body. Also unlike most medication, iodinated contrast media are usually administered in larger quantities and short intervals (as a bolus).

Various agents are marketed as having several properties that will likely affect how well a patient will be able to tolerate the administration of the pharmaceutical compound. Properties that tend to influence how well a patient will tolerate the administration of the contrast are based on the following:

- Ionic vs. nonionic
- Osmolality
- Chemotoxic reaction mechanism
- Idiosyncratic reaction mechanism

Contrast media may be classified as either nonionic or ionic. Ionic agents dissociate into two charged particles (called ions) when introduced to a solution, like water or the patient's bloodstream. Ionic media break down into cations, positively charged particles, and anions, negatively charged particles. Because ionic agents dissociate into ions there will be many little particles (ions) entering into the patient's bloodstream. For every three iodine molecules present in an ionic media, one cation and one anion are produced when ionic contrast agents enter the blood. Therefore, ionic contrast agents are often referred to as 3:2 compounds. Nonionic agents, on the other hand, do not dissociate into particles when in a solution (like the patient's blood).This results in a whole molecule passing through the patient's body and is excreted in the same form by the kidneys. For every three iodine molecules in a nonionic solution, one molecule is produced. Therefore, nonionic contrast media are referred to as 3:1 compounds.

The osmolality of a solution is another determining factor of how well the patient is able to tolerate contrast. Osmolality is the concentration of molecular particles in the contrast media solution. IV contrast media may be divided into two categories on the basis of osmolality:

- High osmolar contrast media (HOCM)
- Low osmolar contrast media (LOCM)

Ionic contrast media belong in the HOCM category with concentration of particles approximately 1300 to 1600 mOsm/kg. It should be noted that all IV contrasts have a greater osmolality than blood plasma, which is approximately 285–290 mOsm/kg. Therefore, IV contrast can be referred to as hyperosmolar solutions, or hypertonic, when comparing to blood plasma. Hypertonic solutions cause a net movement of water from within the tissue into the vascular space. This process can cause a patient to become dehydrated. It is important to verify that the patient is hydrated well before the exam and to advise the patient to drink plenty of liquids after the exam.

Nonionic contrast agents are placed in the low osmolar category, with concentration of particles approximately 500–850 mOsm/ kg. Low osmolar contrast media were introduced in the 1980s. At that time, LOCM cost was much higher than the older HOCM. Due to the higher cost, the LOCM were often reserved for patients at higher risk of adverse reactions. As the price of LOCM decreased, the practice of using LOCM increased. Then in 1996, contrast media that are similar to human blood were introduced. These types of contrast media were called iso-osmolar agents and are included in the LOCM category. Today iso-osmolar agents are used in most intravascular procedures.

A final property of IV contrast media is their viscosity. Viscosity is the thickness of a liquid. The thicker or more viscous the contrast agent's solution, the more force the technologist will have to apply to the syringe for the contrast to be administered. Agents with a lower viscosity tend to be tolerated better than those with a higher viscosity. A contrast agent will have a high viscosity if its molecular particles are large. This is significant not only in terms of patient tolerance of the force of the injection, but also because the kidneys have a more difficult time filtering the larger molecules from the blood. The viscosity of the contrast material can be reduced significantly by heating the liquid to body temperature before injection.

Dose

To properly assess the dose of iodinated contrast media to be delivered, both the iodine concentration and the volume must be considered. As stated previously, the beam attenuation abilities of the contrast media given to the patient is dependent on the amount of iodine in the iodinated contrast material. LOCM are measured in milligrams of iodine per milliliter (mgI/mL) of solution; on the other hand, HOCM are measured in terms of percentage weight per volume of concentration of iodine (mg/mL). When comparing the differences between doses of both contrast media it is important to look at the total grams of iodine delivered to the patient. Not only does proper dose of contrast media result in high-quality images, but proper dosage also results in proper safety to the patient. The adverse effects of overdosage of iodinated contrast media can result in deadly reactions affecting the pulmonary and cardiovascular systems. Although rare, death has occurred as a result of 250 to 300 mL of undiluted HOCM contrast media (Katzberg, 1995). Although contrast media should be administered with care to all patients, the American College of Radiology (ACR) has identified special considerations for the pediatric population concerning administration of contrast media.

Pediatric Consideration

Osmolarity is an important factor in pediatric imaging. Pediatric patients are considered to be susceptible to fluid shifts and have lower tolerance for IV osmotic loads than adult patients do. If the fluid shift is large, cardiac failure and pulmonary edema may result. For this reason, many facilities use nonionic (low osmolarity) contrast media when performing exams. In children with significant preexisting cardiac dysfunction, consideration should be given to the use of an iso-osmolarity intravascular contrast agent. Administering hyperosmolality contrast media intravenously can result in migration of fluid from extravascular soft tissues into the blood vessels. For an abdominal scan in CT, the standard dose of IV contrast is 2.0 mL/kg and should not exceed the adult dose of 150 mL. Oral contrast is given for gastrointestinal tract and pelvis examinations. A water-soluble iodine-based contrast agent can also be given instead of barium. The amount of contrast given is based on the patient's age and weight.

Adverse Reactions

Millions of patients are injected with contrast each year. Of these millions 6–8% of these individuals have a reaction to the contrast media. Fortunately, the majority of these reactions are minor or moderate. Moderate adverse reactions may require treatment and close observation, but hospitalization is generally not required.

Mild adverse reactions include:

- Mild hives (urticaria)
- Itching
- Coughing
- Nasal stuffiness
- Dizziness

Moderate adverse reactions to contrast media include:

- Moderate hives (urticaria)
- Difficulty breathing (dyspnea)
- Cold, clammy skin
- Pallor (paleness)
- Low blood pressure (hypotension)
- Elevated blood pressure (hypertension)
- Rapid heart/pulse rate (tachycardia) or slow heart/pulse rate (bradycardia)
- Wheezing

Severe reactions (occur in less than 1% of all patients and require hospitalization) include:

- Cessation of breathing (apnea)
- Dyspnea
- Rapid breathing (tachypnea)
- Prolonged tachycardia
- Convulsions
- Acute arrhythmias (fibrillation)
- Nonpalpable pulse in carotid artery
- Shock (hypotension, cyanosis, pallor, cold skin)
- Unresponsiveness
- Anaphylactic reaction/anaphylactoid reaction (allergic reactions)
- Cardiopulmonary arrest

Anaphylactic reactions to iodinated contrast media are similar to allergic reactions of foreign materials, such as pollen. Anaphylactic reactions are typically minor, such as itching. Some patients, however, may experience difficulty breathing and edema resulting in bronchospasm. If a patient ever states that he/she is having difficulty breathing and his/her skin color is changing (usually a patchy red/white or flushing, since the capillaries are dilating), assume he/she needs help. If the physician in charge is at any significant distance from the room, then the technologist should prepare 1 mL of 1:1000 epinephrine to be delivered as a subcutaneous injection, but *not* as intravenous injection for administration. It may be necessary to begin CPR. The attending physician may decide to administer epinephrine, via IV, and may need to call a code team. An emergency cart should always be available in each department and checked daily.

Possible Drug Interaction with Contrast Media

It is also important to identify specific medications that patients may be taking because certain medications can interfere with or cause contrast media interactions that are undesirable. ß-Adrenergic blocker is a type of drug used in treating patients with hypertension. These drugs decrease the cardiac output, reduce dilation of bronchial smooth muscle, and block the effect of epinephrine. Patients on this type of medication have an increased risk of anaphylactic reactions; therefore, water-soluble contrast should be used in these patients.

Calcium channel blockers are used to treat hypertension. This drug decreases the contraction of the heart and dilates (widens) the arteries. The use of ionic contrast can result in an increased risk for heart block and a sudden decrease in blood pressure. As an example, nonionic contrast media are used during cardiac catherization.

Diabetics may be on a drug called metformin (Glucophage). Patients on this medication should be advised not to take the medication 48 hr before the exam and 48 hr after the use of iodine contrast media. Metformin given to patients too soon after receiving IV contrast can result in lactic acidosis. Lactic acidosis is a life-threatening condition caused by too much lactate in the blood and low blood pH. Low blood pH means that the patient's blood contains too much acid, which can be harmful to the cells of the patient's body.

Minimizing Adverse Reactions

Due to the different chemical compounds of contrast agents, the package insert should always be reviewed to determine the possibility of adverse reactions. The package insert lists precautions and contraindications associated with the particular contrast. Contrast agents with lower osmolality and low viscosity should be given to patients who are suspected to potentially have a reaction or have a history of adverse reactions. Therefore evaluating the patient's history is vital. Conditions such as kidney disease, liver disease, or diabetes usually warrant nonionic contrast media. Warming IV contrast agents close to body temperature reduces the viscosity and makes the injections easier. Some healthcare organizations administer histamines or steroids to lessen or prevent an allergic reaction. In addition to steroids, diphenhydramine (Benadryl) may be used to block the physiologic effects of the release of histamine, therefore reducing the allergic effect of the contrast. Diphenhydramine is an H_1 antihistamine that works by blocking the effects of histamine at H_1 receptor sites. This results in an increase of vascular smooth muscle contraction, thus reducing urticaria, edema, and respiratory symptoms. Diphenhydramine may be given orally or intravenously.

Administration of Medications

Drugs may be identified by their generic or proprietary (brand) names. Radiopharmaceuticals are often referred to by brand name, generic name, or chemical abbreviation. For example, Ceretec (brand name) may also be called exametazime (generic name) or HMPAO (chemical abbreviation). Therefore, it is important for the technologist to be familiar with the various ways drugs and radiopharmaceuticals may be referred to by patients and other practitioners in the clinical setting.

No medication, including radiopharmaceuticals, should be administered without a physician's order. All medication orders must be verified before any drug is administered to a patient. If the technologist keeps the five "rights" of drug administration in mind, errors will be minimized: The *right* dosage of the *right* drug should be given to the *right* patient at the *right* time by the *right* route.

Medication may be administered by a number of different routes (Table 2.1). Not all routes have a nuclear medicine application. Figure 2.1 illustrates the proper needle placement for parenteral injections. Chapter 3 provides detailed information about preparing unit dosages of radiopharmaceuticals for intravenous injection.

Many nuclear medicine examinations involve the administration of interventional drugs. These drugs, unlike diagnostic radiopharmaceuticals, are intended to produce a change in some physiologic function of the body. Therefore, the possibility that a patient may experience an adverse reaction from an interventional drug is significantly greater than that with a radiopharmaceutical. The technologist must be alert to this possibility and should

Table 2.1 Different Types of Medication Administration Routes

Route	Description	Example	Suggested needle size
Oral	Ingested by mouth	^{123}I capsule	NA[a]
Inhalation	Breathed in through the nose or mouth	^{133}Xe gas	NA
Sublingual	Placed under the tongue	Nitroglycerin tablet	NA
Topical	Applied to skin	Scopolamine	NA
Rectal	Inserted into rectum	Suppository for nausea	NA
Intravenous	Injected into a vein	Many radiopharmaceuticals	1–1.5 in., 20–22 gauge
Intrathecal	Injected into the subarachnoid space	Radiopharmaceutical for cisternography	3.5–4.5 in., 16–25 gauge
Subcutaneous	Injected under the skin	Allergy testing	5/8 in., 23–25 gauge
Intramuscular	Injected into a muscle	Vitamin B_{12} "flushing" dose	1–3 in., 19–25 gauge
Intradermal	Injected between layers of skin	Radiopharmaceutical for lymphoscintigraphy	0.5 in., 26–27 gauge

[a]Not applicable.

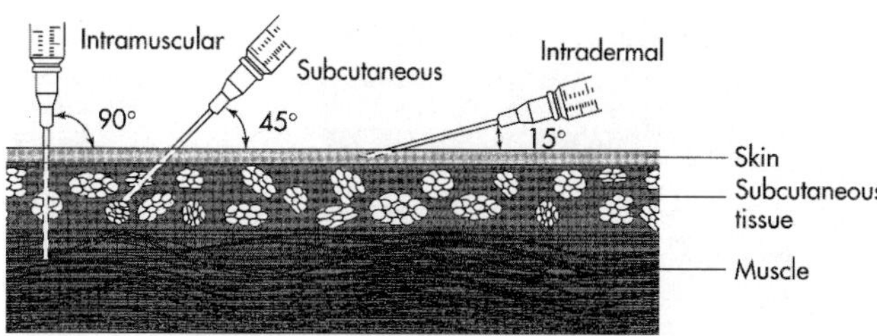

Figure 2.1 Needle placement for parenteral injection. (Reprinted, with permission, from Christian *et al.*, 2004.)

be familiar with the treatment of adverse drug effects. Table 3.5 in Chapter 3 contains a partial listing of the more commonly used interventional agents, their adverse effects, and treatment for those effects.

Infection Control

It is important to take precautions to prevent the transmission of disease from one patient to another and to the technologist and co-workers. Frequent and thorough handwashing is one of the most effective and cost-effective ways to prevent the spread of infection and illness. Hands should be washed before and after contact with each patient and before and after wearing gloves. Prior to washing hands, one should set aside paper towels to use. When washing hands with soap and water, one should wet the hands with clean running warm water. The hands should be rubbed together to make a lather. It is recommended to continue rubbing hands for 15–20 sec or about the length of the "Alphabet Song." The hands should then be rinsed under the running water and dried using a paper towel or air dryer. When possible, the paper towel should be used to turn the faucet off. Soap and water should always be used to clean visibly soiled hands. If soap and water are not available, alcohol-based cleaners may also be used.

Healthcare workers do not always know which patients are infectious. For this reason, it is essential that all technologists follow certain infection control guidelines called "standard precautions." The guidelines assume that all patients are potentially infectious; therefore, the same infection control practices should be applied to all patients. Standard precautions should be used whenever there is a potential for exposure to blood, body fluids, or nonintact skin. Table 2.2 outlines standard precautions guidelines.

Transmission-based precautions should be applied in conjunction with standard precautions whenever infection is suspected or a patient is known to be infectious. Patients with known or suspected communicable diseases are placed in isolation. Transmission-based precautions are intended to minimize the possibility of disease transmission to others and are based on three routes of disease transmission: air, droplet, and direct contact. Table 2.3 outlines precautions to be observed for each route of transmission and identifies some of the diseases for which these precautions are applied.

Table 2.2 Standard Precautions Guidelines

Precaution	Guideline
Handwashing	Wash hands before and after patient contact.
	Wash hands or other skin surfaces immediately if they become contaminated with body fluids.
Gloving	Wear gloves whenever there is a potential for exposure to blood or body fluids or nonintact skin. Wear latex-free gloves if the patient has known latex allergies.
	Remove gloves immediately after each use.
	Change gloves between patients.
Personal protective equipment	Use gloves, fluid-resistant gowns, face masks, protective eyewear, resuscitation masks when contact with body fluids or nonintact skin is possible.
Needle recapping	Do not recap needles or use the one-handed "scoop" technique or a needle-recapping device (in nuclear medicine we do need to secure the needle in some manner to prevent contamination of the radionuclide).
	Discard used needles and other sharps in a puncture-resistant biohazard container.
Biohazardous spills	Clean biohazardous spills immediately.
	Wear appropriate protective equipment.
	Decontaminate the spill area with a bleach solution or other approved disinfectant.

Vital Signs

Vital signs include temperature, pulse, respiration, and blood pressure. They help maintain homeostasis in the body by responding to internal and external stimuli. Normal body temperature remains fairly constant and is a measure of the balance between heat produced in the body and that lost to the environment. The technologist should be certain to use the correct thermometer for whichever area of the body is chosen for measuring body temperature. The pulse is the result of the blood throbbing against the walls of the arteries as the heart beats. The strength and regularity of the pulse, as well as the number of beats per minute, should be noted. The thumb has its own pulse and should never be used to count a pulse. Also, pressing too hard on the area at

Table 2.3 Transmission-Based Precautions

Type of transmission	Precautions
Airborne (tuberculosis, measles)	Standard precautions Private room with negative air pressure ventilation Particulate air filter respirator for caregiver/visitors Door to room closed
Contact (hepatitis A, varicella zoster)	Standard precautions Gloves, gown Decontaminated equipment in contact with patient
Droplet (influenza, pneumonia)	Standard precautions Private room Mask for caregiver

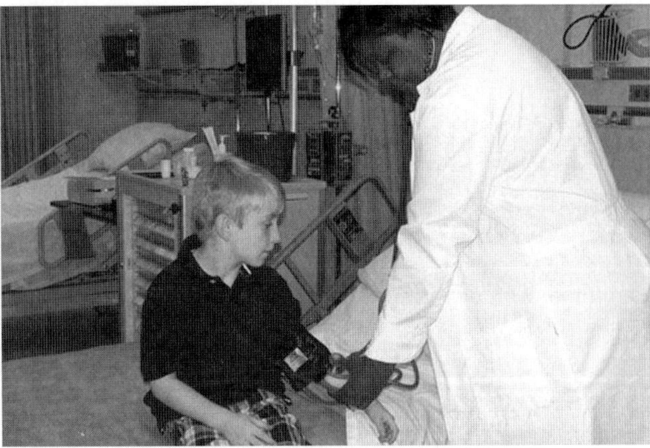

Figure 2.2 A pediatric blood pressure cuff should be used on a young patient when assessing blood pressure. (Courtesy of University of Alabama at Birmingham NMT Program Picture Library.)

which the pulse is being monitored may compress the artery so that the pulse cannot be felt. Respiration refers to the exchange of oxygen and carbon dioxide between the blood and the external environment. One respiratory cycle includes one inspiration and one expiration. The patient should be unaware that respirations are being measured, because he or she may consciously or unconsciously change the breathing pattern. Any signs of respiratory distress or sounds associated with the patient's breathing should be noted along with the number of breaths per minute. Blood pressure measurement assesses the pressure of the blood on the arterial walls during systole and diastole (Fig. 2.2). The upper number of a blood pressure measurement denotes the systolic pressure; the lower figure is the diastolic pressure.

Table 2.4 summarizes the normal limits for adults, measurement sites, and equipment needed for each vital sign. Many factors can affect each of these four signs. Changes in vital signs may indicate a problem or potential problem. In the nuclear medicine area, vital signs are typically monitored before, during, or after an examination involving the administration of interventional drugs; when the physical condition of a patient changes; or when a patient reports nonspecific symptoms of physical distress (feeling "funny" or "different"). It should be noted that taking vital signs does not require a physician's order.

Oxygen Therapy

Oxygen is a drug that must be prescribed by a physician. The order for oxygen therapy may be found in the medical record with other medication orders and identifies the amount of oxygen in liters per minute (L/min) that the patient is to receive and the delivery device. Most patients require a flow rate of 3–5 L/min, but the flow rate should be verified by checking the physician's order. Oxygen may be administered to the patient through a nasal cannula, oxygen mask, oxygen tent/hood, or mechanical ventilator. Oxygen may be available from a wall outlet or a portable tank. The wall outlet is connected to a liquid oxygen supply that furnishes oxygen for an entire facility. It is equipped with an oxygen flow meter to adjust the number of liters per minute the patient is to receive. Portable tanks come equipped with a flow meter and a pressure gauge that indicates the amount of oxygen contained in the tank in pounds per square inch (psi). The regulator valve of a portable tank must be turned on before oxygen will flow out of the tank and before the pressure gauge indicates the amount of oxygen remaining in the tank.

Important safety considerations pertain to oxygen administration. Portable tanks should be secured during transport or when stationary to prevent them from falling. Damage to the regulator may cause the tank to become a dangerous projectile. Oxygen is not explosive, but it does support combustion. Therefore, smoking, open flames, or sparks should be avoided in areas where oxygen is in use.

Cardiac Monitoring

Chapter 9 reviews the normal electrical conduction path through the heart, the normal electrocardiogram (ECG) pattern, and electrode placement. In nuclear medicine, the ECG has two different applications. It may be used to monitor the patient's cardiac status during physical or pharmacologic stress testing or may be interfaced with the scintillation camera to trigger data acquisition. The latter application is referred to as physiologic gating and uses the patient's R wave to control the way in which data are acquired during equilibrium blood pool and myocardial perfusion imaging.

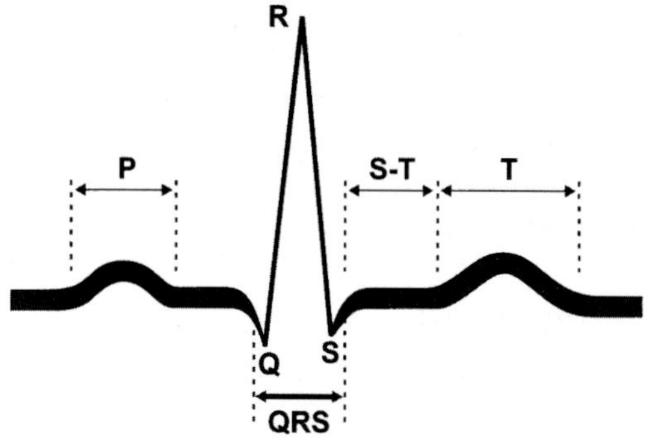

Figure 2.3 Normal electrocardiograph tracing. The P wave indicates atrial depolarization, QRS complex indicates ventricular depolarization, and the T wave indicates ventricular repolarization. (Reprinted, with permission, from Crawford and Husain, 2003.)

Gating can be performed with three ECG electrodes: right arm and left arm leads, placed in the area of the right and left clavicle, respectively, and left leg lead, placed on the left abdomen near the waist. Because the computer needs a strong R wave to initiate data acquisition, it may be necessary to adjust the electrodes to obtain a positive, well-defined R wave. If the patient's heart rate is very irregular, data from different parts of the cardiac cycle may be superimposed, decreasing the accuracy of quantitative information.

A 12-lead ECG provides more information about the heart's electrical activity than a three-lead ECG. This type of monitoring is used to evaluate a patient's cardiac status in preparation for stress testing and to observe changes in the heart rate, rhythm, and conduction pattern during stress. Certain abnormalities identified on a baseline 12-lead ECG may indicate that the patient should not be stressed. Changes in the baseline ECG pattern during stress may indicate that the myocardium is becoming ischemic or that the electrical conduction path is becoming disrupted—signals that the stress test should be terminated.

The ability to recognize certain patterns on an ECG strip is an important skill. Figure 2.3 depicts a normal ECG tracing for one cardiac cycle, where the P wave is the atrial depolarization, the QRS complex is the ventricular depolarization, and the T wave is the ventricular repolarization. Table 2.5 identifies the characteristics of normal sinus rhythm. Recall that the smallest division (or box) on ECG paper represents 0.04 sec and that the larger division (box) is 0.2 sec. Table 2.6 lists the steps in reviewing an ECG tracing. It is essential that the technologist assess the physical condition of the patient as well as the ECG tracing. Two life-threatening rhythms requiring immediate attention are ventricular tachycardia and ventricular fibrillation (Fig. 2.4). Ventricular tachycardia occurs when one strong ectopic focus in the ventricle takes over the conduction system. The heart rate may be 100–250 beats per minute, which the ventricles cannot maintain. Although the rhythm is regular, the cardiac output is too low to be effective, and, if left untreated, the rhythm may progress to ventricular fibrillation. Ventricular fibrillation is an uncoordinated quivering of the ventricles that does not circulate blood. The patient is in cardiac arrest and will need cardiopulmonary resuscitation and defibrillation.

Table 2.4 Vital Signs

Vital sign	Average/normal range	Measurement site(s)	Equipment needed
Temperature	98.6°F (37°C)	Oral	Oral glass thermometer Disposable paper thermometer Electronic probe
		Tympanic membrane	Aural thermometer
	97.6–98°F (36.4–36.7°C)	Axilla	Axillary glass or electronic thermometer
	99.6°F (37.5°C)	Rectal	Rectal glass thermometer
Pulse	60–90 beats/min	Apex of heart Radial artery (at wrist) Carotid artery Femoral artery (groin) Popliteal artery Temporal artery (front of ear) Dorsalis pedis Posterior tibial pulse (inner ankle) Brachial artery (antecubital fossa)	Stethoscope (apical pulse only) Watch with second hand
Respiration	15–20 breaths/min	Chest	Watch with second hand
Blood pressure	120/80 mm Hg	Arm (brachial artery)	Sphygmomanometer and cuff Stethoscope

Table 2.5 Characteristics of Normal Sinus Rhythm

Each cardiac cycle is represented by a P wave followed by a QRS complex followed by a T wave.
All waves and complexes are consistent in shape.
All intervals within normal limits:
P wave: 0.12 sec in duration
PR interval: 0.12–0.20 sec
QRS complex: <0.12 sec in duration
Rate: 60–100 beats/min
Rhythm: regular

Table 2.6 Reviewing an Electrocardiograph Tracing

1. Check P wave for size, shape, and location.
2. Determine atrial rate and rhythm. Rate: Number of P waves in 6 sec × 10 = atrial beats/min.
   Rhythm: Is P wave-to-P wave interval regular?
3. Determine PR interval.
4. Determine ventricular rate and rhythm. Rate: Number of QRS complexes in 6 sec × 10 = ventricular beats/min.
   Rhythm: Is R wave-to-R wave interval regular?
5. Check for QRS complexes after each P wave; determine QRS duration.
6. Is T wave rounded and above isoelectric line?

Emergency Care

When a patient in the nuclear medicine department experiences a medical emergency, the nuclear medicine technologist is often the first medical professional on the scene. The technologist must be observant of changes in a patient's condition and must take appropriate measures swiftly. Whether the event is a minor or major emergency, the technologist should always:

- Stop the nuclear medicine examination
- Stay with the patient
- Call for assistance
- Notify the physician of any changes in a patient's condition
- Prepare to assist with emergency procedures, as needed

Cardiac Arrest

A cardiac arrest is a sudden cessation of blood circulation. A patient in sudden cardiac arrest (SCA) will be unresponsive, have no adequate breathing, and have no signs of blood circulation. Once it is established that the patient is unresponsive, the technologist should call for help (call a *code* in the hospital setting) before beginning cardiopulmonary resuscitation (CPR). Remember the CABs (*c*hest compressions, *a*irway, *b*reathing) of CPR for adults, children, and infants (excluding the newly born). In a team-approach CPR, one rescuer performs chest compressions and another rescuer maintains the airway, monitors the pulse, and performs rescue breathing. It is recommended that barrier devices or bag-mask devices be used to perform rescue breathing in the clinical setting. For a summary of recommendations for healthcare providers see Table 2.7.

Respiratory Arrest

Respiratory arrest is defined as cessation of breathing or slow, shallow, irregular breathing that is inadequate to oxygenate the blood. The patient in respiratory arrest will be unresponsive. Initiate the steps described for CPR. If the patient has a pulse but is not breathing, the rescuer should give one breath every 5 sec for adults and one breath every 3 sec for infants and children (adults = 12 breaths per min and infants and children = 20 breaths per min).

Diabetic Crisis

Diabetes is the body's inability to produce or utilize insulin. Patients who have diabetes control their blood glucose levels with diet, exercise, and medication (insulin or oral medication). Many nuclear medicine examinations require fasting, which can pose a challenge for the patient with diabetes. Low blood sugar (hypoglycemia) is the more common diabetic emergency seen in nuclear medicine settings and has a rapid onset. When the blood glucose level becomes too low, the patient may experience one or more of the following symptoms: sudden weakness, hunger, tremor, sweating, irritability, and blurred vision. The patient may lose consciousness if the low glucose level is not quickly reversed. Treatment for a hypoglycemic episode involves administering a source of sugar—hard candy, fruit juice, or regular soda works well. However, this treatment should be used only if the patient is conscious. Nothing should ever be given by mouth to a semiconscious or unconscious patient. High blood sugar (hyperglycemia) has a slow onset. Patients may experience excessive thirst, increased urine output, loss of weight and/or a fruity-smelling breath. Treatment may involve the administration of insulin, but the technologist should seek immediate medical assistance for the patient.

Seizure

A seizure is a sudden discharge of electrical activity in the brain. It may begin without warning, although some patients may be able to sense the onset of a seizure. Patients may exhibit muscle spasms, confusion, nonresponsiveness, or loss of consciousness. Technologists should take whatever measures are necessary to protect the patient from injury or falling and to prevent aspiration of stomach contents. The patient should not be restrained in any

Table 2.7 BLS CPR Summary of Recommendations for Healthcare Providers (American Heart Association 2011 Guidelines)

	Adults	Children	Infant (excluding newly born)
Recognition	Unresponsiveness No breathing or no normal breathing (i.e., only gasping)	Unresponsiveness No breathing or only gasping	Unresponsiveness No breathing or only gasping
	No pulse palpated within 10 sec for all ages		
CPR sequence	C–A–B (Chest compressions, airway, breathing)		
Compression rate	At least 100/min	At least 100/min	At least 100/min
Compression depth	At least 2 in. (5cm)	About 2 in. (5cm) (At least 1/3 anterior-posterior diameter)	About 1 1/2 in. (At least 1/3 anterior-posterior diameter)
Chest wall recoil	Allow complete recoil between compressions and rotate compressors every 2 min		
Compression interruptions	Minimize interruptions in chest compressions and attempt to limit interruptions to <10 sec		
Airway	Head tilt–chin lift; if trauma is suspected, use jaw thrust		
Compression-to-ventilation ratio (until advanced airway is placed)	At least 100 compressions per min with breaths asynchronous with chest compressions		
Ventilations: when rescuer is untrained or trained and not proficient	Compressions only		
Ventilations with	1 breath every 5 sec; visible chest rise	1 breath every 3 sec; visible chest rise	1 sec per breath; visible chest rise
Defibrillation	Attach and use AED as soon as available. Minimize interruptions in chest compressions before and after shock; resume CPR beginning with compressions immediately after each shock		

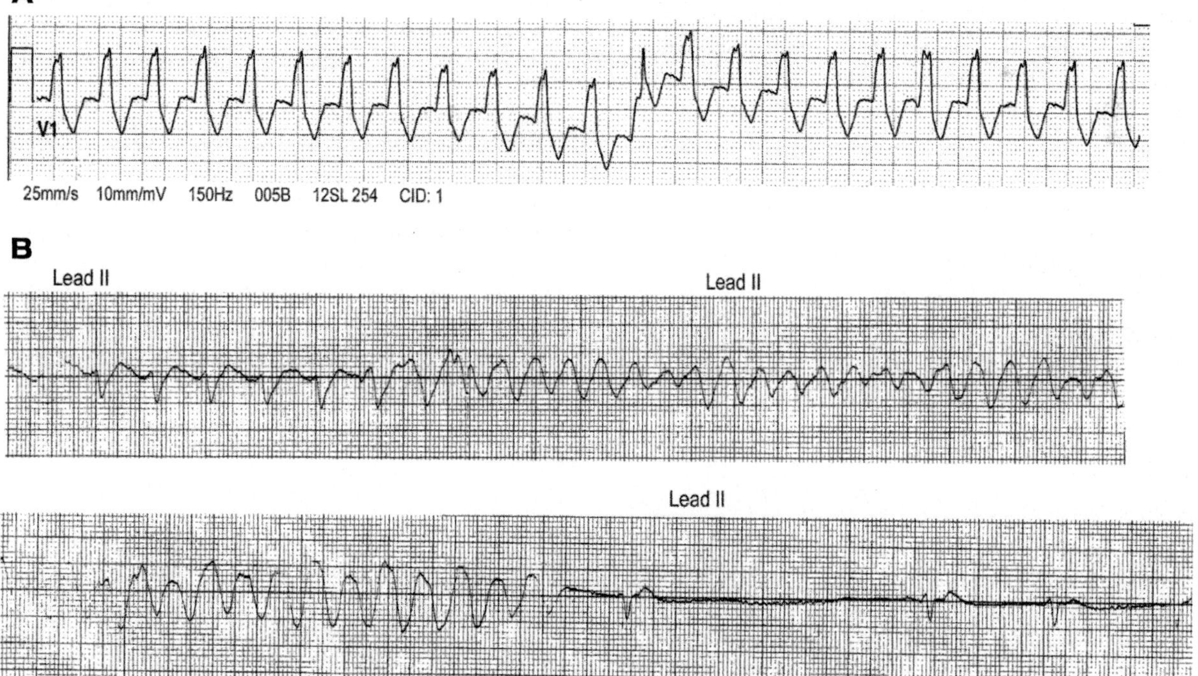

Figure 2.4 Ventricular tachycardia and fibrillation. (A) Example of ventricular tachycardia shows QRS complexes in rapid sequence. (B) Both strips are examples of ventricular fibrillation. In the second strip, the ventricular fibrillation is followed by asystole. (Reprinted, with permission, from Crawford and Husain, 2003.)

way, because this may cause injury. The behavior of the patient during the seizure and the duration of the seizure should be noted.

Cerebral Vascular Accidents (Stroke)

A stroke is a blocked vessel (ischemic stroke) in the brain or a ruptured vessel (hemorrhagic stroke) in the brain. Signs and symptoms of a stroke include one-sided weakness, facial droop on one side, sharp acute pain in the head, blurred vision, difficulty speaking, and/or sudden onset of dizziness. The key factor is identifying whether it is an ischemic or hemorrhagic stroke. A computed tomography scan is needed to identify which type. For ischemic stroke, a patient will be put on thrombolytic therapy immediately. For hemorrhagic stroke, which would be a ruptured blood vessel in the brain, immediate surgery is needed to repair the blood vessel. If thrombolytics are given before it is determined which type of stroke, then a patient who is suffering from a hemorrhagic stroke could internally hemorrhage to death.

Syncope

Fainting (syncope) occurs when there is a sudden, brief loss of consciousness as a result of inadequate blood flow to the brain. It may be caused by a variety of different factors, including hunger, heart disease, fatigue, and orthostatic hypotension, or it may be an emotional response to the medical experience. Signs that the patient may be about to faint include dizziness, pallor, nausea, tachycardia, and cold, clammy skin. Assist the patient into a secure position sitting or preferably lying down. With the patient in the supine position, elevate the feet and legs.

Shock

Shock is a general term that describes a condition of decreased blood flow and oxygen delivery to body tissues, usually as a result of inadequate blood pressure. It may be caused by a large blood loss, cardiac failure, obstruction of blood flow to the vital organs, or massive infection, to name a few. Symptoms of impending shock include: restlessness, pallor, weakness, confusion/lethargy/loss of consciousness, increased pulse rate, and falling blood pressure. The symptoms may occur suddenly and without warning. Immediate medical intervention is essential. The technologist should call for emergency assistance quickly. Until medical personnel arrive, the technologist should assess the patient's vital signs and be ready to initiate CPR.

References and Further Reading

Adler AM, Carlton RR, 2007. *Radiologic Sciences and Patient Care.* 4th ed. St. Louis, MO: W.B. Saunders; 139–344.

Balliger P, 1991. *Merrill's Atlas of Radiographic Positions and Radiologic Procedures.* 7th ed. St. Louis, MO: Mosby.

Christian PE, Bernier DR, Langan JK, eds., 2004. *Nuclear Medicine and PET Technology and Techniques.* 5th ed. St. Louis, MO: Mosby; 211–234, 272–273, 417–418, 428–429.

Crawford ES, Husain SS, 2003. *Nuclear Cardiac Imaging: Terminology and Technical Aspects.* Reston, VA: Society of Nuclear Medicine; 70–71, 77, 109–119.

deWit SC, 2001. *Fundamental Concepts and Skills for Nursing.* Philadelphia, PA: W.B. Saunders; 272–278.

Ehrlich RA, McCloskey ED, Daly JA, 1999. *Patient Care in Radiography with an Introduction to Medical Imaging.* 5th ed. St. Louis, MO: Mosby; 95–106, 132–135, 157–159, 220–223.

Katzberg RW, 1995. *The Contrast Media Manual.* Baltimore, MD: Lippincott Williams & Wilkins; 68.

Potter PA, Perry AG, 2003. *Basic Nursing: Essentials for Practice.* 5th ed. St. Louis, MO: Mosby; 176–213.

Stapleton ER, Aufderheide TP, Hazinski MF, et al., eds., 2001. *Fundamentals of BLS for Healthcare Providers.* Dallas, TX: American Heart Association; 4–34.

Steves AM, Dowd SB, 1999. Patient education in nuclear medicine technology practice. *J Nucl Med Technol.* 27:4–13.

Torres LS, Norcutt TL, Dutton AG, 2003. *Basic Medical Techniques and Patient Care in Imaging Technology.* 6th ed. Philadelphia, PA: Lippincott Williams & Wilkins; 67–70, 138–157, 346–348.

CHAPTER 3 **Radiopharmaceuticals, Interventional Drugs, and Introduction to Pharmacology**

Vivian Loveless, Ann Steves, Norman Bolus, and Amy Byrd Brady

Most, if not all, of the radiopharmaceuticals compounded onsite by the nuclear medicine technologist are labeled with technetium-99m (^{99m}Tc). Therefore, most of the concepts presented in this chapter are applied to the molybdenum-99 (^{99}Mo)/^{99m}Tc generator and ^{99m}Tc radiolabeling. The principles of unit dose preparation discussed at the end of the chapter pertain to any radiopharmaceutical administered to a patient.

Radionuclide Generators

Radionuclide generators provide a convenient source of short-lived radionuclides. In a radionuclide generator, a longer-lived radionuclide, called the parent, decays to a shorter-lived radionuclide, called the daughter. The daughter can be removed periodically as it is replenished by decay of the parent. Examples of parent–daughter systems used in radionuclide generators include germanium-68 (^{68}Ge)/gallium-68 (^{68}Ga), strontium-82 (^{82}Sr)/rubidium-82 (^{82}Rb), and ^{99}Mo/^{99m}Tc. Some of these systems have been developed commercially and are supplied as sterile, shielded, automatically operated devices.

^{99}Mo/^{99m}Tc Generator

A ^{99}Mo/^{99m}Tc generator consists of a column containing aluminum trioxide (alumina) onto which the parent radionuclide, ^{99}Mo, is adsorbed (Fig. 3.1). A porous glass disk holds the alumina in place but allows saline to pass through it. The daughter radionuclide, ^{99m}Tc, is removed or eluted from the column when a sterile, evacuated vial is placed at the opposite end of the saline eluant. The vacuum in the collection vial causes the saline to be pulled through the alumina column, which removes the loosely bound ^{99m}Tc. Because of the different chemical properties of the parent and daughter, ^{99}Mo remains on the column and ^{99m}Tc is collected as the generator eluate in the form of ^{99m}Tc–sodium pertechnetate.

A ^{99}Mo/^{99m}Tc generator is designated as either a "wet" or "dry" column type. A wet column generator contains a supply of sterile saline within the generator itself. To elute this type of generator, the technologist chooses the appropriate size collection vial (usually 5, 10, 20, or 30 mL) to obtain the volume and activity concentration desired. Because no air follows the saline as it flows over the column, the column remains wet. A dry column generator requires that saline be added to the column for each elution. A vial of sterile saline, provided by the generator manufacturer, is placed on the charging port, a needle connected to tubing that carries the saline to the alumina column.

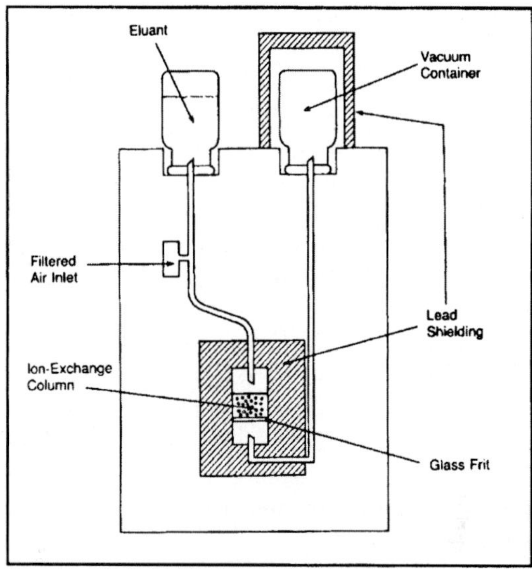

Figure 3.1 Cross-section of a typical commercial radionuclide generator. (Reprinted, with permission, from Chilton and Witcofski, 1986.)

An evacuated vial is then placed onto the needle on the collection port. The vacuum pulls the saline over the column, removing the ^{99m}Tc activity. Using an evacuated vial with a volume larger than the saline volume causes air to be pulled over the column, completely removing any saline, hence the name dry column generator. With this type of generator, the activity concentration of the eluate depends on the volume of saline used to elute the generator. After eluting a wet or dry column generator, the eluate activity and volume should be recorded.

All commercially available ^{99}Mo/^{99m}Tc generators contain ^{99}Mo produced from the fission of uranium-235 (^{235}U). The advantage of using fission ^{99}Mo (FM) is its high specific activity. Specific activity refers to the amount of radioactivity per unit mass of a radionuclide or radiopharmaceutical and is expressed in units such as millicuries per milligram (mCi/mg), megabecquerels per milligram (MBq/ mg), curies per mole (Ci/mol), or gigabecquerels per mole (GBq/mol). Because of its high specific activity, large amounts of ^{99}Mo (FM) can be bound onto a small ion-exchange column, which leads to higher activity concentration in the eluate.

It is extremely important to maintain the sterility of a generator. Manufacturers may place 0.22-μm (micrometer) membrane filters between the column and the collection vial to ensure sterility, but aseptic technique must be observed during the elution process. The septa of eluate and saline vials should be swabbed with alcohol, because the plastic flip tops covering the septa really serve only as dust covers. Before each elution, needles used to collect eluate should be replaced with new, sterile needles (if the generator has the option of replacing needles and if not, then the collection port and charging port should be covered with a sterile vial between use).

The shielding surrounding commercially manufactured generators (which can include lead, tungsten, or depleted uranium) is designed to meet U.S. Department of Transportation requirements. This means that generators are adequately shielded for transport purposes. Additional shielding may be necessary to reduce radiation exposure to personnel responsible for eluting the generator. In addition, the eluate collection vial also should be shielded. Standing at a distance from the generator after the elution has been initiated will further reduce radiation exposure.

Generator Yields

The amount of ^{99m}Tc activity eluted from a generator is proportional to the amount of ^{99}Mo activity present on the column and to the time elapsed since the last elution. After an elution, the amount of ^{99m}Tc activity on the column increases as a result of ^{99}Mo decay. When the ^{99m}Tc in a generator is eluted once a day, the maximum ^{99m}Tc activity is obtained approximately every 24 hr, as shown in Table 3.1. A second or third elution may be performed without severely decreasing the yield of the next morning's elution, depending on the length of time since the last elution. In determining ^{99m}Tc yields, the elution efficiency of the generator also should be considered. The entire ^{99m}Tc activity present on the column will not be eluted. A typical elution efficiency is 85–95%.

The amount of ^{99m}Tc eluted from a generator may vary for several reasons. A mechanical problem, such as an air leak in the tubing, may prevent the saline from being drawn out of the column into the collection vial. In addition, "channeling" of the alumina column causes only a portion of the column to be exposed to saline, leaving ^{99m}Tc on that part of the column not washed with eluant. Finally, chemical reduction of ^{99m}Tc from the +7 (VII) valence state to other reduced states occurs when reducing agents are formed by the radiolysis of water. The reduced ^{99m}Tc remains bound onto the column and is not eluted. This does not happen to a great extent.

Table 3.1 Percentage of ^{99m}Tc Activity Present on Generator Column at Selected Times after Elution

Time since elution (hr)	^{99m}Tc activity (% ^{99}Mo activity)
1	9.4
2	18
3	26
4	32
5	39
6	44
7	49
8	54
9	58
10	61
11	65
12	68
18	80
24	87

Eluate Assay and Quality Control

Concentration

Immediately after elution, the eluate is assayed in a dose calibrator to determine the total ^{99m}Tc activity in the collection vial. The eluate concentration (^{99m}Tc–pertechnetate) is calculated using the formula

$$\text{concentration} = \frac{\text{total } ^{99m}\text{Tc activity (mCi)}}{\text{elution volume (mL)}}$$

The total eluate activity, time of assay, and elution volume should be recorded in the appropriate logbook or recording media.

^{99}Mo Content

Although ^{99}Mo is tightly bound to the alumina column, a very small quantity of ^{99}Mo will be present in the generator eluate. The appearance of ^{99}Mo in generator eluate is called "molybdenum (or moly) breakthrough." Because ^{99}Mo is a radionuclide other than the one desired (^{99m}Tc), the ^{99}Mo in the eluate is considered a radionuclidic impurity. In contrast to ^{99m}Tc, ^{99}Mo has a much longer physical half-life (66 hr) and emits beta particles as well as higher-energy gamma photons. When administered to patients, ^{99}Mo is taken up by the parenchymal cells of the liver and delivers an unnecessary radiation dose to that organ. For this reason, limits have been established for allowable quantities of ^{99}Mo in generator eluate.

The U.S. Nuclear Regulatory Commission states that the first elution of each generator must be assayed for ^{99}Mo content to ensure that maximum allowable limits are not exceeded. The amount of ^{99}Mo in ^{99m}Tc generator eluate may not exceed 5.55 kBq (or 0.15 μCi) per 37 MBq (or 1 mCi) ^{99m}Tc at the time of administration to the patient. The most common method for assaying ^{99}Mo content in ^{99m}Tc eluate is the lead shield method.

Lead Shield (or Moly Shield) Method

The total ^{99m}Tc activity in the eluate should first be measured in a dose calibrator on the ^{99m}Tc setting. Then the generator eluate is placed in a lead container, called a moly shield, and assayed in a dose calibrator on the ^{99}Mo setting. The shield is designed to absorb ^{99m}Tc photons (140 keV) as well as to permit the passage of higher-energy (740, 780keV) ^{99}Mo photons. Sometimes it is necessary to apply a correction factor to the ^{99}Mo assay. Instructions supplied with the moly shield should be consulted. To determine the amount of ^{99}Mo contamination in the eluate, divide the ^{99}Mo assay results by the total number of millicuries of ^{99m}Tc in the eluate measured with the dose calibrator:

$$\text{concentrated ion} = \frac{\mu\text{Ci } ^{99}\text{Mo}}{\text{mCi } ^{99m}\text{Tc}}$$

Radionuclidic purity changes with time. Because ^{99}Mo ($t_{1/2}$ = 66 hr) decays more slowly than ^{99m}Tc ($t_{1/2}$ = 6 hr), the ^{99}Mo-to-^{99m}Tc ratio increases with time. The time at which ^{99}Mo contamination in the ^{99m}Tc eluate will exceed acceptable limits can be calculated using the following equation (this time may be shorter than the generator manufacturer's stated expiration time of the ^{99m}Tc eluate),

$$t = \frac{-\ln \text{Mo}_0/\text{Tc}_0}{0.1052} - 18.03$$

where t is the time in hours after the initial ^{99}Mo assay and Mo_0/Tc_0 is the the initial number of microcuries of ^{99}Mo divided by the initial number of millicuries of ^{99m}Tc.

Example

The initial ^{99}Mo contamination in an eluate of ^{99m}Tc was determined to be 1.3 MBq (35 μCi) ^{99}Mo in 18.5 GBq (500 mCi) ^{99m}Tc immediately after elution at 0700 hr. At what time will the eluate contain a ^{99}Mo level exceeding the established limits?

$$\text{Mo/Tc} = \frac{35\ \mu\text{Ci } ^{99}\text{Mo}}{55\ \text{mCi } ^{99m}\text{Tc}} = 0.07$$

$$t = \frac{-\ln \text{Mo}_0/\text{Tc}_0}{0.1052} - 18.03$$

$$t = \frac{-\ln(0.07)}{0.1052} - 18.03$$

$$t = \frac{(2.66)}{0.1052} - 18.03$$

$$t = 7.26 \text{ hr.}$$

The eluate will contain ^{99}Mo levels exceeding the limit of 5.55 kBq ^{99}Mo/37 MBq ^{99m}Tc (0.15 μCi ^{99}Mo/mCi ^{99m}Tc) at 1415 hr, approximately 7.26 hr after elution.

Aluminum Ion Content

Aluminum (Al^{3+}) from the generator column appearing in the ^{99m}Tc eluate is a chemical impurity, and this impurity can affect the biodistribution of radiopharmaceuticals. The U.S. Pharmacopeia has established a concentration limit for Al^{3+} to be not greater than 10 μg/mL of eluate.

Commercially available test kits for determining Al^{3+} concentration contain specially treated indicator paper and a standard Al^{3+} solution (10 μg/mL). Similar size drops of ^{99m}Tc eluate and the standard Al^{3+} solution are placed adjacent to one another on the indicator paper. The color intensities of both spots are compared. As long as the intensity of the eluate sample is less than that of the standard, the eluate contains less than 10 μg Al^{3+}/mL of eluate.

Preparation of ^{99m}Tc-Labeled Radiopharmaceuticals

Commercially prepared kits are available for compounding a wide variety of ^{99m}Tc-labeled radiopharmaceuticals. Such kits have a long shelf life and can be kept in the nuclear medicine department until a specific ^{99m}Tc-labeled agent is required. ^{99m}Tc–sodium pertechnetate eluted from a ^{99}Mo/^{99m}Tc generator is combined with the appropriate kit reagents to form a tissue-specific compound after a brief incubation period.

Kit instructions include specific information about the amount of activity and volume of generator eluate to be added. Depending on the day's schedule, a range of activities and volumes may be prepared to meet specific scheduling needs. It is, however, important to add only those activities and volumes within the ranges stated in the directions. Failure to do so may affect the stability of the compound and alter its distribution in the body. Information about incubation periods and special procedures (such as heating) necessary to ensure complete radiolabeling are also included in the package insert.

Example

What activity and what volume should be added to the following pentetate kit at 0800 hr if four patients will receive 555 MBq (15 mCi) each, sometime between 0800 and 1200 hr?

Pentetate Kit:
Maximum ^{99m}Tc activity to be added: 11.1 GBq (300 mCi)
Reconstituting volume: 2–10 mL

^{99m}Tc–pertechnetate:
Concentration: 925 MBq/mL (25 mCi/mL)
Total volume: 20 mL
Calibration time: 0800 hr.

Solution

^{99m}Tc–pentetate is prepared by adding the appropriate volume and activity of ^{99m}Tc to the lyophilized ("freeze-dried") pentetate reagent supplied in the sterile reaction vial. To ensure that there will be sufficient activity, assume that all four injections will be given at noon. How much activity will be needed at the time of preparation (0800 hr) if 2.22 GBq (60 mCi) will be needed at 1200 hr?

$$\frac{\text{activity at noon}}{\text{4-hr decay factor}} = \text{activity at 0800 hr}$$

$$\frac{60 \text{ mCi}}{0.63} = 95 \text{ mCI (or 3.51 GBq)}.$$

Calculate the volume of ^{99m}Tc–pertechnetate to be added to the kit at 0800:

$$\frac{95 \text{ mCi}}{25 \text{ mCI/mL}} = 3.8 \text{ mL}.$$

Therefore, 3.51 GBq (95 mCi) in 3.8 mL should be added to the pentetate kit. (Keep in mind that this falsely assumes that all the radioactivity can be withdrawn from the vial, so a slight excess of activity should be added to the kit to compensate for what remains in the vial.)

Labeling of most ^{99m}Tc-labeled compounds, with the exception of ^{99m}Tc–sulfur colloid, requires that ^{99m}Tc be in a more chemically active form, such as the 4+ valence state. When ^{99m}Tc is eluted from the generator, it is in the form of pertechnetate (7+). For this reason, ^{99m}Tc labeling is accomplished in the presence of a stannous compound, a reducing agent. The stannous ion (Sn^{2+}) reduces the valence state of the technetium in the pertechnetate ion from 7+ (VII) to 4+ (IV) or another reduced valence state. The reduced valence state of ^{99m}Tc is more reactive, capable of combining with a variety of compounds, such as macroaggregated albumin (MAA), medronate (MDP), pentetate (DTPA), and disofenin. To prepare kits such as this, the technologist injects the appropriate activity and volume of ^{99m}Tc–pertechnetate into the reaction vial and agitates the vial to dissolve the lyophilized reagent. Some kits may require a brief incubation period or heating for complete labeling to occur.

^{99m}Tc–MAA is prepared with reduced ^{99m}Tc. There is, however, one additional consideration in preparing ^{99m}Tc–MAA, related to the number of MAA particles that will be administered to the patient. The recommended number of MAA particles for an adult dosage is 200,000–700,000 particles. It is extremely important to observe the volume requirements stated in the kit package insert. The volume added to the kit governs the number of particles in each milliliter of radiopharmaceutical and, therefore, the number of particles a patient will receive. If too few particles are administered, the perfusion lung image may be technically unsatisfactory and may have the appearance of decreased uptake. Administering more than the recommended number of particles may pose a danger to the patient if too many small arterioles are blocked with MAA particles. Likewise, if the recommended number of particles is not to be exceeded, it is important to observe the expiration time of the MAA preparation. As ^{99m}Tc decays, the number of radioactive particles decreases but the total number of particles remains constant. Therefore, as time passes, more particles must be administered to obtain the same amount of activity.

^{99m}Tc–sulfur colloid incorporates ^{99m}Tc in the unreduced, 7+ valence state. Therefore, a reducing agent such as stannous chloride is not required. Instead, sulfur colloid kits contain an acid, sodium thiosulfate, a buffer, and gelatin. The labeled compound is prepared in two steps. First, the ^{99m}Tc–pertechnetate, acid, and sodium thiosulfate are heated in a sterile reaction vial in a shielded, boiling-water bath or heating block for several minutes. During the heating, elemental sulfur precipitates out of the solution, condensing to form colloidal size particles containing $^{99m}Tc_2S_7$. After the vial is vented, buffer is added to neutralize the pH. Gelatin is used to maintain particle size at 0.01–1 μm. Larger particles may become trapped in the lung capillaries before reaching the liver. Undesirably large particles can be caused by excessive heating during precipitation or high levels of aluminum ion in the ^{99m}Tc–pertechnetate used to prepare the labeled colloid.

Radiopharmaceutical Quality Control

In reduced ^{99m}Tc agents, ^{99m}Tc is present in three different chemical forms: (A) bound ^{99m}Tc agent, (B) unbound (free) ^{99m}Tc–pertechnetate, and (C) hydrolyzed, reduced ^{99m}Tc (HR–^{99m}Tc). The proportions of these three chemical forms may vary from one preparation to the next. Because the bound ^{99m}Tc agent is the desired form, the others should be present only in very small quantities.

^{99m}Tc–pertechnetate and HR–^{99m}Tc are radiochemical impurities. Radiochemical purity is defined as the fraction of total radioactivity present in its desired chemical form. If radiochemical impurities exceed certain limits in a given preparation, the distribution of the radiopharmaceutical in the patient will be altered. Free pertechnetate can be visualized on images as increased tracer concentration in the stomach, thyroid, and salivary glands. Unexpected uptake in the reticuloendothelial system, especially the liver, may indicate significant amounts of HR–^{99m}Tc.

After radiolabeling, the radiochemical purity of a preparation can be determined using radiochromatography. In this method, a drop of the radiopharmaceutical to be tested is placed at a point (called the origin) near one end of the paper strip (Fig. 3.2). The strip is then immersed in a solvent. By capillary action, the solvent travels up the strip, carrying with it the soluble components in the sample. Insoluble components remain at the origin. As the solvent nears the top of the strip, the strip is removed, dried, and cut in half. Each half is counted in a well counter or dose calibrator, and the labeling or tagging efficiency (the fraction of radioactivity incorporated into the desired radiolabeled agent) is calculated (Fig. 3.3).

The labeling efficiency is determined as follows:

labeling efficiency = 100% − (% free ^{99m}Tc–pertechnetate + %HR − ^{99m}Tc).

As shown in Figure 3.3, each half of the strip contains the labeled compound and/or one of the radiochemical impurities. The solvent and support media required vary with the radiopharmaceutical to be tested. Table 3.2 shows examples of solvent/support media systems for certain radiopharmaceuticals. The R_f value is the distance the component travels from the origin compared with the distance traveled by the solvent (Fig. 3.4):

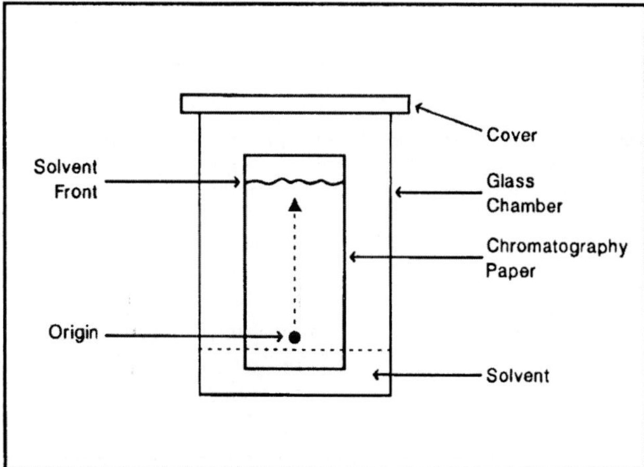

Figure 3.2 Radiochromatography apparatus for determining radiochemical purity.

$$R_f \text{ value} = \frac{\text{distance component travels from origin}}{\text{distance of solvent front from the origin}}$$

Therefore, an R_f value of 0 indicates that the component remains at the origin; an R_f value of 1 indicates that the component is at the solvent front. These values are characteristic for a given radiochemical component in a given solvent/support media system (Table 3.2).

Minimum radiochemical purity values for selected radiopharmaceuticals are given in Table 3.3.

Unit Dose Preparation

When liquid radiopharmaceuticals are received in multidose vials, the technologist must determine the volume containing the desired amount of radioactivity to be administered. The first step in preparing a unit dose is to carefully examine the label on the radiopharmaceutical vial and note the following information:

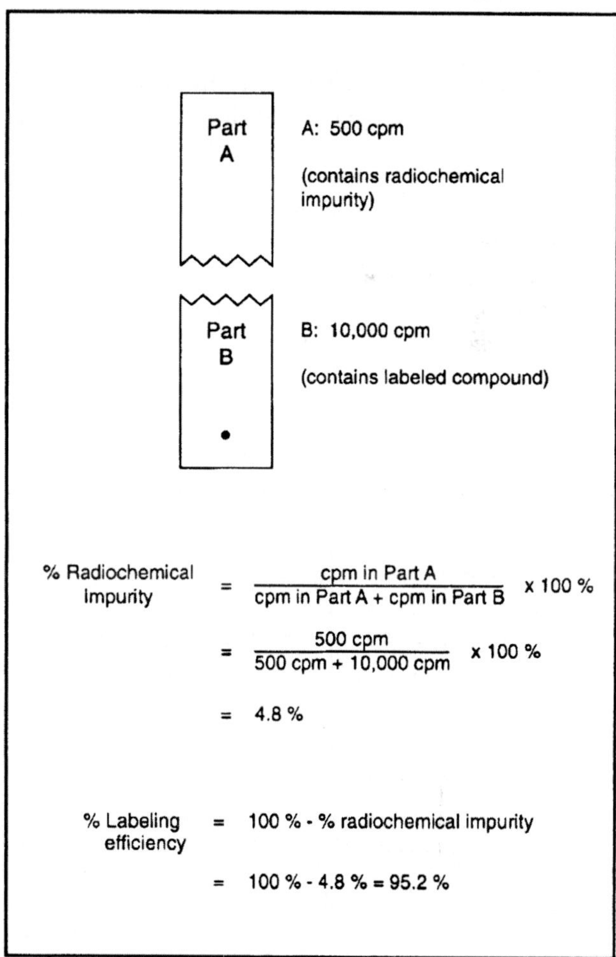

Figure 3.3 Calculation of labeling efficiency or radiochemical purity.

Table 3.2 Radiochromatography Techniques for Selected ^{99m}Tc-Labeled Radiopharmaceuticals

			R_f value[a]		
Radiopharmaceutical	Support media	Solvent	Radiopharmaceutical	Free $^{99m}TcO_4$	HR–^{99m}Tc[b]
^{99m}Tc–sulfur colloid	Gelman ITLC-SG	0.9% NaCl	0.0	0.9	NA
^{99m}Tc–macroaggregated albumin (MAA)	Gelman ITLC-SG	0.9% NaCl	0.0	0.9	NA
^{99m}Tc–sodium pertechnetate	Whatman 31 ET	Acetone	0.0[c]	0.9	0.0
^{99m}Tc–pentetate (DTPA)	Whatman 31 ET	Methyl ethyl ketone	0.0	0.9	0.0
	Gelman ITLC-SG	0.9% NaCl	1.0	1.0	0.0
^{99m}Tc–pyrophosphate	Whatman 31 ET	Methyl ethyl ketone	0.0	1.0	0.0
	Gelman ITLC-SG	0.9% NaCl	1.0	1.0	0.0
^{99m}Tc–medronate (MDP)	Whatman 31 ET	Methyl ethyl ketone	0.0	0.9	0.0
	Gelman ITLC-SG	0.9% NaCl	1.0	1.0	0.0
^{99m}Tc–oxidronate (HDP)	Whatman 31 ET	Acetone	0.0	0.9	0.0
	Gelman ITLC-SG	0.9 NaCl	1.0	1.0	0.0
^{99m}Tc–succimer (DMSA)	Gelman ITLC-SA	Acetone	0.0	1.0	0.0
^{99m}Tc–2,6-diisopropyl IDA (disofenin)	Gelman ITLC-SA	Saturated NaCl	0.0	1.0	0.0
	Gelman ITLC-SA	Distilled H_2O	1.0	1.0	0.0

[a]Distance component travels from origin/distance of solvent from origin.
[b]Hydrolyzed, reduced ^{99m}Tc and includes all colloidal species of reduced ^{99m}Tc.
[c]Methyl ethyl ketone may be used in place of acetone and vice versa.
Reprinted, with permission, from Chilton and Witcofski (1986).

1. Radionuclide and chemical form of radiopharmaceutical: a radionuclide such as ^{99m}Tc may be tagged to a variety of compounds (medronate, pentetate, MAA), so care should be taken to choose the correct radiopharmaceutical for each nuclear medicine procedure.
2. Expiration time/date: the time at which the radiopharmaceutical should no longer be administered to patients.
3. Volume (in milliliters): the total amount of liquid in the vial.
4. Total activity (in millicuries, megabecquerel, microcuries, or kilobecquerel): the total amount of radioactivity present in the vial at the time of assay or calibration.
5. Concentration (in millicuries per milliliter, megabecquerel per milliliter, microcuries per milliliter, or kilobecquerel per milliliter): the amount of activity per unit volume at the time of assay or calibration. Concentration is obtained by dividing the total activity in the vial by the total volume:

$$\text{concentration} = \frac{\text{total activity}}{\text{total volume}}$$

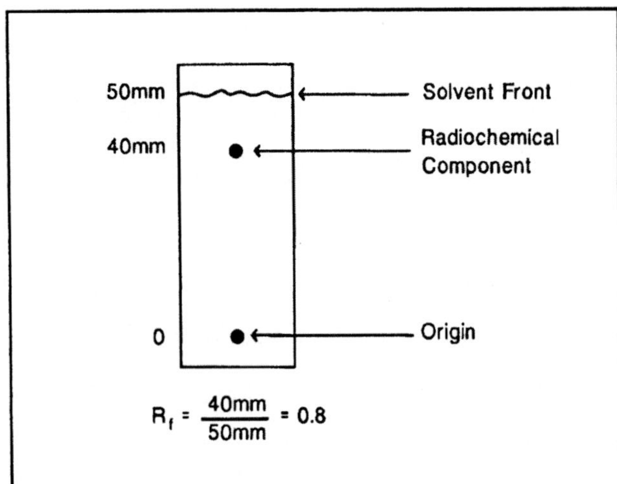

Figure 3.4 Calculation of R_f value.

Table 3.3 Minimum Radiochemical Purity Values for Selected Radiopharmaceuticals (from the U.S. Pharmacopeia)

Minimum purity (%)[a]	Radiopharmaceutical
85	^{99m}Tc–DMSA
90	^{99m}Tc–DTPA
	^{99m}Tc–sodium pertechnetate
	^{99m}Tc–pyrophosphate
	^{99m}Tc–MAA
92	^{99m}Tc–sulfur colloid

[a]Values shown are minimum percentages of radioactivity present in desired radiochemical form. Many radiopharmacy standards for purity are higher than these.

6. Assay or calibration time/date: the time and/or date when the total activity and concentration were determined.
7. Specific activity (in millicuries per milligram, megabecquerel per milligram, μ microcuries per milligram, or kilobecquerel per milligram): the amount of activity per unit mass of a radionuclide or radiopharmaceutical. Do not confuse specific activity with concentration. A specific activity may not appear on all radiopharmaceutical labels.
8. Lot number: a number assigned by the manufacturer to each batch of radiopharmaceutical. The number can be used to trace problems with the radiopharmaceutical.

After the technologist secures the correct radiopharmaceutical and ascertains that the expiration time has not passed, the amount of radioactivity to be administered to the patient is determined. For adults, a standard dosage range has usually been established by the nuclear medicine physician. Occasionally, an adult dosage may be based on the patient's body weight. Several methods can be used to calculate pediatric dosages (Table 3.4). To achieve images of quality and counting statistics similar to those of adults, the method based upon body surface area is recommended. For example, on the basis of this method, a child weighing 30 kg should receive 62% of the recommended adult dosage. Therefore, if the adult dosage is 740 MBq (20 mCi), a child weighing 30 kg should receive 0.62 × 20 mCi or 459 MBq (12.4 mCi).

Next, the initial radiopharmaceutical concentration is decay corrected for the time of administration, and the volume to be administered is determined as follows:

$$C_0 \times \text{DF} = C_t\,,$$

where C_0 is the initial concentration, DF is the decay factor, and C_t is the concentration at time t, so that

$$\frac{\text{patient dose}}{C_t} = \text{volume to be administered.}$$

Example 1

A technologist needs to administer 111 MBq (3 mCi) ^{99m}Tc–MAA to a patient at 1000 hr. If the concentration of the radiopharmaceutical is 555 MBq/mL (15 mCi/mL) at 0600 hr, what volume should be administered to the patient?

Solution 1

Decay correct the initial concentration for 1000 hr. From a table of decay factors for ^{99m}Tc, the decay factor for 4 hr (0600–1000) is 0.631:

$$C_0 \times \text{DF} = C_t\,,$$

or

$$15\ \text{mCi/mL} \times 0.631 = 9.5\ \text{mCi/mL (351 MBq/mL).}$$

Determine the volume to be administered:

$$\frac{\text{patient dose}}{C_t} = \text{volume to be administered,}$$

or

$$\frac{3\ \text{mCi}}{9.5\ \text{mCI/mL}} = 0.32\ \text{mL}$$

Example 2

A technologist needs 129 MBq (3.5 mCi) of ^{201}Tl–thallous chloride to perform myocardial imaging on September 6. If the concentration of the radiopharmaceutical is 74 MBq/mL (2 mCi/mL) on September 8, what volume should be administered to the patient?

Solution 2

Decay correct the September 8 concentration for September 6. From a table of decay factors for ^{201}Tl, the decay factor for 2 days (September 6–8) is 0.634. In this example, the radiopharmaceutical is being administered before the calibration time. Therefore, the initial concentration is the unknown:

$$C_0 \times \text{DF} = C_t\,,$$

or

$$C_0 = C_t/\text{DF},$$

or

$$C_0 = \frac{2.0\ \text{mCi/mL}}{0.634} = 3.2\ \text{mCi/mL (or 118 MBq/mL) on September 6.}$$

Determine the volume to be administered:

$$\frac{\text{patient dose}}{C_t} = \text{volume to be administered,}$$

or

$$\frac{3.5\ \text{mCi}}{3.2\ \text{mCi/mL}} = 1.1\ \text{mL.}$$

Pertinent information, such as the name of the radiopharmaceutical, lot number, activity and volume administered, time, date, person administering the dose, route of administration, and patient's name, should be entered into the appropriate records.

With the appropriate size syringe and a 20- to 22-gauge needle, the technologist withdraws the calculated volume into the syringe in accordance with aseptic and radiation protection techniques. Aseptic technique includes maintaining the sterility of the needle hub as it is

Table 3.4 Methods for Calculating Pediatric Radiopharmaceutical Dosages

1. Clark's rule (weight)	2. Webster's rule (age)	3. Young's rule (age)
$\frac{\text{weight in pounds} \times \text{adult dosage}}{150\text{ lb}}$	$\frac{\text{age (years)} + 1}{\text{age} + 7} \times \text{adult dosage}$	$\frac{\text{age (years)}}{\text{age} - 7} \times \text{adult dosage}$

4. Body surface area[a]

Weight			
kg	lb	Surface area (m^2)	Fraction of adult dose
2	4.4	0.15	0.09
4	8.8	0.25	0.14
6	13.2	0.33	0.19
8	17.6	0.40	0.23
10	22.0	0.46	0.27
15	33.0	0.63	0.36
20	44.0	0.83	0.48
25	55.0	0.95	0.55
30	66.0	1.08	0.62
35	77.0	1.20	0.69
40	88.0	1.30	0.75
45	99.0	1.40	0.81
50	110.0	1.51	0.87
55	121.0	1.58	0.91

[a]Based on average adult surface area of 1.73 m^2.
Reprinted, with permission, from Chilton and Witcofski (1986).

attached to the syringe and the needle itself and sanitizing the top of the radiopharmaceutical vial with alcohol. Radiation protection includes wearing disposable gloves, using syringe and vial shields, working behind a lead shield, and using tongs as appropriate. Working quickly and efficiently minimizes radiation exposure as well. The stability of the radiopharmaceutical can be prolonged if the technologist refrains from injecting air into the radiopharmaceutical vial.

The syringe containing the radiopharmaceutical should then be assayed in a dose calibrator to ascertain that the activity is within the prescribed dosage range. To prevent misadministration, the technologist should label the syringe with the patient's name or identification number, radiopharmaceutical name, initials, activity, and time and date of assay.

Interventional Drugs

Interventional drugs or agents are used in conjunction with radiopharmaceuticals in some nuclear medicine procedures for the purpose of enhancing the information obtained. Unlike radiopharmaceuticals, these pharmaceuticals are not radioactive. These interventional agents possess pharmacologic action, and so are not without the possibility of adverse drug effects. Healthcare professionals administering these pharmaceuticals must be knowledgeable in monitoring patients as well as providing treatment when necessary.

Table 3.5 lists commonly used interventional agents as well as some of the adverse effects and antidotes. This list is not intended to be all-inclusive but may be used as a guide for obtaining more information on the use of these pharmaceuticals. The reader is also referred to other chapters in this book that discuss how these agents are used in various clinical examinations.

Introduction to Pharmacology

Pharmacology includes all aspects of a radiopharmaceutical and/or an interventional drug as it interacts within the body. It includes the pharmacokinetics, pharmacodynamics, and pharmacotherapeutics of the pharmaceutical aspect of radiopharmaceuticals or the interventional drug itself. Once a radiophamaceutical or interventional drug is administered, the way it interacts in the body is a factor of some aspect of pharmacology. The first concept is the drug concentration within the body. A lethal dose would be a dose so large that it becomes toxic to the body. Anything in high enough concentration can be toxic. A therapeutic range is the range of dose that is effective for a particular pharmaceutical or drug. Subthera-

Table 3.5 Nonradioactive Pharmaceuticals Used in Nuclear Medicine

Pharmaceutical	Indication	Dose	Adverse effects	Antidote
ACD Solution	Anticoagulant used in blood labeling	See package insert for labeling	None known	
Acetazolamide (Diamox)	Brain perfusion imaging	1 g in 10 mL sterile water, IV over 2 min	Tingling sensations in extremities and mouth, flushing, lightheadedness, blurred vision, headache	
Adenosine (Adenoscan)	Cardiac stress imaging	140 μg/kg/min for 6 min, or 0.84 mg/kg	Chest discomfort; throat, jaw, or neck discomfort; headache, flushing, dyspnea, ECG change	Discontinue infusion, administer aminophylline if needed
Ascorbic acid	RBC labeling and HDP preparation	See package insert for labeling	May cause temporary faintness or dizziness	
Bethanechol (Urecholine)	Gastric emptying	2.5–5 mg subcutaneously	Abdominal discomfort, salivation, flushing, sweating, nausea, drop in blood pressure	Atropine
Captopril (Capoten)	Renovascular hypertension evaluation	25–50 mg PO 1 hr before study	Orthostatic hypotension, rash, dizziness, chest pain, tachycardia, loss of taste	Saline infusion
Cholecystokinin (Kinevac)	Hepatobiliary imaging	0.02 μg/kg	Abdominal pain, urge to defecate, nausea, dizziness, flushing	
Cimetidine (Tagamet)	Meckel's diverticulum	300 mg/kg for adults; 20 mg/kg IV for children	Diarrhea, headache, dizziness, confusion, bradycardia	
Dipyridamole (Persantine)	Cardiac stress imaging	0.57 mg/kg IV over 4 min	Chest pain, nausea, headache, dizziness, flushing, tachycardia, shortness of breath, hypotension	Aminophylline
Dobutamine (Dobutrex)	Cardiac function	Incremental dose rate over 3 min (adult): 15 μg/kg/min up to 40 μg/kg/min	Angina, tachyarrhythmia, headache, nausea, vomiting	Esmolol
Enalaprilat (Vasotec)	Renovascular hypertension evaluation	Adult: 0.04 mg/kg (max. 2.5 mg) in 10 mL saline, IV over 5 min	Orthostatic hypotension, dizziness, chest pain, headache, vomiting, diarrhea	Saline infusion
Famotidine (Pepcid)	Ectopic gastric mucosa (ulcers)/GERD	Adult: 20 or 40 mg	Headache, dizziness, constipation, diarrhea, arrhythmia, nausea	
Furosemide (Lasix)	Renal imaging	Adult: 20–40 mg IV over 1 min Pediatric: 0.5–1 mg/kg given IV over 1–2 min	Nausea, vomiting, diarrhea, headache, dizziness, hypotension, dehydration	
Glucagon	Meckel's diverticulum	Adult: 0.5 mg (range 0.25–2 mg) Pediatric: 5 μg/kg, given IV or IM	Nausea, vomiting	
Heparin	Anticoagulant	Depends on prothrombin activity	Hemorrhage	
Insulin	FDG-related PET studies	Depends on blood sugar level, generally given if blood sugar is greater than 200 mg/dL	Hypoglycemia	Glucose
SSKI Super saturated potassium iodide (Lugol's Solution)	Block radioactive iodine uptake in thyroid gland as a radioprotectant	Adult:130 mg Child: 65 mg	Skin rash, nausea, angioedema, diarrhea	
Morphine (Astramorph, Duramorph)	Hepatobiliary imaging	0.04 mg/kg,diluted in 10 mL saline, IV over 2 min (range 2–4.5 mg)	Respiratory depression, nausea, sedation, lightheadedness, dizziness, sweating	Naloxone

(continued)

Table 3.5 Nonradioactive Pharmaceuticals Used in Nuclear Medicine (*continued*)

Pharmaceutical	Indication	Dose	Adverse effects	Antidote
Pentagastrin (Peptavalon)	Meckel's diverticulum	6 μg/kg subcutaneously	Abdominal discomfort, urge to defecate, nausea, flushing, headache, dizziness, tachycardia, drowsiness	
Phenobarbital (Luminal)	Hepatobiliary imaging	5 mg/kg/day orally for 5 days	Respiratory depression, nausea, vomiting, dizziness, drowsiness, headache, paradoxical excitement in children	
Ranitidine (Zantac)	Ectopic gastric mucosa	100–150 mg twice daily	Constipation, diarrhea, nausea/vomiting, abdominal discomfort/pain, rash, tachycardia, bradycardia, atrioventricular block, and premature ventricular beats	
Regadenoson (Lexiscan)	Cardiac stress imaging	Adult dose 5 ml (0.4 mg)	Dyspnea, flushing, chest discomfort, angina pectoris, dizziness, chest pain, nausea, abdominal discomfort, and dysgeusia	Aminophylline
rhTSH	Scintigraphy for differentiated papillary and follicular thyroid cancer	Given as two injections of 0.9 mg intramuscularly on each of two consecutive days	Mild adverse reactions such as nausea and headache	
Vitamin B_{12} (Cyanoject, Cyomin)	Schilling's test	1 mg IM	Hypersensitivity reactions, transitory exantherma	

Modified from Table 1 in Park and Duncan (1994). IV, intravenously; IM, intramuscularly.

peutic level of a drug is a dose that is too small and is ineffective. All drugs have a peak onset of maximum therapeutic dose, which is the duration of the drug in the therapeutic range and a half-life time of expected effectiveness within the body.

Routes of delivery of a drug can be via inhalation, IV, IM, spinal cord, orally, transdermal, topically, or rectally. In nuclear medicine, the main ways of delivery are inhalation and IV, while there are some applications for orally, IM, and via the spinal cord (intrathecal) (Table 3.6). What happens to a drug after it is administered is considered part of pharmacokinetics. These include absorption, distribution, metabolism, and elimination from the body:

- Absorption depends on the transport of drug either as an active or passive process, the pH of the drug, and physical factors such as blood flow, surface area, and contact time.
- Distribution depends on blood flow, capillary permeability, and protein binding as well as transport capability such as the blood–brain barrier or a lipophilic vs. a hydrophilic aspect. Bioavailability of a drug is the fraction of a drug that reaches systemic circulation after a particular route of administration and is affected by the firstpass metabolism, solubility, and instability.
- Drug metabolism can affect delivery to target tissues. Pathological conditions can greatly affect metabolism. A prime example would be a sulfur colloid shift when liver disease is in an advanced stage for a liver–spleen study. The spleen and bone marrow will show up more prevalently than the liver. Another example would be a poor renal scan for advanced stages of renal disease. Often overlooked are drug metabolism issues with geriatric or pediatric patients. Smaller doses can be as effective as normal adult doses for these populations due to decreased or increased metabolism, respectively.
- The last aspect of pharmacokinetics is drug elimination. The most important route is usually via the kidneys and can be directly linked to renal filtration, secretion, and reabsorption. The second most important route of elimination of a drug is the gastrointestinal system.

Many aspects make up a pharmacokinetic profile of a drug that depends on mode of administration (oral, IV infusion, IV injection) and whether it is delivered as a single or multiple dose.

Table 3.6 Mechanisms of Localization in Nuclear Medicine

Mechanism	Definition	Example
Capillary blockade	Mechanical obstruction of capillaries or precapillary arterioles in the lung	^{99m}Tc–MAA
Active transport	Cellular metabolism concentrates RP in organ or tissue	^{123}I NaI (sodium iodide) for thyroid function and imaging
Simple diffusion	Movement of RP from area of higher concentration to area of lower concentration	Breakdown of BBB allowing water-soluble RP to penetrate brain in area of affected tissue
Cell sequestration	Removal of damaged or old RBCs from the circulation by the spleen; uptake of WBCs in infection sites	^{51}Cr RBCs taken up by spleen; ^{111}In WBCs, sites of infections
Compartmental localization	Introduction of RP into well-defined body compartment where it remains for an extended period	^{99m}Tc DTPA aerosol; ^{133}Xe
Antigen–antibody complex formation	Radiolabeled antibody binds to tumor-associated antigen	Using tumor-specific labeled antibodies to detect cancer or stage therapy

References and Further Reading

Adenoscan [package insert], 1997. Deerfield, IL: Fujisawa USA.

Chilton HM, Witcofski RL, 1986. *Nuclear Pharmacy: An Introduction to the Clinical Application of Radiopharmaceuticals.* Philadelphia, PA: Lea & Febiger; 26–28, 54–66, 71–82.

Facts and Comparisons, 1999. *Drug Facts and Comparisons.* St. Louis, MO: Wolters Kluwer Health.

Early PJ, Sodee DE, 1995. *Principles and Practice of Nuclear Medicine.* 2nd ed. St. Louis, MO: Mosby; 56–59, 96, 104–117, 747–749.

Eliot AT, 1990. Radionuclide generators. In: Sampson CB, ed. *Textbook of Radiopharmacy: Theory and Practice.* New York, NY: Gordon and Breach Science Publishers; 33–51.

Kowalsky RJ, Falen S, 2004. *Radiopharmaceuticals in Nuclear Pharmarcy and Nuclear Medicine.* 2nd ed. Washington DC: American Pharmacists Association Publications.

Kowalsky RJ, Perry JR, 1987. *Radiopharmaceuticals in Nuclear Medicine Practice.* Norwalk, CT: Appleton & Lange; 59–74.

Marchant T, ed., 1985. *A Guide to Radiopharmaceutical Quality Control.* North Billerica, MA: DuPont.

Park HM, Duncan K, 1994. Nonradioactive pharmaceuticals in nuclear medicine. *J Nucl Med Technol.* 22:240–249.

Phan T, Ling M, Wasnich R, 1987. *Practical Nuclear Pharmacy.* 3rd ed. Honolulu, HI: Banyan Press.

Ponto JA, 1981. Expiration times for ^{99m}Tc. *J Nucl Med Technol.* 9:40–41.

Ponto JA, Swanson DP, Freitas JE, 1987. Clinical manifestations of radiopharmaceutical formulation problems. In: Hladik WB III, Saha GP, Study KT, eds. *Essentials of Nuclear Medicine Science.* Baltimore, MD: Williams & Wilkins; 268–289.

Robbins PJ, 1984. *Chromatography of Technetium-99m Radiopharmaceuticals: A Practical Guide.* Reston, VA: Society of Nuclear Medicine.

Saha GB, 1998. *Fundamentals of Nuclear Pharmacy.* 4th ed. New York, NY: Springer-Verlag.

Schwarz SW, Anderson CJ, Donner JB, 1997. Radiochemistry and radiopharmacology. In: Bernier DR, Christian PE, Langan JK, eds. *Nuclear Medicine Technology and Techniques.* 4th ed. St. Louis, MO: Mosby; 160–183.

Steves AM, 1995. *Nuclear Medicine: Radiopharmacy Series (Six Computer-Assisted Instruction Programs).* Edwardsville, KS: Educational Software Concepts.

Thrall JH, Ziessman HA, 2001. *Nuclear Medicine: The Requisites.* 2nd ed. St. Louis, MO: Mosby.

U.S. Pharmacopoeia Convention, 2000. *United States Pharmacopeia 24* and *The National Formulary 19.* Rockville, MD: U.S. Pharmacopoeial.

Wells P, 1999. *Practical Mathematics in Nuclear Medicine Technology.* Reston, VA: Society of Nuclear Medicine.

CHAPTER 4 Math and Radiation Physics Primer

Liliana Navarrete

Powers and Exponents

Exponents are shorthand for the number of repetitions a quantity is multiplied. This shorthand notation is also used in physics when working with units. For instance, to find the volume of a box, first measure the length, depth, and width. Then multiply each quantity. Imagine that all three quantities are equal to 2 ft. Then the expression for volume would be 2 ft × 2 ft × 2 ft. It can be written as 2^3, where the number 2 is called the base and 3 is called the exponent. Therefore, we have $2 \times 2 \times 2 = 2^3 = 8$. Also, the units used in this case, the feet, can be written using exponential form as ft^3 (cubic feet). Therefore, the volume of the box is 8 ft^3.

In solving mathematical operations with exponents, we have to follow a few rules:

- A quantity to the power zero equals one (example, $5^0 = 1$).
- A quantity to the −1 power is equal to the reciprocal of the quantity (example, $5^{-1} = \frac{1}{5}$).
- To multiply exponent expressions with the same base, keep the base number and add the exponents (example, $5^4 \times 5^3 = 5^7$).
- To divide exponent expressions with the same base, keep the base number and subtract the exponents (example, $5^6 / 5^2 = 5^4$).
- When an exponent expression is raised to a power, then multiply the exponents (example, $(5^4)^2 = 5^8$).

When dealing with exponents, remember that these sets of rules apply not only for numbers but for variables or units as well. For example, to simplify the expression: $(10^8\ m^3)/(10^6\ m^2)$, keep the base number and the base unit, then subtract the exponents (i.e., $10^{(8-6)}\ m^{(3-2)}$), which equals 10^2 m or 100 m.

Scientific Notation

Scientific notation is a standard notation that allows us to handle very large or very small numbers. A number written in scientific notation is a number between 1 and 10 and multiplied by a power of 10. Any number can be written in scientific notation. Numbers greater than 1 have positive exponents (example, $53{,}000 = 5.3 \times 10^4$) and numbers less than 1 have negative exponents (example, $0.0021 = 2.1 \times 10^{-3}$).

Algebra Concepts

Algebra is a generalized math in which letters (called variables) are used in place of numbers. It provides a language in which we can predict outcomes. Before reviewing the equation-solving techniques, it is necessary that you familiarize yourself with different ways of expressing algebraic operations. For instance, there are different ways of expressing multiplication (i.e., $A \times B = A * B = (A)(B) = A \cdot B = AB$) but all are equivalent. There are also different ways of expressing division (i.e., $\frac{1}{x} = 1/x = {}^{1}\!/_{x} = x^{-1}$) but all are equivalent.

Here are some equation-solving techniques. Recall that there is an order in which we perform the operations when they are combined in a single equation:

- First do anything that is in the parentheses.
- Second do any multiplication and/or division.
- Third do any addition and/or subtraction.

Therefore, to undo operations tying up the variable you need to work backward using that order of operations.

When solving a problem, the goal is to convert the equation into the form: variable = number. For instance, let's solve for °C the following equation: °F = (9/5)°C + 32.

To isolate the variable:

- First collect all terms containing the variable on one side of the equation (by subtracting 32 from both sides of the equation, you eliminate 32 from the variable side and get °F − 32 = (9/5)°C.
- Next, undo any operations that are tying up the variable by applying the inverse operation (by multiplying by 5 and dividing by 9 both sides of the equation, you eliminate (9/5) from the variable side and get (°F − 32)(5/9) = °C.

So the answer is °C = (°F − 32)(5/9). The important thing to remember when solving equations is that any operation performed on one side of an equation must be performed on the other side also.

General Atomic and Nuclear Structure

Atomic Components

Atoms are composed of three fundamental particles: electrons, protons, and neutrons. Electrons have a negative electric charge, protons have a positive electric charge, and neutrons have no electric charge. Atoms are naturally electrically neutral, which means they may have the same number of protons and electrons. Neutrons and protons have similar mass, which is almost 2000 times bigger than that of the electrons. The nucleus contains the protons and neutrons, which are also referred to as nucleons. Virtually 99+% of the mass of the entire atom is concentrated in the nucleus since it contains the protons and neutrons. In terms of its size the atomic diameter is about 10^{-8} cm and the nuclear diameter about 10^{-12} cm. This difference of 10^4 (or 10,000) between atomic size and nuclear size indicates the presence of a large amount of empty space within the atom.

When an atom has lost (or gained) an electron, it is no longer electrically neutral, because it has more of one charge than another, and it is called an ion. When electrons are lost, the atom has an excess positive charge, and it is called a positive ion. When electrons are gained, the atom has an excess negative charge, and it is called negative ion.

The mass number, or A-number, represents the number of protons plus neutrons within the nucleus. It is called the mass number because 99+% of the mass of the atom is given by the sum of protons and neutrons.

The atomic number, or Z-number, represents the number of protons in the nucleus. It is called the atomic number because the elemental identity of an atom is determined by the number of protons in the nucleus. In other words, when the Z-number changes (i.e., the number of protons changes), the identity of the atom changes (i.e., it becomes a different element).

These two values are used as subscripts and superscripts of the atomic symbol to indicate the relative numbers of protons and neutrons within an atom. The A-number is displayed as a superscript to the top left of the atomic symbol and the Z-number is displayed as a subscript to the bottom left of the atomic symbol. For instance, ${}^{12}_{6}C$ indicates that carbon's A-number is 12 (i.e., 6 protons plus 6 neutrons within the nucleus) and its Z-number is 6 (i.e., 6 protons in the nucleus, which identifies uniquely this atom as carbon). Since the Z-number is unique for the chemical symbol, it is often omitted (i.e., ${}^{12}C$). The element can have more or fewer neutrons and still be carbon, like ${}^{14}_{6}C$ (the famous carbon-14). Those forms of an element that have the same Z-numbers but different A-numbers (i.e., differing only in the number of neutrons) are called isotopes. Recall that if the Z-number changes the atom becomes a different element (i.e., it is not carbon anymore in our example).

Electronic Shell Transitions

Electron Shells

Electrons are located in orbitals or shells that surround the atomic nucleus. Going from innermost shell outward these shells are designated by the letters K, L, M, N, etc., as shown in Figure 4.1.

Each electron is bound to the atom by an electronic binding energy, usually expressed in the energy unit known as the electron volt (eV). The closer the electron is to the nucleus, the greater the electronic binding energy. The electronic binding energy is unique to each individual element and it is usually expressed as a negative quantity since this energy must be supplied from an outside source to physically remove an electron from the atomic orbital. If an electron is removed from the atom and then an ion is produced, this is called an ionization event.

Characteristic X Rays

When an electron moves between energy shells, the movement is referred to as an electronic transition. Energy must be absorbed from an outside source to move an electron to a higher energy state. Once the electron is in a higher energy state, it will move to fill in any lower energy vacancies that may exist. For instance, if an electron vacancy occurs in a K shell, an electron from a higher energy shell like the M shell could fall to fill up the vacancy as shown in Figure 4.2.

This transition to a lower energy state will result in a release of energy, in other words, the emission of a photon (a massless particle that has no electric charge). Photons' energy can vary, in the electromagnetic spectrum, from infrared light to gamma rays. When the emitted photons come from electron transitions between energy shells, their energy falls into the X-ray portion of the electromagnetic spectrum and is therefore referred to as X rays. The energy of these X rays is just the difference in

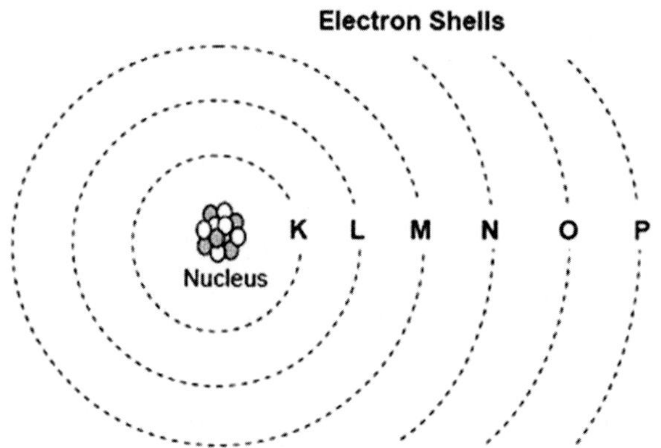

Figure 4.1 Electron shell designations.

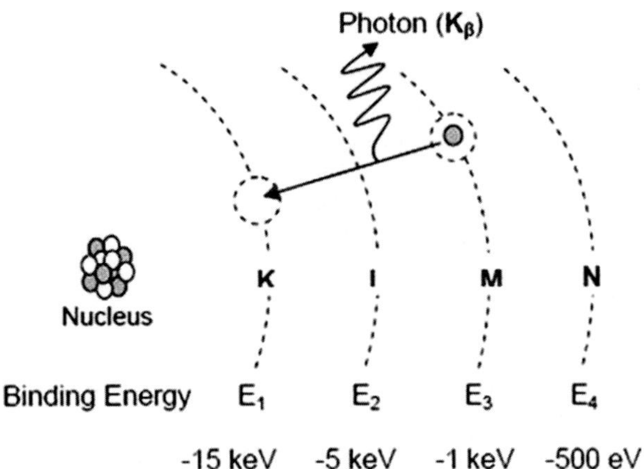

Figure 4.2 X-ray emission by the transition of an outer-shell electron (M shell) into an inner-shell vacancy (K shell). The emitted radiation energy is equal to the difference in binding energies of the electron shells (14 keV).

the binding energies between the two shells involved (14 keV from Fig. 4.2 example). Since electronic binding energies are unique to each individual element, these X rays will have energy signatures that are characteristic of the element from which they originate, hence the name "characteristic X rays."

Characteristic X rays are identified by the letter that indicates the shell to which the electron falls (K in Fig. 4.2), and a Greek subscript (β in Fig. 4.2) that indicates from how many shells away that electron has fallen (i.e., α from one shell away, β from two shells away, γ from three shells away, etc.).

Factors Affecting Nuclear Stability

An element is radioactive when its nucleus will spontaneously emit radiation to achieve nuclear stability. That radiation can be emitted in the form of particles, photons, or both. The two factors that directly influence whether a specific nuclear configuration will be stable or radioactive are the proton-to-neutron ratio and the binding energy per nucleon.

The Proton-to-Neutron Ratio

In the periodic table, as elements build up, more protons are added to the nucleus (i.e., the Z-number increases). As a result strong electrical forces of repulsion result inside the nucleus due to the repulsive force that exists between the like positive charges. The addition of neutrons to the nucleus adds a degree of stability because they are uncharged particles that take up space and allow the positive charges of the protons to be placed further from each other to lower the repulsive forces between protons. Generally, the same number of neutrons and protons form a stable nuclear configuration for elements up to $Z = 20$. For $Z > 20$, there must be more neutrons than protons in order to have a stable nuclear configuration. However, there can be too many neutrons or too many protons in a nucleus, which will cause the nucleus to become unstable (or radioactive). For instance, carbon-13 (i.e., 6 protons plus 7 neutrons) is a stable isotope of carbon that has an extra neutron, but just the addition of one more neutron produces carbon-14, which is radioactive.

Nuclear Binding Energy per Nucleon

The nuclear binding energy is the energy that holds nuclear components together. Recall that, by the law of conservation of matter, matter can be converted into energy. It is this mass–energy conversion process that provides the energy that holds the nucleus together (i.e., the nuclear binding energy). It is important to note that the binding energy per nucleon alone cannot be used to determine whether a particular nuclear configuration will be stable or radioactive. However, when we compare the binding energies per nucleon of two different isotopes of an element, the one having the greater binding energy per nucleon will most likely be stable and the one having the lower binding energy per nucleon will most likely be radioactive. In summary, the greater the nuclear binding energy per nucleon, the more likely a particular nuclear configuration will be stable (or not radioactive).

Radioactive Decay Modes

When the nucleus has excess protons and/or neutrons it will try to get rid of its excess through the emission of particle radiation. When the nucleus has excess energy it will try to get rid of its excess through the emission of a photon of electromagnetic radiation. Often an unstable nucleus will need to emit only energy sufficient to bring it to an almost stable state. When this condition occurs and the nucleus remains in an excited state for a prolonged period, the unstable nucleus is said to be in a metastable state. This condition of the nucleus is designated by the superscript "m" (i.e., ^{99m}Tc). In general, when a nucleus is unstable, it will try to remove that instability by one of the following radioactive decay modes.

Alpha Decay

If an unstable nucleus has too many protons and too many neutrons, it will most likely emit alpha (α) radiation. An α-particle is identical to a helium nucleus (i.e., two protons and two neutrons). This particle carries a highly ionizing electric charge (+2), which means that as the particle travels through tissue it creates many ion pairs and free radicals (i.e., atoms with an unpaired number of electrons) that could be damaging to biological tissue. Even though an α-particle is capable of dumping large amounts of energy into the biological tissue, it is not considered an external hazard because it has very low penetrating abilities (i.e., loses its energy very quickly). Note that each time an α-particle is emitted, a new element is formed (known as the daughter product) since the Z-number changes. For instance, when thorium-232 emits an α-particle, the daughter product is radium-228 (i.e., ${}^{232}_{90}\text{Th} \rightarrow {}^{228}_{88}\text{Ra} + \alpha +$ energy). In α-decay the Z-number of the parent product is reduced by 2 and the A-number by 4 (i.e., two protons plus two neutrons).

Beta Decay

Unstable nuclei having an excess number of neutrons (i.e., neutron rich) will tend to decay by negative beta (β) particle emission. In general, one of the excess neutrons is converted into a proton, an electron or β-particle, and an anti-neutrino. The proton remains in the nucleus of the daughter product while the negative β-particle (β^-) and the anti-neutrino ($\bar{\nu}$) are ejected from the unstable nucleus. β-particles are more penetrating than α-particles but the penetration depth depends upon energy. Low-energy betas cannot be detected with a standard Geiger counter and a more sensitive counter like the liquid scintillation detector must be used in this case. When a β-particle is emitted, the Z-number of the daughter product is increased by 1 (i.e., a neutron is converted into a proton). For instance, when carbon-14 emits a β-particle the daughter product is nitrogen (i.e., ${}^{14}_{6}\text{C} \rightarrow {}^{14}_{7}\text{N} + \beta^- + \bar{\nu} +$ energy). In β-decay the Z-number of the parent product is increased by 1, but the A-number is not changed.

Positron Emission

Unstable nuclei having an excess number of protons (i.e., proton rich) will tend to decay by positron emission and/or electron capture. In positron emission, one of the excess protons is converted into a neutron, a positive electron or positron, and a neutrino. The neutron remains in the nucleus of the daughter product while the positron (β^+ or e^+) and the neutrino (ν) are ejected from the unstable nucleus. For the positron to be formed, the parent nucleus must have at least 1.02 MeV of energy available for the decay process to occur. A positron particle (e^+) interacts almost immediately with an electron (e^-) to create an annihilation event. Both particles annihilate each other and produce two 511-keV photons that travel out 180° from each other as shown in Figure 4.3.

When a positron (β^+) is emitted, the Z-number of the daughter product is decreased by 1 (i.e., a proton is converted into a neutron). For instance, when oxygen-15 emits a β-particle the daughter product is nitrogen-15

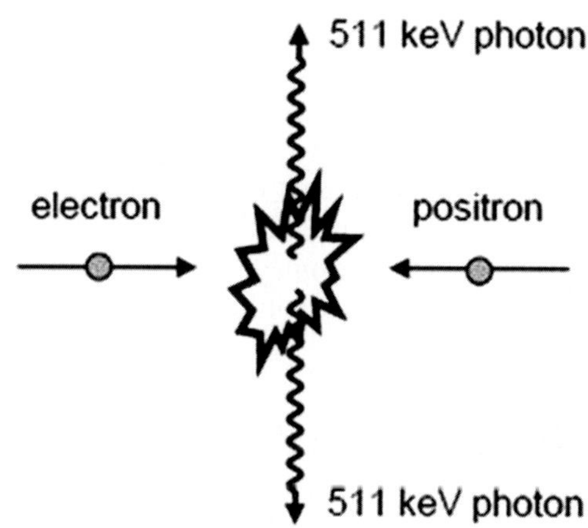

FIGURE 4.3 Annihilation radiation in which electron and positron particles annihilate each other and produce two 511-keV photons that travel out 180° from each other.

(i.e., ${}^{15}_{8}\text{C} \rightarrow {}^{15}_{7}\text{N} + \beta^+ + \nu +$ energy). In positron emission the Z-number of the parent product is decreased by 1, but the A-number remains unchanged.

Electron Capture

Electron capture (EC) is an alternative mode of decay if a proton-rich nucleus cannot meet the 1.02 MeV of energy required for a positron emission. In this decay mode, typically an inner-shell electron is captured by the unstable nucleus. The captured electron combines with an excess proton to produce a neutron and a neutrino. The neutron remains in the nucleus of the daughter product while the neutrino (ν) is ejected from the unstable nucleus. The captured electron creates a vacancy in the inner electron shell of the atom giving rise to the production of characteristic X rays. For instance, when the iodine-125 nucleus captures an inner-shell electron, the daughter product is tellurium-125 (i.e., ${}^{125}_{53}\text{I} + e^- \rightarrow {}^{125}_{52}\text{Te} + \nu +$ energy). In EC the Z-number of the parent product is decreased by 1, but the A-number remains unchanged. Note that positron decay and electron capture produce the exact same daughter product in the end. Overall, radionuclides that are proton rich may decay by positron emission only, electron capture only, or both positron emission and electron capture.

Gamma Decay

Gamma (γ) emission is the decay mode for those unstable nuclei that just need to rid themselves of excess energy. Often one of the other decay processes will leave the nucleus in an excited state, which will be followed by the emission of a γ-photon (i.e., γ-rays). For instance, technetium-99m emits γ-radiation (i.e., ${}^{99m}_{43}\text{Tc} \rightarrow {}^{99}_{43}\text{Tc} +$

γ). In γ-emission the Z-number of the parent product and the A-number remain unchanged. It is important to remember that all types of electromagnetic photons carry neither mass nor charge. They are pure electromagnetic energy that can be very penetrating, depending upon the energy. For the above reasons, to interact with matter they must have a direct hit. Recall also that there is no difference between an electromagnetic photon, a γ-photon, and an X-ray photon except for their origins.

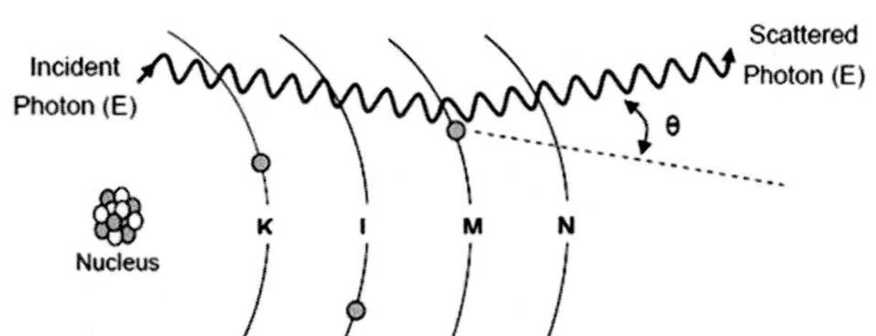

FIGURE 4.4 Classical scattering in which the incident photon experiences only a slight change in its direction and essentially no energy change.

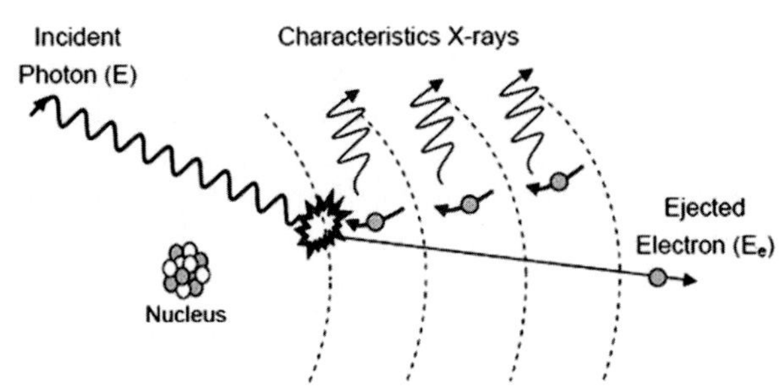

FIGURE 4.5 Photoelectric absorption in which the ejection of a shell electron results in the emission of characteristic X rays.

Radiation's Interaction with Matter

Radiation may be of two general types: particulate and electromagnetic. Particulate radiation refers to particle radiation having mass like α-, β-, and neutron radiation. Electromagnetic radiation, also known as photon radiation, refers to radiation that carries neither mass nor electric charge like γ-rays and X rays. When a charged particle or photon of radiation interacts with matter multiple things can happen: the radiation will expend some of its energy as it excites a passing atom's electrons; the radiation will expend some of its energy as it interacts with a passing nucleus; and the radiation will expend enough of its energy to create a complete ionization event (i.e., an ion pair). The method by which radiation interacts with matter is determined by whether the radiation carries any electrical charge, the energy of the radiation, and the type of matter it travels through. Since nuclear medicine mainly deals with photon radiation, we focus on photon interactions with matter.

Whenever a photon interacts with matter of any type, it can transmit through the material unaffected, it may be totally absorbed, or it may be scattered. The exact way a photon interacts is primarily determined by its energy. Ordered from low to high energy, a photon will interact in one of the following ways.

Classical Scattering

Classical scattering is typically a low-energy nonionizing interaction in which the photon is momentarily absorbed either by a shell electron or by the atom as a whole, and then reemitted with only a slight change in its direction and essentially no energy change (see Fig. 4.4). This type of interaction occurs in only about 5–10% of interactions of diagnostic energy photons in tissue.

Photoelectric Absorption

This process occurs when the incident photon has energy that is just a little greater than the binding energy of an inner-shell electron. When the incident photon interacts directly with the inner-shell electron, it gives up its entire energy to the inner-shell electron and ejects it with a certain amount of kinetic energy. Therefore, photoelectric absorption is an ionizing type of interaction that represents the complete absorption of the incident photon. The ejection of a shell electron results in the emission of characteristic X rays. The whole process is shown in Figure 4.5.

Compton Scattering

Compton scattering is a medium-energy photon interaction in which the incident photon ejects an outer-shell electron having a lower binding energy (see Fig. 4.6). In addition to the ejected electron, a lower-energy scattered photon is produced. This lower-energy scattered photon will most likely be photoelectrically absorbed in its next interaction. Compton scattering is also an ionizing type of interaction, and it tends to be the predominant mode of interaction of diagnostic energy photons in soft tissue.

Pair Production

Pair production is high-energy photon interaction in which the incident photon interacts with the intense electromagnetic field of the nucleus. The photon disappears and in its place an electron–positron pair appears (i.e., pair production); the process is shown in Figure 4.7.

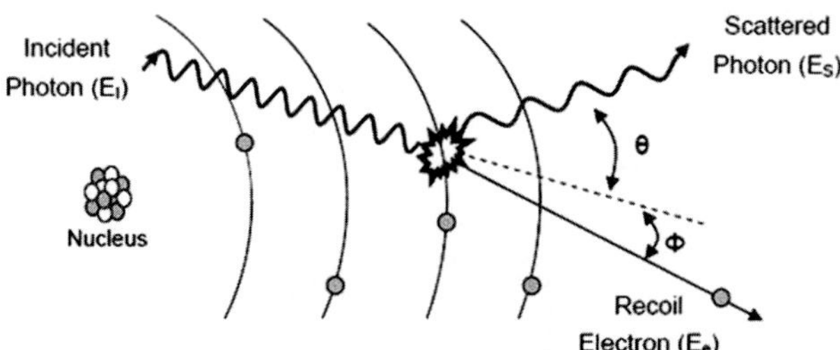

FIGURE 4.6 Compton scattering in which the incident photon ejects an outer-shell electron and also a lower-energy scattered photon is produced.

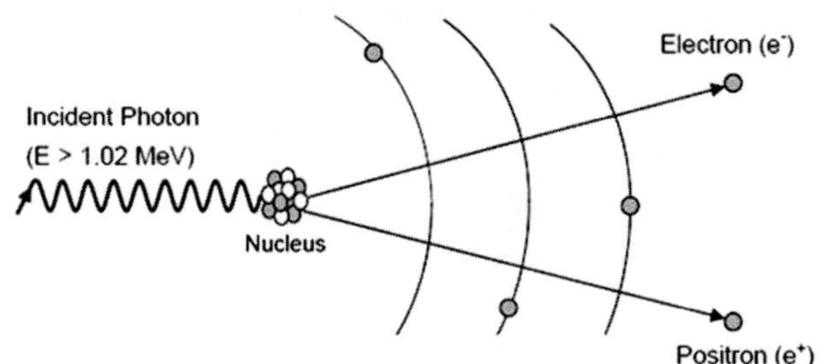

FIGURE 4.7 The incident photon interacts with the nucleus producing an electron–positron pair.

References and Further Reading

Bushberg JT, Seibert JA, Leidholdt EM, Boone JM, 2002. *The Essential Physics of Medical Imaging.* 2nd ed. Philadelphia, PA: Lippincott Williams & Wilkins.

Cherry SR, Sorenson JA, Phelps ME, 2003. *Physics in Nuclear Medicine.* 3rd ed. Philadelphia, PA: Saunders.

Christian PE, Waterstram-Rich KM, 2007. *Nuclear Medicine & PET/CT: Technology & Techniques.* 6th ed. St. Louis, MO: Mosby.

Thompson, MA, 2006. Notes from class: Medical Radiation Physics. University of Alabama at Birmingham.

CHAPTER 5 **Instrumentation and Basic Counting Statistics**

Patricia Wells, Remo George, Amy Byrd Brady, and Norman Bolus

Nuclear medicine uses a number of instruments to detect and quantify radiation. This chapter deals with selecting the appropriate instrument and instrument parameters for a task. Chapter 6 covers quality control testing of these instruments.

Instrument Selection

Survey Meters

Survey meters are used to measure radiation exposure rates. A Geiger–Mueller (G–M) counter is used for surveys to detect contamination (Fig. 5.1). It is appropriate for this purpose because it has a rapid response time. It can also detect a wide range of exposure rates because it uses multiple scales. The U.S. Nuclear Regulatory Commission requires that facilities have a survey meter capable of detecting exposure rates from 1 μSv/hr (0.1 mrem/hr) to 1 mSv/hr (100 mrem/hr). G–M counters meet this requirement.

G–M counters may be fitted with an end-window probe or a pancake probe. The pancake probe allows the technologist to survey a larger area. The end window must be pointed directly at the source for accurate detection.

G–M counters are not as accurate as portable ionization meters ("cutie pies," the code name inspired by its diminutive size given to this instrument when developed for the Manhattan Project during World War II), but they are more sensitive. The cutie pie has a longer response time, so the exposure rate calculation is based on more data and is therefore more accurate. It is superior to the G–M counter in measuring high dose rates. The portable ionization chamber is most useful for accurately determining the exposure rate being produced by a patient who has received a radionuclide, particularly a therapeutic dosage.

Well Counter

The well counter uses a thallium-activated sodium iodide (NaI [Tl]) crystal to detect very low activities of radioactivity. It is significantly more efficient than a gamma camera, because the radioactive sample is actually placed into a well that has been bored into a thick cylinder of crystal. The well counter's sensitivity also limits the instrument's use, because activities much greater than 74 kBq (2 μCi) can cause coincidence loss. When too many photons strike the crystal, counts are lost while the instrument is in deadtime. If the counting rate is very high, the well counter may experience perpetual deadtime (paralysis).

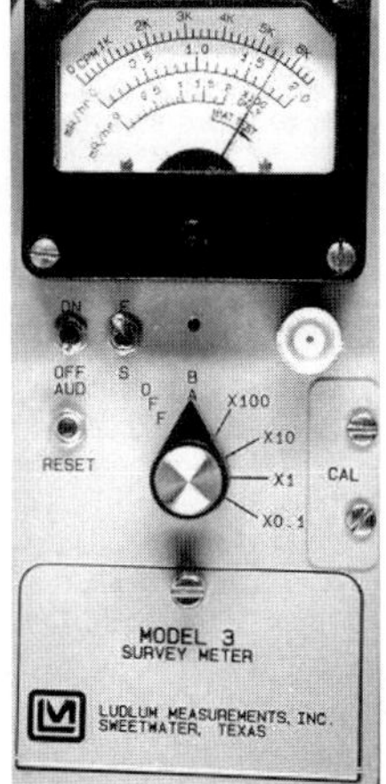

Figure 5.1 Typical G–M detector survey meter showing battery check deflection. (Courtesy of University of Alabama at Birmingham NMT Program Picture Library.)

The well counter is used for wipe tests to detect very low levels of removable contamination. It can detect activities that are below the background levels seen with a G–M counter. It is also used to count blood, plasma, and urine samples from patients who are having non-imaging studies, such as blood volumes and, historically, Schilling tests. The standards used for such tests must be diluted to a known percentage of the original patient dosage so as not to produce coincidence loss or paralysis.

Uptake Probe

An uptake probe uses an NaI(Tl) crystal to quantitate activity within a patient. It may be connected to the same spectrometer used by the well counter. A toggle switch allows the technologist to select between the two detectors. The uptake probe is not as sensitive as the well counter because of detector-to-source geometry. A cylinder-shaped collimator, often called flat-field collimation, limits the area "seen" by the crystal and eliminates much of the background activity. The patient is usually positioned several inches from the end of the collimator to ensure that the entire organ of interest is within the field of view. Commonly used for thyroid uptakes, this can result in some loss of counts if the organ of interest is too large or too close to the probe, because some photons will miss the collimator opening. As long as the thyroid or other organ of interest is a standard distance away and is positioned at the same distance from the collimator each time it is counted (referred to as being on the same iso-response curve), then a true comparison of counts can be made with it and a standard.

The standard used for thyroid uptake studies is the patient's capsule or another capsule prepared at the same time and activity. It does not require dilution, because the uptake probe can accept much higher counting rates than the well counter. The uptake probe is also used for splenic sequestration studies.

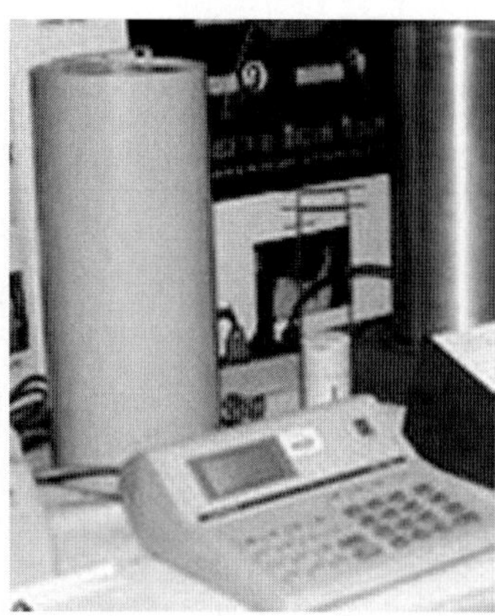

Figure 5.2 Typical dose calibrator used to assay doses in nuclear medicine. (Courtesy of University of Alabama at Birmingham NMT Program Picture Library.)

Dose Calibrator

The dose calibrator is an ionization chamber that measures radioactivity in curies or becquerels rather than in counts per unit time (Fig. 5.2). It can accurately measure dosages as low as 0.01 μCi, as well as activities in the curie range. Dose calibrators readily detect γ photons but are less sensitive for β radiation, because only high-energy β radiation can pass through the glass chamber walls. Correction factors are usually required for measuring β radiation.

Gamma Camera

Gamma cameras come in a variety of configurations, including single-, double-, and triple-head models (Fig. 5.4). Some models allow for whole-body imaging or portable use. Many models are capable of performing tomographic (single-photon emission computed tomography [SPECT]) imaging.

The choice of planar vs. SPECT imaging is based on the purpose of the study and time constraints. Planar imaging is appropriate for many studies. However, SPECT allows for greater sensitivity and resolution in imaging of tissues deep within the body or in areas where other structures interfere. Because SPECT images an organ or tumor from many angles, the exact location and size can be better determined.

SPECT acquisitions are not as time consuming in modern cameras as in the past. However, consideration should be made if the patient must maintain an uncomfortable position for a prolonged period of time, in which case the possibility of patient motion artifacts increases.

Patient-to-detector distance affects resolution for whole-body, planar, and SPECT imaging. It may be necessary to adjust the distance as the camera moves along a patient's body during whole-body imaging. Patient-to-detector distance can be a problem during SPECT, because the camera may be very close to the patient's body at some projections and distant at others. The distance from the center of rotation must remain constant or the image reconstruction will be erroneous. Some tomographic cameras can acquire data using an elliptical (or body-contouring) orbit, allowing the camera to remain closer to the body at the anterior and posterior aspects as well as the lateral positions (Fig. 5.3).

Positron Emission Tomography Camera

Positron emission tomography (PET) technology has developed rapidly, with a variety of crystals being used (Fig. 5.5). Crystals must be thicker and denser than those used in gamma cameras to stop the 511-keV photons produced during positron annihilation. PET cameras produce studies with higher resolution than SPECT cameras, particularly when the area of interest is deep within the body.

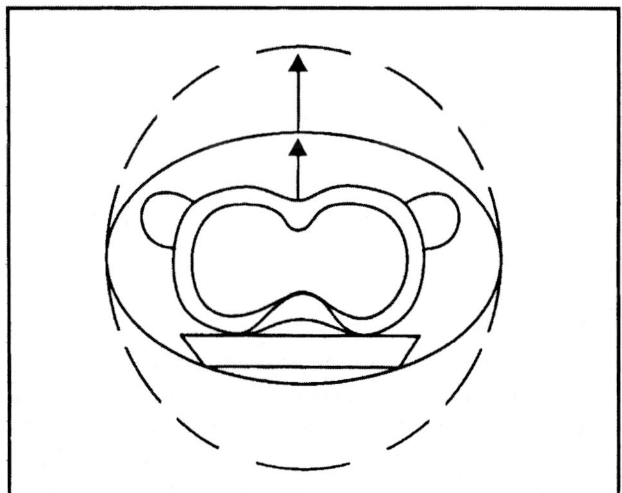

Figure 5.3 Comparison of distance between patient and detector with circular and elliptical orbits.

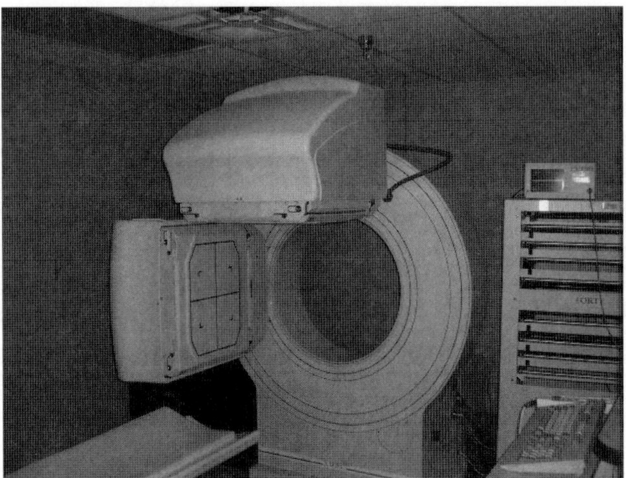

Figure 5.4 Typical dual-head gamma camera, in cardiac imaging 90° orientation mode. (Courtesy of University of Alabama at Birmingham, West Birmingham, AL.)

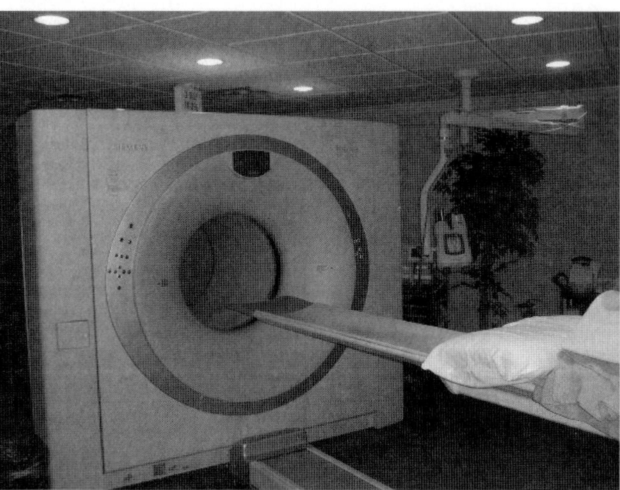

Figure 5.5 Typical PET/computed tomography (CT) camera. (Courtesy of Image South, PET Center of Birmingham, Birmingham, AL.)

Instrument Operating Parameters

Counting Statistics Primer

Three important types of counting statistics errors that one should be familiar with can occur. They are *mistakes*, which we should work to avoid and can cause grossly inaccurate results. Often referred to as "user error," these can be simple mistakes like leaving the γ camera set for ^{57}Co instead of ^{99m}Tc after calibrating with a ^{57}Co sheet. *Systematic errors*, which are consistent but inaccurate, can be difficult to detect unless we use statistical analysis of results to determine. Tests such as chi-square analysis can reveal that a systematic error is occurring. The last type of error is *random errors*. Random error will always exist and is impossible to totally eliminate. It can be minimized and an amount of random error can be predicted using statistics, which is often called precision. Therefore, systematic errors can be precise but not accurate, while random error, which is expected because of the randomness of the decay of radioactivity, can be precise and accurate as long as it is predicted and expected (Fig. 5.6).

Energy spectrums are exhibited in mono- or polyenergetic curves, which depend on the overall spectrum of a radionuclide. Every peak and valley of an energy spectrum has some meaning; however, a photopeak of interest for imaging purposes is always displayed as a Poisson or Gaussian distribution by nature. This is due to the nature of the counting system technology used in nuclear medicine technology. The best-case scenario would be a spike at the peak of interest; however, usually this is a distribution of energy signals around a main photopeak (Fig. 5.7). The randomness of these energy signals (in kilo-electron volts) that are counted as a part of a window around a main photopeak can be predicted

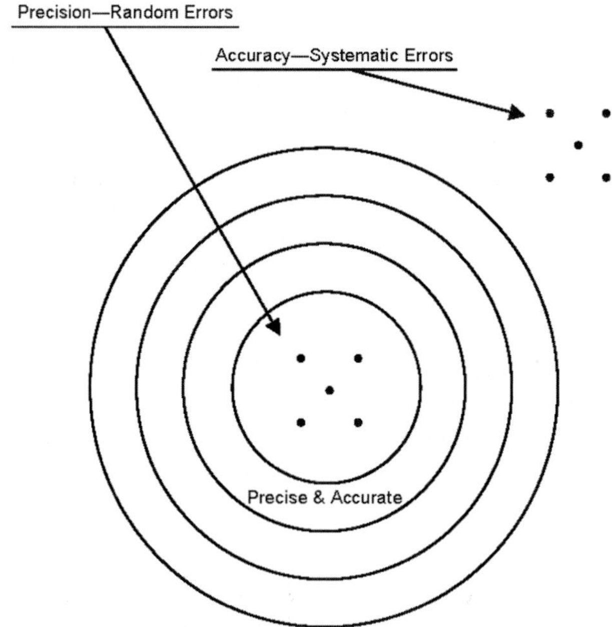

Figure 5.6 Comparison of precision vs. accuracy concerning counting errors. Precise targeting allows one to hit the middle of the bull's-eye, but some random error occurs with not all points being exactly in the same spot. Accurate targeting can still be precise but involve a systematic error that misses the bull's-eye entirely.

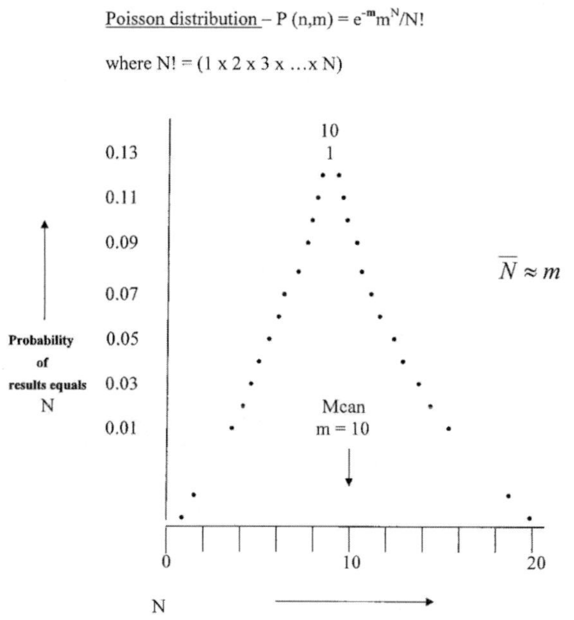

Figure 5.7 Example of a Poisson or Gaussian distribution, which is considered a normal distribution around a mean (average) number. Poisson distribution: $P(n,m) = e^{-m}m^N/N!$, where $N! = (1\times2\times3\times\ldots\times N)$.

to ensure the accuracy of the counting instrument. This is usually done by calculating the percentage error and keeping the error as low as possible; generally at or below 1% error is considered acceptable and optimal.

Calculating Percentage Error

Percentage error is also known as percentage uncertainty. The most common way to calculate this is by taking 100% and dividing it by the square root of the average or a single count in counts per minute:

$$V = \frac{100\%}{\sqrt{N}},$$

where V is the uncertainty and N is either the average count or a single count per minute.

Using this equation for a 10,000 count one obtains a 1% error. It is a general rule of thumb that any nuclear medicine procedure or wet lab test should not be done with less than 10,000 counts since this is the threshold amount for a 1% counting error due to random error.

The following equation can be used to determine how long to count for a certain counting error; this depends on the count rate

$$\text{Time (minutes)} = \frac{R_s + 2R_b}{(R_s)^2}\left(\frac{100\%}{v}\right),$$

where R_s is net count rate sample in counts per minute, cpm (net count rate sample cpm = gross cpm—background cpm), R_b is the background cpm, and v is the desired percentage uncertainty.

Confidence Intervals

Often it is necessary to determine if a counting system is operating according to expected random error. The expected confidence intervals can be used to compare expected vs. observed counts from a nuclear counting system. An expected confidence interval is a calculated range from a normal distribution surrounding an average based on the expected standard deviation. To determine expected confidence intervals, take the average of a number of samples greater than 10,000 cpm; generally at least 10 samples are used. For example, if the average number is 12,555 cpm, then the square root of this number would be the expected standard deviation of the count or 112 cpm, and 1 standard deviation confidence interval range would be 112 of 12,555 or 12,443 to 12,667. By convention, we would then say that of the 10 samples done, 68% would be expected to fall in this 1 standard deviation confidence interval. Observed amounts may be different, which could mean that a systematic error is occurring with the counting system and you would then want to perform a chi-square test to see whether this is the case. Likewise, the second (95%) and third (99.9%) standard deviation would be 2 times 1 standard deviation and 3 times 1 standard deviation, respectively, and the corresponding ranges (confidence intervals) would be 224 of 12,555 and 336 of 12,555 (Table 5.1).

Semilog Graphing

Semilog graphing is important for mathematically and graphically calculating half-life or whenever the natural decay of radionuclide is needed in a time–activity curve (sometimes referred to as TAC). By using semilog graphing, the natural curve associated with the decay of radioactivity becomes a straight line. The slope of the line can be determined and used mathematically to aid in half-life determination, half-value layer determination, and other time–activity equations.

Semilog graph paper is designed so that the *y*axis of the graph has a logarithmic scale and the *x*-axis a linear scale. The *y*axis of a semilog graph is defined in terms of the number of cycles. The entire length of the *y*-axis could be one cycle, that is, from 1 to 10, or two cycles from 1 to 10 to 100. To know how many cycles to use, you should know the logarithmic range of the values. For example, the data ranges from 1000 to 100,000 counts. Therefore, 1000 to 10,000 would be one cycle and 10,000 to 100,000 would be one cycle. A total of 2 cycles would be used for data ranging from 1000 to 100,000 counts. Figure 5.8 displays semilog graph paper with a total of 3 cycles.

Table 5.1 Example of 1, 2, and 3 Expected Confidence Interval for an Average Count of 12,555 cpm with 10 Samples

Standard deviation	Square root of 12,555 cpm = 1 standard deviation	Lower confidence interval limit	Upper confidence interval limit	Expected no. of samples that should fall in CI	Observed no. of samples that fall in CI
1 × 112	112	12,443	12,667	6–7/10	Depends
2 × 112	224	12,331	12,779	9–10/10	Depends
3 × 112	336	12,219	12,891	10/10	Depends

For average count of 12,555 cpm with 10 samples counted.

Well Counter and Uptake Probe Parameters

Minimum Counts

Samples and standards should be counted for a time interval that results in a minimum of 10,000 counts. The total count is divided by the time to provide cpm, which is the data used in most calculations. Because each count is converted to cpm, variable counting times can be used.

Geometry

The standard used for thyroid uptake studies must be counted with the same geometry as the patient to ensure that counting is done at the same iso-count contour curve. A positioning bar is often used to ensure that the distance is consistent. For instance, when the uptake probe is used for splenic sequestration, the positioning must be identical for each uptake interval.

Geometry also affects the results obtained when counting samples in a well counter. To achieve accuracy, all of the following parameters must be identical for a particular study: sample volume, sample container, and sample placement. Samples containing high activities must be diluted, and a dilution factor must be included in the calculation. If both samples and standards contain high activities, they can all be counted on top of the well instead of within it. As long as the same geometry is used for each, the results will be accurate and reproducible.

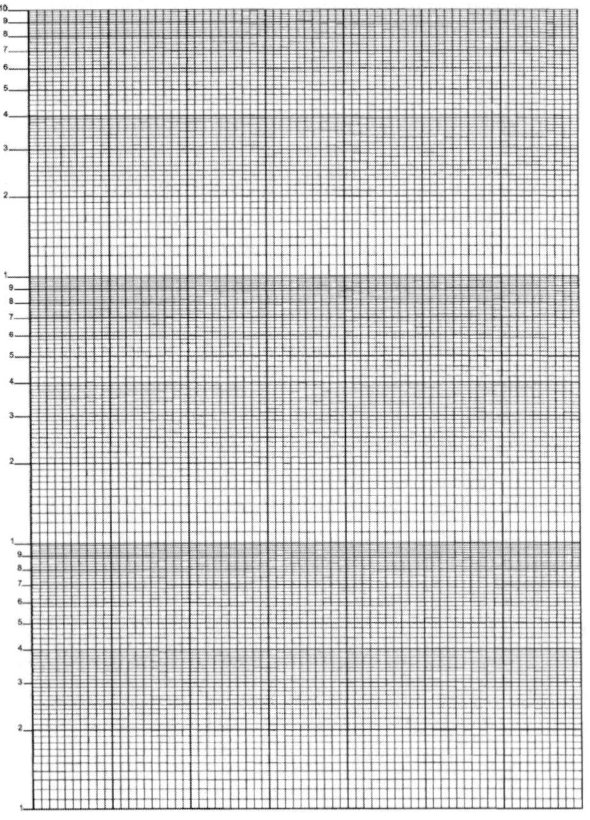

Figure 5.8 Three-cycle semilog graph paper.

Pulse-Height Analyzer Settings

Both well counters and uptake probes use a spectrometer to select the energies that are to be accepted by the pulse-height analyzer. A spectrometer uses one of two methods for selecting the energies. The first employs an upper- and lower-level discriminator (ULD and LLD, respectively). A specific energy is selected for each using the potentiometer dials on the instrument. The second method uses an LLD or threshold and a window above it. The window is expressed in kilo-electron volts. For example, if a 10% window for cesium-137 (^{137}Cs) (662 keV) is desired, the spectrometer must be set to accept energies between 629 and 695 keV. If the spectrometer uses the first method, the LLD will be set for 629 keV and the ULD will be set for 695 keV. If the second method is used, the threshold will be set for 629 keV and the window will be set for 66 keV (10% of 662 keV).

Gamma Camera Parameters

Collimators

Image resolution, sensitivity, and magnification can be enhanced by using various collimators. The energies produced by a radionuclide also affect collimator selection. The characteristics that determine the function of a collimator include: hole size, thickness of the septal walls, length of bore, and slant of the holes. Figure 5.9 shows four standard collimator configurations and how each affects the size of the image created on the crystal. The parallel-hole configuration has several variations, such as low-energy all-purpose (LEAP, also called general all-purpose [GAP]) and high-resolution and high-sensitivity collimators. The high-resolution collimator has narrow holes and a long bore, so photons entering the collimator at even a moderate angle will be stopped when they strike a septum. This improves the quality of the image by eliminating scatter but decreases sensitivity (the number of photons striking the crystal). A high-sensitivity collimator has holes that are larger than those of a LEAP collimator. The bore is also shorter. This allows more photons to reach the crystal but at the expense of resolution. The LEAP collimator is designed to optimize resolution and sensitivity.

When medium-energy radionuclides (indium-111 [^{111}In], iodine-131, and gallium-67) are used, a collimator with thicker septal walls and a longer bore is required. High-energy nuclides (511-keV positron emitters) require even thicker walls and an even longer bore. Without these modifications, the energetic photons would penetrate the septa, causing increased scatter and decreased resolution. The longer bore increases the probability that a partially attenuated photon will strike the septa to be stopped before it strikes the crystal. Medium- and high-energy collimators provide lower sensitivity and resolution than low-energy collimators because more of the crystal is covered with lead. It is important to note that the terms low, medium, and high energy are relative. For example, collimators from different manufacturers may be labeled as medium-energy collimators, but, because each collimator may have a slightly different design, the actual photon energy range for a specific medium-energy collimator will be different.

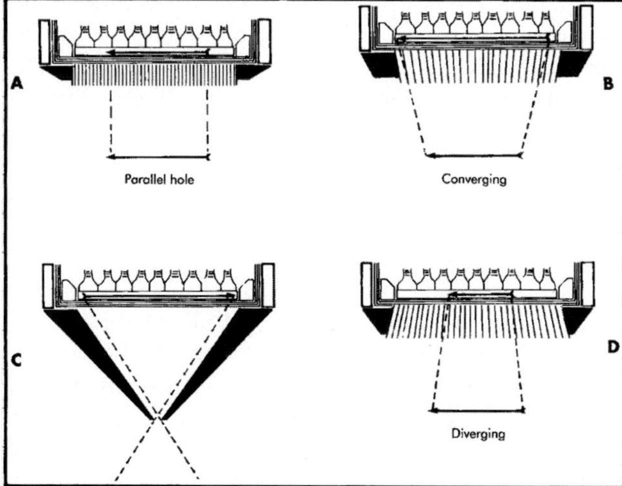

Figure 5.9 Four standard collimator configurations. A. Parallel hole, B. Converging hole, C. Pinhole, D. Diverging hole. (Reprinted, with permission, from Christian *et al.*, 2003.)

The source-to-collimator distance affects resolution, sensitivity, and magnification, depending upon the type of collimator involved. Table 5.2 summarizes these effects.

Pulse-Height Analyzer Settings

Gamma cameras use a centerline and window to select the energies that will be accepted. The photopeak energy is used as the centerline, and the size of the window is determined by a percentage of the centerline energy. For example, a 20% window for ^{99m}Tc would utilize a centerline of 140 keV and include energies that fall between 126 keV (−10% of 140) and 154 keV (+10% of 140). The window would be 28 keV wide. A 20% window for the 245-keV γ radiation from ^{111}In would be 48 keV wide (245 keV ± 10% = 221–269 keV).

The wider the window, the greater the sensitivity. However, if the window is widened so that it includes more Compton scatter, resolution will decrease. Window width is selected on the basis of resolution and sensitivity requirements of a specific study.

Matrix Size and Memory Mode

Most scintillation cameras used today are interfaced with a computer. The counts collected during image acquisition are stored in the computer's memory. The camera crystal is electronically divided into a matrix consisting of many small areas called pixels (picture elements). Each

Table 5.2 Effect of Increasing the Source-to-Collimator Distance

Collimator type	Resolution	Sensitivity	Magnification
Parallel hole	Decreases	Slight decrease	No magnification at any distance
Diverging	Decreases	Decreases	Decreases
Converging	Decreases	Increases slowly, then decreases beyond the focal plane	Increases
Pinhole	Decreases	Increases	Depends on distance of source organ to pinhole aperture (b) and distance from the aperture to the crystal face (focal length = f)*

*If b = f, then there is no magnification or reduced image size (1:1). If b < f, then magnification increases. If b > f, then image size is reduced.

pixel is assigned a separate storage location in the computer memory. At the beginning of an acquisition, all of the storage locations are set to 0. When a count is detected in a particular location in the crystal, the storage location in computer memory corresponding to that location in the crystal is incremented by 1. At the conclusion of an acquisition, each storage location contains a number indicating the number of counts that have been registered at that location in the crystal.

The matrix size describes the number of pixels that will be used to acquire an image. To determine the total number of pixels being used in an acquisition, one simply multiplies. For example, the number of pixels in a 64 × 64 matrix is 4096. Matrix size influences the spatial resolution of an image. In general, the larger the matrix (the greater the number of pixels), the better the spatial resolution within the limits of the camera and collimator resolution.

The maximum number of counts that can be contained in a pixel is related to the number of bits in each pixel, which is related to memory mode. Each bit is essentially an on/off switch. The number of on/off combinations determines the number of counts that can be recorded in a single pixel. This is calculated using 2^x, where x is the number of bits and 2 represents the switching being either on or off. Memory may be either byte mode or word mode. One byte contains 8 bits and 1 word contains 16 bits. One word, therefore, equals 2 bytes. A byte can contain a maximum of 2^8 or 256 counts, and a word can contain 2^{16} or 65,536 counts. Byte mode is used when no more than 256 counts will be acquired in a pixel. If this limit is likely to be exceeded, then word mode must be used. If the maximum counts per pixel are exceeded, the additional counts that should have been recorded are lost, resulting in inaccurate data.

Computers can save data in byte mode or word mode. In byte mode, each byte of information requires 1 byte of memory. The amount of memory required for a study is equal to the number of pixels if the study is acquired in byte mode. If the study is acquired in word mode, twice as much memory is required, because 1 word equals 2 bytes. Table 5.3 shows commonly used matrix and mode settings, the memory required for each, and examples of when each may be used.

Table 5.3 Matrix, Mode, and Memory[a]

Matrix size/mode	Pixels in matrix	Bytes of memory	Studies
64 × 64 byte	4,000	4,000	First pass
64 × 64 word	4,000	8,000	Low-count SPECT (^{201}Tl)
128 × 128 word	16,000	32,000	High-count SPECT (^{99m}Tc)
256 × 256 byte	65,000	65,000	Low-count planar
256 × 256 word	65,000	128,000	High-count planar
512 × 512 byte	262,000	262,000	Whole-body scan
512 × 1024 byte	524,000	524,000	Whole-body scan

[a]Data are rounded.

Acquisition Mode

Studies can be acquired in either frame mode (most common) or list mode. In frame mode, all counts are collected into one storage matrix in a given time period. The matrix size and framing rate are selected before acquisition. The framing rate is the length of time each image is acquired. For example, a "spot" view bone image will have only one frame of data collected for either a total number of counts or for a fixed length of time. A renal function study, a dynamic frame-mode acquisition, may have a framing rate of 20 sec/frame for 25 min for a total of 75 frames of data. After acquisition, the matrix and framing rate cannot be adjusted, although frames can be added together.

Two factors must be considered when selecting the frame rate for a dynamic study: the purpose of the study and the count rate. A quantitative study will usually be performed for a shorter framing rate to provide more data points, whereas a qualitative study requires adequate counts per frame to provide the desired resolution. The higher the count rate, the shorter the frame rate can be. For example, a first-pass cardiac study for ejection fraction calculation is acquired at 0.2–0.5 sec/frame, whereas the first-pass portion of a three-phase bone scan of the feet is acquired at 2–4 sec/frame.

In list mode, counts are stored sequentially as x and y coordinates. Other parameters may be stored along with the x and y coordinates such as time markers and the R wave from an ECG. One advantage of the direct storing of the x and y coordinates as digital information in the system as well as the additional information is that after acquisition, this information may used to enhance the image or change it by processing the data in a different way. Also, the matrix and framing rate are selected and if necessary, these can be changed until the optimum parameters are identified.

Zoom Mode

Zoom mode may be used when a small organ occupies only a portion of the field of view. Acquiring in zoom mode (analog zoom) increases resolution. Postacquisition zoom makes the image larger and easier to see but does not improve resolution. With a significant postacquisition zoom factor, resolution actually decreases.

When zoom mode is used, the matrix size remains the same but is spread over a smaller area, usually the middle of the field of view, so each pixel is smaller. When zoom mode is used during a SPECT acquisition, a uniformity correction flood that is acquired in the same zoom mode must be applied, so the pixel size is matched.

Information Density

Information density, the number of counts per square centimeter, directly affects resolution. There must be adequate counts in a frame to resolve differences between activities in adjacent pixels (contrast). Increasing the counts decreases the signal-to-noise ratio and improves the quality of the image. Background subtraction can be used to further increase the target-to-background ratio.

General Gamma Camera Signal Processing

With digital processing of image acquisition signals, signal processing of the data is very important to modern nuclear medicine instrumentation and image production. Various aspects of the digital information can be manipulated to form the final image; these include drawing regions of interest, developing time–activity curves, normalizing the image, filtering the signal, and reconstructing the image using all of the available data.

Region of Interest (ROI)

A closed boundary surrounding an area for which statistics are desired. Two methods are generally used for creating ROIs: *manual method* in which the operator visually identifies edge of organ and *automatic edge detection method* in which the computer identifies organ edge through use of one of several edge-detection algorithms.

Time–Activity Curves (TAC)

The total number of counts in ROI placed on an organ at various frames of a dynamic study plotted as function of time. TAC curves provide information on the physiological functioning of the organ.

Normalization

Normalization is performed when comparing two different regions or images. *Image or frame normalization* is used when adjusting display intensities of two different images or frames with different maximum counts, respectively. This is done by taking all the pixels in the image or frame with lowest maximum count and multiplying each pixel with the same multiplication factor so that its maximum count matches that of the second image or frame, thus making it easier to compare the data sets. *Area normalization* is usually performed when trying to compare two regions of interest of unequal size as when employing background subtraction with a relatively smaller background ROI than the actual organ ROI. Normalized background counts are obtained by multiplying the total counts in the background ROI by a correction factor. The correction factor for normalization is calculated by taking the ratio of the number of pixels in larger ROI (usually the organ ROI) and dividing it by the number of pixels in the smaller ROI (usually the background ROI).

Filters

Filters, which are mathematical algorithms, are used to decrease statistical noise in an image or to enhance edges by removing or reducing the frequencies that make up an image. SPECT studies must be filtered to help eliminate the star artifact produced by the backprojection process and to decrease the effects of noise. The star artifact is found in the low frequencies, whereas data from the target (the activity in the tissue) are primarily found in the low and medium frequencies. Statistical noise occurs across the whole frequency spectrum but is most apparent in the high frequencies where there is less activity (Fig. 5.10).

A ramp filter (or high-pass filter) is used to suppress the star artifact and enhance edges. It is used only in filtered backprojection image reconstruction. Low-pass filters are used to decrease the effects of high-frequency noise (statistical count fluctuations). The two most frequently used low-pass filters are the Butterworth and Hanning filters.

The Butterworth filter has two variable parameters: the critical frequency (or cutoff frequency) and the power factor (or order). The critical frequency may be defined in two ways: (1) the frequency at which the filter magnitude drops to zero, or (2) the frequency at which the filter magnitude drops below a given value. When discussing filters, it is important to know which definition is being used. When a high critical frequency is used, more high frequencies are retained in the image. If the study is underfiltered (that is, if the critical frequency is set too high), the images will appear grainy or pixelated. If the critical frequency is set too low and the study is overfiltered, the images will become overly "smoothed" and lesions may actually become hidden.

The power factor is related to how fast the filter is cut off or how quickly the transition is made between fre-

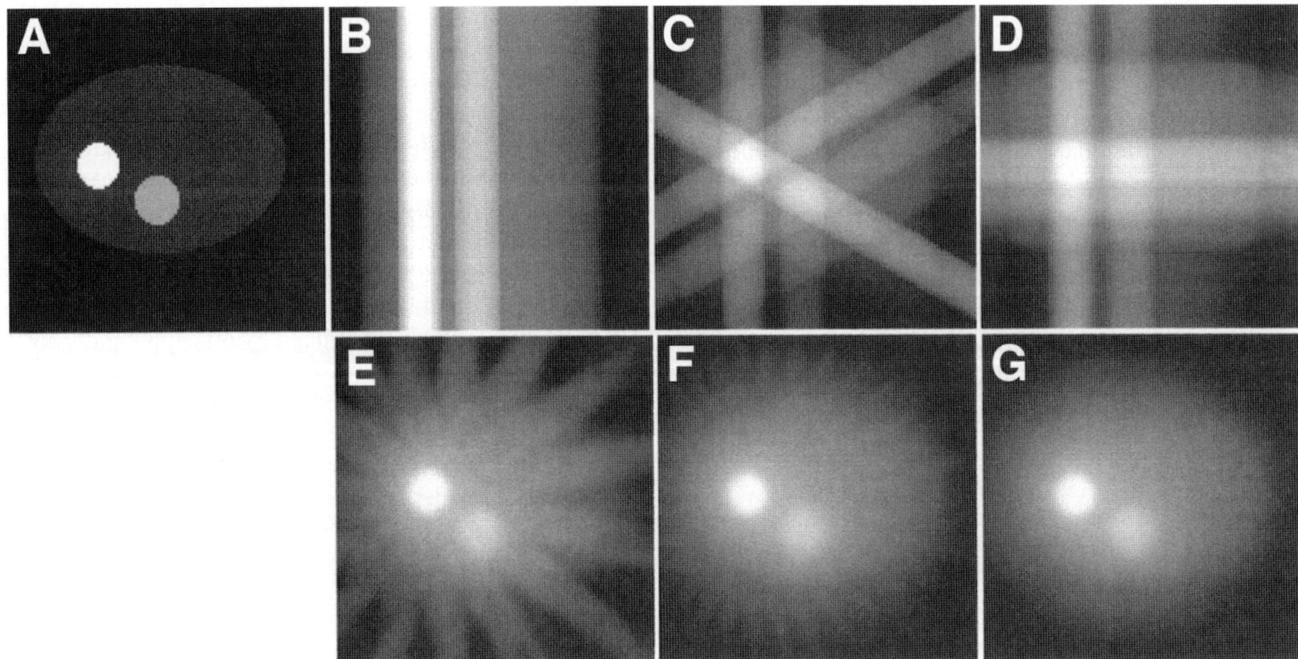

FIGURE 5.10 Illustration of star (or streak) artifact. (A) Slice used to create projections. (B–G) 1, 3, 4, 16, 32, and 64 projections equally distributed over 360° are used to reconstruct slice using backprojection algorithm. Activity in reconstructed image is not located exclusively in original source location, but part of it is also present along each line of backprojection. As number of projections increases, star artifact decreases. (Bruyant, 2002, p. 1347.)

quencies that are kept and those that are eliminated from the image. Changing the power factor produces much more subtle changes in the images than changing the critical frequency. However, the higher the power factor, the steeper the slope and the more high frequencies removed. The lower the power factor, the more high frequencies are preserved (see Fig. 5.11).

The Hanning filter uses a single parameter: the cutoff frequency. This is the frequency at which the filter reaches zero. Frequencies above the cutoff are eliminated, so the lower the cutoff, the smoother the image. Over- and underfiltering will have the same effects as seen with the Butterworth filter.

Image Reconstruction

Nuclear medicine produces 2D "projections" of the 3D radionuclide distribution inside the body or organ. Image reconstruction is the process of transforming a set of 2D projections into a 3D image. One important benefit of this technique is that it facilitates improved contrast and easier interpretation of radioactivity distribution pattern by eliminating (or minimizing) overlapping organ tissue below and above the slice of interest.

Simple backprojection reconstruction is the simplest image reconstruction method and it makes no assumptions about the form of the image before reconstruction. The major problem with simple backprojection reconstruction is that it leaves "extra" counts on the image in the wrong places creating a "Star" or "Spoke" artifact.

Filtered backprojection (FBP) reconstruction is used to remove the "star" or "spoke" artifact from the simple backprojection reconstructed images. This can be done before backprojection (prefiltering) or after backprojection (postfiltering). FBP is usually done in the frequency space domain (where a mathematical operation like Fourier synthesis is used to change a projection's actual data from being a function of amplitude vs. "counts/pixel" to a completely equivalent function of amplitude vs. "cycles/pixel" or in the spatial domain (using a process called convolution). Images are then mathematically reconstructed from these collected "transformed projections" of activity. One drawback of FBP is that it assumes no "attenuation" of activity by the surrounding tissue and hence has no mechanism for attenuation correction.

Iterative reconstruction methods are very computer intensive and until recently the computer power needed to perform this reconstruction hadn't been available in the clinic. This is a successive approximation technique in that the final image is achieved after successive algebraic iterations (or approximations) of the obtained projection data to match the projection data of an estimated "guess image." Iterative reconstruction methods can correct for attenuation, depth, and scatter effects. *Ordered-subset expectation maximum (OSEM)* is a type of iterative algo-

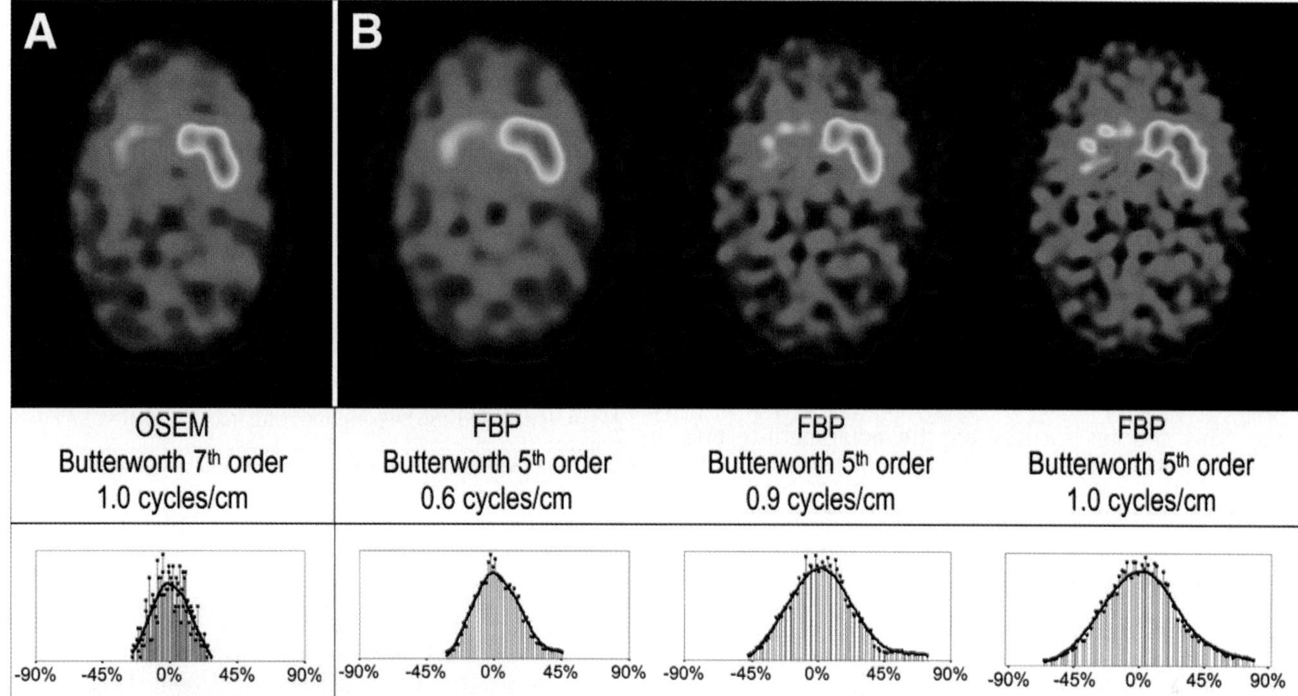

Figure 5.11 Example of differentiation between caudate and putamen in OSEM-reconstructed images (A) and in images reconstructed by filtered backprojection (FBP) with various filter parameters (B) for phantom scan. Histograms show activity distribution within occipital reference region expressed as percentage difference from mean counts per voxel. (Koch *et al.*, 2005, p. 1807.)

rithm used in modern PET systems that is faster and more efficient than conventional iterative methods. Instead of using all of the data in each iteration, OSEM uses only selected subsets of the projection data, which results in fewer iterations and substantially faster reconstruction. A high-quality image is achieved with a balance of iterations and a high number of subsets.

References and Further Reading

Bruyant PP, 2002. Analytic and iterative reconstruction algorithms in SPECT. *J Nucl Med.* 43(10):1343–1358.

Cherry SR, Sorenson JA, Phelps ME, 2003. *Physics in Nuclear Medicine.* 3rd ed. Philadelphia, PA: Saunders; 89–98, 100–106, 115–117, 218–226.

Christian PE, Bernier DR, Langan JK, eds, 2003. *Nuclear Medicine and PET: Technology and Techniques.* 5th ed. St. Louis, MO: Mosby; 56–79, 98–122.

Christian P, 2001. Nuclear counting systems. In: Fahey F, Harkness B. *Basic Science of Nuclear Medicine* [book on CD-ROM]. Reston, VA: Society of Nuclear Medicine.

Cooke CD, 1998. *How Shall I Filter?: Let Me Count the Ways* [videotape]. Reston, VA: Society of Nuclear Medicine.

Early PJ, Sodee DB, 1995. *Principles and Practice of Nuclear Medicine.* 2nd ed. St. Louis, MO: Mosby; 139–144, 177–188, 216–249.

English RJ, 1995. *Sngle-Photon Emission Tomography: A Primer.* Reston, VA: Society of Nuclear Medicine; 49–55, 61–69.

Harkness B, 2001. Factors affecting high quality SPECT. In: Fahey F, Harkness B. *Basic Science of Nuclear Medicine* [book on CD-ROM]. Reston, VA: Society of Nuclear Medicine.

Koch W, Hamann C, Welsch J, Pöpperl G, Radau PE, Tatsch K, 2005. Is iterative reconstruction an alternative to filtered backprojection in routine processing of dopamine transporter SPECT studies? *J Nucl Med.* 46(11):1804–1811.

Lee K, 1991. *Computers in Nuclear Medicine: A Practical Approach.* Reston, VA: Society of Nuclear Medicine; 7–11, 87–98, 147–220.

Madsen M, 1994. Computer acquisition of nuclear medicine images. *J Nucl Med Technol.* 22:3–11.

Madsen M, 2001. The gamma camera. In: Fahey F, Harkness B. *Basic Science of Nuclear Medicine* [book on CD-ROM]. Reston, VA: Society of Nuclear Medicine.

Powsner RA, Powsner ER,1998. *Essentials of Nuclear Medicine Physics.* Malden, MA: Blackwell Science; 78–91, 126–131, 144–147.

Wells P, 1999. *Practical Mathematics in Nuclear Medicine Technology.* Reston, VA: Society of Nuclear Medicine; 81–82, 140–146, 154–158.

Yester M, 2001. Collimators. In: Fahey F, Harkness B. *Basic Science of Nuclear Medicine* [book on CD-ROM]. Reston, VA: Society of Nuclear Medicine.

CHAPTER 6 Instrumentation Quality Control

Patricia Wells, Ann Steves, and Norman Bolus

The standard of practice and, in some cases, regulatory agencies require that quality control testing be performed on instruments to ensure patient safety and diagnostic accuracy. The term *quality control* refers to the tests that are performed to identify equipment problems and is only one part of quality assurance, a system designed to identify problems, propose solutions, and monitor results to achieve the desired level of performance. This chapter focuses on the equipment-testing segment of a quality assurance system.

Table 6.1 Scintillation Camera Quality Control

Test[a]	Recommended testing frequency[b]
Field uniformity	Daily
Spatial resolution	Weekly
Spatial linearity	Weekly
SPECT center of rotation	Weekly
SPECT uniformity correction	Monthly

[a]These tests should also be performed after repair or preventive maintenance.
[b]Camera manufacturers may recommend other testing frequencies.

Scintillation Camera

Table 6.1 lists the quality control tests to be performed on scintillation cameras and the optimal testing frequency according to the current standard of practice.

Field Uniformity

Field uniformity is the ability of a scintillation camera to produce a uniform image when the source provides a uniform distribution of photons over the detector (Fig. 6.1). Clinically, it is the ability of the instrument to produce accurate images of a radionuclide distribution in patients. Common sources of nonuniformity are seen in Figure 6.2.

Field uniformity measurements may be intrinsic or extrinsic. Intrinsic testing monitors the condition of the sodium iodide crystal and electronics associated with the scintillation camera detector and is performed without a collimator attached to the detector. The extrinsic method, performed with a collimator in place, assesses the instrument as it is used clinically. Both methods have advantages and disadvantages. However, once a specific method is adopted, it should be used consistently by everyone performing quality control testing in the nuclear medicine department to ensure that day-to-day comparisons can be accomplished. Table 6.2 compares the testing procedures for the two methods.

Uniformity images should be inspected carefully for areas of nonuniformity and compared with previous flood images (Fig. 6.3). The possibility of subtle changes requires comparison of current images with those acquired several weeks or months previously. Causes of field nonuniformity are listed in Table 6.3, along with the common appearance and action required in each case. Figures 6.4, 6.5, and 6.6 are examples of three of the causes of field nonuniformity listed in Table 6.3.

Figure 6.1 Homogeneous distribution of activity on a uniformity flood. Uniformity images should be inspected carefully for areas of nonuniformity and compared with previous flood images. (Courtesy of Children's Hospital of Alabama, Birmingham, AL.)

Spatial Resolution

Spatial resolution is the ability of a scintillation camera to separate small objects in space, or how much each point in an image is blurred. Clinically, resolution affects the ability to visualize small defects. As with field uniformity, spatial resolution can be measured intrinsically or extrinsically with an appropriate bar or multihole phantom (Fig. 6.6). The smallest bar and space width or hole size should be matched to the resolution limits of the camera system specified by the camera manufacturer.

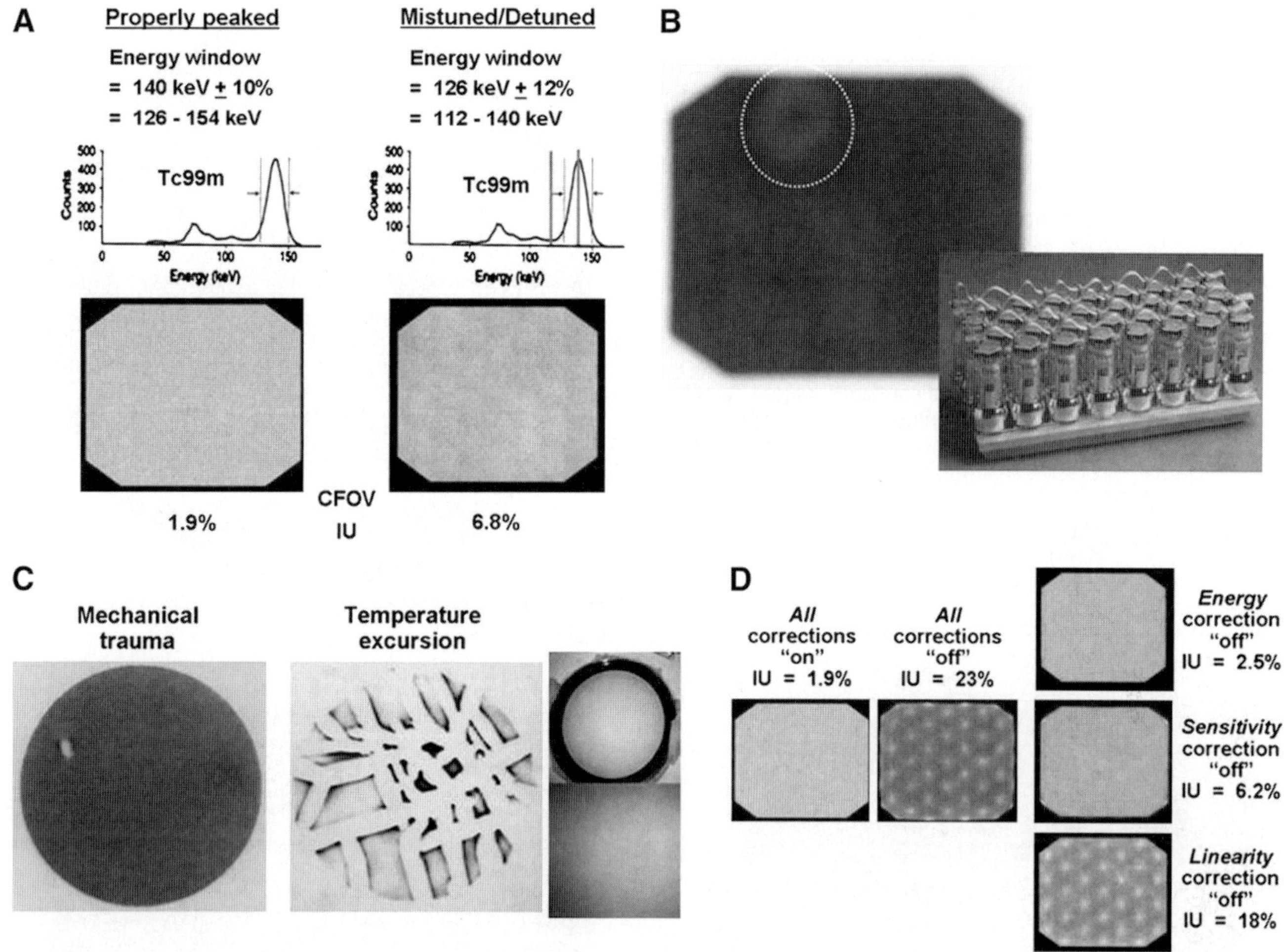

Figure 6.2 Sources of gamma camera nonuniformity. (A) Mistuning (or detuning), meaning that the photopeak of the radionuclide does not coincide with the photopeak energy window of the camera, perhaps because the energy window (as shown) or high voltages of PMTs are not set correctly. (B) Uncoupling of PMT from crystal, resulting in loss of all or part of light signal in resulting air gap between the PMT entrance window and crystal. (Courtesy of Dr. Barbara Binkert, New York Presbyterian Hospital, New York, NY.) (C) Cracked crystal, either because of mechanical trauma (impact) or temperature excursion (i.e., temperature increase or decrease at a rate faster than 5°C/hr, causing crystal to expand or contract, respectively, to the point of cracking). Note that it is the rate of temperature change that is critical. Photographs on the right show cracked crystal that produced corresponding image. Even though the cracks are grossly imperceptible, artifacts produced are dramatic. (Courtesy of Dr. Barbara Binkert, New York Presbyterian Hospital, New York, NY.) (D) Corrupted, deleted, or switched-off software correction tables. Even perfectly functioning gamma cameras have some nonuniformity due to point-to-point variations in energy spectra, greater sensitivity at and lower sensitivity between PMTs, and residual nonuniformity due to ill-defined factors such as variations in crystal thickness. Associated nonuniformities are measured and used to create energy, linearity, and uniformity (or sensitivity) correction tables. Note that the linearity correction table has the biggest effect on uniformity: if corrupted, deleted, or switched off, PMT pattern becomes grossly apparent, and IU approaches 20%. Fortunately, in contrast to the uniformity correction table and, to a lesser extent, the energy correction table, the linearity correction table rarely needs to be updated once the gamma camera is installed; if updating becomes necessary, it is almost always done by field-service personnel of the manufacturer, not by the end user (Zanzonico, 2008, p. 1120).

Hine–Duley Phantom

The Hine–Duley phantom consists of lead bars and spaces of three different widths; the bars are embedded in plastic (Fig. 6.7A). Because resolution is not measured equally over all areas with this phantom, multiple images must be acquired to assess resolution for the entire detector area using the minimum bar spacing.

Four-Quadrant Bar Phantom

The four-quadrant bar phantom contains spaces and lead bars of four different widths (Fig. 6.7B). The spaces and bars in each quadrant are of equal width. Four images, acquired at 90° to one another, are required to assess resolution over the entire detector.

Table 6.2 Comparison of Intrinsic and Extrinsic Scintillation Camera Quality Control

Method-specific factor	Intrinsic	Extrinsic
Collimator	None	Low-energy, parallel hole
Radiation source	^{99m}Tc point source	^{99m}Tc refillable sheet source
Radiation source	^{99m}Tc refillable sheet source	^{57}Co sealed sheet source
Radiation source	^{57}Co sealed sheet source	
Source position	Point source placed in open-topped lead container at 4–5 crystal diameters away from detector	Sheet sources placed directly on collimator or supported several inches above face
Source position	Sheet sources placed directly on crystal face or supported several inches above face	

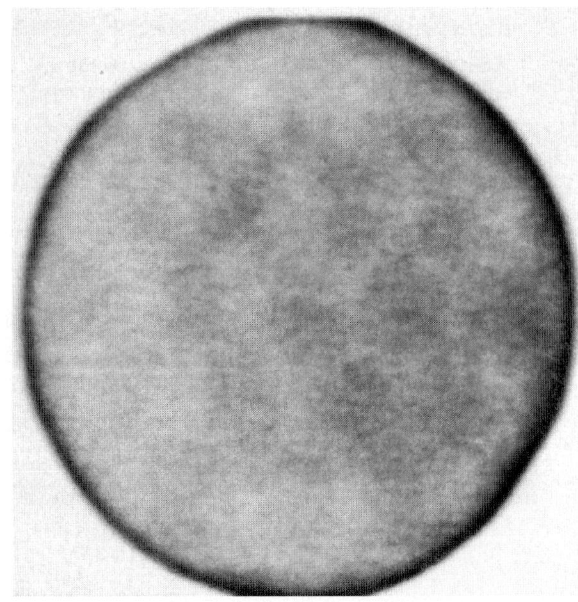

Figure 6.4 Incorrect or misadjusted photopeak showing photomultiplier tubes.

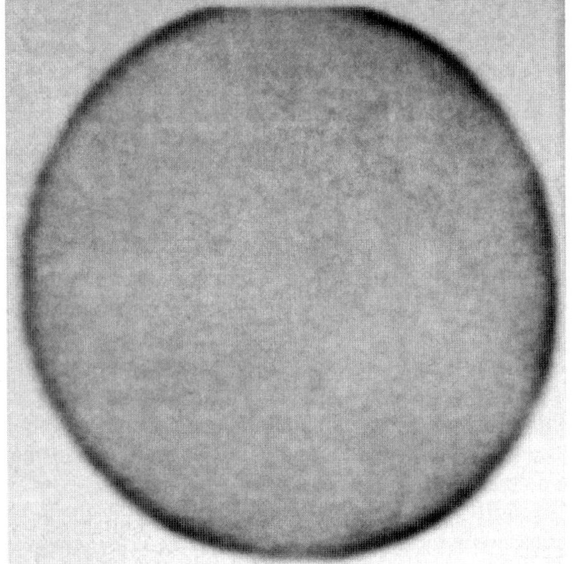

Figure 6.3 Nonhomogeneous distribution of activity on a uniformity flood.

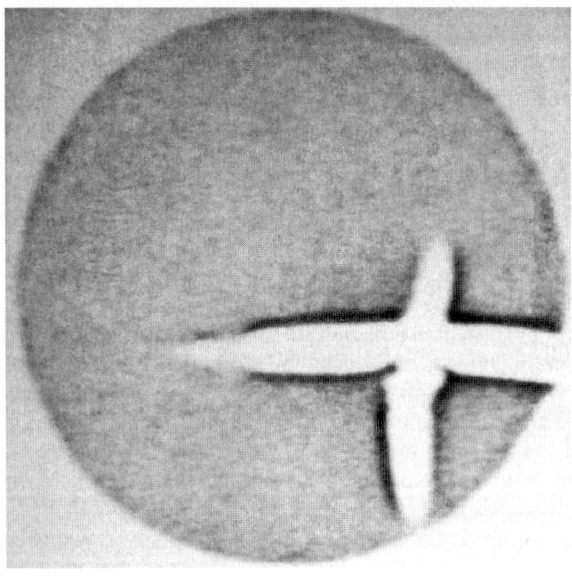

Figure 6.5 Cracked crystal.

Parallel-Line Equal-Space Phantom

All lead bars and spaces are of equal width in the parallel-line equal-space (PLES) phantom (Fig. 6.7C). Two images acquired at 90° to one another are necessary to monitor resolution over the entire crystal.

Orthogonal-Hole Phantom

The orthogonal-hole phantom consists of a lead sheet containing holes of equal diameter arranged at right angles to one another (Fig. 6.7D). Only one image is needed to determine resolution over all areas of the detector. These phantoms may also be designed as a circle of pie-shaped wedges, with each wedge containing rows of holes set at different intervals. If the pie-shaped wedge phantom is used then multiple images are required, placing the wedge with the smallest spacing over each portion of the crystal.

Resolution phantom images should be carefully examined to detect changes in resolution by comparing current images with previous ones. As with uniformity testing, sudden changes from one day to the next are usu-

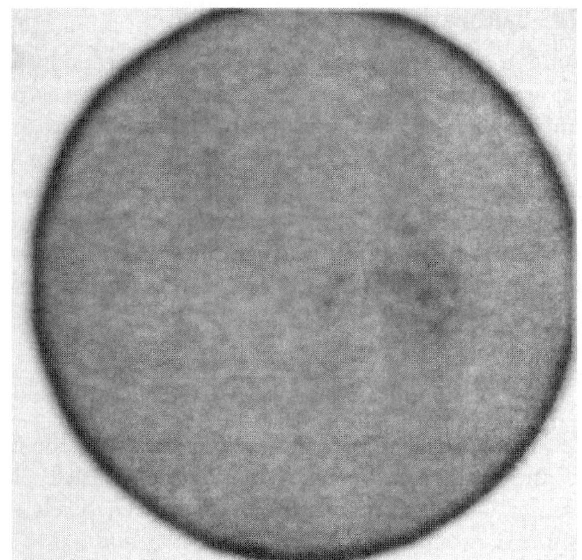

Figure 6.6 Radioactive contamination seen on uniformity flood as ill-defined area of increased activity.

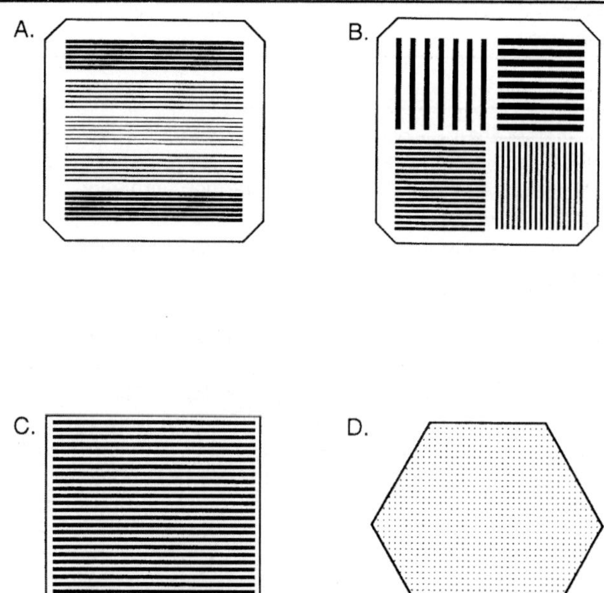

Figure 6.7 Transmission phantoms used to measure the spatial resolution of a scintillation camera. (A) Hine–Duley phantom. (B) Four-quadrant bar phantom. (C) Parallel-line equal-space (PLES) phantom. (D) Orthogonal-hole phantom.

Table 6.3 Causes of Scintillation Camera Field Nonuniformities

Cause	Common appearance	Action to be taken
Incorrect or misadjusted photopeak	Hot or cold tubes, or generalized nonuniformity (see Fig. 6.2)	Select correct peak or adjust photopeak
Broken crystal	Cold spiderweb defect, or cold spots possibly with a hot edge (see Fig. 6.5)	Crystal must be replaced by service engineer
Collimator defect	Cold spots possibly with a hot edge	Collimator must be rebored or replaced
"Mistuned" photomultiplier tube (PMT)	Circular cool area, larger than actual diameter of PMT	Autotune camera (if design allows); request service if camera cannot be autotuned
PMT failure	Circular cold or hot spot, larger than actual diameter of PMT	Must be replaced by service engineer
Radioactive contamination on crystal	Warm to hot focal or diffuse activity (see Fig. 6.6)	Decontaminate using proper procedures or collimator
X,Y misalignment	Image misshapen	Must be repaired by service engineer
Hydroscopic (water) damage to crystal	Dark "measles" most readily seen when image is acquired slightly off-peak to the left (into backscatter peak)	Crystal must be replaced by service engineer
Historically, film processing artifacts on silver-based film	"Roller marks" or films too dark or too light	Rollers require cleaning, chemical adjusted, or solution temperatures adjusted
Scratched or dirty cathode ray tube screen or multiformatter lens	Irregular cold spot in same location on every image	Screen must be replaced if scratched; clean dirt away with soft brush
Static artifacts on silver-based film	Black streaks of branched "lightning" or fingerprint artifacts	Reprint images if necessary; avoid banging cassettes and touch only edges of films

Table 6.4 Factors Affecting Scintillation Camera Spatial Resolution

Factor	Effect
Off-peak or poor uniformity	Decreased resolution
Pulse-height analyzer window width	Decreased resolution with wider window
Source-to-detector distance	Decreased resolution with increased distance
γ-ray energy	Decreased resolution with higher energy or with very low energies
Collimator type	Increased with high-resolution collimator; decreased with high-sensitivity collimator
Crystal degradation	Resolution decreases with age and various environmental conditions

ally caused by improper photopeak adjustment. Subtle changes over time are expected as the crystal ages. Factors that can affect spatial resolution are listed in Table 6.4.

Spatial Linearity

Spatial linearity is the ability of a scintillation camera to produce a uniform image with straight lines corresponding to straight lines in a phantom. Clinically, it is the accurate portrayal of true organ shape. Linearity can be assessed along with resolution by examining the straightness of a set of parallel bars or, in the case of the orthogonal-hole phantom, the straightness of parallel rows of holes. Current images should be compared with those obtained when the scintillation camera was installed.

Sensitivity

Sensitivity is the ability to detect ionizing events in a sodium iodide crystal expressed in counts per second per microcurie (cps/μCi). It can be measured simultaneously when uniformity is performed if the activity of the source and the room background are known. The activity in the source must be carefully measured and corrected for decay; then the count rate obtained per unit activity can be calculated. The calculated sensitivity is then compared with previous values. Sensitivity can be affected by incorrect energy settings, incorrect collimation (if extrinsic sensitivity is performed), or improper detector-to-source distance.

Testing frequency depends upon the facility's protocol and the manufacturer's recommendations. A change in sensitivity can be a useful indicator of minor or slow degradation of the system that may be corrected by scheduled preventive maintenance long before effects are seen on patient studies.

Pixel Calibration

To obtain accurate measurements of organ or lesion size, pixel size must be determined. Pixel calibration is performed by placing two point sources about 30 cm apart on the camera surface. The exact distance between the sources is measured, and an image of the sources is acquired. An activity profile is generated by the computer, and the number of pixels between the two activity peaks is determined. The following equation is used to determine the pixel size:

$$\text{pixel size} = \frac{\text{distance between sources}}{\text{no. of pixels between activity profile peaks}}$$

Pixel size will change with matrix size: the larger the matrix, the smaller the pixel. For example, if each pixel measures 6 × 6 mm in a 64 × 64 matrix, pixels will measure 3 × 3 mm in a 128 × 128 matrix and 1.5 × 1.5 mm in a 256 × 256 matrix.

Single-Photon Emission Computed Tomography

Cameras used for single-photon emission computed tomography (SPECT) acquisitions require additional quality control testing procedures beyond the standard tests performed for all gamma cameras.

Uniformity Correction Map

Nonuniformities across the field of view caused by crystal imperfections, photomultiplier tube (PMT) response, and collimator construction must be corrected for both planar and tomographic imaging. However, because the effects of these variations are multiplied by the number of projections acquired during tomographic acquisition, SPECT tolerates a much smaller variance in field uniformity. Even small nonuniformities introduce artifacts into reconstructed images.

A high-count uniformity flood is used as a map when the computer applies a correction algorithm to every pixel in the SPECT images. A correction map must be acquired for each collimator used for SPECT acquisitions and for each matrix size. A sealed sheet source that is guaranteed to have less than 1% variation in activity uniformity is required. Because it is very difficult to achieve this level of uniformity in a refillable source, these should not be used. The flood should be acquired for a period of time that will result in at least 10,000 counts per pixel, so that the data exhibit only a 1% error. Therefore, at least 30 million counts should be acquired for a 64 × 64 matrix and 120 million counts for a 128 × 128 matrix. Because these are very long acquisitions, they will usually be set up at the end of the day and allowed to run overnight.

The uniformity map used for a specific tomographic reconstruction must match the collimator and the matrix that were used for the acquisition. Failure to use the correct map or to keep maps current can result in ring artifacts in the reconstructed images (see Fig. 6.8).

Maps should be acquired frequently enough to assure that any changes in the instrument are accounted for. The frequency of testing depends on the manufacturer's recommendation and the condition of the camera. Weekly, biweekly, or monthly testing may be employed. Newer gamma camera models are less prone to variation than older models, so the age of the system may affect the frequency. As a system ages, the maps may need to be performed more frequently as components become less reliable. Any suspected damage to the collimator requires that a new map be acquired immediately.

Center of Rotation Correction

The center of rotation (COR) evaluation is used to correct for slight variations in the position of the camera head as it rotates. When the rotation is perfect, the reconstruction matrix will always place a given pixel in the same location within a three-dimensional matrix. If the camera head does not remain true to its position, then data from a particular projection will be attributed to a different pixel in the matrix. In other words, the computer will "think" the pixel is in a different place or match it to an electronic mechanical center.

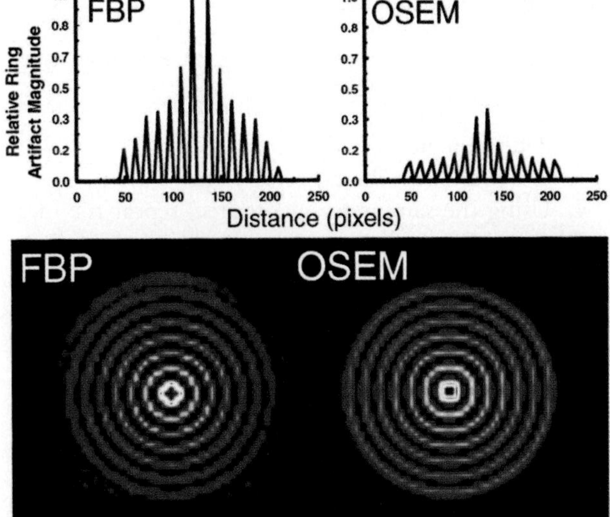

Figure 6.8 Appearance of ring artifacts in filtered backprojection reconstruction (FBP) and ordered subset expectation maximum (OSEM) reconstructions. One-pixel-thick profiles taken through the center of each image are shown above. Each profile was divided by mean counts in its corresponding uncorrupted transaxial slice and expressed as a fraction of the maximum value of the FBP profile (Leong, 2001).

The COR is acquired using a point source or line source that is placed off center on the imaging pallet. Generally, a 360° acquisition is performed using the camera's COR protocol. The computer will calculate correction factors for various head positions as necessary. A separate COR value should be acquired for each collimator used for SPECT acquisitions, because weight and fit may cause variations in rotation that are specific to that collimator.

If data are shifted as little as 0.5 pixels, the resolution of the reconstructed image will be affected. Gross changes in camera head position may not allow for adequate correction, and repair may be necessary. COR values should be acquired on a weekly or biweekly basis, depending upon the age and construction of the camera or manufacturer's instructions.

Positron Emission Tomography

This section serves as an introduction to positron emission tomography (PET), which is also covered in more detail in Chapter 7.

Blank Scan

The blank scan is performed on a PET scanner each day before it is used for patient studies. The acquisition uses a long-lived source, such as germanium-68, to produce sinograms for every possible detector pair in each detector ring. The sinograms consist of lines of response that represent the coincidence events that have been detected by various pairs of detectors. The technologist reviews the sinogram to determine if all detectors are operating properly. Using the sinogram as a map, computer software determines correction factors that account for variations in response caused by individual detector blocks. These data are used to correct the transmission study (Fig. 6.9).

Background Counting Rate

The background counting rate should be acquired on a daily basis to identify certain mechanical malfunctions as well as the presence of contamination.

Normalization

Normalization calibration is performed monthly or quarterly. It uses a long-lived source to evaluate differences in sensitivity of the crystals in each pair of detectors. Correction factors are determined and applied to each emission scan during reconstruction. Because this procedure requires very high counting statistics (like a uniformity correction map), the acquisition is usually performed overnight.

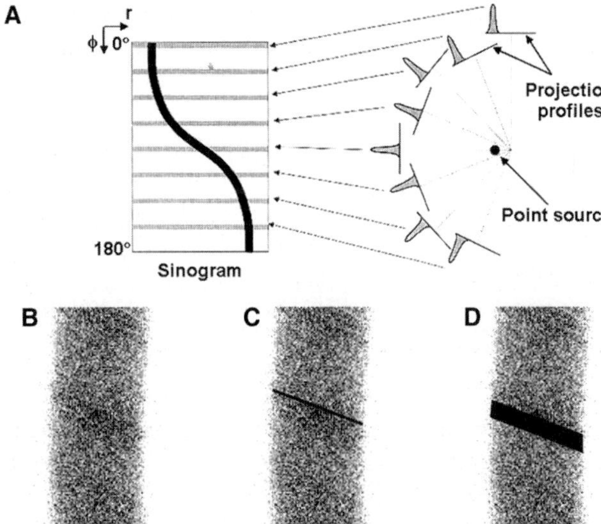

Figure 6.9 (A) Sinogram (i.e., histogram) presentation of emission tomography (i.e., SPECT or PET) data. (B–D) PET sonograms of uniform-cylinder source without any visually perceptible discontinuities or other artifacts (B), with blank diagonal line indicative of faulty detector (crystal) element (C), and blank diagonal band indicative of faulty detector block (D) (Zanzonico, 2008, p. 1125).

Table 6.5 Dose Calibrator Quality Control

Test[a]	Testing frequency
Constancy	Daily before use
Linearity of activity	Quarterly
Accuracy	Annually
Geometry dependence	At installation

[a]All tests should be performed at installation, after adjustment, and after repair.

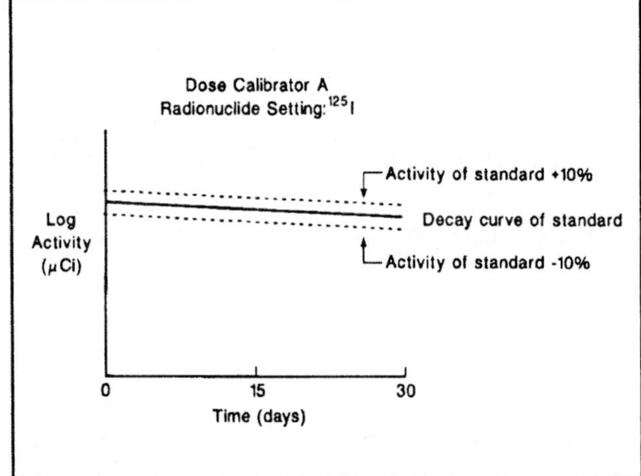

Figure 6.10 Graph of dose-calibrator constancy.

Dose Calibrator

The U.S. Nuclear Regulatory Commission (NRC) requires licensees to perform quality control tests on dose calibrators according to recognized standards of practice and to retain calibration records for 3 years. The records must include the model and serial number of the instrument, the date of calibration, the results, and the name of the individual who performed the test. Table 6.5 lists the dose-calibrator quality control tests and testing frequency. As a "rule of thumb," ±10% is used as a threshold action level for necessary repairs; however, the NRC specifically states that the manufacturers' recommended percent error be used for determination of repair, which may be less than ±10% but rarely more.

Constancy

Constancy (or precision) testing determines the reproducibility of measurements of a source of known activity from day to day. A long-lived standard of known activity, such as cobalt-57 (^{57}Co) or cesium-137 (^{137}Cs), is measured at each of the commonly used radionuclide settings. Each measurement is compared with the expected (decay-corrected) value for the standard at that setting on that day. A graph or chart noting the expected values and the acceptable range is usually used to track instrument performance (Fig. 6.10). The acceptable range is usually ±10% of the expected value; however, some manufacturers suggest ±5% of expected value. If your radioactive license states that these are done according to the manufacturer's recommendations then you would need to confirm that you are in compliance. An outline of the constancy testing procedure includes:

1. Count a long-lived standard on the appropriate dose-calibrator setting.
2. Obtain a background count at the same setting to determine net activity.
3. Compare with the expected value.
4. Using the same reference source, repeat the measurement for all commonly used radionuclide settings.
5. Correct each for background.
6. Compare actual readings with expected readings using a graph, chart, or the following equation:

$$\text{percentage error} = \frac{\text{actual value}}{\text{expected value}} \times 100\%.$$

If the constancy error is greater than 10%, the instrument usually must be repaired or replaced.

Linearity of Activity

A linearity test ascertains how accurately a dose calibrator measures activities over a wide range, from millicurie to microcurie amounts. The test involves assaying a source with a relatively short half-life over a period of several days and comparing the predicted and measured results.

The starting activity should approximate the highest activity that will be administered to a patient. The starting activity should be assayed until it reaches at least 1.1 megabecquerel (MBq) (30 μCi). It could be lower than 30 μCi depending on manufacture recommendations or license requirements. Measured activities should be within at least ±10% of expected activities. Linearity testing is conducted as follows:

1. Assay an aliquot of technetium-99m (^{99m}Tc) at 2- to 3-hr intervals over 3 or more days.
2. Correct all measurements for background.
3. Using decay factors, calculate the expected activity for each time the sample was measured.
4. Plot both the expected and measured activities on semilog paper (activity vs. time), as shown in Figure 6.11.
5. If linearity errors exceed at least 10%, calculate correction factors using the following equation:

$$\text{correction factor} = \frac{\text{expected activity}}{\text{measured activity}}$$

Correction factors should be clearly displayed on the dose calibrator. The appropriate correction factor should be applied whenever activities are measured in ranges subject to unacceptable variations in linearity. The correction factor is applied as follows:

$$\text{true activity} = \text{measured activity} \times \text{correction factor.}$$

An alternate method of performing an activity linearity test is to use the commercially available Calicheck (Calcorp, Cleveland, OH) or Lineator (Biodex Medical Systems, Shirley, NY) systems. These systems consist of a series of lead tubes that absorb ^{99m}Tc photons by a known amount. After the source is assayed initially, it is measured several more times after each of the lead tubes is placed in sequence around the source. Measurements of the shielded source simulate radioactive decay. This method saves time and decreases personnel exposure.

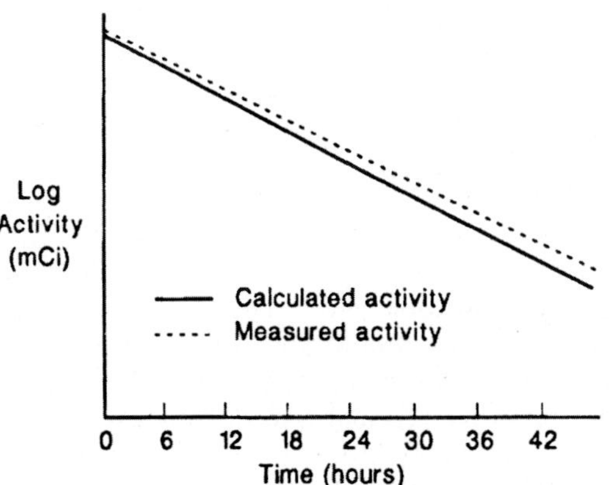

Figure 6.11 Dose-calibrator activity linearity graph.

Accuracy

Accuracy testing assesses the ability of a dose calibrator to provide a true measure of the activity of radionuclides of different gamma energies. At least two different long-lived standards of known activity should be used, one of which should have a photon energy between 100 and 500 keV. The instrument must produce readings that are within ±10% of the expected value. Accuracy testing is performed as follows.

1. Determine the expected value for each source using decay factors and determine the acceptable range for each (±10%).
2. Assay each standard in the dose calibrator three times at the appropriate radionuclide setting.
3. For each standard, average the three readings and subtract the background to obtain the net activity.

If the accuracy error is greater than 10%, the dose calibrator usually must be repaired or replaced.

Geometric Variation

Evaluation of geometric variation determines the effect of sample volume and configuration on the measurement of a sample's activity. For example, 0.74 gigabecquerels (GBq) (20 mCi) contained in a 1-mL volume in a syringe and 0.74 GBq (20 mCi) contained in a 10-mL volume in a glass vial may yield significantly different measurements when assayed in the same dose calibrator. To ascertain the error in measuring activity of varying volumes in a vial, the following procedure may be used:

1. Assay 37–74 MBq (1–2 mCi) ^{99m}Tc in a minimal volume (1–2 drops) in a 20- to 30-mL vial. Correct reading for background.
2. Increase the volume in the vial by adding water in 2-mL aliquots until the maximum volume is reached.
3. Assay the vial after each addition of water and correct for background.
4. Using the activity for the 4-mL volume as a standard, compare all other readings with this activity.
5. Calculate correction factors for volumes that exceed 10% of the expected activity using the equation shown previously.

Correction factors should be clearly displayed on the dose calibrator. The appropriate correction factor should be applied whenever activities are measured in volumes subject to unacceptable variations.

Each type of syringe that is used for administering radioactive dosages should also be tested for geometric variation at commonly used volumes. The following method may be used to measure geometric variation for syringes:

1. Place 74–740 MBq (2–20 mCi) of ^{99m}Tc in a vial.
2. Measure the activity.
3. Withdraw a commonly used volume containing a commonly used activity into the syringe being tested.
4. Measure the activity in the syringe.
5. Calculate the expected activity using the following equation:

   expected activity = vial activity before withdrawal − vial activity after withdrawal.

6. Calculate the percentage error as described in the constancy procedure.
7. Repeat process for each type of syringe used to administer radiopharmaceuticals to patients. Several common volumes and activities should be tested for each.
8. Correction factors should be calculated for any geometric variations causing measurements to vary by more than 10% from the expected activity.

Scintillation Spectrometer

A scintillation spectrometer is an instrument (such as an uptake probe or scintillation well-counting system) that uses pulse-height analysis to determine which pulses will be counted. Table 6.6 contains a list of quality control tests and the frequency with which they should be performed on scintillation spectrometers.

Voltage Calibration

Calibration of a scintillation spectrometer involves determining the appropriate operating high voltage and amplifier gain. The *operating voltage* is the high voltage applied to the dynodes of the PMT. The high voltage can be adjusted so that the arbitrary units on the pulse-height analyzer dials, upper- and lower-level discriminators (ULD and LLD, respectively), correspond to meaningful energy (voltage) units. Typically, the dials are divided into 1000 units. The gain setting will determine the increments for each unit. The approximate operating voltage for commonly used radionuclides will usually be supplied by the manufacturer of the instrument. Most modern scintillation spectrometers are purely digital and require manipulation of these numbers using drop-down windows, etc., instead of physical dials.

The optimal high-voltage setting should be checked for drift using a long-lived sealed source, such as ^{137}Cs, and the following procedure:

1. Set the ULD and LLD for a narrow window, usually 3%.
2. Select the established gain and high-voltage settings.
3. Place the source in the well or at a preset distance from the uptake probe.
4. Obtain a 1-min count on the established high-voltage setting.
5. Obtain 1-min counts at high-voltage settings several units above and below this setting.
6. Record all counts and graph, if desired, or record electronically.
7. The voltage setting at which the highest count rate is obtained is the operating voltage, with decreasing count rates found on settings just above and below the optimal setting.

The high-voltage setting should not vary significantly from day to day. A constant drift or marked variations indicate problems with the high-voltage supply.

Table 6.6 Scintillation Spectrometer Quality Control

Test[a]	Testing frequency
Voltage calibration	Daily
Background check	Daily
Constancy	Daily
Chi square for precision	Variable depending upon age and condition of unit
Energy dependence	Annually

[a]All tests should be performed at installation, after adjustment, and after repair.

Constancy

A long-lived sealed source of known activity should be counted each day to evaluate constancy. ^{137}Cs is frequently used. A graph of the expected values (corrected for decay) ±10% can be used for comparison. The counting rate should not fall outside of these values. The following method is used to assess constancy:

1. Determine the optimal high-voltage setting.
2. Obtain a 1-min background count.
3. Compare the background counting rate with previous values to detect variations or contamination.
4. Count source and correct for background.
5. Compare the counting rate with the expected value.

Energy Resolution

If a sodium iodide detector could convert light photons to an electrical pulse perfectly, the photopeak in a gamma spectrum would look like a narrow line. Instead, pulse heights of varying amplitudes, representing a range of energies around the photopeak energy, form the familiar bell-shaped peak. The width of the photopeak is an indicator of the accuracy of the conversion from light to electrical energy, or the energy resolution of the instrument.

A ^{137}Cs source is typically used to measure energy resolution in the following way:

1. Using the proper operating voltage and a narrow window, measure the counts for a preset time at 10-keV increments around the photopeak.
2. Plot counts per 10-keV interval vs. the midpoint of the counting interval (Fig. 6.12).
3. Calculate the full width at half maximum (FWHM) as follows: (a) divide the maximum photopeak count by 2 to obtain the half maximum; (b) draw a line across the photopeak at the half-maximum level; and (c) drop perpendicular lines to the *x*axis where the half-maximum line intersects the two edges of the photopeak. The distance between the two perpendicular lines (in energy units) is the FWHM.
4. Calculate the percentage energy resolution as follows:

$$\text{percentage energy resolution} = \frac{\text{FWHM (keV)}}{\text{midpoint of photopeak (keV)}} \times 100\%.$$

A typical range for ^{137}Cs is 8–12%. The energy resolution will degrade (that is, the value will become larger) as the crystal ages or if a problem develops with the amplifier or PMT.

Chi-Square Test for Precision

The chi-square test is a procedure that checks for random errors greater than those that would be predicted. Random errors affect the reproducibility (or precision) of measurements. These are always present in radiation counting because of the random nature of radioactive decay. If a source is counted 10 times for 1 min, each measurement will be different, even though the same activity is counted each time. The question then becomes whether the variations in the measurement are a result of the randomness of radioactive decay or are a malfunction of the counting instrument. To answer that question, a chi-square test is conducted as follows:

1. Using a long-lived standard (^{137}Cs or ^{57}Co), determine the time required to acquire at least 10,000 counts. Use this as the preset time.
2. Collect a series of measurements (usually 10), each for the preset time (Fig. 6.13).
3. Compute the mean (average) value.

$$\bar{N} = \frac{\Sigma N_i}{n},$$

where N_i is an individual measurement and n is number of measurements.

4. Calculate the chi-square (χ^2) value as follows:

$$\chi^2 = \frac{\Sigma(N_i - \bar{N})}{\bar{N}}.$$

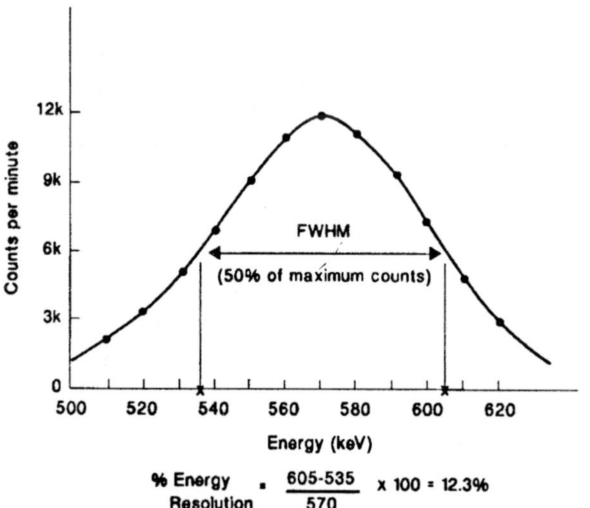

Figure 6.12 Energy resolution determination.

N_i	$(N_i - \bar{N})^2$
10150	17956
9988	784
9899	13689
10060	1936
9954	3844
10099	6889
9999	289
10005	121
10027	121
9979	1369
$\bar{N}$ = 10016	Sum = 46,998

$$\chi^2 = \frac{46{,}998}{10{,}016} = 4.692$$

Figure 6.13 Chi-square calculation. Using the tables in the appendices to this book, find 9 degrees of freedom (degree of freedom is the result after you subtract 1 from the total number of observations—in this example, 10 observations minus 1 equals 9 degrees of freedom, $n - 1$), and 4.692 falls between an acceptable probability of 0.90 and 0.50, indicating that the variations in counts are probably the result of the randomness of radioactive decay and not an instrument malfunction.

5. Using the chi-square table (Appendix B), find the probability (*P*) for the number of measurements and calculated chi-square value. The *P* value denotes the probability that random variations observed in a series would equal or exceed the calculated chi-square value (see Fig. 6.13).

Acceptable *P* values are between 0.1 and 0.9. Values greater than 0.9 or less than 0.1 indicate that the variations in the measurements do not match the expected and that the instrument should be checked.

Survey Meter

Table 6.7 lists the quality control steps that should be performed on survey meters and the calibration frequency required by the NRC. Daily reference checks are performed by measuring a long-lived source using constant geometry before each use to verify instrument calibration. Acceptable readings are within ±20% of the calibrated exposure rate, which should be posted on the survey instrument. Records of daily reference checks do not need to be kept; however, the NRC does require that survey meter calibration records be maintained for 3 years.

Table 6.7 Survey Meter Quality Control

Test[a]	Testing frequency
Battery check	Before each use
Reference check (with dedicated source)	Before each use
Calibration	Annually

[a]All tests should be performed at installation, after adjustment, and after repair.

References and Further Reading

Christian PE, Bernier DR, Langan JK, eds. 2003. *Nuclear Medicine and PET: Technology and Techniques.* 5th ed. St. Louis, MO: Mosby; 26–27, 79–95, 300–302.

Botti J, 2001. Gamma camera performance evaluation and QC. In: Fahey F, Harkness B, eds. *Basic Science of Nuclear Medicine* [book on CD-ROM]. Reston, VA: Society of Nuclear Medicine; 243–252.

Cherry SR, Sorenson JA, Phelps ME, 2003. *Physics in Nuclear Medicine.* 3rd ed. Philadelphia, PA: Saunders; 182–183, 227–251, 321–324.

Christian P, 2001. Nuclear medicine counting systems. In: Fahey F, Harkness B, eds. *Basic Science of Nuclear Medicine* [book on CD-ROM]. Reston, VA: Society of Nuclear Medicine; 179–189.

Chu RYL, Simon WE, 1996. Quality control testing of dose calibrators. *J Nucl Med Technol.* 24:124–128.

Early PJ, Sodee DB, 1995. *Principles and Practice of Nuclear Medicine.* 2nd ed. St. Louis, MO: Mosby; 150–175, 211–215, 257–281, 296–313.

English RJ, 1995. *Single-Photon Computed Tomography: A Primer.* 3rd ed. Reston, VA: Society of Nuclear Medicine; 35–47.

Graham LS, 2001. SPECT data acquisition and quality control. In: Fahey F, Harkness B, eds. *Basic Science of Nuclear Medicine* [book on CD-ROM]. Reston, VA: Society of Nuclear Medicine; 261–268.

Groch MW, Erwin WD, 2001. Single-photon emission computed tomography in the year 2001: instrumentation and quality control. *J Nucl Med Technol.* 29:12–18.

Keim P, 1994. An overview of PET quality assurance procedures: Part I. *J Nucl Med Technol.* 22:27–34.

Keim P, 1994. An overview of PET quality assurance procedures: Part II. *J Nucl Med Technol.* 22:182–187.

Kirchner PT, Siegel BA, eds., 1996. *Nuclear Medicine: Self-Study Program II: Instrumentation.* Reston, VA: Society of Nuclear Medicine; 5–9, 29–31.

Klingensmith WC, Eshima D, Goddard J, 2003. *Nuclear Medicine Procedure Manual: 2003–05.* Englewood, CO: Wick Publishing; 16.1–21.4.

Leong LK, Kruger RL, O'Connor MK, 2001. A comparison of the uniformity requirements for SPECT image reconstruction using FBP and OSEM techniques. *J Nucl Med Technol.* 29(2):81.

Madsen M, 2001. The gamma camera. In: Fahey F, Harkness B, eds. *Basic Science of Nuclear Medicine* [book on CD-ROM]. Reston, VA: Society of Nuclear Medicine; 243–252.

Moses W, 2001. PET data acquisition and processing. In: Fahey F, Harkness B, eds. *Basic Science of Nuclear Medicine* [book on CD-ROM]. Reston, VA: Society of Nuclear Medicine; 261–267.

Ruhlmann J, Oehr P, Bierscak HJ, 1999. *PET in Oncology: Basics and Clinical Application.* New York, NY: Springer-Verlag; 26–33.

Thrall JH, Ziessman HA, 2001. *Nuclear Medicine: The Requisites.* 2nd ed. St. Louis, MO: Mosby; 27–30, 42–43.

Von Schulthess GK, ed., 2000. *Clinical Positron Emission Tomography: Correlation with Morphological Cross-Sectional Imaging.* Philadelphia, PA: Lippincott Williams & Wilkins; 20–21.

Wells P, 1999. *Practical Mathematics in Nuclear Medicine Technology.* Reston, VA: Society of Nuclear Medicine; 113–137, 159–160.

Zanzonico P, 2008. Routine quality control of clinical nuclear medicine instrumentation: a brief review. *J Nucl Med.* 49:1114–1131.

CHAPTER 7 Positron Emission Tomography and Computed Tomography Operating Principles

William Hubble and Norman Bolus

The growth of positron emission tomography (PET) and computed tomography (CT) for applications in oncology, cardiology, and neurology has created a demand for technologists that are knowledgeable in performing PET/CT studies. Anatomical localization, attenuation correction, and assistance with intensity-modulated radiation therapy are all significant benefits to direct coregistration of PET and CT images. It is essential that nuclear medicine technologists have a thorough understanding of operating principles and characteristics of PET/CT scanners. This chapter covers the fundamentals for both imaging devices.

Positron Emission Tomography Systems

Positron Emission

PET images are produced by recognizing events created by the annihilation reaction of proton-rich radionuclides. Positron decay or emission results when a proton is converted to a neutron, a positron, a neutrino, and energy. When a positron is emitted from the nucleus, it travels a few millimeters and ionizes many atoms before pairing with an electron (positronium) and undergoing an annihilation interaction, which produces a pair of 511-keV annihilation photons that travel in opposite directions at approximately 180° apart.

Positron radionuclides used in PET imaging are listed in Table 7.1. The most widely used radiopharmaceutical is 2-[^{18}F]-fluoro-2-deoxy-D-glucose (^{18}F-FDG). ^{18}F-FDG is a nonphysiological compound with a chemical structure very similar to that of naturally occurring glucose. ^{18}F-FDG is a good reflection of the distribution of glucose uptake in the body and phosphorylation by cells in the body. The phosphorylation of the ^{18}F-FDG within the cell "traps" the molecule for the duration that it is useful for diagnostic imaging. The ability to noninvasively image cellular glucose metabolism is important in oncological applications because cancer cells use glucose at higher rates than normal cells. PET/CT imaging has major clinical applications for studying patient diseases in oncology, cardiology, and neurology.

PET Detectors

Many scintillation crystals have been utilized for PET detection. They are listed, along with their properties in Table 7.2. Ideal PET scintillation crystals should be dense, have a high atomic number, have high relative light yield in comparison to thallium-activated sodium iodide (NaI[Tl]), and a short-light decay time. NaI(Tl) is not the ideal scintillation crystal for PET due to its lower density, lower atomic number, and long-light decay time when compared to the other PET detector materials. Bismuth germinate (BGO) was first employed in the late 1970s and has historically been the most widely used PET detector crystal. BGO limitations are in its relatively low light yield and long-light decay time. PET scanners using BGO employ septa to reduce the number of scatter and random events. This technique of using lead or tungsten septa, positioned between the rings of the detectors, is classified as 2D mode. Lutetium oxyorthosilicate (LSO), lutetium yttrium oxyorthosilicate (LYSO), and gadolinium oxyorthosilicate (GSO) are three new materials gaining wide acceptance in modern PET scanners. Both GSO and LSO are doped with cerium to improve their scintillation efficiency. LSO and LYSO are dense and have relatively high atomic numbers and short light decay times. LSO, LYSO, and GSO scanners do not employ the use of septa and image in what is classified as 3D mode. PET scanners that operate only in 3D mode rely solely on "electronic collimation" and often employ narrow coincidence timing windows to reduce random events. 3D mode acquires significantly more events, and reconstruction algorithms are more

Table 7.1 Common and Experimental PET Radionuclides and Half-Lives ($T_{1/2}$)

PET radionuclides	$T_{1/2}$
^{11}C	20.4 min
^{13}N	9.96 min
^{15}O	123 sec
^{18}F	110 min
^{64}Cu	12.7 hr
^{68}Ga	68 min
^{76}Br	16.2 hr
^{82}Rb	76 sec
^{86}Y	14.74 hr
^{124}I	4.2 days

Table 7.2 Properties of Scintillation Crystals Used for PET Imaging[a]

Property	NaI(Tl)	BGO	LSO (Ce)	LYSO	GSO	BaF_2	$LaBr_3$
Linear attenuation coefficient at 511 kev ($cm^{(1)}$)	0.341	0.950	0.866	0.83	0.698	0.454	0.476
Attenuation Length[b]	2.88	1.05	1.16	1.20	1.43	2.2	2.1
Energy resolution at 511 kev	6.6%	10.2%	10%	14%	8.5%	11.4%	N/A
Relative light yield[c]	100%	15%	75%	−75%	25–30%	5–12%	160%
Decay time in nanoseconds	230	300	40	42	60	0.6–0.8	15–25
Hygroscopic?	Yes	No	No	No	No	No	Yes
Chemical composition[d]	NaI:Tl	$Bi_4Ge_3O_{12}$	Lu_2SiO_5:Ce	$Lu_{1.9}Y_{0.5}SiO_5$:Ce	Gd_2SiO_5:Ce	BaF_2	$LaBr_3$

[a]Reprinted with permission from Prekeges (2011, Table 14–2, p. 192).
[b]Attenuation length is the average crystal thickness needed to stop 511-keV photons.
[c]Relative light yield is stated relative to NaI(Tl) at 100%.
[d]The elements listed after the colon are impurities that contribute to more efficient scintillation.

complex and require more corrections for 3D randoms and scatter than 2D mode. In 3D mode a significant overlap of scanned area is necessary to compensate for the reduced sensitivity at the ends of the field of view (FOV) of the detectors.

LSO, LYSO, and GSO have fast enough light decay times to perform time of flight PET (TOF-PET) analysis. TOF-PET allows the system to determine, along the line of response (LOR), where the event happened. The advantage of TOF-PET is that it improves image contrast with fewer events than conventional LOR PET systems (see Fig. 7.1).

PET Scanner Design

PET scanners have 8000 to 25,000 or more crystals, which are laid out to form several rings of detectors. PET crystals are about 4 mm in size and 10–30 mm in depth. The spatial resolution of PET is significantly better than that of SPECT (4 mm vs. 12 mm). Each crystal is too small to have its own photomultiplier tube (PMT); therefore, a group of crystals is put together in a detector block. Typically four PMTs are used on a detector block. Detector blocks may be further grouped into buckets or cassettes, which may be treated as a unit. PET scanners have higher sensitivity than their gamma camera counterpart. PET scanners are about 50 to 100 times more sensitive than the gamma camera.

The gantry bore (hole through which the patient and table must pass) for commercially available systems is 56–70 cm. PET scanners typically have 18–40 consecutive rings of crystals and create a FOV of 15–18 cm. An oncological PET image typically consists of individual FOV images called "bed positions," which are appended together in the reconstruction process to create a continuous 3D image matrix (five to eight bed positions or eyes to thighs). Some organs, such as the brain or heart, can be imaged in a single bed position. Spatial resolution of PET scanners is determined primarily by the size of the crystals and their separation.

Coincidence Detection

Annihilation events striking opposing detectors create a LOR within the PET detector. The total number of events detected by the coincidence circuit in a PET scanner is referred to as prompt coincidences. These events are typically classified as trues, randoms, and scatters. A pair of annihilation photons, from a single annihilation interaction, striking two detectors at the same time is termed a true count or true coincidence annihilation event (Fig. 7.2). When two atoms decay at nearly the same time, photons from two different annihilation events may be detected. When this happens, a false event referred to as a random is created. Randoms are essentially accidental coincidences in which the detected photons arise from unrelated annihilation reactions (Fig. 7.2). Random events increase with more activity or when the scanner is in 3D mode. A scatter event originates from a single annihilation interaction, but because one or both of the annihilation photons undergoes Compton scattering within the object, the LOR is incorrect (Fig. 7.2). Scatter is affected by the distribution of radioactivity, size, and density of the object or objects and their locations relative to the detectors. Approximately 50% of photons scatter within the body. The goal in PET imaging is to increase the number of true events (signal) while decreasing the random and scatter events (noise). The signal-to-noise ratio (SNR) is then the true coincidence count rate (the signal) divided by the randoms and scatters (noise). The most appropriate quantitative expression of a PET scanner's performance is the noise-equivalent count rate (NECR) (see Sample Calculation on page 72). The NECR is the square of the SNR. It is recommended that the PET scanner be operated at or below the activity concentration to the peak NECR (Fig. 7.3).

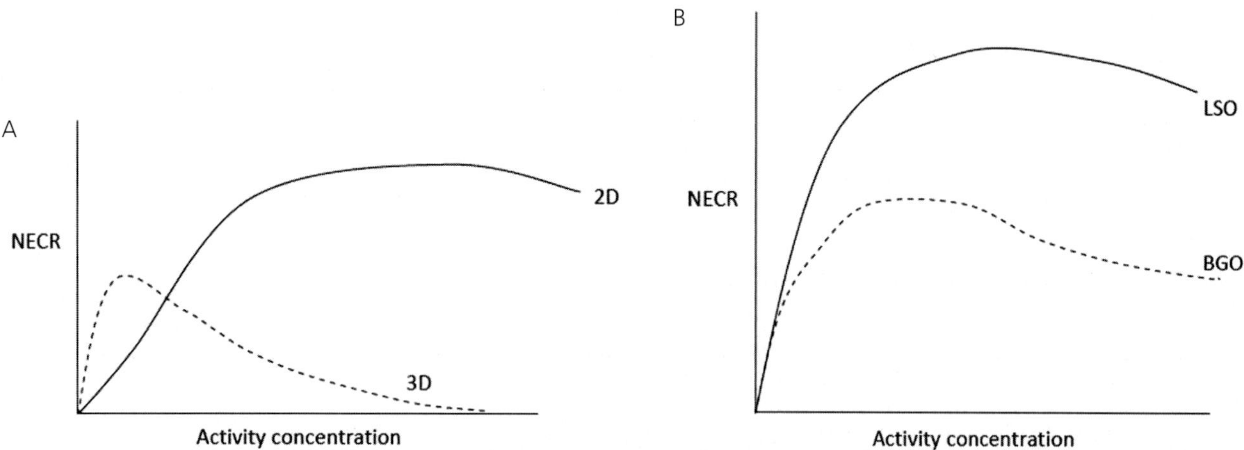

Figure 7.1 (A) 2D vs. 3D noise-equivalent count rate (NECR) comparison. (B) Benefits of LSO vs. BGO concerning NECR. (Re-created/modified from Prekeges, 2011, Fig. 16–4.)

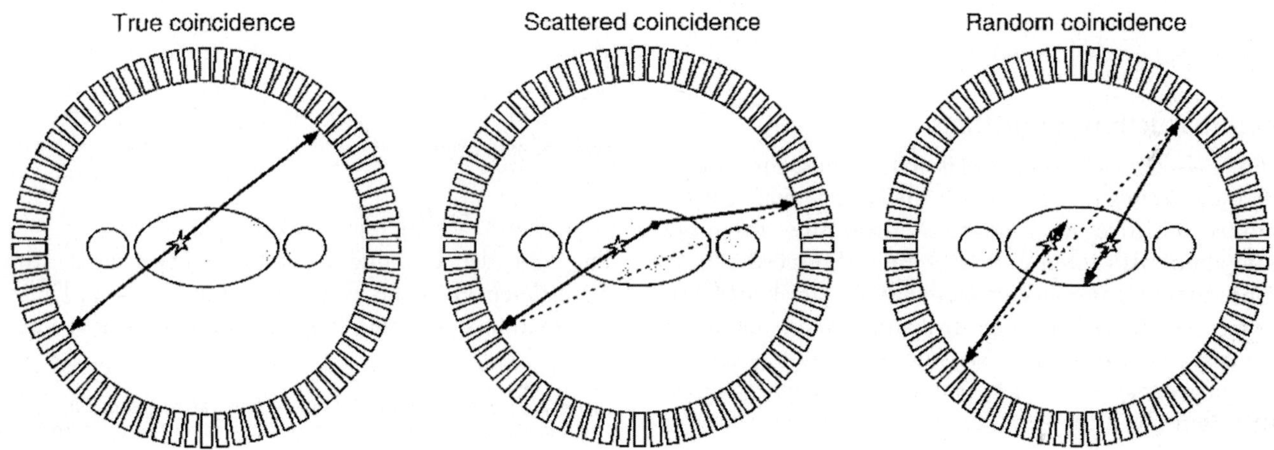

Figure 7.2 PET coincidence detection showing true, scatter, or random events that can contribute to image. (Reprinted, with permission, from Cherry *et al.*, 2003.)

Data Acquisition

PET/CT scanners require the CT scan to be performed first so the reconstructed attenuation correction map from the CT scan can be used for PET reconstruction with attenuation correction. It should be noted that dedicated PET scanners used ^{68}Ge or ^{137}Cs radioactive rod sources. The advantages of CT-generated attenuation correction include: essentially noiseless attenuation maps, reduced acquisition time, and improved anatomic information.

Millions of LORs will be acquired and stored for use in the reconstruction of the 3D distribution of radiotracer. If two photons are from the same annihilation interaction, they should be detected by opposing crystals at about the same time. Coincidence window timing sets a narrow window to ensure that accepted pulse pairs are detected within about 4 to 12 nsec or less. Data acquisition may also include acquisition of delayed events

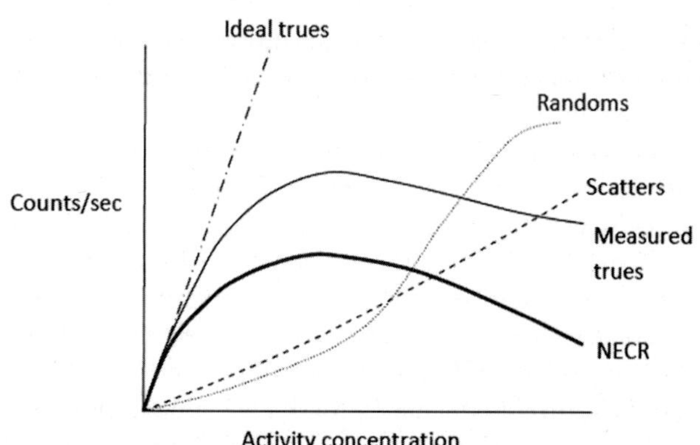

Figure 7.3 Components of the NECR. It is best that a tomography be operated at or below the activity concentration corresponding to the peak NECR. (Re-created/modified from Prekeges, 2011, Fig. 16–3.)

(those that are definitely random events, using a delayed timing window, usually 60–100 nsec). Information gathered by the delayed timing window can be used to estimate the random rate. Estimation from single count rates can also be used to estimate random coincidences. This method measures the single event at each detector. These estimation methods can be used as a means for noise reduction caused by random events. A prompt sinogram is created and must be corrected for several factors, including subtraction of random coincidences, attenuation, scatter, dead time, and radioactive decay. In PET, data are stored in sinogram matrices. The most common choice of matrix size for reconstructed PET images is 128 × 128. Quality control (QC) images are often reconstructed in 256 × 256 to provide better resolution for QC. Visual assessment and comparison of the nonattenuated corrected PET images, attenuation corrected PET images, and CT attenuation images permit the technologist the opportunity to identify artifacts and patient motion that may occur during imaging.

Reconstruction Algorithms

Filtered backprojection (FBP) is no longer used in clinical PET and reconstruction is performed using iterative algorithms. Iterative reconstruction algorithms are more computationally intense and therefore are somewhat time consuming but produce images with less streak artifacts. These algorithms create repeatedly improved estimates of the data to create images. Maximum-likelihood expectation maximization (MLEM) was one of the first iterative algorithms available. A faster and more efficient version was created called ordered-subset expectation maximization (OSEM). Row-action maximum-likelihood algorithm (RAMLA) is a vendor-specific algorithm that provides results similar to those of OSEM.

PET Calibrations and Quality Control

PET scanner QC is essential to ensure the acquisition and creation of high-quality diagnostic patient images. PET QC is composed of two types of calibrations: characterization and correction calibrations. Characterization calibrations are those fundamental to the operation of the PET scanner, such as energy, position, PMT gain, and coincidence timing window. Correction calibrations compensate for inherent variations in the scanner and perform meaningful scaling of image, such as normalization, blank scan, and absolute activity (well-counter) calibrations. The PET community has collaborated on identification of standards for PET tomography performance, the most recent publication of which is the NEMA Standard NU 2–2001, *Performance Measurements of Positron Emission Tomographs.* A recommended quality assurance testing for PET scanners is included in Table 7.3. Much of the routine QC needed for PET can be done in an automated fashion and requires only the verification that the system is functional.

Energy Window Calibration

PET scanners operate at one energy (511 keV). Energy window calibration is typically performed only after repair, during quarterly (or as recommended by manufacturers) preventive maintenance (PM) service, or just before normalization is done. This is typically performed by a service engineer.

Gain Settings

The calibration and adjustments of amplifier gains from PMTs are fundamental to ensuring that a uniform sensitivity response from the individual detectors and modules is maintained. Gain settings should be adjusted to compensate for temperature changes that affect the performance and stability of the electronics. Gain update calibration procedures should be run at least weekly or even daily to keep systems in top performance and to prevent sensitivity drift.

Coincidence Timing Calibration

The coincidence timing calibration adjusts for the timing differences in the event detection circuitry. Timing information is analyzed (a histogram may be generated)

Table 7.3 Recommended Quality Assurance Testing for Dedicated PET Tomographs[a]

Frequency	Quality control tests
Daily	• PMT baseline check and gain adjustment • Blank scan • Uniform cylinder or point source scan
Weekly	• Uniformity check • Well-counter calibration check • Coincidence timing check • Energy window calibration
Quarterly	• Preventive maintenance • Detector efficiency/normalization scan • Cross-calibration

Annually	• NMEA NU-2 testing
	  • Spatial resolution
	  • Sensitivity
	  • Intrinsic scatter fraction
	  • Scatter correction
	  • Count rate performance
	• Update of normalization factors and well-counter calibration, which may be required more frequently.

[a]Reprinted with permission from Prekeges (2011, Table 17–1, p. 233).

to determine timing differences from various detector circuits. Coincidence timing checks should be performed weekly.

Normalization Calibration

Normalization is performed to ensure that individual detectors display the same response to a uniform source of radioactivity. The normalization calibration is used much like a high-count uniformity correction in the scintillation camera. It is performed with radioactive rod sources or a ^{68}Ge cylindrical phantom. Very high statistics are required and the normalization takes at least 6 hr. The normalization calibration table is used to correct for sensitivity from all detectors. Normalization calibrations are performed quarterly or after repair.

Absolute Activity Calibration (Cross-Calibration or Well-Counter Calibration)

Absolute activity calibration factors are used to convert pixel values into a measure of absolute activity per voxel. This calibration is performed by taking a precisely known amount of activity and loading a water-filled phantom whose volume is accurately known. The phantom is imaged, reconstructed, and processed into a set of correction factors that allows the conversion of a patient scan into a representation of the percentage of injected dose per volume or gram of tissue. This conversion creates an image that represents a quantitative image for measurement of standard uptake values (SUVs) of tissue or tumors. Absolute activity calibrations are performed only after all other calibrations have been performed and they should be done quarterly or after major service.

Blank Scan (Air Scan or Reference Scan)

Blank scans are performed daily to provide accurate transmission scan data for the attenuation correction of images. This is done through quick acquisition using the rod source(s) or a ^{68}Ge cylinder. Blank scans are used as a reference uniformity measure for the transmission scan used in attenuation correction. Blank scans should be evaluated visually for any abnormal streaks that show specific crystal or module variations and changes in regional sensitivity (Fig. 7.4). Broad diagonal bands will be seen on the sonogram when PMT problems arise or when a signal is lost from a module. In some respects, the blank scan may be thought of as viewing a daily uniformity flood image on a scintillation camera, providing an overall indicator of scanner performance.

PET Artifacts

The source of PET artifacts can be tracked to three sources: operator, scanner, and patients.

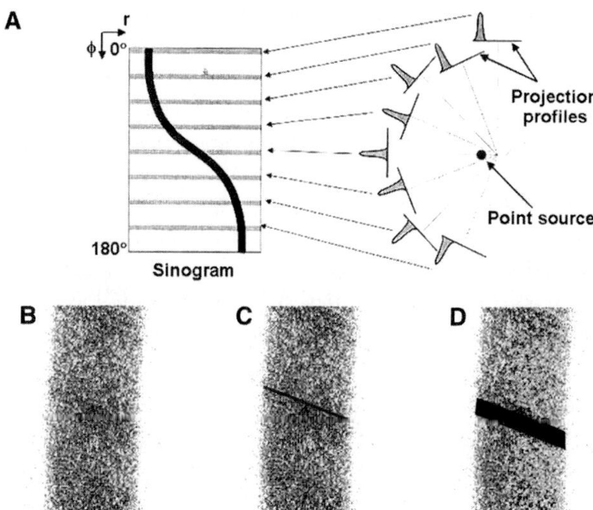

Figure 7.4 (A) Sinogram (i.e., histogram) presentation of emission tomography (i.e., SPECT or PET) data. (B–D) PET sonograms of uniform-cylinder source without any visually perceptible discontinuities or other artifacts (B), with blank diagonal line indicative of faulty detector (crystal) element (C), and blank diagonal band indicative of faulty detector block (D) (Zanzonico, 2008).

Operator

Artifacts caused by the operator are a result of the parameters and settings selected by the operator for the study as well as poor-quality control practices. Calculation of the standardized uptake value requires an exact measurement of the dosage administered. It should be noted that PET generally requires much less operator interaction than SPECT. Most of the choices are simply part of the acquisition protocol.

Scanner

Examples of PET scanner artifacts can be traced to electronic malfunctions of detector blocks, detector boards, coincidence processing, and event sorting electronics, etc. Mechanical misregistration due to misalignment of the PET and CT images is another example of potential scanner-related artifacts.

Patient

Examples of patient-related artifacts can be associated with patient motion, patient size, metallic objects with the body, and poor preparation prior to the exam.

Computed Tomography Systems

X rays were discovered by Wilhelm Conrad Roentgen on November 8, 1895. The CT scanner (which employs a rotating X-ray tube) was developed by Godfrey

Hounsfield in the very late 1960s. By the late 1970s, many hospitals had CT scanners installed and they came into widespread use. The PET/CT scanner was introduced at the turn of the 21st century and has become the accepted standard for performing state-of-the-art PET imaging. A low-dose CT scan is used for attenuation correction and anatomical localization in PET/CT imaging procedures. CT not only achieves minimal superimposition of tissues, but also has improved contrast differences over planar X-ray techniques. A high-quality CT is commonly referred to as a diagnostic CT study or scan.

X-Ray Physics

X rays are produced in the electron shell structure of the atom while γ rays are created by the nuclear forces at the center of the atom. In X-ray tubes, there are two different types of reactions that produce X rays: bremsstrahlung radiation (braking radiation) and characteristic radiation. Bremsstrahlung radiation occurs when energetic electrons pass very near the nucleus of the atom. The strong force of the positively charged atom causes the negatively charged electron to decelerate; the path of the electron is significantly changed and some of the kinetic energy of the electron is lost and converted into X rays. Bremsstrahlung produces continuous spectrum of X-ray energies. Characteristic X rays are produced following the ionization of an atom that leaves an inner shell. Empty outer-shell electrons that drop in to fill the inner-shell vacancy must lose energy, which is released as X rays.

X-Ray Tube Design

CT uses X rays produced in an X-ray tube as its imaging photons. The X-ray tube rotates and X rays that pass through the object being imaged are registered in detectors opposite the X-ray tube. The number of X rays detected, when compared to the number of X rays produced, provides a measure of the attenuation that has occurred in the object. An X-ray tube is an evacuated glass container containing a negatively charged cathode (filament or coil of wire, which becomes a source of electrons when a current is applied) and a positively charged rotating anode, which is composed of titanium/zirconium/molybdenum (TZM) or graphite due to the excessive heat generated (Fig. 7.5). A tube warm-up is typically required before generating X rays to prevent damage to the anode. Only about 1% of the energy applied to the system is converted to X rays that exit the tube window; the remaining 99% of energy creates heat. Activation of the cathode filament circuit heats the filament wire due to its electrical resistance, causing it to release electrons by thermionic emission. The negatively charged electrons are then accelerated toward the positively charged anode striking the focal spot of the anode

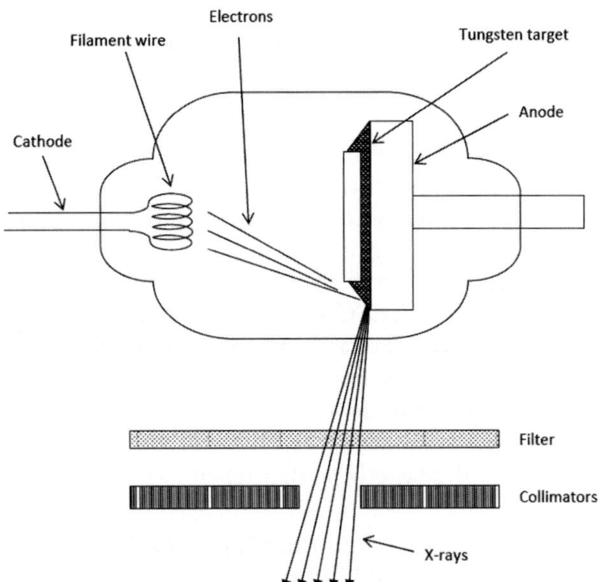

Figure 7.5 Diagram of an X-ray tube that produces X rays via direct ionization interactions and through bremsstrahlung interactions. (Re-created from Prekeges, 2011.)

producing X rays. The operator controls the potential difference between the cathode and the anode and the cathode filament current. The potential difference (kilovolt peak or kVp) determines the kinetic energy given to the emitted electrons, which in turn designate the maximum X-ray energy. The cathode filament current determines the number of electrons released at the cathode and therefore the number of X rays created. It is measured in milliamperes (mA).

CT Filters

An X-ray tube produces billions of X rays per second and their energies are polychromatic (having many different energies). X rays leaving the anode are filtered through aluminum to absorb the low-energy X rays, which will only contribute to the radiation dose received by the patient.

CT Collimation

CT scanners use collimators to protect the patient and limit the beam to the size of the detector array active during acquisition. They are constructed of lead and permit an opening for necessary radiation to pass through. It is important to understand that they are not constructed like collimators used on gamma cameras. A pre-collimator (used before X rays enter the patient) defines the beam shape and width (usually fan or cone shape) and protects the patient from excess radiation and a post-collimator (used to reduce scatter after leaving the patient) is used before the radiation strikes the CT detectors. Advantages of thinner collimation include less volume averaging, increased spatial resolution, and fewer streaking artifacts from high-density objects. Disadvantages of thinner collimation include increased quantum mottle (noise) and increased scanning time.

CT Data Acquisition System

The CT data acquisition system (DAS) transmits data from the detectors to the computer. Each slice needs its own DAS channel and each individual detector has an input into the DAS.

CT Detector Array

CT scintillation detectors are made of ultrafast ceramic materials from rare elements such as silicon, germanium, cadmium, yttrium, or gadolinium. The detectors used in CT are solid state and can number in the hundreds or thousands in a single CT system. A photodiode takes the place of the PMT. A semiconductor junction creates an interface where an electronic signal is easily generated when radiation is detected by the junction. The more radiation detected, the larger the electrical signal produced. Ceramic solid-state detectors are very fast, can be extremely stable, and are produced from an array of very small, efficient detectors that can cover a large area. The detectors are aligned in rows and the number determines whether a scanner is classified as an 8-, 16-, 40-, 64-, 128-, etc., slice scanner. Adaptive detector arrays can have several different size detectors with smaller detectors in the center of the array and larger detectors elements at the edges.

CT Acquisition

In CT, the gantry rotates continuously in one direction on the slip-ring system while the patient table moves at a constant speed through the gantry to quickly perform the scan (Fig. 7.6). The rotation speed is the time required for the gantry to make one revolution. Common gantry rotation speeds of 0.3–1.0 sec with a table motion of about 10–20 mm/sec are used in oncological PET/CT acquisitions. All CT scans begin by performing a scout scan (topogram) so the region of the body to be covered by the CT scan can be defined. Scout scan parameters are built into imaging protocols and used only for localization.

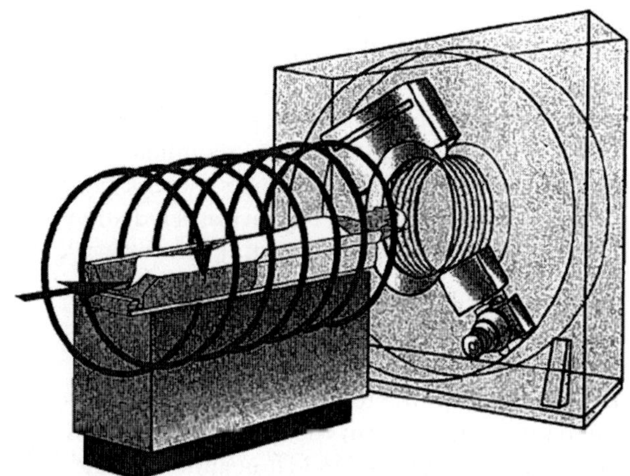

Figure 7.6 Multislice helical CT detector motion creates a spiral pattern along the patient as both the gantry and imaging table move during acquisition to cover a large area of the body. The more slices obtained by the scanner, the faster the imaging table motion. (Reprinted, with permission, from Christian and Waterstram-Rich, 2007.)

Pitch

Pitch is the ratio of the patient's movement through the gantry during one 360° beam rotation relative to the beam collimation. Pitch is entered as a parameter that is set in defining the procedure for the acquisition of patient data. It is sometimes called volume pitch or beam pitch in multislice CT. It can be calculated with the following equation:

$$\text{pitch} = \text{table movement per rotation (mm)}/ (\text{number of slices})(\text{slice width in mm}).$$

Increasing the pitch decreases the number of views per linear scan distance, which in turn decreases radiation exposure. Decreasing the pitch increases the number of views per linear scan distance, which in turn increases improved spatial resolution. Diagnostic CT images typically use lower pitch, including overlapping of images during acquisition to improve diagnostic capabilities. PET/CT studies are typically performed with higher pitch, 1 or greater, since the study is primarily for attenuation correction and anatomical localization.

Kilovolt Peak

Recommendations for the kilovolt peak settings for low-dose CT scans will be department and manufacturer specific and can be adjusted by the operator. Typically they range from 80 to 140 kVp. Factors to determine the appropriate kilovolt peak can depend on the body part being imaged, size of the patient, and the position of the patient's arms during the acquisition. Increasing kilovolt peak increases the penetration of the object being X-rayed (increases the energy of the X rays), decreases noise, and creates fewer beam-hardening artifacts, but increases the dose to the patient and reduces attenuation differences in tissue.

Milliampereseconds

Recommendations for the milliampere seconds (mAs) settings for low-dose CT scans will be dependent on the age, size, height, and weight of the patient. Typically they range from 20 to 120 mAs. Increasing milliampere seconds decreases image noise (produces more X rays) and increases contrast resolution, but increases radiation dose to the patient. The effects of adjusting kilovolt peak and milliamperes are shown in Figure 7.7.

Noise

Quantum mottle is the term used in radiography to describe noise resulting from the finite number of X rays used to make an exposure. In CT, quantum mottle is directly related to the number of X rays detected by each detector. Fewer X rays result in more noise.

CT Dose Index

The radiation dose to the patient is of considerable concern with CT imaging because it is the highest exposure in medical imaging, with the possible exception of fluoroscopy. CT parameters (particularly peak kilovoltage and milliampere seconds) should conform to guidelines specified and recommended by the manufacturer and approved by the interpreting physician. Information on the estimated radiation exposure from an individual CT examination is available to the operator immediately before the scan is started. The information is displayed as the CT dose index (CTDI) measured in milligray (mGy). The CTDI sums the dose from each gantry revolution on the basis of the parameters for peak kilovoltage, milliampere seconds, collimation, and rotation speed. The dose may be further specified by the term $CTDI_w$ for the "weighted" measurement or $CTDI_{vol}$ for the average dose over the total "volume" scanned.

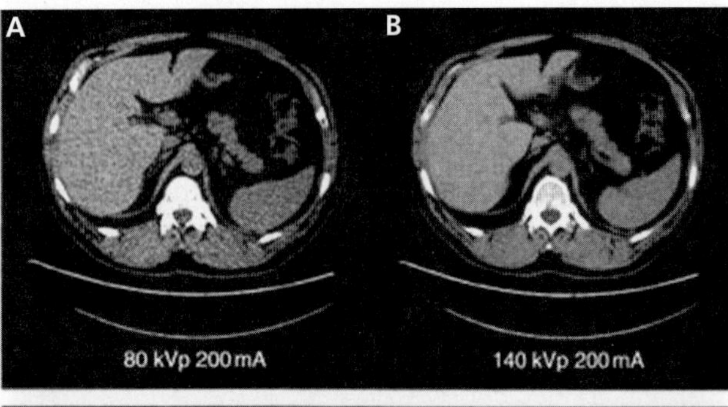

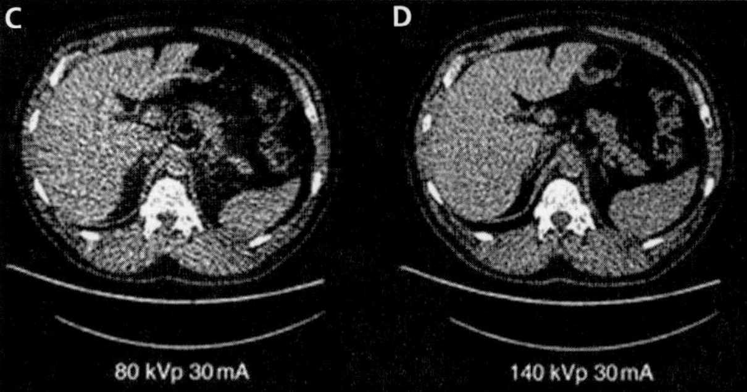

Figure 7.7 Peak kilovoltage and milliamperes have a significant influence on image quality. (A) A noisy image at 80 kVp and 200 mA. (B) More detail of vertebrae at 140 kVp and 200 mA. (C) A very poor-quality image with ring artifacts at 80 kVp and 30 mA. (D) 140 kVp and 30 mA eliminates artifacts from image C. (Reprinted, with permission, from Christian and Waterstram-Rich, 2007.)

CT Image Reconstruction

CT Numbers

The pixel values assigned in the CT image are called CT numbers (Hounsfield units). They are computed by calculating the relative difference between the linear attenuation coefficient of tissue and that of water. The equation used is $CT_{tissue} = (u_{tissue} - u_{water})/u_{water} \times 1000)$, where u_{tissue} is the attenuation coefficient of the area examined and u_{water} is the known value for the attenuation coefficient of water. The CT number for water has a value of 0. The CT number for air has a value of -1000.

CT Display

The allowable numbers for CT numbers in most systems is -1024 to $+3071$, for a total of 4096 (2^{12}). The CT numbers for various tissues in Hounsfield units (HU) or CT numbers are set values as shown in Table 7.2 (on page 72). The range of CT numbers possible is more than 4000. The human eye is thought to be able to discern only 30–100 different shades of gray; therefore, only a limited range of values are displayed in the image. The appearance of CT images thus depends on the window and level set by the user. A window centerline and window width allow the desired tissue to be displayed while allowing CT values below or above the window to be out of the viewable intensity range. A narrower window increases contrast. Examples of preset window/level combinations in CT would be for lung, soft tissue, and bone.

CT FOV

The reconstruction diameter, which acts like a software zoom on the data, may be defined. The full FOV may be 700 mm or a 70-cm gantry bore; this would include the imaging table and patient extremities and leave plenty of space around the patient. This full reconstruction FOV may be needed if this reconstructed data set is to be used to attenuation-correct a SPECT or PET study. Smaller FOVs may be used for diagnostic CT studies or studies where the CT will be simultaneously displayed with PET or SPECT. A reconstruction diameter of 500 mm is commonly used for whole-body PET/CT studies; a reconstruction diameter of 300 mm or smaller may be desired if only the head or neck region is to be reviewed. The reconstruction FOV will be set into a matrix size, and therefore, the smaller the reconstruction FOV, the greater the magnification of the image and the finer the detail that may be seen. Most often a 512 × 512 matrix size will be used. The pixel size within the image may be calculated by: pixel size (mm) = FOV (mm)/(matrix × zoom). For example, an FOV of 500 mm into a 512 × 512 matrix with a zoom of 1.0 will have a pixel size of 0.97 mm.

Reconstruction Kernel

Each vendor's CT scanner will have a variety of reconstruction kernels. The kernel is an algorithm that, in the case of CT reconstruction, defines the clinical application and amount of smoothing applied in the reconstruction process. The kernels are typically identified by body area and followed by a number: the higher the kernel number, the sharper the image. A reconstruction protocol may allow predefining of several reconstructions, each using a different kernel, which will be automatically executed upon completion of data acquisitions.

CT Attenuation Map

Attenuation correction CT studies will need to be adjusted for patient size and thickness and special adjustments will be needed for pediatric patients. The reconstruction diameter of low-dose CT for SPECT or PET attenuation correction must include the full body width so the CT is generated over the full width of the patient. It is often set to the maximum diameter of the gantry bore to ensure that there is no truncation of any part of the body, which may cause a truncation artifact. Prior to using the CT image as an attenuation map it needs to be converted to attenuation at 511 keV. The CT-generated attenuation correction map can be used to create attenuation correction factors that are applied to each LOR of the emission sonogram. The PET and CT images are displayed on either side of a workstation screen, with coregistered slices in the middle. The PET images are displayed in color and CT images are displayed in black and white, allowing the viewer to visualize the information from both studies in a single image.

CT Quality Control

CT scanners require performance assessment on a regular basis. Daily QC tests include warm-up of the X-ray tube, verification of tube output and detector response at various peak kilovoltage and milliampere settings, and evaluation of tomographic uniformity, CT number accuracy, and image noise at clinical scanning parameters. Imaging of a water-filled cylindrical phantom is a standard practice.

Other QC tests, such as image slice thickness, spatial resolution, linearity of CT numbers, and low- and high-contrast resolution, are required on a less frequent basis. Alignment of the lasers between PET or SPECT and CT scanners should be verified. A complete list of CT quality control standards is available from the American College of Radiology.

Tube Warm-Up

Daily tests will begin with an X-ray tube warm-up. The results of this warm-up test are automatic on modern systems and the computer screen will display a message that the system is acceptable for use or report results and possible service recommendations if warranted.

Cylindrical Water-Filled Phantom

A water-filled cylindrical phantom is provided to test CT number values, noise level in a test scan, and perhaps a resolution pattern testing with either visual or computer-generated analysis. Images of the QC phantom should be reconstructed and evaluated visually and quantitatively. Images of the QC phantom should appear uniform without any streaks or rings.

Common CT Artifacts

The common sources of CT artifacts can be tracked to three possible sources: operator, scanner, and patients.

Operator

Examples of operator-caused artifacts are a result of the parameters and settings selected by the operator for the study. Artifacts can be the result of inappropriate settings of peak kilovoltage, milliamperes, slice width, increment, kernel, etc.

Scanner

Scanner artifacts are those generated by the electrical or mechanical operation of the scanner. They may include ring artifacts from mismatched detector performance, streaks, incorrect mechanical motion, image distortion, partial volume effects, and so on.

Patients

Patient-generated artifacts commonly come from patient motion, beam hardening, or metallic artifacts (commonly causing streak artifacts).

Sample Calculation 7.1 Noise Equivalent Count Rate (NECR) Sample

Equation to use is:

$$NECR = N^2_{trues} / N_{trues} + N_{scatters} + (k)(N_{randoms})$$

Where N_{trues} = counts/voxel of true accepted events; $N_{scatters}$ = counts/voxel of scatter accepted events; $N_{randoms}$ = counts/voxel of random accepted events; and k = 1 or 2 (1 = randoms estimated from single event rates or 2 = randoms from online correction factor event rates).

Therefore, as an example: If activity = 33 kBq/mL versus 13 kBq/mL, the following information from a phantom could be determined:

	33 kBq/mL	*13 kBq/mL*
Trues	290 kcps/voxel	136 kcps/voxel
Scatters	160 kcps/voxel	66 kcps/voxel
Randoms	433 kcps/voxel	61 kcps/voxel

Using the equation above, the following results for each would be:

	33 kBq/mL	*13 kBq/mL*
k = 1	~95 kcps/voxel	~70 kcps/voxel
k = 2	~64 kcps/voxel	~57 kcps/voxel

Thus, this shows that even though there is approximately a 254% increase in activity from 33 kBq/mL to 13 kBq/mL, there is only about a 36% increase in kcps/voxel for the k = 1 calculations and about a 12% increase for the k = 2 calculations. This shows that the final reconstructed tomographic image is unable to effectively use most of the extra counts of the higher activity concentration.

Re-created/modified from Prekeges, 2011, Fig. 16–3.

Table 7.2 Set CT Numbers for Various Tissues in Hounsfield Units (UN) or CT Numbers.

Air	−1000
Lung	−850 to −200
Fat	−30 to −250
Water	zero
Heart	10 to 60
Brain	20 to 40
Blood	20 to 80
Liver	20 to 80
Muscle	35 to 50
Spleen	40 to 60
Bone	150 to 500
Dense bone	350 to 1000
Metal	>2000

(Re-created/modified from Christian and Waterstram-Rich, 2007, box 11–1.)

References and Further Reading

Cherry SR, Sorenson JA, Phelps ME, 2003. *Physics in Nuclear Medicine*. 3rd ed. Philadelphia, PA: Saunders.

Christian PE, Waterstram-Rich, KM, 2007. *Nuclear Medicine and PET/CT Technology and Techniques*. 6th ed. St. Louis, MO: Mosby.

Prekeges J, 2011. *Nuclear Medicine Instrumentation*. Sudbury, MA: Jones & Bartlett Learning.

Zanzonico P, 2008. Routine quality control of clinical nuclear medicine instrumentation: a brief review. *J Nucl Med*. 49:1114–1131.

CHAPTER 8 **Health Informatics and Introduction to Research Methods**

Pamela Paustian, Crystal Botkin, and Norman Bolus

Medical Informatics

Medical informatics is an area of information technology that includes medical, nursing, and allied health informatics. The American Medical Informatics Association (AMIA) defines medical informatics as the profession that focuses on all uses and aspects of data organization, data analysis, data management, and use of information technology in healthcare. Health informatics, a classification within medical informatics, utilizes information technology in healthcare facilities and focuses on the implementation and use of clinical information systems including data entry, data analyses, data management, and future system development (AMIA, 2010).

In a clinical setting medical informatics relies on healthcare standards to ensure the protection of patient information. All healthcare organizations are required by federal law to follow the Health Insurance Portability and Accountability Act standards to protect private health information of patients. Additionally, if a healthcare organization is accredited by the Joint Commission, the organization must also utilize the Joint Commission Standards for protecting patient information. It is imperative that employees of the healthcare industry recognize the different information systems used in the healthcare setting and manage patient information appropriately.

Joint Commission

The Joint Commission is a private not-for-profit accrediting body for healthcare organizations in the United States whose goal is to increase quality and improve the delivery of healthcare to the public. The Joint Commission provides accountability for the protection of patient information and requires healthcare organizations to responsibly manage all healthcare information. The Joint Commission divides gathered healthcare data into four major categories: patient-specific information, aggregate information, knowledge-based information, and comparative information. All healthcare organizations accredited by the Joint Commission must provide education to healthcare providers and personnel regarding policies, patient rights, and responsibilities (Joint Commission, 2010).

The Joint Commission Information Management Standards

On the basis of the Joint Commission accreditation standards, an accredited healthcare organization is required to maintain information privacy and confidentiality of all health information data. These standards include information security, data integrity, continuity of information, data storage, data retrieval, and dissemination of clinical and nonclinical data. Accredited organizations must have complete and accurate medical records for every patient who is cared for, treated, or served by the organizations' providers or personnel. A medical record must contain only patient-specific information related to patient care, treatment, and services rendered to the patient (Joint Commission, 2010).

Consent and authorization are required to be provided by all patients being cared for, treated by, or served by a healthcare organization. Copies of consent and authorization forms for treatment, surgery, and release of information must be maintained as part of the medial record. These forms are considered legal documents and must be part of the medical record. The provider who delivers care to the patient must obtain signed informed consent documents prior to the delivery of treatment. Standardized forms that require authorization of the release of patient information must also be signed by the patient before any healthcare documentation or information can be released to outside parties (Brodnik *et al.*, 2009).

Healthcare providers and personnel must maintain the confidentiality of patient health information and protect patient privacy. Professional standards, such as those set forth by the Joint Commission, address professional conduct and the need to hold patient information private. All providers and personnel associated with a healthcare organization must thoroughly understand the policies, rights, and responsibilities of maintaining patient data and also be able to educate patients concerning their individual rights and entitled privacy.

Health Insurance Portability and Accountability Act

In 1996 the United States Congress federally enacted the Health Insurance Portability and Accountability Act (HIPAA). The purpose of the act is to federally regulate and offer protection of private health information maintained by healthcare organizations. The act is composed of two primary titles. Title I focuses on healthcare access and portability, which offers protection to individuals who change jobs or health insurance policies. Title II establishes privacy and security regulations for identifiable health information related to individuals, which includes the HIPAA Privacy Rule. The goal of HIPAA-Title II is to improve the effectiveness, efficiency, privacy, and security of health information utilized by the healthcare organizations by establishing boundaries, security, consumer control, accountability, and responsibility (HIPAA Privacy Rule's Right of Access and Health Information Technology, 2009).

The HIPAA Privacy Rule addresses uses and disclosures of Protected Health Information (PHI). PHI relates to patients' physical or mental health status in any form, which includes paper-based information, electronic information, and oral information. This rule requires that all organizations provide patients with a notice of the organizations' privacy practices as well as access to their individual health information (HIPAA, 2009).

Under HIPAA regulations, healthcare organizations must designate an information privacy official who handles all HIPAA training in the organization, receives and investigates HIPAA complaints, and also enforces the penalties against personnel of the organizations who fail to comply with privacy requirements established by HIPAA.

Noncompliance or wrongful disclosure of private health information by healthcare providers and personnel will result in penalties, which includes fines and imprisonment.

Patient Information

Patient information includes all types of patient records, physical or electronic health records, the content of the patient records, and ownership and release of those health records. Patient health records are maintained using information technology systems such as hospital information systems, radiology information systems (RIS), picture archiving and communications systems (PACS), radiopharmacy information systems, and telemedicine systems.

Information Systems and Standards

There are several different types of information systems and standards utilized in healthcare organizations. These systems vary on the basis of the type of healthcare organization, type of healthcare delivery system, or physician practice. Hospital information systems are composed of two primary types of systems: administrative information systems and clinical information systems (Wager *et al.*, 2009).

Administrative information systems utilized in healthcare organizations contain administrative information related to personnel, materials and supplies, equipment, and financial data used to support general operations of the healthcare organization. Clinical information systems exist at the hospital and departmental levels and contain clinical and health-related information used by providers to treat and document patient care. Clinical systems at the hospital level include electronic medical record systems, medication administration systems, computerized order-entry systems, and clinical decision support systems. Departmental clinical information systems include radiology information systems, radiopharmacy information systems, pharmacy information systems, and laboratory information systems. As an example, a radiology information system is a departmental system utilized to store, evaluate, and transmit patient data and radiological images. This type of information system is usually composed of an image tracking and reporting system, which links to patient tracking and scheduling. Many wired healthcare organizations have the ability to link the radiology information system to the organization's electronic medical record. Another system found in this area may include a picture archiving and communications system (PACS). A PACS is a system that acquires, presents, stores, and displays filmless digital medical images via network communications from equipment sources such as X-ray, ultrasound, nuclear medicine, magnetic resonance imaging, and computed tomography scans. This information can be viewed from a designated workstation or via a web-based interface (Wager *et al.*, 2009).

Through the advancement of major technology infrastructure implementation, telemedicine has had a major impact on the access to quality healthcare. Telemedicine utilizes telecommunication technology for clinical care and enables providers to deliver healthcare services to patients geographically distant from the provider's location. Through the use of teleradiology providers are able to securely transmit radiological images to another provider for review rather than the patient having to travel to other specialists or locations.

Medical Record Content

For a medical record to be considered accurate and complete it must contain the patient's identification and demographic information, complaint, personal and family history, allergies, informed consent, complete history of patient's current ailment and physical examination, special examinations, such as radiography, clinical laboratory, other consultations, patient's initial diagnosis and condition, medical treatment, medications prescribed/administered, progress notes, final diagnosis, condition on discharge, and follow-up (Brodnik *et al.*, 2009).

A patient's health record is the document all healthcare providers use to collect and store clinical documentation generated by the delivery of treatment or service to the individual patient. The health record protects the legal interests of the patient, healthcare provider, and the healthcare organization. Proper documented information justifies the care plan, treatment, and delivered services to the patient, and promotes the continuity of care among different providers treating the patient. A patient's health record, paper or electronic, is the official business record created by the healthcare organization. While the information maintained in the patient record relates to the individual patient and the patient has access to the information, all health records and other health-related documentation related to the care of a patient are the property of the hospital or the healthcare provider who created the record. Information documented in a patient record is admissible as evidence in legal proceedings and may be used in liability lawsuits, criminal cases, workers' compensation claims, and malpractice lawsuits (Wesley *et al.*, 2009).

Introduction to Basic Research Methods

Scientific research is necessary to keep up with the ever-changing environment in nuclear medicine. Many questions and/or problems arise in daily practice and may be answered only through systematic investigation. According to the Webster's Dictionary, scientific method is defined as "principles and procedures for the systematic pursuit of knowledge involving the recognition and formulation of a problem, the collection of data through observation and experiment, and the formulation and testing of hypotheses." The following paragraphs provide a brief overview of research design and medical decision-making.

Research design is commonly thought of as the structure of a research project. There are several different design types, which include but may not be limited to experimental, quasi-experimental, and observational. In an experimental study design, the investigator randomly allocates study participants to two or more groups, whereas in a quasi-experimental study design the investigator assigns study participants to two or more groups—there is no randomization. An observational study design is used when the investigator passively observes how things happen in the natural, unchanged environment. These study designs can be further broken down into subtypes. Examples are provided in Table 8.1. A study design is chosen on the basis of several factors including cost, practical and ethical considerations, the hypothesis, and the significance of the research topic.

A literature review is also an important part of the research process. According to DePoy and Gitlin (2005), there are four main reasons to review the literature:

1. Determine previous research on the topic of interest
2. Determine level of theory and knowledge development
3. Determine relevance of current knowledge base to problem area
4. Provide rationale for selection of research strategy

Table 8.1 Differences between Experimental, Quasi-experimental, and Observational Studies

Experimental	Quasi-experimental	Observational
Randomized control trial (RCT)	Pre-test/post-test with controls	Cohort
Group randomized trial (GRT)	Pre-test/post-test w/out controls	Case control, cross-sectional

Online databases for periodicals, books, and documents are great places to start for the search for relevant literature. The amount of information obtained might be overwhelming; therefore, some discrimination should be used when determining if each piece is of importance to the topic of interest. This review allows the development of a knowledge base about the topic of interest and provides an understanding of how your study fits into the knowledge of the topic area.

Collection of data and information for the topic of interest can be very daunting. There are many different ways to collect the data depending on the topic that is being studied. Quantitative data are usually considered numerical and generate statistics, while qualitative data may describe experiences through interviews and/or focus groups. It takes much more time and usually fewer people take part in qualitative research; therefore, it is perceived that quantitative research may reach many more people and is quicker than qualitative. Some other examples of ways to collect data may include observation, written questionnaires, record review, instrumentation, tests, and measures.

Many terms are used to describe the effectiveness of a particular test, instrument, or measure. Some of these terms are used in medical decisionmaking. See Table 8.2 for descriptions.

Dissemination of your research findings is very important in expanding the breadth of knowledge and the future of the profession. Several components should be included in a written publication of the research topic. These include an abstract, introduction, materials and methods, results, discussion, and references. The abstract allows for a quick review of scientific publications and should be in the first section of the publication. The abstract offers a brief, single-paragraph description of the research study that mentions the hypothesis, methods, and results. The introduction section should provide the reader with the rationale behind the study and should introduce the objectives of the study. The material and methods section describes the specialized equipment and general procedures used in the study. The results portion presents the findings of your study and usually includes statistical figures if appropriate for the topic being studied. Some common statistics that are used are the chi-square test, standard deviation, coefficient of variance,

Table 8.2 Common Research Method Terms and Definitions

Term	Definition	Calculation
Validity	Strength of conclusions, inferences or propositions: was the conclusion correct?	NA
Reliability	Consistency of measurement: degree to which an instrument measures the same way each time	NA
Reproducibility	Pertains to a group of studies that can consistently get similar results	NA
True positive (TP)	Person with a positive test who is truly ill	NA
False positive (FP)	Person with a positive test who is not ill	NA
True negative (TN)	Person with a negative test who is truly well	NA
False negative (FN)	Person with a negative test who is not well	NA
Sensitivity	Percentage or fraction of ill patients who have a positive test	(TP/[TP + FN])
Specificity	Percentage or fraction of well patients who have a negative test	(TN/[TN + FP[)
Prevalence	Percentage or fraction of ill people in a population at a specific time (number of existing cases)	([TP + FN]/[TP + FN + TN + FP])
Incidence	Measure of the risk of developing a new condition or disease in a specific time frame (number of new cases)	(No. of new cases)/ (Total population at risk)
Positive predictive value	Probability of having the disease given a positive test result in people who are truly ill	(TP/[TP + FP])
Negative predictive value	Probability of not having the disease given a negative test in people who are truly well	(TN/[TN + FN])

and the *t*test. These values assist in providing information to the reader about the significance of the study. The discussion section allows an opportunity to provide information about the interpretation of the results and shows support for the conclusions that are made. This section may also include any limitations that affected the research that was done. References are always important. All literature that was used for information about the topic should be cited according to the guidelines of the journal to which the publication is being submitted.

References and Further Reading

American Medical Informatics Association (AMIA), 2010. https://www.amia.org/, accessed May 14, 2010.

Bolus NE, 2001. Epidemiology for the nuclear medicine technologist. *J Nucl Med Technol.* 29(3):143–147.

Brodnik MS, McCain MC, Rinehart-Thompson LA, Reynolds R, 2009. *Fundamentals of Law for Health Informatics and Health Information Management.* Chicago, Il: American Health Information Management Association.

Christian PE, Waterstram-Rich, KM, 2007. *Nuclear Medicine and PET/CT Technology and Techniques.* 6th ed. St. Louis, MO: Mosby.

DePoy E, Gitlin LN, 2005. *Introduction to Research: Understanding and Applying Multiple Strategies.* 3rd ed. St. Louis, MO: Elsevier Mosby.

HIPAA Privacy Rule's Right of Access and Health Information Technology, 2009. http://www.hhs.gov/ocr/privacy/hipaa/understanding/special/healthit/index.html/.

Joint Commission, 2010. http://www.jointcommission.org/, accessed May 14, 2010.

Personal Health Records and the HIPAA Privacy Rule, 2009. http://www.hhs.gov/ocr/privacy/hipaa/understanding/special/healthit/index.html

Wager KA, Lee FW, Glaser JP, 2009. *Healthcare Information Systems: A Practical Approach for HealthCare.* San Francisco, CA: Jossey-Bass Publishing.

Wesley-Odom B, Brown D, Meyers C, 2009. *Documentation for Medical Records.* Chicago, Il: AHIMA.

CHAPTER 9 **Cardiovascular System**

Kathleen Murphy, Timothy Baker, Amy Byrd Brady, and Norman Bolus

Nuclear imaging of the cardiovascular system is a major component of day-to-day work in most nuclear medicine departments. An understanding of all aspects of nuclear cardiology is essential in the preparation of nuclear medicine technologists.

Cardiac Anatomy and Physiology

The heart is a muscular organ that rests in the center of the chest in an area called the mediastinum. Two-thirds of the heart lies left of the midline next to the base of the left lung. The heart is angled away from the midline with the apex being approximately 30°–50° from the sternum (Fig. 9.1).

A sac called the pericardium surrounds the heart and holds it in place. The wall of the heart is divided into three layers: the epicardium (or external layer), the myocardium (or cardiac muscle), and the endocardium (or inner layer). The heart is divided into four chambers: left and right atria and ventricles (Fig. 9.2). Deoxygenated blood enters the right atrium from the superior and inferior vena cavae. The right atrium and ventricle are separated by the tricuspid valve. During ventricular diastole (relaxation or filling phase), the tricuspid valve opens, allowing the blood to flow from the right atrium into the right ventricle. The blood exits the right ventricle during ventricular systole (contraction phase) and travels through the pulmonary valve into the pulmonary artery, which leads into the lungs. Carbon dioxide and oxygen are exchanged in the alveoli of the lungs. As a result of this exchange, the blood becomes oxygen rich. The newly oxygenated blood enters the left atrium by way of the pulmonary veins. The blood then passes across the mitral valve into the left ventricle during ventricular diastole. The oxygenated blood is introduced into the systematic circulation during ventricular systole by passing through the aortic valve and into the aorta.

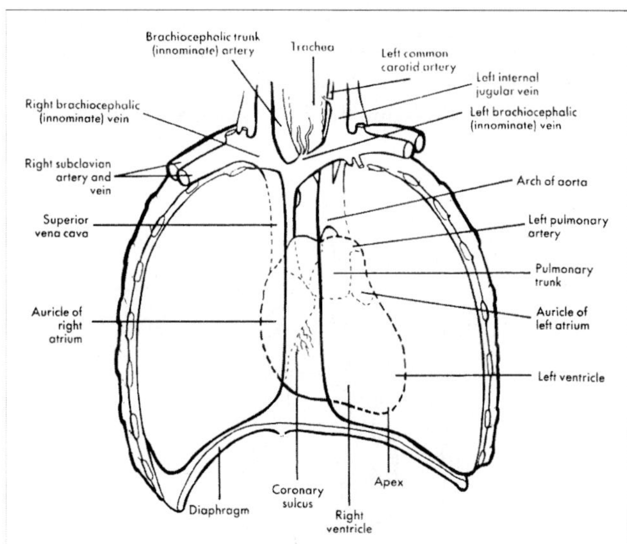

Figure 9.1 Anterior schematic of the anatomy of the heart and great vessels.

Coronary and Systemic Circulation

Perfusion of blood into the heart muscle itself is through coronary circulation. Coronary circulation begins at the base of the aorta where the right and left coronary arteries (RCA and LCA, respectively) originate. The RCA exits the aorta, usually follows the right posterior sulcus, and branches posteriorly (posterior descending artery [PDA]) toward the apex. The RCA supplies the posterior and inferior areas of the myocardium. In some patients, the RCA also supplies the apex. The LCA exits the aorta at the level of the left coronary sinus. The LCA branches into the left anterior descending artery (LAD) and the left circumflex artery (LCX). The LAD usually traverses down the anterior surface of the heart to provide blood to the septal and anterior walls of the myocardium. In most patients, the LAD also provides blood to the apex.

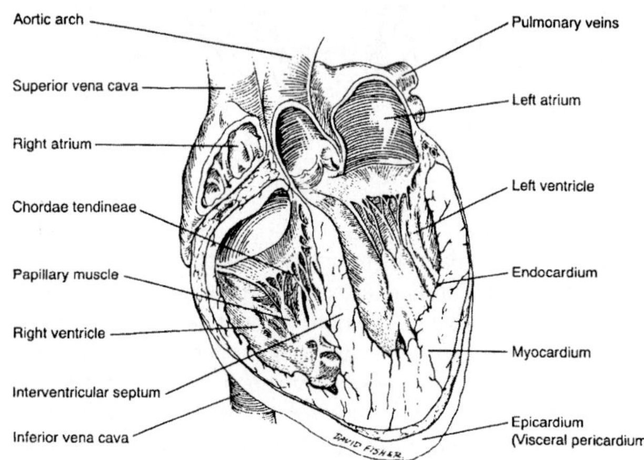

Figure 9.2 The human heart is divided into four chambers with walls of varying thickness.

Note: Nuclear cardiology has almost become a separate modality within nuclear medicine itself. This chapter covers base material for review. The editors refer you to Part II, Chapter 1, "Advanced Nuclear Cardiology" of this review guide for more in-depth information.

The LCX and its branches service the lateral free wall (Fig. 9.3). The perfusion of oxygenated blood away from the heart to the rest of the body and the return of deoxygenated blood to the heart is called systemic circulation.

Conduction System

A cardiac cycle is the period from the end of one heart contraction (systole) to the end of the next. Between the two contractions is a period of relaxation, or diastole. Each cardiac cycle is initiated by electrical stimulation in the heart, preparing it to contract.

The electrical impulse that initiates contraction begins in the sinoatrial (SA) node, a small mass of specialized tissue located in the right atrium near the entrance of the superior vena cava (Fig. 9.4). The SA node is the pacemaker for the heart and generates regular impulses at the rate of 60–100 beats per minute. The impulses from the SA node are directed to the atrioventricular (AV) node, where the impulse transmission is slowed. The AV node serves as a gatekeeper for the ventricles and, as such, allows only 40–60 impulses per minute to pass on to the ventricles. From the AV node, impulses travel through the bundle of His to the right and left bundle branches, which carry the impulses to the tips of both ventricles. (The bundle of His, known as the AV bundle or atrioventricular bundle, is a collection of heart muscle cells specialized for electrical conduction that transmits the electrical impulses from the AV node [located between the atria and the ventricles] to the point of the apex of the fascicular branches.) The terminal branches for the two bundle branches are called the Purkinje fibers. These fibers carry impulses to the individual myocardial cells, resulting in the simultaneous contraction of both ventricles.

The electrocardiogram (ECG) is a graphical representation of the electrical activity of the heart. A normal ECG pattern is composed of a P wave, a QRS complex, and a T wave (Fig. 9.5). (The QRS complex consists of the Q wave, which is the first negative deflection of the complex, the R wave, which is the first upward deflection, and the S wave, which is the rest of the complex.) Each of these is related to an event in the cardiac cycle. The P wave represents atrial depolarization (activation) of the atria. Atrial depolarization is initiated by the SA node and immediately precedes contraction of the atria. The slowing of impulse transmission at the AV node is indicated by the interval between the P wave and the QRS complex, known as the PR interval. The blood flows from the atria into the ventricles during this interval. The QRS complex indicates depolarization of the ventricles. As these chambers contract, the blood flows from the ventricles into the pulmonary artery and aorta. The ST segment represents a rest period between depolarization and repolarization (relaxation) of the ventricles. Repolarization of the ventricles is delineated by the T wave. The contraction and relaxation of the atria and ventricles are 180° out of phase with one another; that is, the atria are contracting when the ventricles are relaxing and vice versa. Repolarization of the atria is not seen in the ECG, because it is obscured by the QRS complex.

In a healthy individual, the normal heart rate is 60–100 beats per minute. The cardiac rhythm is regular, and the P wave, PR interval, and QRS complex occur at constant intervals.

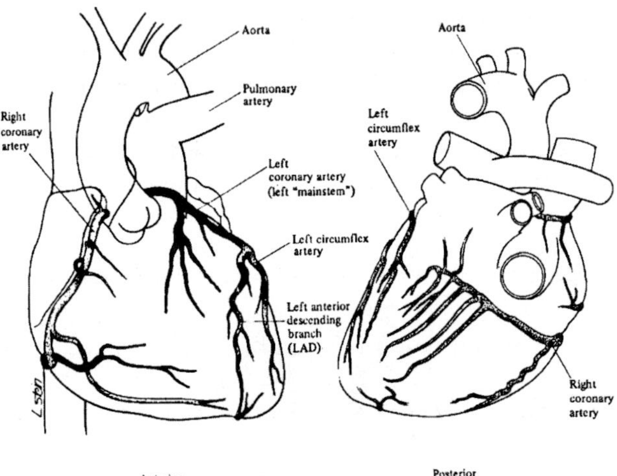

Figure 9.3 Two main vessels arising directly from the aorta—the right and left coronary arteries—supply nutrients and oxygen to the myocardium. The right coronary artery supplies the right atrium and ventricle as well as the inferior part of the left ventricle. The left circumflex artery supplies the posterior wall of the left ventricle and a portion of the inferior and lateral walls. The left anterior descending artery supplies much of the left myocardium and the interventricular septum. (Reprinted, with permission, from English *et al.* 1993, p. 11).

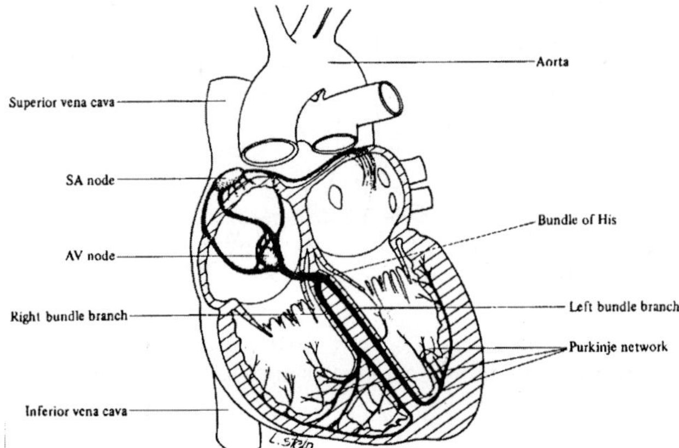

Figure 9.4 The cardiac conducting system is responsible for initiating and transmitting the electrical impulse that causes the heart to contract. (Reprinted, with permission, from English *et al.* 1993, p. 14.)

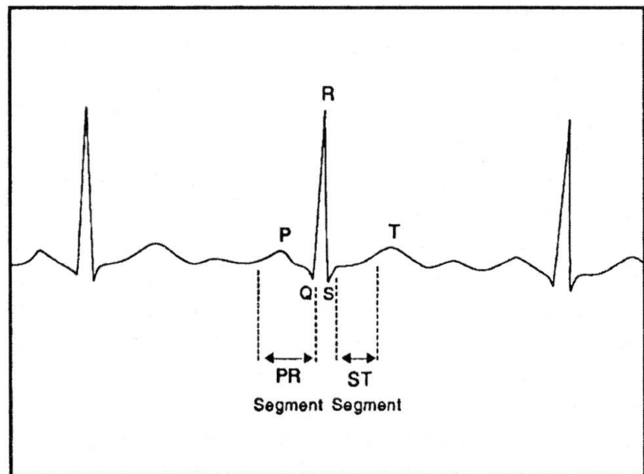

Figure 9.5 A normal electrocardiogram pattern.

Decreased blood flow to the myocardium may be demonstrated by a depression of the ST segment below the isoelectric baseline. This is of particular interest to nuclear medicine practitioners, because, during a stress study, the patient's ECG may exhibit ST segment depression, indicating that the patient is experiencing myocardial ischemia.

Coronary Artery Disease

Nuclear cardiology procedures are ordered for a variety of indications. Coronary artery disease (CAD) and the pathologic events that may result are the most common indications for performance of a cardiac radionuclide study.

Myocardial ischemia is defined as decreased blood flow to the myocardium as a result of narrowing or occlusion of a coronary artery. Angina pectoris (chest pain) is the major symptom associated with myocardial ischemia and may result in ST segment depression on an ECG. As the narrowing of the arterial lumen worsens, symptoms will usually become more severe. Patients with stable angina may not experience ischemia at rest. However, when the myocardial oxygen demand is increased, ischemia occurs because the atherosclerotic arteries are unable to keep up with demand.

Myocardial infarction (MI) usually results from total occlusion of a narrow coronary artery by a blood clot. Because of the lack of blood flow, this occlusion causes necrosis of the myocardium fed by the blocked vessel. The infarcted or necrotic tissue may be surrounded by an area of injury, or ischemic myocardium. The injured and ischemic areas of the myocardium are viable and may benefit from therapeutic intervention, such as coronary artery bypass graft (CABG) surgery or percutaneous transluminal coronary angioplasty (PTCA). The signs and symptoms of an acute MI may include unstable angina, diaphoresis, belching, nausea, dyspnea, ashen coloration, hypotension, elevated ST segment, deep Q wave, fever, and tachycardia. Complications of MI include arrhythmias, pulmonary edema, cardiogenic shock, ventricular aneurysm, mitral valve insufficiency, ventricular septal defect, and cardiac rupture.

The assessment of myocardial viability is an important indication for the performance of myocardial perfusion imaging. Viable myocardium may be at risk for infarction, but myocardial perfusion imaging may help determine whether the patient can benefit from an invasive interventional treatment such as CABG or PTCA. Hibernating myocardium is severely, chronically ischemic tissue that is viable but appears to be nonfunctioning and has decreased perfusion. It is important to differentiate between hibernating and infarcted myocardium, because hibernating myocardium is viable and has a high likelihood of benefiting from revascularization.

Myocardial stunning is a phenomenon that may occur after a patient experiences an acute episode of severe ischemia or an MI that is terminated by thrombolysis or revascularization. When the myocardium is stunned, it is deprived of blood flow. Timely restoration of perfusion results in salvage of viable myocardium. Patients who have stunned myocardium after the interruption of an acute cardiac event usually do not require additional intervention, because the stunning is a temporary response to the occlusion and revascularization has already occurred. Stunning can also occur in patients with severe CAD who experience ischemia after prolonged exercise, followed by a return of normal or near normal perfusion at rest. Patients who have stunned myocardium as a result of prolonged exercise are good candidates for revascularization.

Myocardial Perfusion Imaging

Myocardial imaging can be used to demonstrate myocardial ischemia, MI, and hibernating and stunned myocardium. Myocardial imaging can be performed with thallium-201 (^{201}Tl)–thallous chloride, technetium-99m (^{99m}Tc)–sestamibi, ^{99m}Tc–tetrofosmin, rubidium-82 (^{82}Rb)–chloride, nitrogen-13 (^{13}N)–ammonia, and fluorine-18 (^{18}F)–fluorodeoxyglucose (FDG). Clinical indications for performing myocardial perfusion imaging include:

1. diagnosis of CAD (presence, location, extent),
2. assessment of coronary artery stenosis,
3. assessment of myocardial viability,
4. prognosis post-MI,
5. monitoring of the effects of treatment.

Treadmill Exercise Testing

In many cases, individuals with CAD do not know they are at risk, because the symptoms of CAD become obvious only during exertion. A bicycle ergometer or the more common treadmill can be used to perform exercise stress testing. Exercise increases the heart rate, which, in turn, causes the myocardium to demand more blood from the coronary circulation. In patients with CAD, the coronary circulation cannot meet the increased demand. This inadequate perfusion or ischemia may result in chest pain (angina pectoris), neck or jaw pain, arm pain, or shortness of breath.

The purpose of exercise testing is to evaluate patients with possible CAD in a controlled setting by re-creating symptoms experienced on exertion. With the aid of a 12-lead ECG, these clinical symptoms can be correlated with electrical data to determine whether ischemic changes occur. Nuclear imaging can be added to the test by the administration of a radiopharmaceutical during peak exercise to visualize ischemic areas in the myocardium induced by exercise. The patient must continue to exercise for 1–2 min after tracer administration to maintain the maximum myocardial oxygen demand while the tracer is being taken up by the myocardium.

Patient History and Preparation

Patients should be hemodynamically stable for at least 48 hr before undergoing an exercise test. Contraindications to exercise stress include unstable angina, acute MI (within 2–4 days), uncontrolled hypertension (systolic >220 mm mercury (mm Hg); diastolic >120 mm Hg), pulmonary hypertension, untreated life-threatening arrhythmias, uncompensated congestive heart failure, advanced atrioventricular block (in a patient without a pacemaker), acute myocarditis, acute pericarditis, severe mitral or aortic stenosis, severe obstructive cardiomyopathy, and acute systemic illness. The patient should fast for at least 3 hr before the exercise test. A physician must be consulted to determine the optimum diet on the day of the study for insulin-dependent patients with diabetes. The patient should also be instructed to wear comfortable clothing and footwear and should not undergo any unusual physical exertion for at least 12 hr before the stress test.

Pertinent patient history includes family history, lifestyle (smoking, alcohol consumption, exercise, etc.), recent symptoms, previous history of heart disease or hypertension, and current medications. Beta- and calcium channel-blockers adversely affect the patient's ability to reach an adequate level of myocardial demand during treadmill exercise by altering the heart rate and blood pressure response to exercise. These medications may be withheld before the stress test at the discretion of the attending physician. A physical or pharmacologic limitation that may affect the patient's ability to reach the target heart rate must be brought to the attention of the physician in charge of the stress procedure. Physical exercise is preferred, but pharmacologic stress may be indicated in patients who are unable to exercise adequately. Table 9.1 lists some of the medications that can affect exercise response.

In treadmill testing, a certain level of exercise must be reached for adequate evaluation of the patient. This level is usually 85% of the patient's maximum predicted heart rate based on the patient's age (220 − patient's age). Other reasons for terminating exercise include: marked ST segment depression (>3 mm), ischemic ST segment elevation (>1 mm in a lead without a pathologic Q wave), ventricular or supraventricular tachycardia, progressive decrease in blood pressure, and abnormal elevation of blood pressure (>250/130 mm Hg).

For myocardial perfusion imaging, the technologist must ensure that a large-bore intravenous catheter is securely placed to allow injection of the radiopharmaceutical at peak exercise. Radiation safety procedures should be practiced during the stress test. For the technologist, this would include the use of gloves, protective clothing, and a syringe shield. All other personnel involved in the test should also wear gloves to prevent the possible spread of radioactive contamination in case of a spill or leaking catheter.

For ECG monitoring, electrodes are placed on the patient's chest using a modified 12-lead setup (Fig. 9.6). The right- and left-arm electrodes are placed at the midclavicular line, just below the clavicle. The right- and left-leg electrodes are placed just below the rib cage in the right and left lower quadrants of the abdomen. The skin should be cleansed with alcohol to remove any skin oils and should be lightly abraded to achieve good electrical contact. Excess hair may prevent adequate electrical contact and may necessitate dry shaving small areas where the electrodes will be attached. Patients should be advised not to apply any moisturizer or powder on the day

Table 9.1 Drugs That Can Affect Exercise Response

Drug	Discontinue before test
Nitroglycerin	1 hr
Long-acting nitrates	12 hr
Tranquilizers/sedatives	1 day
Antiarrhythmic agents	2 days
Beta-blockers	72 hr
Diuretics	4 days
Antihypertensives	4–7 days
Digitalis	1–2 weeks
Calcium channel blockers	48–72 hr

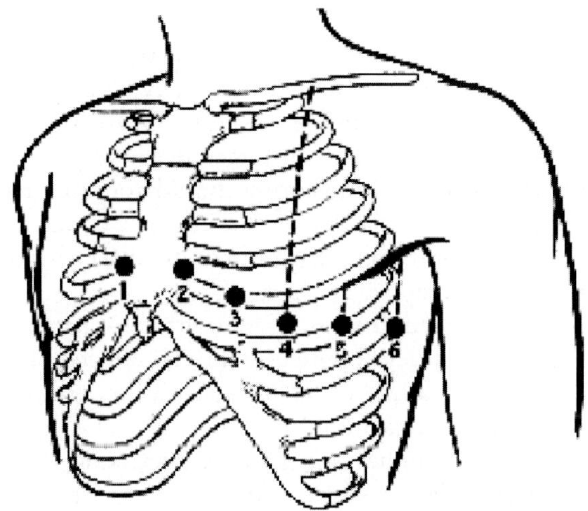

Figure 9.6 Sites of electrode placement for cardiac stress testing. (1) Fourth intercostal space at right margin of sternum, (2) fourth intercostal space at left margin of sternum, (3) midway between positions 2 and 4, (4) fifth intercostal space at junction of left midclavicular line, (5) at horizontal level of position 4 at left anterior axillary line, (6) at horizontal level of position 4 at left midaxillary line. (Reprinted, with permission, from Zakus *et al.* 1990.)

of the stress test. Securely attaching the electrodes will ensure a quality ECG.

Exercise Protocols

The physician can choose from a variety of exercise protocols when deciding which protocol is best suited for an individual patient. The two most commonly used protocols are the Bruce and modified Bruce protocols. In the Bruce protocol, the speed and elevation of the treadmill increases every 3 min. Each 3-min interval is called a stage and represents an increase in the patient's workload, thereby increasing the heart rate. The modified Bruce protocol is a variation in which the elevation increases slightly every 3 min, but the speed remains slow. This is generally reserved for patients with limited exercise capacity.

Pharmacologic Stress Agents

Many patients cannot perform a treadmill or bicycle stress test because of physical limitations, poor motivation, or medications that hinder an adequate increase in myocardial oxygen demand. These patients benefit from the use of a pharmacologic stress agent.

Dipyridamole (Persantine)

Intravenous administration of dipyridamole indirectly increases the level of exogenous adenosine in the patient's blood by deactivating adenosine deaminase. The increased blood level of adenosine results in vasodilation of the coronary arteries. Adenosine activates the A2 receptors on the cell membrane of smooth muscle. This creates a "myocardial steal" phenomenon that diverts blood away from myocardium that is fed by stenotic coronary arteries, resulting in an increased uptake in myocardium supplied by healthy arteries and decreased or absent uptake in myocardium that receives its blood supply from atherosclerotic or stenotic coronary arteries. When used in conjunction with myocardial perfusion imaging agents, differences in perfusion become apparent during imaging.

Patient History and Preparation

A thorough patient history or a full review of the patient's medical record is essential. The patient should have nothing by mouth (NPO) for a minimum of 4 hr before dipyridamole infusion. Administration of xanthine derivatives (aminophylline, theophylline, caffeine, etc.) must be discontinued for 12–24 hr before testing. Caffeine and other xanthine derivatives compete with adenosine for binding sites on the walls of the coronary arteries and may result in a false-negative exam. Caffeinated products include coffee, tea, chocolate, some soft drinks, and some medications. Decaffeinated products should also be avoided, because they contain a small amount of caffeine.

Contraindications and Adverse Effects

Contraindications for dipyridamole infusion include history of bronchospasm or pulmonary disease, active wheezing, hypotension (systolic <90 mm Hg), and severe mitral valve disease. Other contraindications include MI within 2 days, unstable angina within 48 hr, severe aortic stenosis, severe obstructive hypertrophic cardiomyopathy, and severe orthostatic hypotension.

Adverse side effects include chest pain, headache, dizziness, ECG changes, nausea, flushing, tachycardia, dyspnea, and hypotension. Aminophylline can be administered to alleviate or reverse these effects, typically at dosages of 125–250 mg intravenously. The administration of aminophylline reverses the vasodilatory effects and may result in a false-negative exam if it is given before the tracer has had a chance to be taken up by the myocardium. If at all possible, the aminophylline should not be administered until 1–2 min after the injection of the tracer. Nitroglycerine can be administered to relieve chest pain if the injection of aminophylline does not alleviate the patient's angina.

Administration Protocol

The dosage of intravenous dipyridamole given over a 4-min time interval is 0.142 mg/kg/min (0.56 mg/kg diluted in 50 mL of saline); therefore, an accurate weight must be obtained before calculating the dosage to be administered. A baseline heart rate, blood pressure, and 12-lead ECG are obtained before the infusion begins. These parameters are acquired continuously during the administration of the dipyridamole and are recorded every minute. The peak effect takes place at approximately 2–3 min after the infusion has ended. The tracer is injected 3–5 min after the 4-min infusion of dipyridamole has ended. The patient should be monitored for at least 15 min after administration of the dipyridamole or until the heart rate, blood pressure, and ECG have returned to baseline.

Adenosine (Adenocard)

The intravenous infusion of adenosine directly increases the level of adenosine in the patient's blood. As mentioned previously, adenosine is a potent coronary vasodilator.

Patient History and Preparation

The patient's history and preparation would be treated the same for the adenosine infusion as for administration of dipyridamole.

Contraindications and Adverse Effects

The contraindications for adenosine administration include the same conditions listed for dipyridamole, as well as second- or third-degree AV block (without a pacemaker) because of the negative dromotropic (SA and AV node) effect that occurs with the infusion of adenosine. Adenosine should not be given to patients who are taking oral dipyridamole.

The adverse effects associated with adenosine infusion include flushing, chest pain, dyspnea, ST segment depression, dizziness, nausea, and hypotension. Because of the short half-life of adenosine (<2 sec), side effects will usually dissipate within 1–2 min of the discontinuation of the infusion. Aminophylline can be administered if the cessation of the adenosine infusion does not reverse the adverse effects.

Administration Protocol

Patient preparation is the same as for dipyridamole infusion. The dosage is 240 μg/kg and is administered at a rate of 140 μg/kg/min for 6 min. The tracer is injected at 3 min into the infusion. Two intravenous lines must be established (or a dual-port catheter used) to allow for the continuous infusion of adenosine while the tracer is being administered. Adenosine's short plasma half-life (<2 sec) requires a continuous infusion to ensure the continuation of vasodilation while the tracer is being taken up by the myocardium. Also, administering the tracer through its own port avoids giving the patient a bolus of adenosine. A baseline heart rate, blood pressure, and 12-lead ECG are obtained, continuously monitored, and recorded every minute during the infusion. Monitoring should continue for at least 5 min after cessation of the infusion or until the patient's heart rate, blood pressure, and ECG have returned to baseline.

A 7-min titrated dosage can be utilized for patients at increased risk for development of adverse effects. The infusion begins at a rate of 50 μg/kg/min for 1 min, followed by increases each minute to 75, 100, and 140 μg/kg/min. The radiopharmaceutical is injected at the end of the fourth minute.

Regadenoson (Lexiscan)

Regadenoson is an A_{2A} adenosine receptor that is a coronary vasodilator. Intravenous administration of regadenoson activates the A_{2A} adenosine receptor and produces coronary vasodilation, which, in turn, increases coronary blood flow. The maximal plasma concentration of regadenoson is accomplished within 1–4 min after injection.

Patient History and Preparation

A thorough patient history or a full review of the patient's medical record is essential. Patients should avoid any products containing methylxanthines for at least 12 hr prior to administration of regadenoson. Methylxanthines include caffeinated coffee, tea, or other caffeinated beverages, caffeine-containing drug products, and theophylline. Also, dipyridamole should be withheld for at least 2 days prior to administration of regadenoson.

Contraindications and Adverse Effects

Contraindications for regadenoson include patients who have second- or third-degree AV block or sinus node dysfunction unless the patient has a functioning artificial pacemaker. Contraindications also include patients with bronchospasm. The safety of regadenoson in patients with bronchospasm has not been established. Patients with a systolic blood pressure <90 mm Hg and patients with a known hypersensitivity to regadenoson should also avoid this drug.

Adverse side effects include dyspnea, headache, flushing, chest discomfort, angina pectoris, dizziness, chest pain, nausea, abdominal discomfort, and dysgeusia. Aminophylline can be administered to alleviate or reverse these effects, typically at dosages ranging from 50 to 250 mg by slow intravenous injection (50 to 100 mg over 30–60 sec).

Administration Protocol

The dosage of intravenous regadenoson is 5 mL or 0.4 mg. Regadenoson is injected rapidly over 10 sec into a peripheral vein using a 22-gauge or larger catheter or needle. Following the regadenoson injection, a 5-mL saline flush is administered immediately. After the saline flush is complete, wait 10–20 sec and then administer the radionuclide or tracer. The radionuclide may be injected directly into the same catheter as regadenoson. The patient may be imaged 45–60 min following the regadenoson injection when using ^{99m}Tc-based cardiac radiopharmaceuticals.

Use of Low-Level or Isometric Exercise with Vasodilator Infusion

A combination of low-level or isometric exercise with the administration of dipyridamole, adenosine, or regadenoson has been shown to decrease side effects and subdiaphragmatic uptake and increase the target-to-background ratio. Many protocols that utilize walking, bicycle stress, or isometric exercise during or immediately after the infusion of a pharmacologic agent have been proposed. This technique is not universally accepted, and if a patient has left bundle branch block (LBBB), you would not exercise them.

Dobutamine (Dobutrex)

Dobutamine is a positive inotropic and chronotropic pharmaceutical. This pharmacologic stress agent actually enhances the force of the heart's contractions and increases the heart rate, thus increasing the myocardial oxygen demand. Dobutamine stimulates the β-1 receptors in the myocardium, resulting in an increase in the force and frequency of the contractions, and is the pharmacologic agent that most closely mimics the effects of physical exercise on the heart. Dobutamine administration is indicated for patients who are unable to exercise and who cannot undergo pharmacological vasodilator stress infusion because of the presence of severe bronchospastic disease.

Contraindications and Adverse Effects

Beta-blockers are the primary contraindication for dobutamine administration. These antihypertensives should be discontinued for 24 hr before testing. Other contraindications include recent MI (<1 week), unstable angina, hemodynamically significant left ventricular outflow tract obstruction, critical aortic stenosis, atrial tachyarrhythmias with uncontrolled ventricular response, ventricular tachycardia, uncontrolled hypertension, aortic dissection, or large aortic aneurysm. Reasons for early termination of the dobutamine infusion are the same as for exercise stress. The most common adverse effects include chest pain, palpitations, headache, flushing, dyspnea, paresthesia, and ischemic ST segment depression. Dobutamine should be discontinued if these symptoms become too severe, and a beta-blocker (esmolol) should be administered to reverse the adverse effects.

Administration Protocol

The patient should be NPO for a minimum of 4 hr before the test, and beta-blocker therapy must have been discontinued for 24–48 hr. Dobutamine administration is broken down into stages very similar to those of a treadmill test. Dobutamine has a serum half-life of 2 min, so it must be infused continuously during the tracer administration. Therefore, a dual-port catheter or the insertion of two intravenous lines is recommended to avoid giving a bolus of dobutamine while injecting the tracer.

Intravenous infusion begins at a rate of 5 μg/kg/min for 3 min. The dobutamine is diluted in 50 mL of normal saline or 5% dextrose/water. Stepped increases follow at 3-min intervals to infusion rates of 10, 20, 30, and 40 μg/kg/min. At the beginning of the last stage, the radiopharmaceutical is injected. A baseline heart rate, blood pressure, and 12-lead ECG should be obtained before the infusion begins. These parameters should be monitored continuously and recorded every minute during the administration of the dobutamine and for at least 5 min after completion of the infusion or until the patient's heart rate, blood pressure, and ECG return to baseline.

Planar Myocardial Perfusion Imaging

Image Acquisition

The patient should be placed supine on a table that will allow exact duplication of the positioning for stress and rest imaging. The angles of the camera head and/or yoke should be recorded to assist in the accurate reproduction of the same views. The camera must be positioned as close as possible to the patient to ensure adequate resolution and count statistics. A zoom factor of 1.2–1.5 should be applied during acquisition if using a large-field-of-view camera.

Three standard views are obtained (Fig. 9.7). The left anterior oblique (LAO) view is usually obtained at 45°. The anterior view is acquired with the camera head 45° back from the LAO angle. The left lateral view is obtained with the patient lying on the right side (right lateral decubitis) and the camera head angled at 90° or until the best long axis of the left ventricle is acquired. The patient is placed in the decubitis position in an effort to decrease the diaphragmatic attenuation that occurs when lying

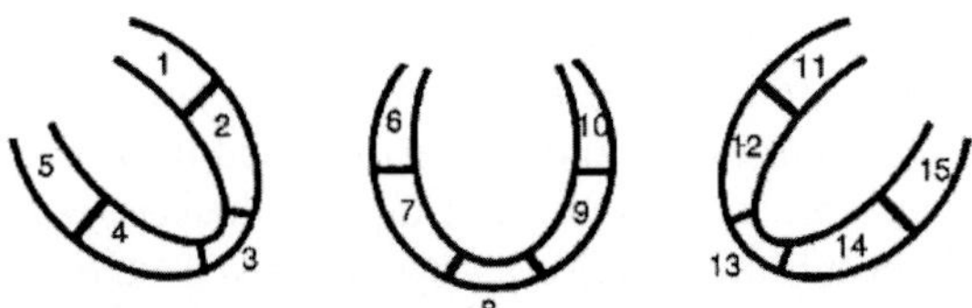

Figure 9.7 Planar myocardial perfusion segments. (1) Basal anterolateral, (2) midanterolateral, (3) apical, (4) midinferoseptal, (5) basal inferoseptal, (6) septal, (7) inferoseptal, (8) inferoapical, (9) inferolateral, (10) lateral, (11) basal anterior, (12) midanterior, (13) apex, (14) midinferior, (15) basal inferior. (Reprinted, with permission, from Port, 1999, p. 6:G79.)

supine. Diaphragmatic attenuation may cause a false-positive defect in the inferior wall of the left ventricle.

Breast tissue is another possible source of attenuation, and each set of images should be acquired with the breast in the same position (i.e., if the patient has her bra off during the stress images, she should also have it off during the redistribution images). A flexible radioactive line source can be used to outline the breast while a 1-min image is acquired. This allows the physician to see where the breast lies in relation to the myocardium.

It is very important to acquire both sets of images (immediate poststress and rest or redistribution) in a reproducible fashion. The angles and patient position relative to the camera must be reproduced exactly during the second set of images. This ensures that any changes visualized on the redistribution images reflect physiologic changes and are not the result of positioning errors.

Processing

Image processing usually consists of side-by-side displays of the background-subtracted and smoothed stress and rest or redistribution images. Circumferential profile analysis is performed on each planar image to provide quantitative myocardial perfusion information. The percentage washout of ^{201}Tl and the heart-to-lung ratio may also be calculated. The regions of interest (ROIs) used to calculate the lung-to-heart ratio are the same shape and size. The myocardial ROI should not be placed on the anterior or anterolateral wall because of heart/lung overlap in those regions.

Image Findings

Normal myocardial perfusion images consist of uniform distribution throughout the left ventricle (Fig. 9.8). The normal right ventricle may or may not be visualized, because the muscle is relatively thin compared with that in the left ventricle. Areas of MI will appear as fixed defects that are present on the stress and redistribution or rest images. A cold defect that is present on stress and demonstrates filling-in on the redistribution or rest images is indicative of myocardial ischemia (Fig. 9.9).

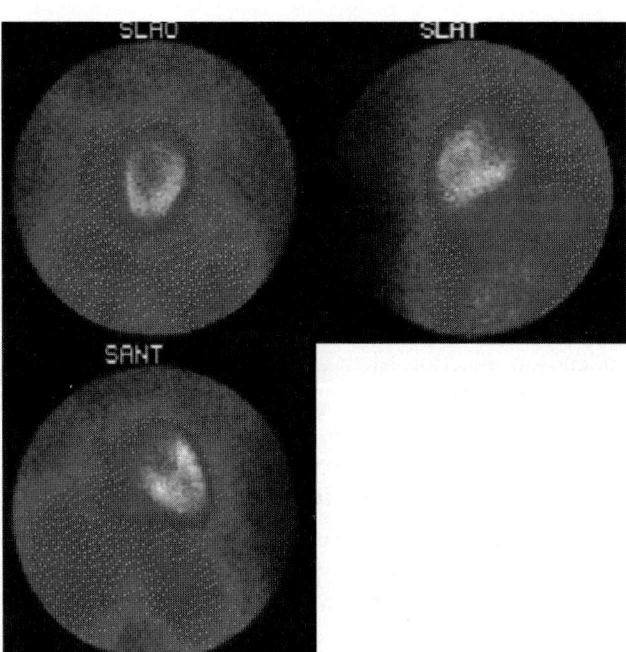

Figure 9.8 Normal planar ^{201}Tl myocardial perfusion scan. (Courtesy of Frans J. Th. Wackers, MD, Yale Cardiovascular Nuclear Imaging Laboratory, New Haven, CT.)

SPECT Myocardial Perfusion Imaging

Acquisition

Myocardial perfusion single-photon emission computed tomography (SPECT) imaging can be acquired over 180° or 360°, using a circular or noncircular orbit with continuous or step-and-shoot motion. The step-and-shoot method consists of either 32 or 64 stops for a 180° rotation, or 64 or 128 stops for a 360° rotation. Each stop is separated by approximately 3°–6°. The recommended pixel size is 6.4 ± 0.2 mm for a 64 × 64 matrix acquisition.

The patient is positioned with both arms or only the left arm up over the head. The patient should be made as comfortable as possible in an effort to minimize motion resulting from discomfort. A variety of devices, such as armrests, wedges, and Velcro straps, have been used to provide patient comfort and stability. Myocardial perfusion SPECT studies can also be acquired in the prone or decubitis position in patients who are likely to move if imaged in the supine position. Prone imaging is sometimes used for patients who are likely to have diaphragmatic attenuation of the inferior wall of the left ventricle.

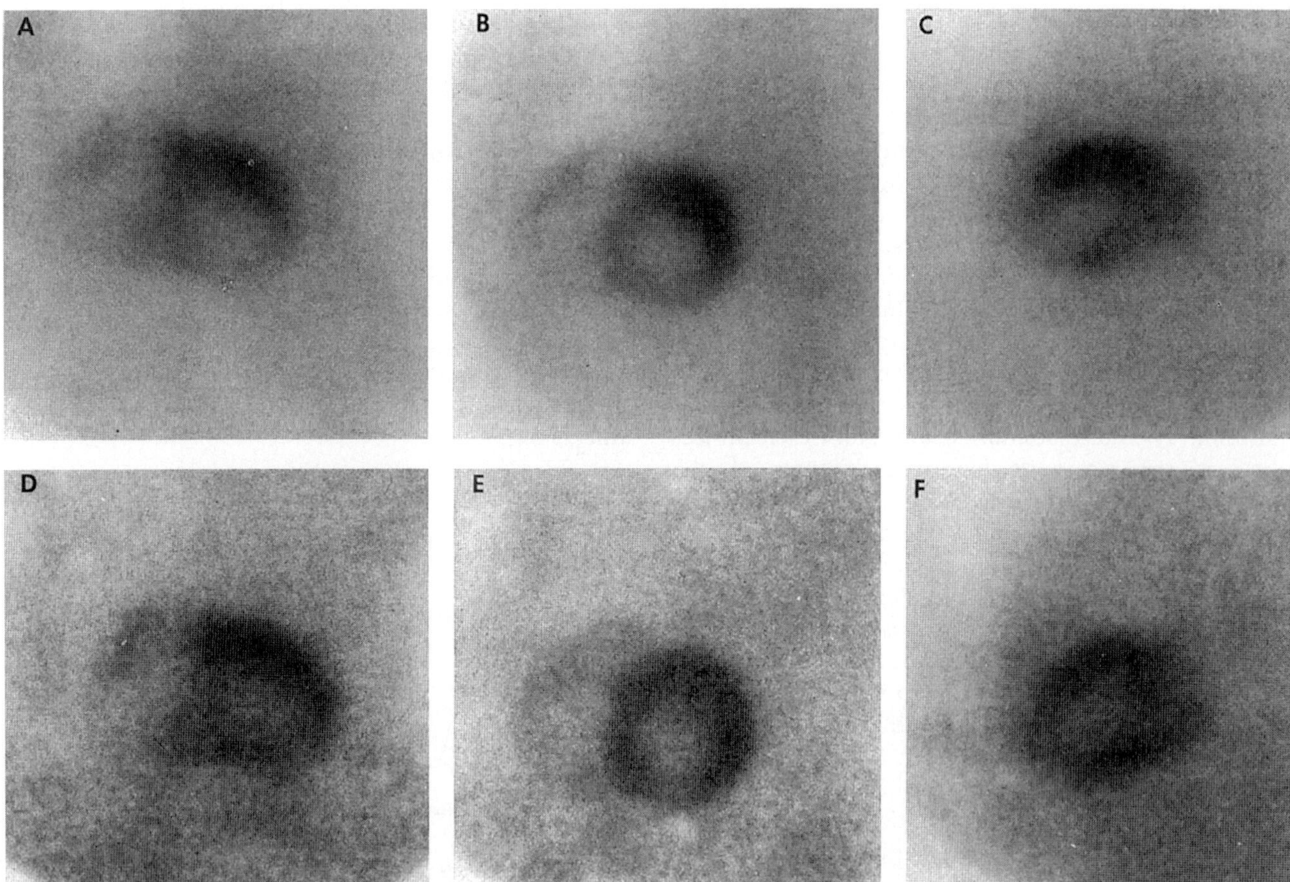

Figure 9.9 Abnormal planar thallium images in the anterior, 40° LAO and 70° LAO projections. Stress images (A–C) show perfusion defects in the inferior, septal, and apical areas of the left ventricle. Delayed images (D–F) demonstrate tracer redistribution in these areas, a pattern consistent with exercise-induced ischemia. (Courtesy of the Department of Veterans Affairs Medical Center, Buffalo, NY.)

The technologist should explain the importance of remaining still to the patient before the acquisition begins. The patient should be closely monitored for motion during the acquisition, and, if the patient moves dramatically, the study should be terminated. A new SPECT study can be initiated, or planar images can be acquired instead if it is determined that the patient will not be able to remain still for the duration of the SPECT study. Motion artifacts can appear as blurred or cold areas on the SPECT slices.

ECG gating of the planar or SPECT studies can be obtained with the placement of nonattenuating electrodes in the standard lead II configuration and a 100% acceptance window. Gated SPECT images allow the interpreting physician to assess wall motion and thickening, and ejection fraction (EF) can be estimated as well. This functional assessment helps the physician to evaluate areas of the myocardium with decreased uptake that may be caused by attenuation or a true perfusion defect. For example, an area of fixed decreased uptake is seen in the anterior wall of a female patient. Is this indicative of an area of necrosis, or is the decreased uptake the result of breast attenuation? The physician can confidently interpret the study as being normal with an attenuation artifact if the area in question demonstrates normal wall motion and thickening.

Processing

The raw data should be reviewed in cine format in an effort to identify any sources of attenuation or artifacts. Artifacts caused by small movements can be removed by using motion correction software.

Attenuation from the breast and/or diaphragm is a problem that is frequently encountered while performing myocardial perfusion imaging. Attenuation correction software and hardware are available. The creation of an attenuation map from the acquisition of a transmission scan allows for the correction of attenuation artifacts.

The raw data are usually corrected for uniformity and center-of-rotation offset errors on the fly (during acquisition). Filtering of the raw SPECT data is performed to enhance resolution and suppress noise in the images. A low-pass filter is usually applied to the raw data before reconstruction. Low-pass filters suppress high-frequency noise and result in smoothing of the images with some loss in resolution. The Butterworth filter is the most commonly used low-pass filter for myocardial perfusion SPECT studies. Filtering may be performed before or after image reconstruction.

Reconstruction of the planar projections may be performed with either the filtered backprojection technique or the iterative technique. These techniques use a mathematical algorithm to estimate the distribution of the tracer in the images. Backprojection creates transaxial slices from the multiple projections acquired during acquisition. The corresponding counts from each projection are smeared back toward the center of the reconstruction space for the creation of each slice. The "smear" of counts from each projection is called a ray. When the ray from every image is backprojected, the end result is a transaxial slice surrounded by a star artifact caused by the smearing of the counts toward the center. A high-pass ramp filter is applied during reconstruction to reduce the star artifact. The ramp filter suppresses the low frequencies and enhances the high frequencies, resulting in images with sharp edges. A smoothing filter, such as the Butterworth filter, is applied to decrease high-frequency noise and improve resolution.

The iterative reconstruction technique involves an estimation of the tracer distribution through a series of approximations. The estimations are made repetitively until the desired result is obtained. This is a more accurate reconstruction method but has not been utilized until recently, because the processing time was prohibitive. However, today's computer systems are fast enough to make iterative reconstruction a clinical reality. Iterative reconstruction must be used if attenuation correction software is to be applied to the data.

Background subtraction is performed on the raw data to enhance the visualization of the myocardium and to improve image contrast. Myocardial perfusion images acquired with ^{99m}Tc or ^{201}Tl agents must be normalized to activity in the heart, using a standardized method, before they are quantified and displayed for interpretation. A number of normalization techniques can be used. One method normalizes to the average counts per pixel in the hottest region of the myocardium. The images may be displayed in gray or color scales. The excessive use of contrast should be avoided, because areas of normal perfusion may appear as cold defects, resulting in false-positive interpretations.

Finally, the selection of the angles that will be used to generate the short-axis, horizontal long-axis, and vertical long-axis slices are critical steps in the processing of myocardial perfusion SPECT studies. Some software packages automate this selection, but, in some cases, the axis for oblique slice generation is determined by the technologist processing the study. Midventricular transverse and vertical long-axis slices are used when choosing the long and short axis of the left ventricle. Choosing incorrect angles for the reorientation of the slices can introduce artifacts that can be mistaken for pathologic defects.

The rest and stress images are displayed together for comparison and should be displayed in a standard format that includes stress/rest or stress/redistribution short-axis, vertical long-axis, and horizontal long-axis slices (Figs. 9.10 and 9.11). Gated SPECT slices should be displayed as summed images in the standard format and in cine format for the assessment of wall motion and thickening.

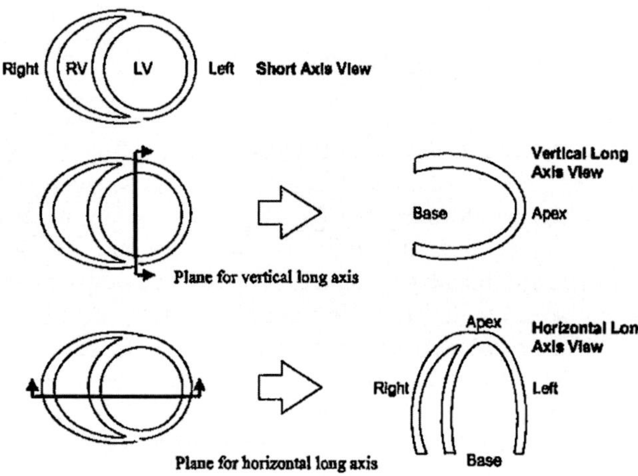

Figure 9.10 Orientation for display of myocardial perfusion tomographic slices. (Reprinted, with permission, from Guidelines and Communications Committee, Commission on Health Care Policy and Practice, 2001, p. 12.)

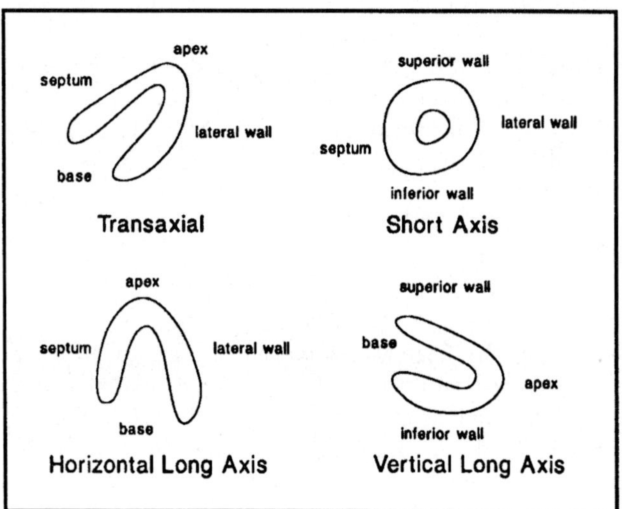

Figure 9.11 Orientation of cross-cardiac sections.

Quantitative processing provides the physician with objective data related to the presence, size, and severity of defects in the myocardium. An ROI is placed around the myocardium. It is very important to include only myocardial counts in the ROI. The counts in the regions of the patient's myocardium can be compared with a normal database (Fig. 9.12).

A polar map (bull's-eye) is a graphical representation of the myocardial perfusion and is derived from the short-axis slices for the anterior, inferior, lateral, and septal information. The vertical long-axis slice is used to obtain the apical data for inclusion in the polar map (Fig. 9.13).

Myocardial Perfusion Radiopharmaceuticals

^{201}Tl-Thallous Chloride

Thallium is an analog of the element potassium (K), which is used by the myocardium during contractions. Thallium does not collect in the myocardium permanently but is constantly being pumped in and out of the myocardial cells via the sodium–potassium pump. This phenomenon makes ^{201}Tl an ideal agent for assessing the extent of CAD and for determining the viability of affected myocardium.

Coronary arteries that are stenotic or narrow provide decreased blood flow to the areas of the myocardium that they supply. This condition is intensified during exercise, when the myocardium's demand for oxygen is greater. The partially blocked or atherosclerotic coronary artery, however, cannot respond normally by dilating to increase the blood flow to the myocardium. Because the amount of ^{201}Tl uptake is based on the amount of blood flow to that area of the myocardium, ischemic regions will concentrate less ^{201}Tl and appear as areas of decreased activity on the images. When the patient is at rest and the myocardium's need for oxygen has lessened, blood flow in the diseased artery may be adequate. Because ^{201}Tl is constantly being pumped in and out of the myocardial cells into the circulation, ^{201}Tl redistribution into previously ischemic areas can occur and is visualized on delayed images (2–4 hr after injection), resting ^{201}Tl images, 24-hr delayed images, or re-injection images. In the case of stress-induced ischemia, defects visualized on the stress images appear to fill in with tracer on redistribution images. The patient must be imaged within 5–10 min after cessation of stress, because the defects present at peak myocardial oxygen demand may begin to fill in rapidly, resulting in a false-negative scan if the images are acquired after redistribution occurs. Infarcted or necrotic areas will not accumulate tracer during rest or stress imaging, because the myocardial cells in these areas are no longer functional. Such data provide a highly accurate picture of the amount of viable or salvageable myocardium.

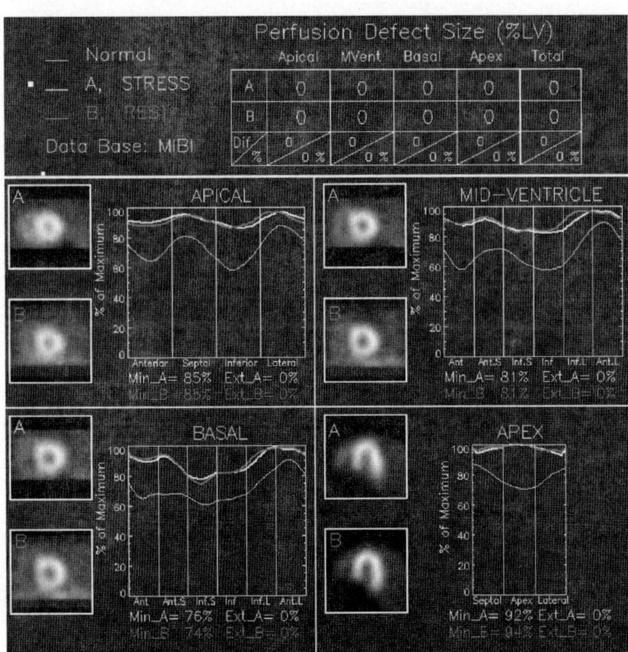

Figure 9.12 Normal ^{99m}Tc–sestamibi SPECT quantitation. (Courtesy of Frans J. Th. Wackers, MD, Yale Cardiovascular Nuclear Imaging Laboratory, New Haven, CT.)

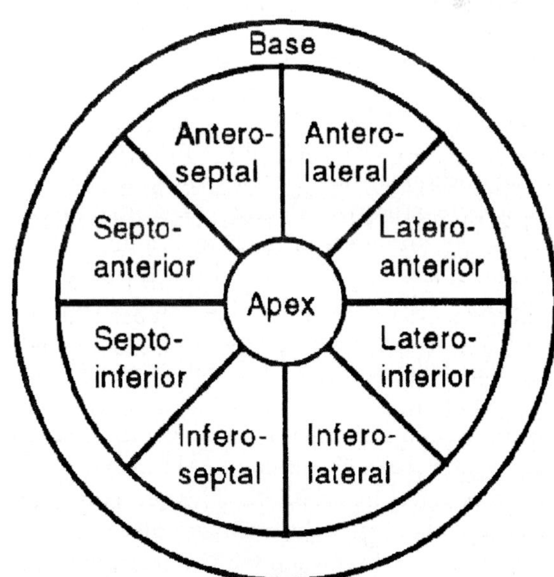

Figure 9.13 Ten myocardial segments on a polar or bull's-eye map. (Reprinted, with permission, from Van Train *et al.*, 1994.)

^{201}Tl Stress/Redistribution Image Acquisition

The choice between planar and SPECT image acquisition depends on the patient's ability to lie still during the acquisition. SPECT imaging is the preferred and more commonly performed acquisition method, but at times planar image acquisition is necessary.

^{201}Tl Planar Imaging

Imaging should begin 10 min after the administration of 74–148 megabecquerels (MBq) (2–4 mCi) of ^{201}Tl. Mercury X rays in the 68–80 keV range are emitted during the decay of ^{201}Tl, and a 30% window is centered over 72 keV. The use of a second 20% window centered on the 167-keV γ-ray emissions is optional. The images are typically acquired with a low-energy all-purpose collimator and a matrix size of 128 $\times$ 128-word mode. A minimum of 600,000 counts in the total field of view or 8 min of acquisition time is necessary to obtain high-quality images.

After the stress images are acquired, the patient should be instructed to return for delayed imaging in 3–4 hr. The patient may be instructed not to eat during this time, or may be permitted a light snack, and to avoid caffeine, sugar, and carbohydrates, because glucose ingestion results in accelerated clearance of ^{201}Tl from the myocardium.

^{201}Tl SPECT Imaging

The ^{201}Tl SPECT study should be obtained using a low-energy all-purpose collimator. Each image is acquired for 40 sec. Planar images may be acquired before the SPECT acquisition. The planar images can be used to calculate lung-to-heart ratio and to assist in the identification of artifacts in the SPECT slices.

Resting ^{201}Tl Imaging

Resting ^{201}Tl studies are sometimes performed to assess the patient who may have suffered an acute MI. Defects seen at rest are indicative of necrotic or scarred tissue, because ^{201}Tl localizes only in viable myocardium. The patient should fast for at least 4 hr before the resting injection of ^{201}Tl. A dosage of 92.5–111 MBq (2.5–3 mCi) of ^{201}Tl is injected intravenously. Imaging begins at 10–15 min, followed by the acquisition of delayed images at 3–4 hr.

Thallium re-injection has been shown to increase the sensitivity of stress/redistribution ^{201}Tl imaging for the detection of viable myocardium. This procedure can be performed at the 3- to 4-hr mark after delayed imaging or even 24 hr later. In this procedure, the patient receives an intravenous injection of 55.5 MBq (1.5 mCi) of ^{201}Tl. Imaging can begin 10–15 min after the ^{201}Tl administration. Planar and/or SPECT images are then obtained just as they were for the earlier image sets. These re-injection images are then compared with the stress and redistribution images to identify any areas of late reversibility. A lack of ^{201}Tl uptake in an area of the myocardium after re-injection indicates a high probability of nonviable tissue.

^{99m}Tc–Sestamibi (Cardiolite)

In the 1980s, researchers worked to find a myocardial perfusion agent with better imaging characteristics than ^{201}Tl. Much of this research centered on finding a ^{99m}Tc-based radiopharmaceutical that would yield high myocardial count rates while delivering a modest radiation dose to the patient.

^{99m}Tc–sestamibi is an isonitrile compound that binds to the mitochondrial membrane inside the myocardial cell. The uptake of sestamibi is proportional to blood flow. Unlike ^{201}Tl, ^{99m}Tc–sestamibi undergoes redistribution at a very slow rate and remains fixed in the myocardium for hours. The increased count statistics associated with the use of ^{99m}Tc myocardial perfusion agents allow for the simultaneous evaluation of perfusion and function. The higher activity administered with the ^{99m}Tc-based perfusion tracers is adequate for the acquisition of a first-pass and/or gated myocardial perfusion study. A major disadvantage of ^{99m}Tc–sestamibi is its hepatobiliary clearance. The liver, gallbladder, and bowel uptake can cause problems when processing ^{99m}Tc–sestamibi SPECT images.

A variety of imaging protocols are available, including:

- 1-day stress/rest or rest/stress,
- 2-day stress/rest or rest/stress,
- dual-isotope protocol.

In a rest/stress 1-day protocol the first injection is the low dosage (296–444 MBq or 8–12 mCi), and the second injection is the high dosage (925–1110 MBq or 25–30 mCi). Generally, the stress/rest 1-day protocol utilizes 370–555 MBq (10–15 mCi) for the first dosage and 925–1110 MBq (25–30 mCi) for the second dosage. For the 2-day protocol, both injections are generally 740–1110 MBq (20–30 mCi). Imaging begins at 15–60 min after the stress injection and 60–90 min after the rest injection. However, images can be obtained up to 4 hr after injection because of the slow redistribution of ^{99m}Tc–sestamibi.

A high-resolution parallel-hole collimator is used when imaging ^{99m}Tc–sestamibi. Planar views can be acquired in as little as 5 min per view (10 min per view, if gated). A 20% window is centered over the 140-keV γ emissions from the decay of ^{99m}Tc. When acquiring a SPECT study, generally, 20–25 sec per stop are required for the higher-dosage administration and 40 sec per stop for the lower-dosage acquisition (Fig. 9.14).

^{99m}Tc–Tetrofosmin (Myoview)

^{99m}Tc–tetrofosmin is a diphosphine that forms a lipophilic, cationic complex with technetium. Tetrofosmin is taken up rapidly by the myocardium, and it is theorized that it localizes in the mitochondria of the myocardial cells. ^{99m}Tc–tetrofosmin clears from the liver and the lung faster than ^{99m}Tc–sestamibi. Like sestamibi, tetrofosmin remains in the myocardium for several hours after injection, resulting in the need for separate injections at rest and stress.

The acquisition and processing protocols for ^{99m}Tc–tetrofosmin are the same as those for ^{99m}Tc–sestamibi. However, because of the rapid uptake and background clearance of ^{99m}Tc–tetrofosmin, imaging can begin earlier.

Dual-Radionuclide Myocardial Perfusion SPECT

This protocol involves the use of 92.5 MBq (2.5 mCi) of ^{201}Tl injected at rest and 814–925 MBq (22–25 mCi) of a ^{99m}Tc-based myocardial perfusion agent administered during stress. Rest/stress imaging can be accomplished on the same day. Acquisition parameters for the SPECT studies are the same as those mentioned for ^{201}Tl- and ^{99m}Tc-labeled perfusion agents, respectively. This method has the advantage of combining the unique characteristics that ^{201}Tl brings to the assessment of myocardial viability with ^{99m}Tc–sestamibi imaging at stress. There are also protocols that allow one to do the ^{201}Tl stress portion first and then 814–925 MBq (22–25 mCi) of a ^{99m}Tc-based myocardial perfusion agent administered during rest. As long as the ^{201}Tl portion is done first, the protocol will not have to be concerned with backscatter radiation from the 140-keV ^{99m}Tc-based agent.

Cardiac PET Imaging

Myocardial perfusion and viability can be assessed using positron-emitting radionuclides. ^{82}Rb is a potassium analog that is produced by a strontium-82/^{82}Rb generator, thus eliminating the need for a cyclotron adjacent to the imaging area. ^{82}Rb has a 75-sec half-life; therefore an infusion system is necessary. ^{82}Rb is taken up by the myocardium via the sodium–potassium adenosine triphosphatase pump. The dosage administered to the patient at rest and at stress is approximately 2220 MBq (60 mCi) for each image set. The images are reconstructed into short-axis, vertical long-axis, and horizontal long-axis slices (Fig. 9.15).

^{13}N–ammonia has a short half-life of 10 min; therefore, its use is limited to imaging centers that have a cyclotron in the vicinity. ^{13}N–ammonia diffuses across the cell membrane of the myocardial cells and is used to quantify regional blood flow of the heart. ^{13}N–ammonia (555–740 MBq or 15–20 mCi) is administered at stress and at rest.

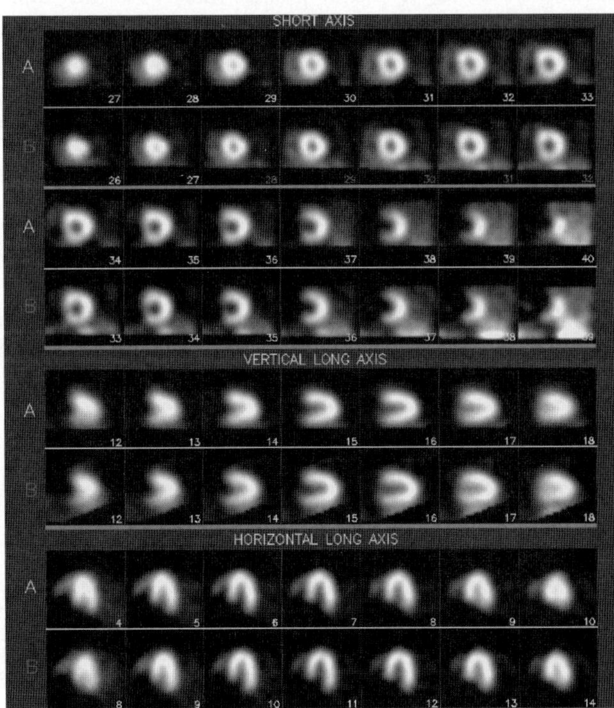

Figure 9.14 ^{99m}Tc–sestamibi SPECT slices. (Courtesy of Frans J. Th. Wackers, MD, Yale Cardiovascular Nuclear Imaging Laboratory, New Haven, CT.)

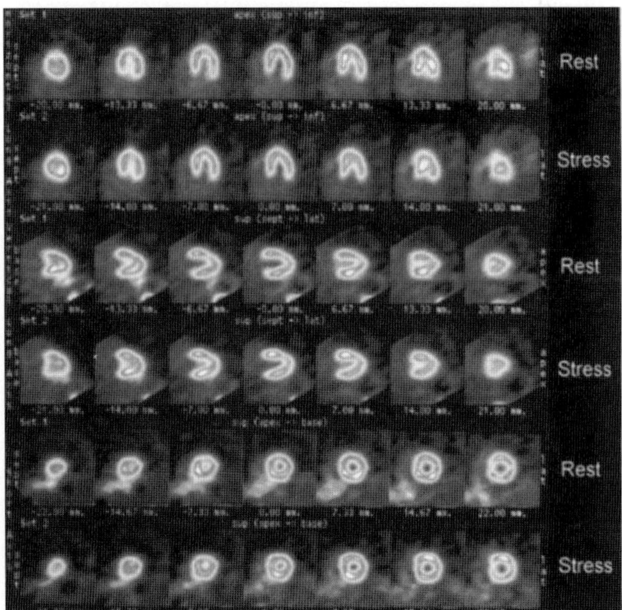

Figure 9.15 Normal rest/stress ^{82}Rb perfusion scans. (Reprinted, with permission, from Crawford and Husain, 2003, p. 100.)

^{18}F-FDG is a glucose analog with a half-life of 110 min. This relatively long half-life enables the delivery of ^{18}F-FDG to imaging centers from remote cyclotrons. Fatty acid is the primary energy source for the myocardium, but glucose is used for energy when the blood level of fatty acid is low. This allows for the metabolic imaging of the myocardium using ^{18}F-FDG. Viable myocardial tissue will demonstrate ^{18}F-FDG uptake, whereas necrotic or infarcted myocardium will appear cold (due to decreased perfusion) on ^{18}F-FDG images. The patient receives a dosage of 85–555 MBq (5–15 mCi) at stress and at rest, and imaging takes place 30–40 min after injection. Uptake of ^{18}F-FDG in the myocardium is minimal when a patient has been fasting. Glucose loading has been used to increase the uptake of ^{18}F-FDG by the myocardium. Tomographic ^{18}F-FDG data are reconstructed into the standard slices (Fig. 9.16).

Equilibrium-Gated Blood Pool Imaging

Gated blood pool imaging has been given a variety of names over the years: multigated blood pool acquisition (MUGA), radionuclide ventriculography (RVG), and equilibrium radionuclide angiography (ERNA or RNA). This test involves labeling the red blood cells (RBC) with ^{99m}Tc–pertechnetate and imaging the blood pool in the heart using a gated acquisition technique. MUGA can be performed at rest or during stress. However, stress blood pool imaging is seldom performed and will not be discussed. Clinical indications for ERNA include:

1. detection or assessment of CAD,
2. MI (acute or remote),
3. detection or assessment of congestive heart failure,
4. assessment of cardiac function in chemotherapy patients,
5. evaluation of cardiac function in patients with valvular disease.

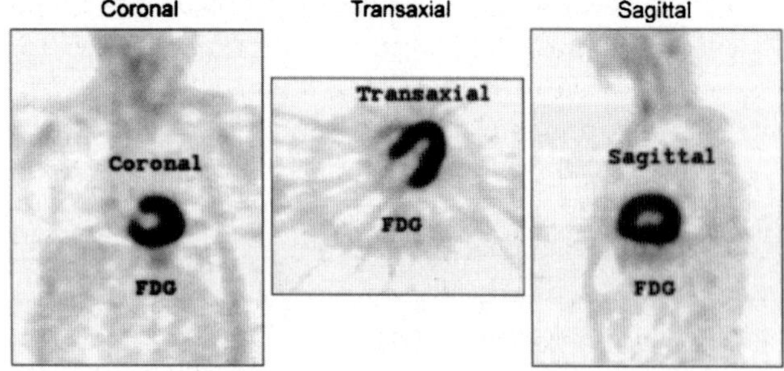

Figure 9.16 Whole-body FDG scan showing normal distribution in the myocardium of a fasting adult. (Reprinted, with permission, from Crawford and Husain, 2003, p. 103.)

Patient Preparation

A resting ERNA does not require any specific patient preparation.

Radiopharmaceuticals

The most commonly used radiopharmaceutical for gated blood pool imaging is 555–1110 MBq (15–30 mCi) of ^{99m}Tc-labeled RBCs. ^{99m}Tc–human serum albumin (HSA) has also been used for ERNA imaging.

Three methods can be used to label RBCs with ^{99m}Tc–pertechnetate: in vitro, in vivo, and modified in vivo/in vitro. The in vitro method involves withdrawing 2–10 mL of blood from the patient, centrifuging and washing the cells, and combining the packed RBCs with a reducing agent, such as stannous pyrophosphate in the presence of an anticoagulant. ^{99m}Tc–pertechnetate is then added and incubated at room temperature for 20–30 min. During this time, the pertechnetate ion is reduced so that it can be transported across the RBC membrane and attach to hemoglobin. The actual incorporation of the pertechnetate ion into hemoglobin is not well understood, but this method yields a very high labeling efficiency. The newly labeled RBCs are then reinjected back into the patient for imaging. This labeling method is extremely stable, and imaging can be performed up to 4 hr later. A single-patient kit that can be used as an alternative to the in vitro method is UltraTag (Mallinckrodt, St. Louis, MO). This kit has a very high labeling efficiency (typically greater than 95%) but does not require that the RBCs be separated by centrifugation.

The in vivo method starts with an intravenous injection of 2–3 mg of stannous pyrophosphate. This material is allowed to circulate for 15–20 min followed by the intravenous injection of ^{99m}Tc–pertechnetate. The labeling efficiency of the in vivo method is lower than that of the in vitro method, typically between 60 and 90%.

To increase the labeling efficiency of the in vivo method, a modified in vivo/in vitro method was developed. The typical labeling efficiency for this method is between 90 and 95%. This involves the intravenous injection of stannous pyrophosphate, followed by a waiting period of approximately 20 min. Whole blood is withdrawn from the patient into a shielded syringe that contains ^{99m}Tc–pertechnetate and an anticoagulant. The syringe is gently inverted to mix the contents and is incubated at room temperature for 10 min. The contents of the syringe are injected into the patient.

Image Acquisition

The patient is placed supine on an imaging table, and three electrodes are placed for a standard lead II ECG. The negative and reference electrodes are placed just below the right and left clavicles, respectively. The posi-

Table 9.2 Definitions Commonly Used in Nuclear Cardiology

Word	Definition	Equation
Stroke volume (SV)	The volume of blood ejected by either ventricle during ventricular systole	
Cardiac output (CO)	The volume of blood that the heart pumps per minute	CO = SV × heart rate
End diastolic volume (EDV)	The capacity of the ventricle after it is completely filled with blood; the largest volume reached by ventricle during a cardiac cycle	
End systolic volume (ESV)	The residual capacity of the ventricle at the end of contraction; the smallest volume reached during a cardiac cycle.	
Ejection fraction (EF)	The percentage of blood ejected from the ventricle during each contraction	EF = [EDV − ESV]/EDV × 100

tive electrode is placed just below the ribs on the left side. The electrodes must be placed out of the field of view to avoid attenuation, and the R waves must be of sufficient amplitude to trigger the data collection. Either a low-energy all-purpose or high-resolution parallel-hole collimator is used. The LAO view is usually obtained at 45° but should be adjusted until the best septal separation is acquired. The anterior view is acquired with the camera head 45° back from the LAO angle. The left lateral view is obtained with the patient lying on the right side (right lateral decubitis) and the camera head angled at 90° or until the best long axis of the left ventricle is acquired. Each view is acquired for 3–7 million counts in the total field of view. If an assessment of right ventricular function is indicated, a gated first-pass study can be obtained in list mode while the labeled RBCs are being injected. The gated first-pass study is acquired in the 10°–15° RAO position.

Data are acquired by dividing the cardiac cycle into 16, 24, or 32 frames (Fig. 9.17). The time that an individual frame will accumulate counts during a single cardiac cycle is dependent on the average length of the patient's R–R interval and is usually calculated by the acquisition software after sampling the patient's ECG. A 20–30% acceptance window is placed around the average R–R interval. When an R wave is accepted, the counts begin to be deposited into the first frame of the acquisition and continue to accumulate until the predetermined time interval is complete. Then the second frame accumulates counts for that time, followed by the third frame, etc. Over the course of a few hundred beats, the cumulative information gathered gives an accurate picture of cardiac wall motion. Because the cardiac cycle is now divided into discrete frames, end-diastolic and end-systolic frames can be identified on the basis of the number of counts in the left ventricle (Table 9.2).

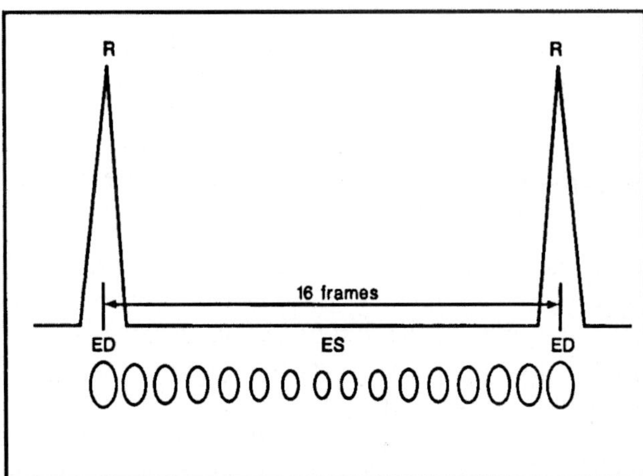

Figure 9.17 Relationship of left ventricular volume and electrocardiographic tracing. A representative cardiac cycle (from which left ventricular ejection fraction is calculated) is generated by adding together data from hundreds of cardiac cycles. ED, end diastole; ES, end systole.

Data Processing

Global EF is the percentage of diastolic volume pumped during a cardiac cycle and is calculated using the following formula:

$$\%EF = \frac{\text{net diastolic counts} - \text{net systolic counts}}{\text{net diastolic counts}} \times 100.$$

Regional EFs can also be generated by dividing the ventricle into segments. A cine loop of each view is created and displayed for qualitative assessment of ventricular wall motion. The cine is a composite of the cardiac cycle, running as a continuous loop of the 16, 24, or 32 frames that were acquired. This display assists the physician in the visualization of wall motion abnormalities, such as akinesis (absence of motion), hypokinesis (decreased motion), and dyskinesis (when a segment of the ventricle bulges out as the remainder of the ventricle contracts, also known as paradoxical motion).

Technical Considerations

A composite cardiac cycle can be produced only if the R–R intervals are of approximately equal length (regular rhythm). Small variations in the R–R interval length are expected and accounted for when setting the R–R interval acceptance window. However, in patients with severe arrhythmias, it may be impossible to obtain adequate data, because the R–R interval length falls outside of the acceptance window and many beats are rejected.

Careful adherence to a standardized RBC labeling procedure will help ensure high labeling efficiency. Excess free ^{99m}Tc–pertechnetate in structures surrounding the heart may obscure cardiac chambers and make it difficult to identify ventricular borders. The RBCs of patients on high dosages of steroids or heparin may be difficult to label with ^{99m}Tc–pertechnetate, although the mechanism of this interference with the labeling process is not completely understood.

FIRST-PASS IMAGING

First-pass radionuclide angiography is a useful tool in the evaluation of patients with left ventricular dysfunction, interventricular shunts, myocardial ischemia, or infarction. This technique is used to record the initial passage of the radiopharmaceutical through the cardiac chambers. An advantage to first-pass analysis is that the tracer activity is limited to one chamber at a time, making it easier to define the ROIs, and background interference is decreased. In addition, this procedure is rapidly completed and does not require that the patient lie still on an imaging table for a prolonged period of time. First-pass imaging can be obtained using any ^{99m}Tc radiopharmaceutical, including ^{99m}Tc myocardial perfusion agents. The use of a ^{99m}Tc-labeled myocardial perfusion agent allows for the assessment of ventricular function with the first-pass study and myocardial perfusion and function with a gated SPECT study.

Patient Preparation

A baseline ECG should be obtained and used to assess the patient's heart rhythm. Because first-pass studies are representative of only two or three beats, a regular rhythm without ectopic beats or premature ventricular contractions (PVCs) is essential for a successful study. If the radiopharmaceutical enters the right ventricle during a spurious beat, the entire study may be technically inadequate. For patients with frequent PVCs, an equilibrium-gated blood pool study with bad beat rejection would be a better choice.

Image Acquisition

A large-bore (18-gauge or larger) catheter is inserted into an external jugular or right medial antecubital vein so that a small bolus of activity can be pushed rapidly without resistance. The choice of radiopharmaceutical is dependent on whether another study will be acquired after the first pass (e.g., myocardial perfusion imaging or MUGA). If the patient is scheduled only for a first-pass study, ^{99m}Tc–pentetate (DTPA) or ^{99m}Tc–pertechnetate are the preferred tracers. The volume of labeled RBCs should be kept to a minimum if a MUGA is planned after the first-pass study, or the in vivo labeling method may be used. Regardless of the radiopharmaceutical, the volume injected must be as small as possible, preferably less than 1 mL. A small volume will help ensure that the injected bolus remains intact as long as possible. The volume to be injected must not exceed the volume of the tubing used to administer the radiopharmaceutical. A large volume will result in the bolus separating. The use of a vein that offers a direct path to the superior vena cava also minimizes the possibility of bolus fragmentation. The bolus is delivered smoothly and rapidly with a saline flush of at least 10 mL.

A multicrystal camera is preferred for first-pass acquisitions because of the increased sensitivity, but such systems are not available in most nuclear medicine departments. A gamma camera can be used to acquire first-pass studies if it has the ability to acquire data at a high count rate (200,000 counts/sec or greater) and is equipped with a high-sensitivity collimator. Positioning is one of the most difficult aspects of first-pass imaging, because it is performed before the radiopharmaceutical is injected. The patient can be positioned supine or upright, with the camera in the anterior or 10°–15° RAO position. A 37-MBq (1-mCi) source can be used to ensure that the sternal notch and the xiphoid process are in the field of view before injection. Alternatively, a ^{57}Co sheet source can be placed behind the patient, resulting in a transmission scan that depicts the lungs with the cardiac shadow. Both methods ensure that the entire heart is in the field of view before beginning the acquisition.

The acquisition is started, the bolus is injected, and the acquisition is terminated once the tracer travels through the right side of the heart, the lungs, and the left side of the heart.

Data Processing

First-pass angiography can be used to assess patients with suspected interventricular shunts. A mix of oxygen-rich and oxygen-poor blood is ejected into the systemic circulation as a result of the shunting of blood from the right ventricle into the left ventricle. This results in poor perfusion of tissues and organs.

The presence of the tracer in the venous blood being shunted into the left ventricle and systemic circulation can be easily detected. An ROI is drawn over the right ventricle, lungs, and left ventricle or nonpulmonary background region. These regions are applied to the dynamic series of images. Peaks representing the bolus of activity are observed by graphing each region over time.

In patients with shunts, the peak of left ventricular or background activity will occur earlier or be superimposed on the lung peak.

Left ventricular EF can be calculated after the creation of a left ventricular ROI. Application of the ROI to the dynamic set of images should give two to three peaks of bolus activity representing ventricular contraction. The apices of these peaks are representative of diastole, whereas the low points represent systole. EF is calculated by obtaining the counts associated with each of these points.

References and Further Reading

Blust JS, Boyce TM, Moore WH, 1992. Pharmacologic cardiac intervention: comparison of adenosine, dipyridamole and dobutamine. *J Nucl Med Technol.* 20:53–59.

Christian PE, 1997. Computer science. In: Bernier DR, Christian PE, Langan JK, eds. *Nuclear Medicine Technology and Techniques.* 4th ed. St. Louis, MO: Mosby; 118–122.

Crawford ES, Husain SS, 2003. *Nuclear Cardiac Imaging: Terminology and Technical Aspects.* Reston, VA: Society of Nuclear Medicine.

DePuey EG, Garcia EV, Berman DS, 2001. *Cardiac SPECT Imaging.* 2nd ed. Philadelphia, PA: Lippincott Williams & Wilkins. 3–16, 41–65, 89–154, 201–204.

DePuey EG, ed., 1994. *Myocardial Imaging with Cardiolite: A Workbook.* 2nd ed. North Billerica, MA: DuPont Pharma Radiopharmaceuticals, Inc..

Early PJ, Sodee DB, eds., 1995. *Principles and Practice of Nuclear Medicine.* 2nd ed. St. Louis, MO: Mosby; 370–442.

English CA, English RJ, Giering LP, Manspeaker H, Murphy JH, Wise PA, 1993. *Introduction to Nuclear Cardiology.* 3rd ed. North Billerica, MA: DuPont Pharma Radiopharmaceuticals.

English RJ, 1995. *SPECT: A Primer.* 3rd ed. Reston, VA: Society of Nuclear Medicine; 23–31.

Faber TL, 1997. Tomographic imaging methods In: Gerson MC, ed. *Cardiac Nuclear Medicine.* 3rd ed. New York, NY: McGraw-Hill Companies, Inc.; 53–80.

Fletcher CF, Balady G, Froelicher VF, Hurtley LH, Haskell WL, Pollock ML (American Heart Association Writing Group), 1995. Exercise standards: a statement for healthcare professionals from the American Heart Association. *Circulation.* 91:580–615.

Garcia EV, 1996. Imaging guidelines for nuclear cardiology procedures: part 1. *J Nucl Cardiol.* 3:G1–G46.

Guidelines and Communications Committee, Commission on Health Care Policy and Practice, 2001. *Society of Nuclear Medicine Procedure Guidelines Manual 2001–2002.* Reston, VA: Society of Nuclear Medicine; 1–14.

Guyton AC, 1979. *Physiology of the Human Body.* 5th ed. Philadelphia, PA: WB Saunders; 127.

Jones S, Hendel RC, 1993. Technetium-99m tetrofosmin: a new myocardial perfusion agent. *J Nucl Med Technol.* 21:191–195.

Lee K, 1991. *Computers in Nuclear Medicine: A Practical Approach.* Reston, VA: Society of Nuclear Medicine; 147–227.

Park HM, Duncan K, 1994. Nonradioactive pharmaceuticals in nuclear medicine. *J Nucl Med Technol.* 22:242, 244–245.

Port SC, ed., 1999. Imaging guidelines for nuclear cardiology procedures: part 2. *J Nucl Cardiol.* 6:G47–G84.

Powsner RA, Powsner ER, 1998. *Essentials of Nuclear Medicine Physics.* Malden, MA: Blackwell Science; 114–135.

Strauss HW, Griffeth LK, Shahrokh FD, Gropler RJ, 1997. Cardiovascular system. In: Bernier DR, Christian PE, Langan JK, eds. *Nuclear Medicine Technology and Techniques.* 4th ed. St. Louis, MO: Mosby; 323–354.

Thrall JH, Ziessman HA, 2001. *Nuclear Medicine: The Requisites.* St. Louis, MO: Mosby; 65–109.

Train KV, Garcia EV, Maddahi J, Areeda J, Cooke CD, Kiat H, Silagan G, Folks R, Friedman J, Matzer L, Germano G, Bateman T, Ziffer J, DePuey EG, Fink-Bennett D, Cloninger K, Berman DS. 1994. Multicenter trial validation for quantitative analysis of same-day rest-stress technetium-99m-sestamibi myocardial tomograms. *J Nucl Med.* 35:609–618.

Wackers FJ, 1992. Artifacts in planar and SPECT myocardial perfusion imaging. *Am J Cardiac Imaging.* 6:42–58.

Wahl RL, Buchanan JW, eds., 2002. *Principles and Practice of Positron Emission Tomography.* Philadelphia, PA: Lippincott Williams & Wilkins; 320–380.

Zakus SM, Eggs DA, Shea MA, 1990. *Mosby's Fundamentals of Medical Assisting: Administrative and Technical Theory and Technique.* 2nd ed. St. Louis, MO: Mosby; 589.

CHAPTER 10 Central Nervous System

Anthony Knight, Robert Gladding, and Norman Bolus

Continued advances in single-photon emission computed tomography (SPECT) along with positron emission tomography (PET), PET/CT, and SPECT/CT imaging, which are now a part of mainstream clinical practice, have resulted in a resurgence of brain imaging in recent years. Regional cerebral blood flow and metabolic imaging studies have become powerful tools in the investigation of a wide array of neurologic disorders. Although SPECT, PET, PET/CT, and SPECT/CT imaging predominate, this review also discusses planar brain imaging and cisternography.

Brain–Blood Barrier Imaging

Brain–blood barrier (BBB) radionuclide imaging alone has become a rarely performed procedure in traditional nuclear medicine because of its limitations and the advancement of other imaging modalities, such as computed axial tomography (CT) and magnetic resonance imaging (MRI). However, with the advent of hybrid imaging using PET/CT and SPECT/CT in tumor viability imaging, staging, and therapy assessment for brain tumor treatment, BBB imaging can still be a useful procedure. This is discussed more under brain perfusion imaging using PET agents. In addition, in certain instances when planar methods of nuclear medicine imaging are the only options available (for example, when a patient's condition requires bedside imaging or when claustrophobia or contrast media sensitivity preclude using MRI or CT), BBB imaging is also used as a means of determining cerebral brain death. This practice, while still used, is falling by the wayside as perfusion agent protocols are becoming more widely accepted in diagnosing brain death.

BBB imaging is most useful when the following pathologies are suspected:

1. primary (e.g., glioma, meningioma) or metastatic disease,
2. intracranial inflammatory disease (e.g., abscess, encephalitis),
3. cerebrovascular disease (e.g., cerebral hemorrhage, vascular occlusion, hemangioma, arteriovenous malformation),
4. complications of head trauma (e.g., subdural hematoma, brain death).

Radiopharmaceuticals

The radiopharmaceuticals used to perform BBB imaging do not normally cross the BBB. The BBB is a defense mechanism that prevents certain undesirable substances from reaching the brain and cerebral spinal fluid (CSF). However, a number of cerebral pathologies result in the disruption of this barrier, which allows these radiopharmaceuticals to enter the area of abnormality.

Technetium-99m (^{99m}Tc)-labeled radiopharmaceuticals can be used to perform BBB imaging. ^{99m}Tc–pertechnetate is probably the least desirable, because it normally accumulates in the choroid plexus of the brain, making it necessary to administer a blocking agent, such as potassium perchlorate. ^{99m}Tc–pentetate (DTPA) is a better agent for planar brain imaging because:

1. Pentetate is rapidly cleared from the circulation by the kidneys, thus providing lower radiation exposure to the patient and increased target-to-nontarget ratios. Imaging can begin sooner with this agent than with ^{99m}Tc–pertechnetate.
2. Pentetate does not accumulate in the choroid plexus, making pretreatment with potassium perchlorate unnecessary.
3. The primary PET agent would be fluorine-18 (^{18}F)-labeled fluorodeoxyglucose (FDG), which concentrates in tumor cells within the brain more readily than surrounding brain tissue, if the tumor is viable through the phosphorylation process of the ^{18}F-FDG, and it will appear "hotter" and can be located with the addition of CT imaging. Thus the dual functional imaging and structural imaging of PET/CT allows for a better diagnosis, staging, and assessment of brain tumors overall as discussed later in the chapter.

Clinical Procedure

Patient Preparation

Patient preparation includes those steps common to all imaging procedures: verify the identity of the patient, confirm the written order for the procedure, and obtain medical information relevant to the patient's condition and to the clinical indications for the test. Potassium perchlorate (0.2–1.0 g) must be administered orally before performing brain imaging with ^{99m}Tc–pertechnetate.

Imaging

Traditional BBB imaging is almost exclusively performed using planar techniques. The scintillation camera is prepared with an appropriate collimator (e.g., low energy, all purpose, converging) and proper energy settings. Although exact protocols vary from institution to institution, BBB imaging is typically a three-phase study consisting of dynamic cerebral blood flow images, followed by static blood pool images and delayed static images performed 30 min to 3 hr after tracer administration. Additional delayed images may be necessary for those patients with poor blood clearance whose initial images suggest an abnormality.

An anterior flow study is routinely performed with the patient sitting in the upright position (if possible). The head is positioned with the forehead and nose touching the collimator. The top of the head should be below the top of the field of view. The anterior neck should also be included to visualize carotid blood flow. Failure to obtain a true anterior position could result in images that may be incorrectly interpreted as indicative of asymmetrical cerebral blood flow, when, in fact, the perceived difference is the result of inappropriate positioning of the head. It is also imperative that the head remain still during imaging. A strip of tape to secure the head to the collimator may be helpful. An intravenous bolus injection of 555–1110 megabecquerels (MBq) (15–30 mCi) of one of the aforementioned ^{99m}Tc-labeled agents is administered. Imaging begins as the tracer is being injected. The flow images are usually obtained at 1- to 3-sec intervals for a duration of 30–60 sec. In patients with suspected cerebellar pathology or in pediatric patients (in whom lesions in the posterior fossa seem to dominate) a posterior blood flow study may be desired. The physician should be consulted before positioning the patient.

Sixty-second blood pool images should be obtained within 5–10 min after completion of the flow study. Typically, both the blood pool and delayed views are obtained in the anterior, posterior, right and left lateral, and vertex positions. Most protocols stipulate that the anterior projection be acquired for 500,000–1,000,000 counts and all subsequent images acquired for that same time. The vertex projection should be obtained with a lead cape draped over the patient's shoulders to prevent interference from activity in the rest of the body. On lateral views, a lead shield can be used to reduce the counts arising from facial activity. It is important to obtain the immediate and delayed static images in the same projections if there is any suspicion of a lesion or other abnormality on the initial images.

Image Findings

Knowledge of the gross anatomy of the brain and the cerebral circulatory system is important to understanding tracer distribution patterns (Fig. 10.1).

Normal Tracer Distribution

Approximately 6 sec after tracer administration, there is symmetric distribution of the radiopharmaceutical in the right and left carotid arteries and visualization of the anterior cerebral artery. Visualization of the superior sagittal sinus after 15 sec indicates that arterial blood has begun to flow into the venous system (Fig. 10.2).

Normal delayed static images usually show symmetric activity around the entire skull border. Increased activity is observed around the face and base of the skull as well as in the sagittal, transverse, and sigmoid sinuses as a result of blood pool activity in these areas.

Abnormal Tracer Distribution

Any disruption of the BBB from a lesion in the brain will result in increased localization of the radiopharmaceutical in the area of the pathology (Fig. 10.3). In the case of brain death, the flow study will demonstrate tracer distribution in the carotids and a complete absence of perfusion in the middle and anterior cerebral arteries (Fig. 10.4).

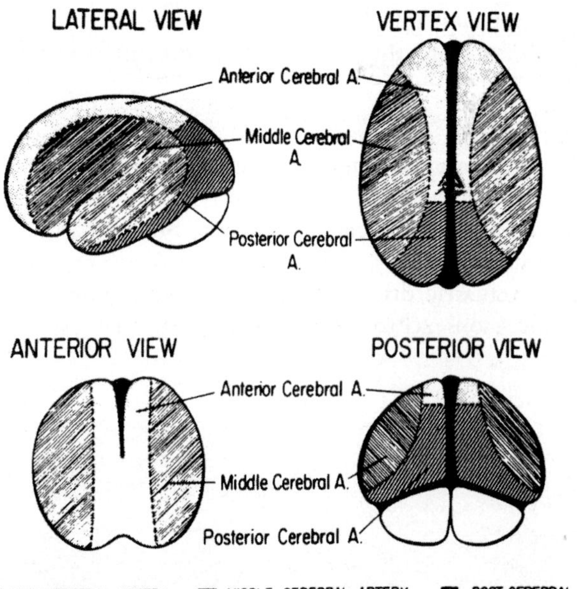

Figure 10.1 Regional cortical distribution of the cerebral arteries. (Reprinted, with permission, from Freeman and Johnson, 1972, p. 295.)

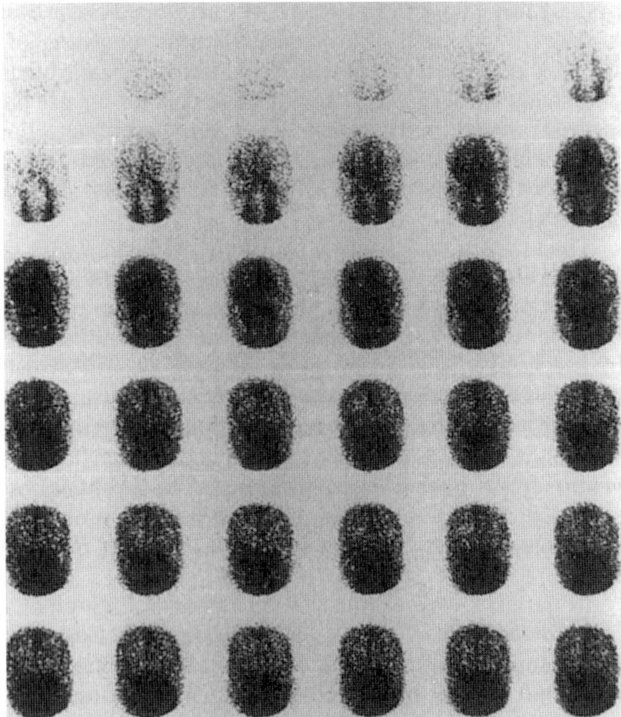

Figure 10.2 Normal anterior cerebral blood flow study. (Courtesy of the Hospital of the University of Pennsylvania, Philadelphia, PA.)

Brain Perfusion Imaging

Brain perfusion imaging has proven to be a very useful method for evaluating functional abnormalities in brain tissue. Brain perfusion imaging is clinically indicated when the following abnormalities are suspected:

1. cerebrovascular disease: acute stroke, transient ischemic attacks
2. dementia: Alzheimer's disease, multi-infarct dementia
3. psychiatric disorders: affective disorders (e.g., depression), schizophrenia
4. seizure disorders: identification and location of sites of focal epilepsy
5. head trauma (e.g., cerebral brain death).

Brain perfusion imaging is generally performed using SPECT, with the exception of brain death studies, which routinely use planar imaging protocols.

Radiopharmaceuticals

The two primary radiopharmaceuticals used for brain perfusion imaging are ^{99m}Tc–exametazime (HMPAO) and ^{99m}Tc–bicisate (ECD). Both tracers are lipid soluble and can, therefore, cross the BBB. Although the exact mechanism is not known, the solubility of each agent changes once inside the cell, making it difficult for the tracer to diffuse back into the circulation. Thus, the agent becomes "fixed" within the brain cells. Tracer uptake is believed to be proportional to cerebral blood flow. Imaging may take place up to 6 hr after tracer injection. The typical adult dosages for the ^{99m}Tc-labeled tracers are 370–740 MBq (10–20 mCi). Use fresh generator eluate (<2 hr old) for optimal results with ^{99m}Tc–HMPAO. Do not use pertechnetate obtained from a generator that has not been eluted for 24 hr or more.

Clinical Procedure: SPECT

Patient Preparation

Explain the entire procedure to the patient. If possible, it is best to place the patient supine in a quiet, dimly lit room for radiopharmaceutical administration. A butterfly needle should be placed into an antecubital vein of either arm. After 5–10 min, the tracer may be administered through the butterfly, followed by a saline flush. Following removal of the butterfly, the patient should remain quiet and unstimulated for at least 10–15 min to allow the tracer to localize in the brain. Because of its rapid blood clearance, ^{99m}Tc–bicisate imaging may begin 15–20 min (45 min may be preferred) after administration. When using ^{99m}Tc–exametazime, imaging should start

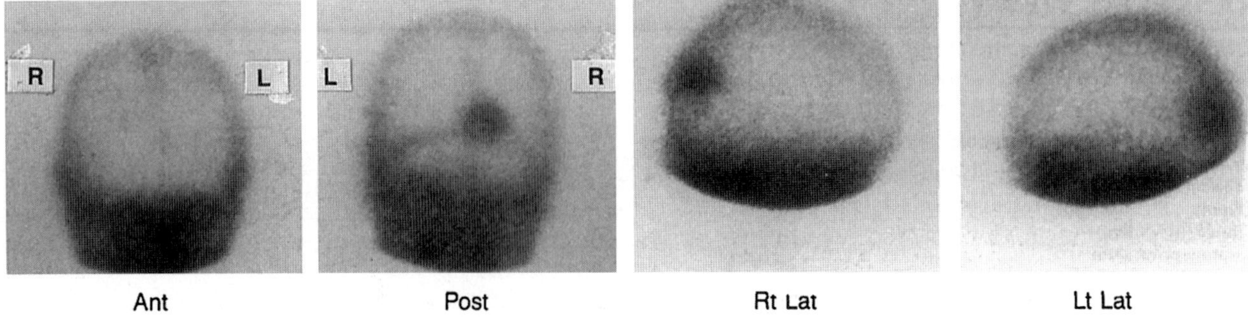

Figure 10.3 Abnormal static brain image depicts a primary brain tumor in the midoccipital region. (Reprinted with permission from the Hospital of the University of Pennsylvania, Philadelphia, PA.)

no earlier than 1 hr (90 min may be preferred) after injection to ensure an acceptable target-to-background ratio. Imaging may be delayed for several hours with either agent, because they undergo little, if any, redistribution. As long as the minimum waiting period has been met, imaging may begin at the time that is most suitable for the patient and the department.

Imaging

A triple-head tomographic camera system with ultrahigh-resolution collimators is the best instrument to use for brain imaging; however, single- and dual-head cameras may also be used. The patient should be resting as comfortably as possible with the head secured to minimize movement. The detectors should be placed as close as possible to the patient's head, which should be positioned far enough into the detector array to image the entire cerebellum.

Image acquisition typically takes 20–40 min, depending on how well the technologist thinks the patient can tolerate the procedure. To begin imaging, position the detector perpendicular to the floor at the side of the head, as if acquiring a lateral view. Adjust the camera to rotate under the patient's head first, before the camera begins to come over the patient's face. This allows 180° of data to be acquired even in those cases where imaging must be stopped because the patient becomes agitated or panics when the camera rotates over the face. Typical acquisition parameters are 64 views, 40 sec per view, for a 360° rotation.

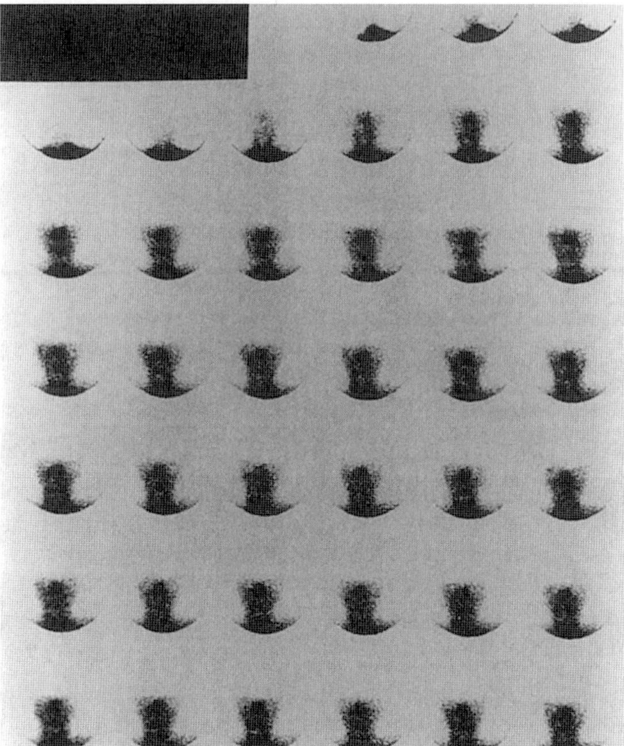

Figure 10.4 Anterior cerebral blood flow study demonstrates brain death. Note the absence of activity over cerebral hemispheres. (Reprinted with permission from the Hospital of the University of Pennsylvania, Philadelphia, PA.)

Image Findings

After the projection images are acquired, computer-reconstructed images in the transaxial, sagittal, and coronal planes are obtained. Knowledge of cross-sectional anatomy is necessary to process the data and present the necessary information to the physician for interpretation (Fig. 10.5).

Normal Tracer Distribution

Distribution of the tracer is usually symmetric in both cerebral hemispheres. Because blood flow to gray matter structures is much greater than to white matter, some structures (such as the basal ganglia and the thalamus) will show greater intensity as a result of increased tracer uptake. White matter typically presents as an area of decreased or no uptake (Fig. 10.6).

Abnormal Tracer Patterns

The site of acute cerebral infarct is usually observed as a photopenic defect (absence of tracer uptake in that area) and is directly related to the cerebral artery affected by the stroke (Fig. 10.7).

Alzheimer's disease findings are usually consistent with decreased perfusion in the parietal, temporal, and frontal lobes of both hemispheres. This contrasts with multi-infarct dementia, which usually shows random areas of decreased or absent uptake as a result of multiple areas of infarction.

Patients diagnosed with schizophrenia typically show areas of decreased perfusion in the frontal lobes. Other significant findings include increased activity in the area of the basal ganglia and temporal lobes. In general, clinically depressed patients tend to show decreased tracer uptake over the entire cerebral cortex, whereas manic patients seem to have greatly increased perfusion overall. During active seizure activity, an area of intense focal uptake of the radiopharmaceutical can be observed.

Pharmacologic Intervention

Acetazolamide (Diamox) stimulation is used in patients with transient ischemic attacks, carotid artery disease, cerebrovascular disease, and other conditions, such as Alzheimer's disease, in which cerebral perfusion is decreased. This test may be used to identify ischemic areas in the brain in much the same way dipyridamole is used to demonstrate the same condition in the heart. Acetazolamide is a drug that induces cerebral vasodilatation.

TRANSAXIAL VIEWS

1. Falx cerebri
2. Body of corpus callosum
3. Putamen
4. Hippocampus
5. Glomus in trigone of lateral ventricle
6. Superior vermis of cerebellum
7. Thalamus
8. Fornix
9. Insula (Isle of Reil)
10. Septum pellucidum

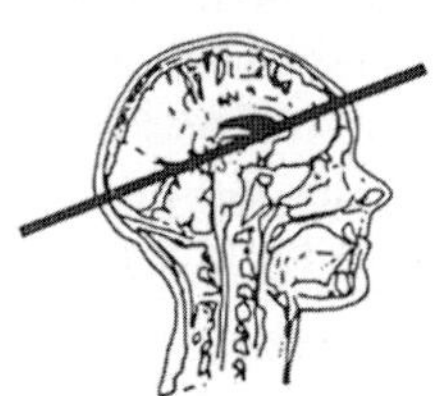

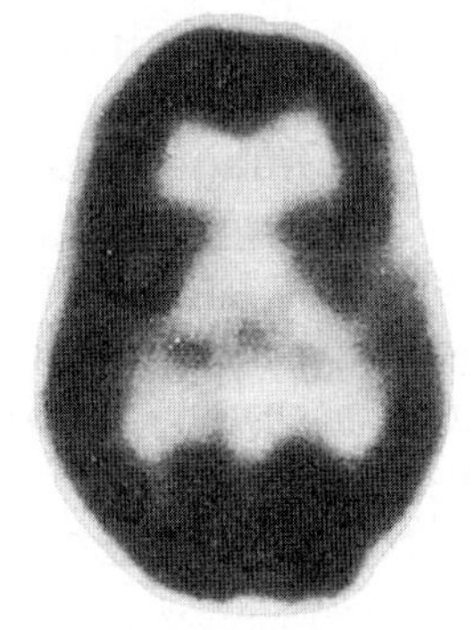

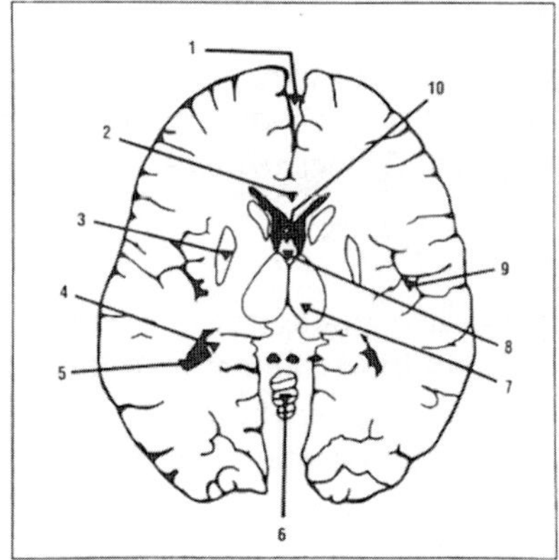

CORONAL VIEWS

1. Caudate nucleus
2. Putamen
3. Temporal lobe of cerebrum
4. Lateral (Sylvian) fissure
5. Genu of corpus callosum

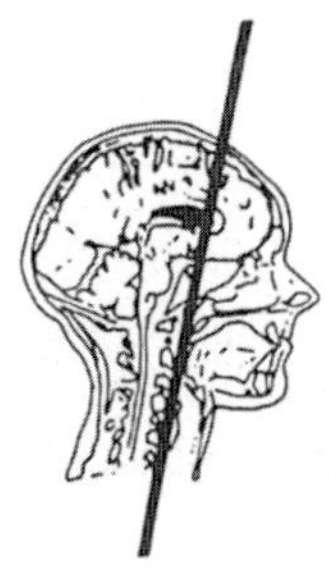

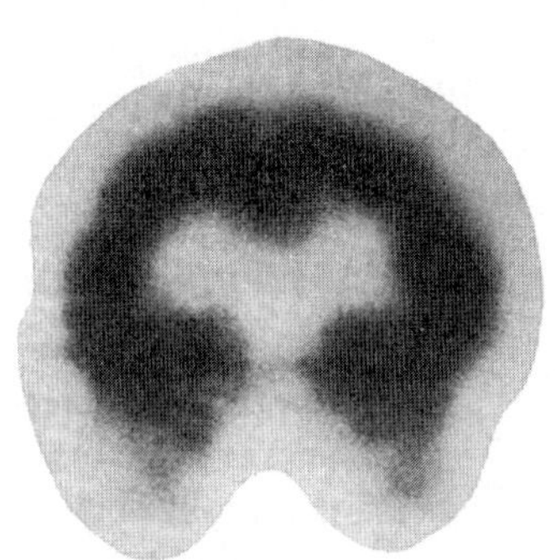

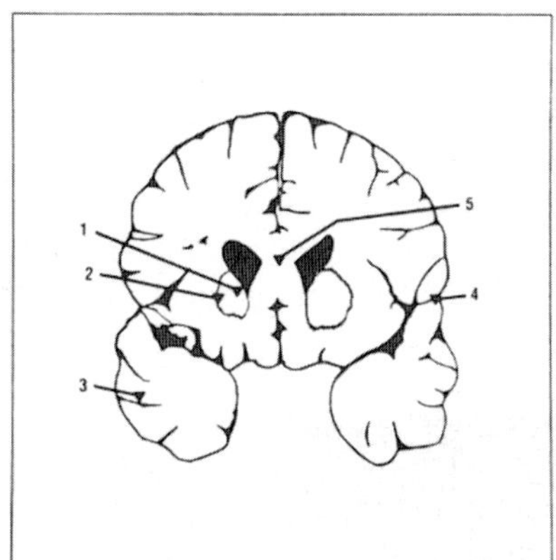

SAGITTAL VIEWS

1. Precentral gyrus
2. Posterior limb of internal capsule
3. Lenticular nucleus
4. Uncinate-fasciculus (frontotemporal)
5. Amygdala
6. Hippocampus
7. Tentorium cerebelli
8. Visual radiations (temporal)
9. Visual radiations (parietal)
10. Central sulcus (of Rolando)

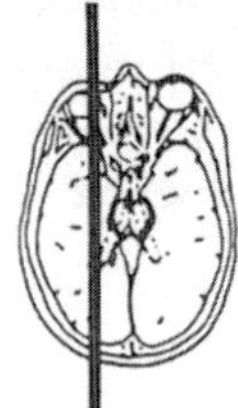

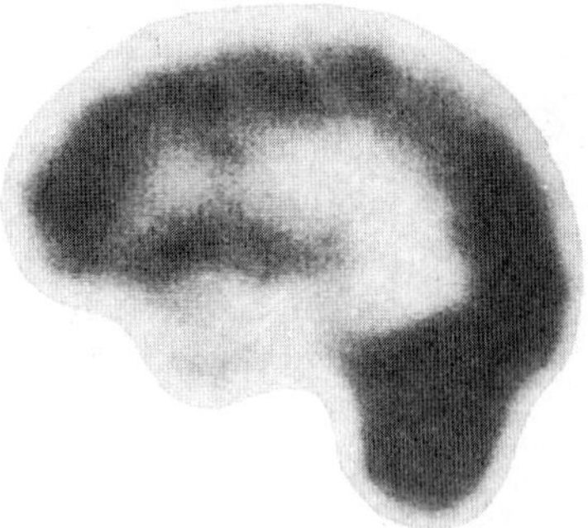

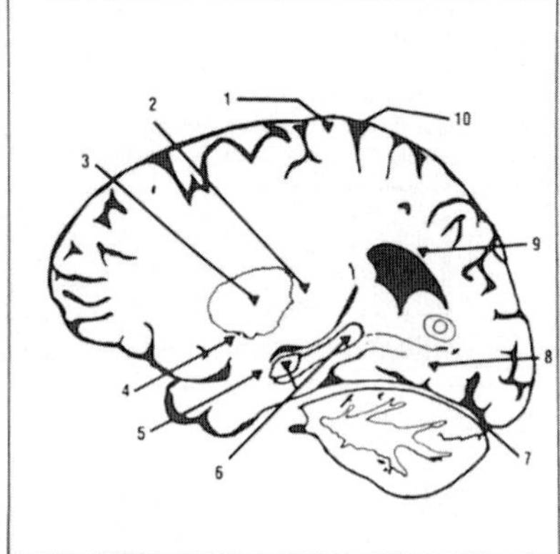

Figure 10.5 Representative anatomical cross-sections of the brain. (Reprinted, with permission, from Karesh *et al.,* 1989. Images courtesy of Nuclear Medicine Services, Harry S. Truman Memorial Veterans Hospital and the University of Missouri Hospitals and Clinics, Columbia, MO.)

1. Genu of corpus callosum
2. Lateral fissure (of Sylvius)
3. Lenticular nucleus
4. Cerebral peduncle
5. Parahippocampal gyrus
6. Cerebellar hemisphere
7. Superior cerebellar vermis
8. Red nucleus
9. Subthalamic nucleus
10. Head of caudate nucleus

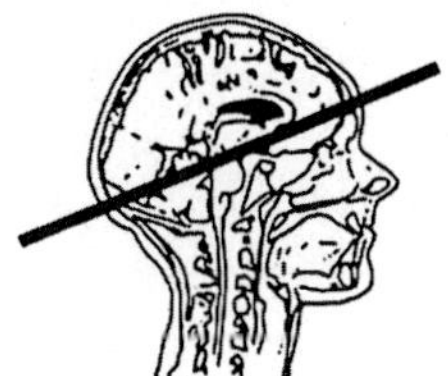

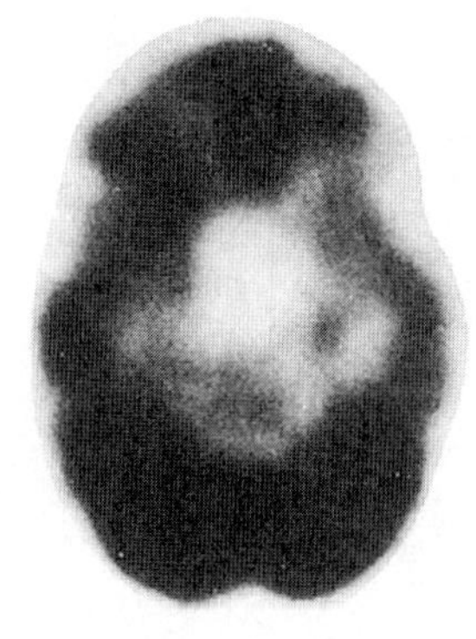

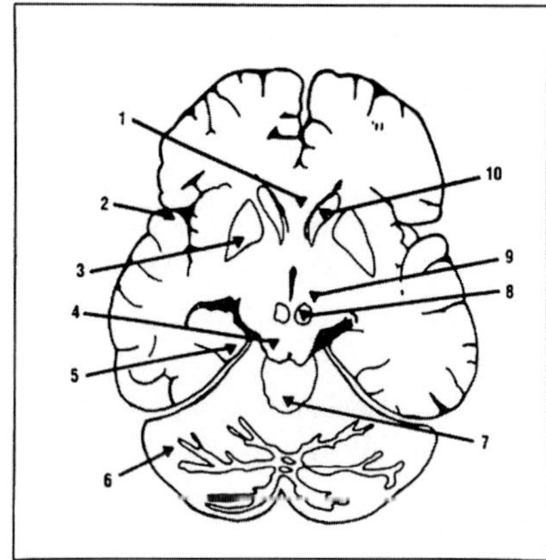

1. Corpus callosum
2. Caudate nucleus
3. Internal capsule
4. Thalamus
5. Lenticular ventricle
6. Hippocampus
7. Substantia nigra
8. Cerebral peduncle
9. Pons
10. Third ventricle
11. Fornix
12. Cingulate gyrus
13. Falx cerebri
14. Superior sagittal sinus

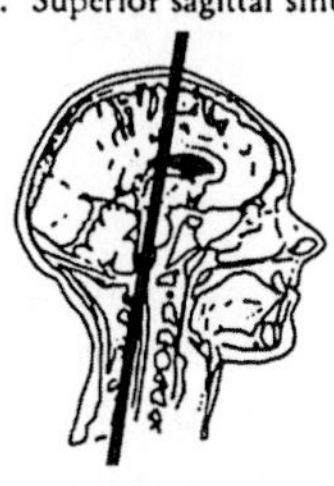

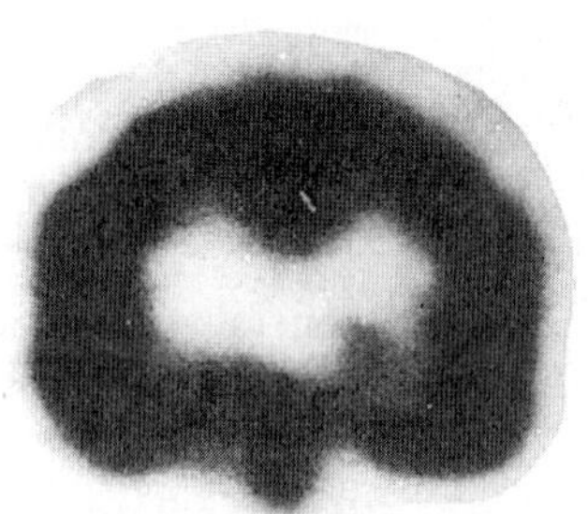

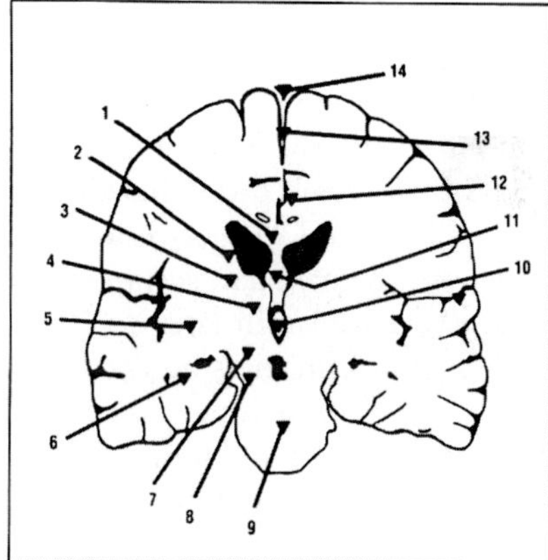

1. Genu of corpus callosum
2. Caudate nucleus
3. Hypothalamus
4. Red nucleus
5. Tectum of mesencephalon
6. Tegmentum of pons
7. Parieto-occipital fissure
8. Paracentral lobule

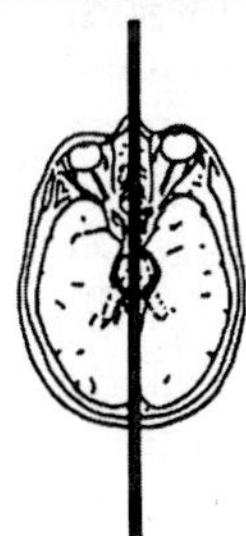

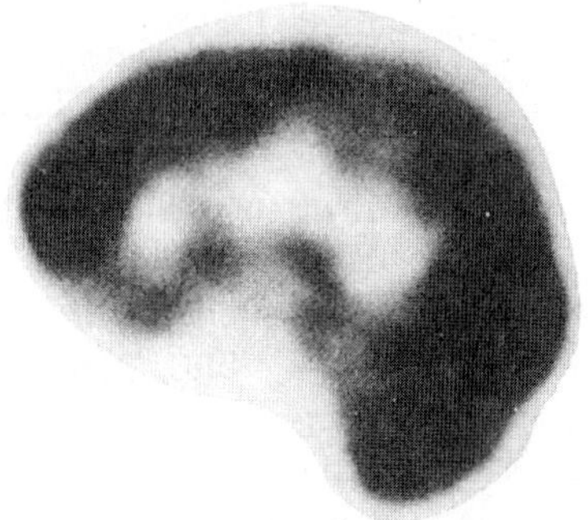

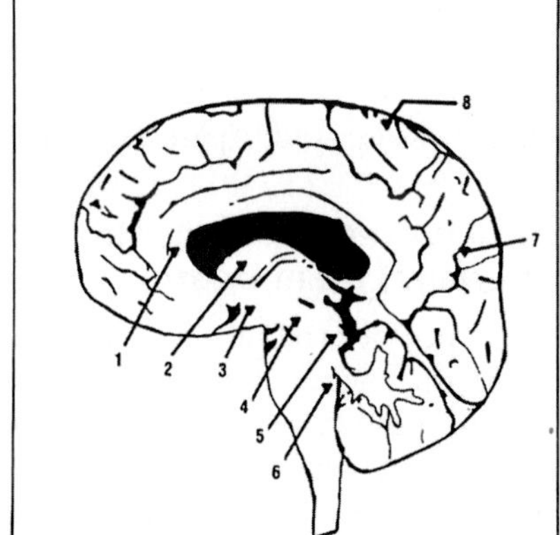

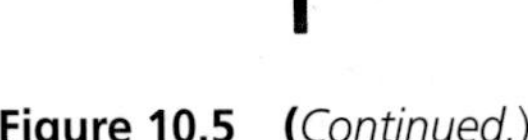

Figure 10.5 (*Continued.*)

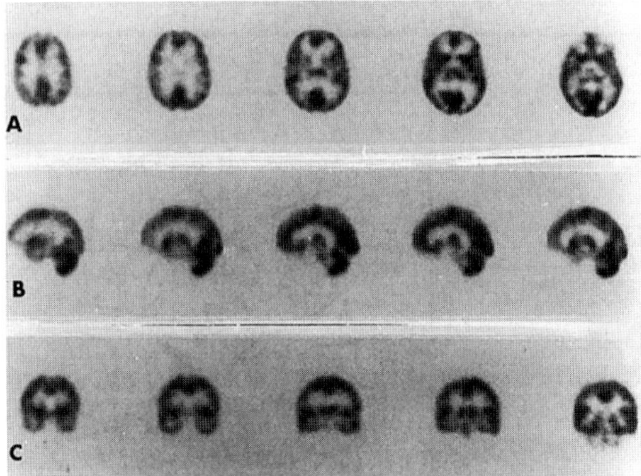

Figure 10.6 Representative transaxial (A), sagittal (B), and coronal (C) slices of a normal brain SPECT study. (Reprinted with permission from the Hospital of the University of Pennsylvania, Philadelphia, PA.)

After oral or intravenous administration of this drug, normal blood vessels dilate, but diseased ones do not.

A baseline brain image without acetazolamide is obtained first. The next day, acetazolamide (1 g) is administered, followed 25 min later by ^{99m}Tc–exametazime or ^{99m}Tc–bicisate. Imaging begins 15 min after tracer administration. The baseline and acetazolamide images are compared. Areas of induced ischemia are visualized as areas of decreased tracer uptake on the acetazolamide images.

Side effects of acetazolamide include flushing, tingling sensations in the extremities and around the mouth, lightheadedness, blurred vision, headache, mild confusion, nausea, and urinary urgency. These effects are usually mild, subsiding within 10–15 min. Administering the drug slowly over a period of 2 min can minimize these effects. Contraindications for acetazolamide administration include allergy to sulfa drugs, increased cerebral pressure, and hepatic cirrhosis.

Clinical Procedure: Planar Imaging for Cerebral Brain Death

The absence of cerebral blood flow is an indication of brain death. The accurate diagnosis of brain death is essential in cases where the discontinuation of life support or organ harvesting for transplantation is being considered. Because the immediate localization of the perfusion brain agents to the cerebral and cerebellar tissue provides an index of blood perfusion, many institutions have established perfusion agent protocols for assessing brain death. Recent research suggests that this technique is generally more accurate than radionuclide cerebral angiography using BBB agents.

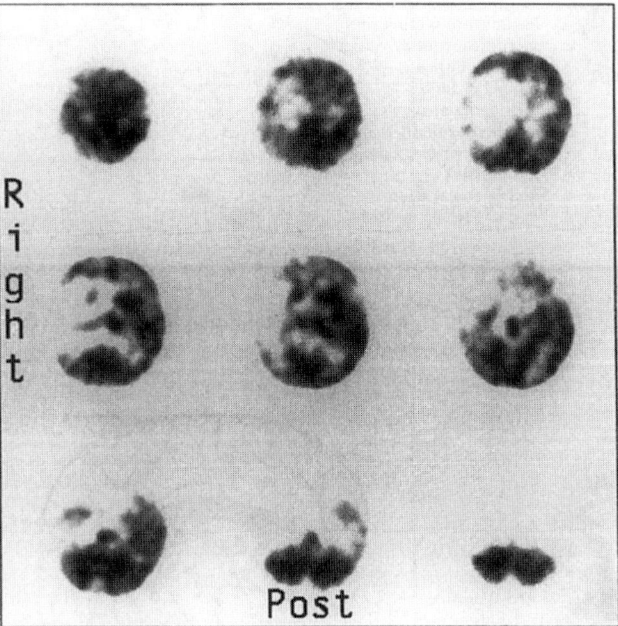

Figure 10.7 HMPAO images of a patient with a history of stroke show significantly reduced blood flow distribution of the middle cerebral artery on the right side. (Reprinted, with permission, from Alavi and Hirsch, 1991.)

Patient Preparation

Because these patients are comatose, consent for the study must be obtained from a surrogate decision maker. A flow study usually is not necessary, so the ^{99m}Tc-labeled agent can be administered in the patient's hospital room.

Imaging

Static planar images are typically obtained in the anterior and lateral views 1–3 hr after injection of ^{99m}Tc–exametazime. (If ^{99m}Tc–bicisate is used, imaging may begin sooner.) A converging collimator or an acquisition zoom is often used when imaging pediatric patients. As with BBB planar imaging, the acquisition is collected for counts on the initial anterior image and then for the same time for any additional images. Imaging rarely takes more than 30 min. Anterior and laterals views are typically all that are needed, but protocols vary from institution to institution.

The condition of patients undergoing a brain death study can change rapidly. Often studies are repeated 1 or 2 days after a negative study was obtained only to find that the patient no longer has cerebral blood flow.

Image Findings

Normal Tracer Distribution

The images should show intense symmetric tracer uptake throughout both cerebral hemispheres and the cerebellum. Unlike SPECT imaging, the planar brain images are unlikely to show much brain detail (Fig. 10.8). If greater detail of specific areas is desired, the patient should be reimaged using SPECT.

Abnormal Tracer Patterns

The total absence of tracer uptake in the brain suggests that the patient is brain dead (Fig. 10.9). Any uptake at all is a negative indication for brain death. It should be noted that a negative study does not necessarily imply normal brain perfusion. Perfusion defects that imply that cerebral blood flow is compromised in specific areas may be seen. The research suggests that the more severe the defects, the greater the probability that the patient eventually will become brain dead.

PET Brain Imaging

PET has a number of advantages over routine nuclear medicine imaging procedures. PET instrumentation routinely provides greater spatial and temporal resolution than can be obtained using Anger scintillation systems. Attenuation is less problematic with PET because of the higher-energy photon emissions (511 keV) of positron-emitting radiotracers. In addition, the uncollimated PET system provides improved sensitivity, which in turn allows easier use of extrinsic sources for attenuation correction. With the introduction of PET/CT systems, where precise CT information serves as the transmission data for attenuation correction, coregistration of both physiologic and anatomic information can be used to accurately define a lesion's position in three-dimensional space. The advantages in resolution and attenuation correction provide increased reliability in the quantitative data obtained using PET.

A possible disadvantage with PET is tracer availability. The short physical half-lives of positron emitters necessitate either an on-site cyclotron, which requires a significant financial investment for construction and maintenance, or close proximity to a regional PET radiopharmaceutical distributor. Another limitation of PET is the inherent variability in spatial resolution, related to the energy of the positron emission. Higher-energy positrons travel farther in tissue before annihilation than lower-energy positrons. The greater the distance between the point of annihilation and the true site of the initial decay event, the greater the drop in image resolution. A PET system's inability to perform simultaneous imaging of two different PET tracers (because of the identical photon energies involved) also can be seen as a disadvantage. Imaging of a second PET tracer is not advised until the near-complete decay of the first. However, because of the short half-lives, rapid sequential studies can be acquired.

PET brain imaging is being used in a variety of situations. The most common indications for PET brain imaging include but are not limited to the evaluation of primary brain tumors, epilepsy, and dementia.

Radiopharmaceutical

^{18}F-FDG is the most widely used tracer for PET brain imaging. FDG is a glucose analog with uptake that is dependent on blood flow and is actively transported into viable cells and irreversibly trapped. It can be used to accurately estimate the rate of use of exogenous glucose (under steady-state serum glucose conditions). At 30–40 min after the intravenous administration of ^{18}F-FDG, acquired images are indicative of the glucose metabolism that has occurred over that time period.

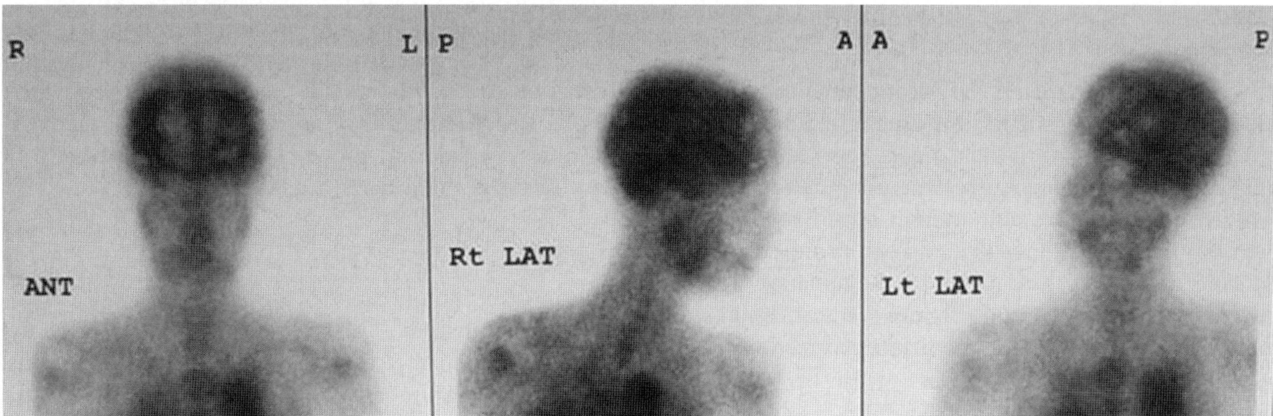

Figure 10.8 Planar brain images demonstrating viable brain tissue evidenced by significant tracer uptake in the cerebral cortex. (Reprinted with permission from the University of Iowa Hospitals and Clinics, Iowa City, IA.)

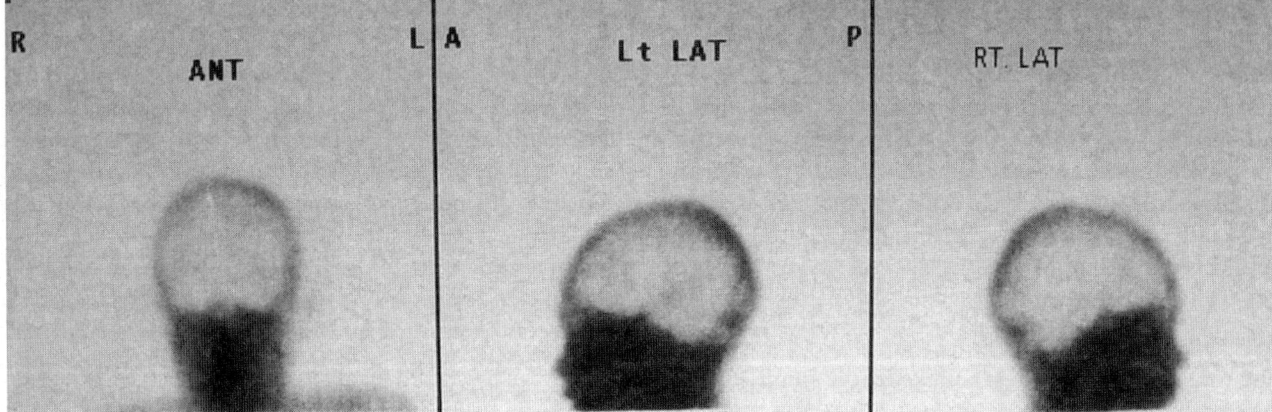

Figure 10.9 Planar brain images demonstrating brain death evidenced by absence of tracer uptake in the cerebral cortex. (Reprinted with permission from the University of Iowa Hospitals and Clinics, Iowa City, IA.)

Clinical Procedure

Patient Preparation

The patient must fast for a minimum of 4 hr before the injection of ^{18}F-FDG to prevent hyperglycemia. If ^{18}F-FDG is administered during hyperglycemia, relatively poor brain uptake results. Because it is so critical that the patient have a stable blood glucose level (especially for quantification accuracy), many centers recommend a much longer period of fasting. If hyperglycemia is suspected, the patient's blood sugar levels should be checked. If the glucose level is greater than 200 mg/dL, small amounts of insulin may be given intravenously to lower the blood glucose level. If insulin is given, the blood levels should be rechecked and reevaluated. (If glucose levels remain high, the patient may be rescheduled.) The tracer should be injected through an intravenous line while the patient is lying in a quiet, dimly lit room. The patient should remain still for the 40-min uptake period but should not go to sleep during that time. The dosage of ^{18}F-FDG typically used for brain imaging is 370–740 MBq (10–20 mCi).

Imaging

Exact imaging parameters vary from system to system. An emission scan of the head is usually acquired for approximately 30 min with the patient in a supine position, but acquisition time may vary depending on the injected activity, organ uptake, and scanner sensitivity. The patient should be encouraged to void before and as often as possible after the scan to minimize the radiation dose to the bladder and surrounding organs. A transmission scan should also be acquired for attenuation correction.

Normal Image Findings

Tracer uptake in gray matter normally is demonstrated in a pattern not unlike that of SPECT brain perfusion agents. Active brain tissue typically will demonstrate relatively intense tracer uptake, whereas inactive tissue will show lesser degrees of uptake (Fig. 10.10).

Abnormal Image Findings

Primary Brain Tumors

Research suggests a positive correlation between ^{18}F-FDG uptake on PET scans and tumor or grade of malignancy. Although ^{18}F-FDG is not a specific tumor marker, a high-grade tumor typically will demonstrate intense ^{18}F-FDG uptake, whereas cell necrosis will show no uptake (Fig. 10.11).

Epilepsy

For patients who have epilepsy and whose seizures cannot be controlled by medication, surgery is often considered. PET has proven to be effective in locating the seizure focus in the brains of many of these patients. The PET scans of patients who are injected with ^{18}F-FDG while in the interictal phase routinely show significant reduction of tracer uptake in the area of the seizure focus (Fig. 10.12). The scans of persons who are injected during the ictal (seizing) phase typically demonstrate focal "hot" areas at the seizure focus (Fig. 10.13).

Dementia

The most common cause of dementia in the elderly is Alzheimer's disease. The accurate classification of this disease can help the clinician determine the best course of patient management. PET imaging with ^{18}F-FDG has demonstrated a pattern unique for Alzheimer's. Images of patients with Alzheimer's disease typically show de-

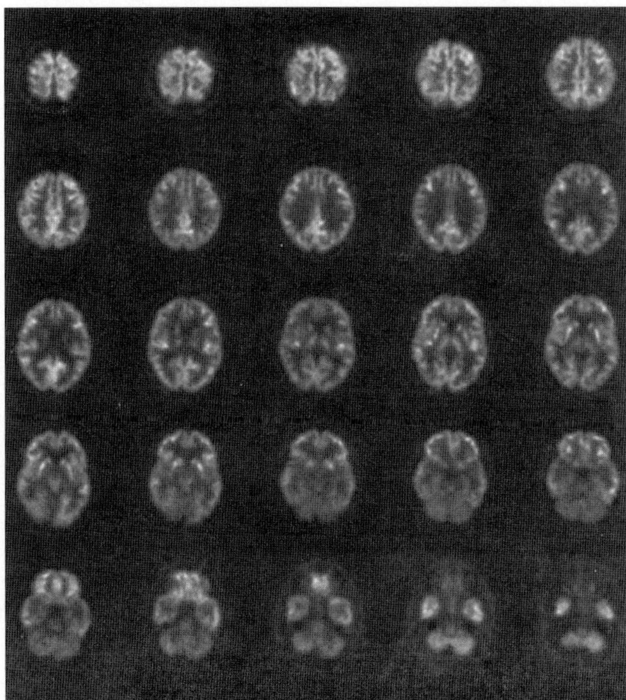

Figure 10.10 Normal ^{18}F-FDG transaxial images. (Reprinted, with permission, from Perlman and Stone, 1998, p. 337.)

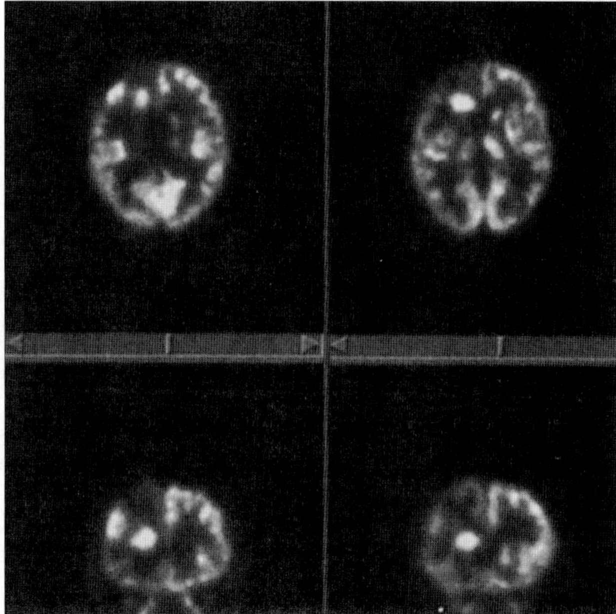

Figure 10.11 ^{18}F-FDG scan (transaxial slices above, coronal slices below) of a patient with glioblastoma multiforme as demonstrated by increased uptake centrally and peripherally. Adjacent areas of decreased uptake are secondary to prior surgery and radiation therapy. (Reprinted, with permission, from Perlman and Stone, 1998, p. 339.)

creased uptake in the parietal, temporal, and frontal cortex, but the sensorimotor and visual regions appear essentially normal (Fig. 10.14). Non-Alzheimer's-type dementias will show considerably different uptake patterns. For example, with Pick's disease (frontotemporal dementia), decreased uptake is typically seen in the frontal lobes only. With Creutzfeldt–Jakob disease (human equivalent of bovine spongiform encephalopathy or "mad cow disease"), PET images demonstrate generalized poor uptake of ^{18}F-FDG throughout the brain.

Cisternography

CSF imaging or cisternography is performed to evaluate the flow of CSF through its normal pathways. CSF circulates around the brain and spinal cord and acts as a shock absorber for the central nervous system. It is produced in the choroid plexus in the ventricles of the brain. The lateral ventricles, located in the cerebrum, connect with the third ventricle, which is located near the thalamus. The third ventricle is connected to the fourth, which lies between the brain stem and the cerebellum. The fourth ventricle empties CSF into the subarachnoid space, where it flows around the spinal cord and brain. CSF is absorbed from the subarachnoid space into the venous circulation (Fig. 10.15). Total CSF volume is 125–140 mL. Under normal conditions, CSF is formed at the same rate as absorption.

Clinical indications for CSF imaging include diagnosis of normal pressure hydrocephalus, detection of CSF leaks, and evaluation of ventricular shunt patency. Cisternography is performed by administering indium-111 (^{111}In)–pentetate intrathecally into the subarachnoid space between the third and fourth lumbar vertebrae. ^{111}In has two major γ emissions, 173 and 247 keV, and a physical half-life of 2.8 days. After introduction of the tracer into the subarachnoid space, the tracer follows the normal pathway of the CSF until it is reabsorbed into the blood from the CSF and is excreted by the kidneys. The major advantage of using ^{111}In for CSF imaging is that its relatively long half-life permits delayed imaging up to 72 hr or longer, if necessary.

Clinical Procedure

Patient Preparation

The radiopharmaceutical is introduced into the subarachnoid space of the spine by lumbar puncture, an invasive procedure that is always performed by a physician. The patient should remain supine for several hours after the lumbar puncture to prevent headache or other side effects resulting from temporary CSF imbalance. If a CSF leak is suspected, cotton swabs should be placed in the nose to rule out rhinorrhea or in the ears to rule out otorrhea. The swabs should be removed approximately

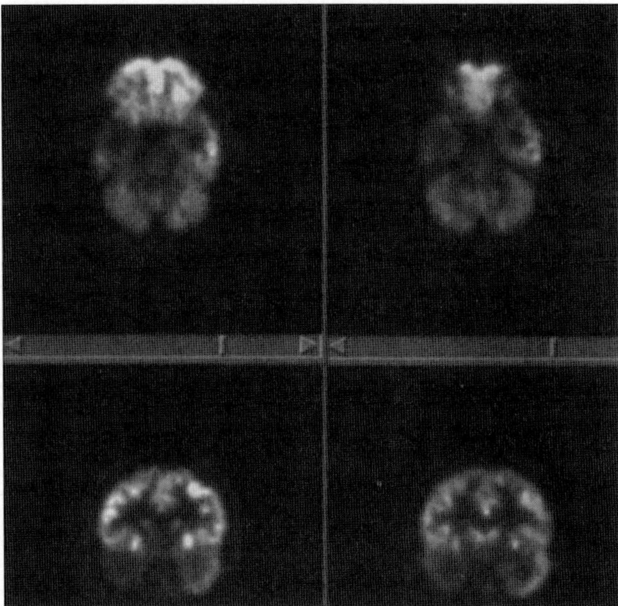

Figure 10.12 ^{18}F-FDG scan (transaxial slices above, coronal slices below) of an epileptic patient being considered for resection of the seizure focus. Since the patient was injected while in the interictal state, the severe reduction of FDG uptake in the right temporal lobe is consistent with a seizure focus in that area. (Reprinted, with permission, from Perlman and Stone, 1998, p. 340.)

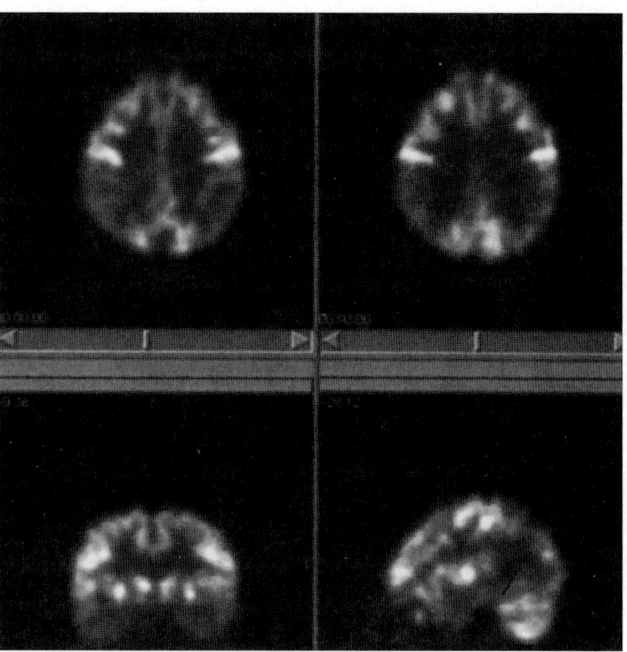

Figure 10.14 ^{18}F-FDG scan (transaxial slices above, coronal slices below) of an elderly patient presenting with dementia. The transaxial, coronal, and sagittal images show reduced FDG uptake in both parietal and temporal cerebral cortices. This distribution pattern is typical for Alzheimer's disease. (Reprinted, with permission, from Perlman and Stone, 1998, p. 341.)

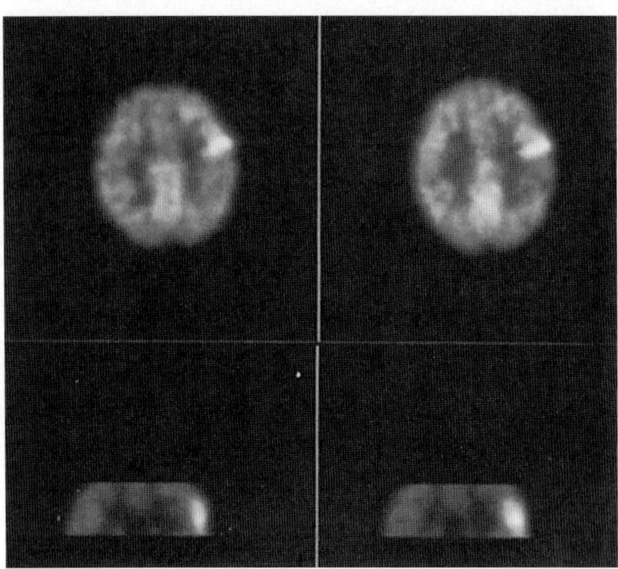

Figure 10.13 ^{18}F-FDG scan (transaxial slices above, coronal slices below) of a patient having seizures secondary to Rasmussen encephalitis. FDG was injected during a seizure episode. The images identify a hypermetabolic seizure focus in the left parietal region. (Reprinted, with permission, from Perlman and Stone, 1998, p. 340.)

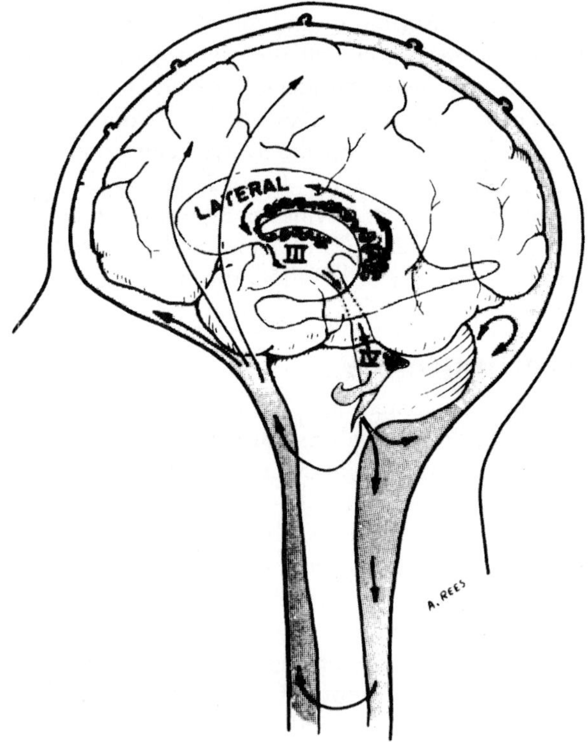

Figure 10.15 Normal cerebrospinal fluid blood flow. (Reprinted, with permission, from Freeman and Johnson, 1975, p. 251.)

every 2 hr after tracer administration and counted in a well counter to detect any CSF leaks.

Imaging

Adjust the energy settings on the scintillation camera for ^{111}In. Use a medium-energy collimator matched to the higher-energy emissions of ^{111}In. Obtain images of the head to include the anterior, posterior, and lateral projections at 4–6 hr after tracer administration. Activity should be seen in the spinal cord ascending into the basal cisterns of the brain. If no activity is observed in the basal cisterns, it may mean that extravasation of the radiopharmaceutical has occurred at the site of the lumbar puncture. Imaging the injection site first can help rule out tracer extravasation. Activity in the kidneys also confirms extravasation into the surrounding soft tissue, which may be cause for terminating the examination.

If introduction of the tracer is successful, acquire additional images at 24, 48, and, if needed, 72 hr after tracer administration. Be certain to include the entire skull and as much of the spinal tract as possible in the field of view.

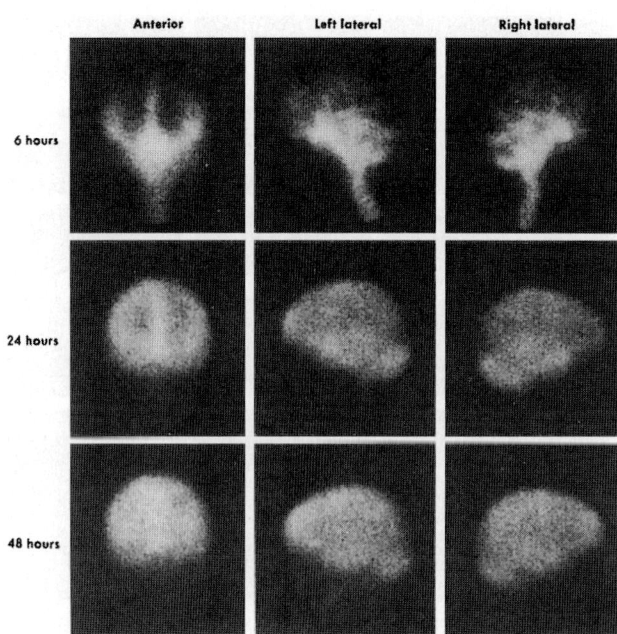

Figure 10.16 Normal cisternogram showing anterior and both lateral views at 6, 24, and 48 hr after intrathecal administration. (Reprinted, with permission, from Bernier *et al.*, 1989, p. 293.)

Normal Image Findings

At 4–6 hr, the radiopharmaceutical should have completed its ascent. At 24 hr, activity should be seen in the subarachnoid spaces surrounding the cerebral hemispheres as well as in the interhemispheric cisterns. Also at this time, the tracer should be visualized in the superior sagittal region, the site at which reabsorption of CSF occurs. Failure of the tracer to complete its ascent by 24 hr indicates the need for delayed images at 48 and possibly 72 hr. Tracer clearance from the basal cisterns also should be observed at 24 hr (Fig. 10.16).

Abnormal Image Findings

Normal Pressure Hydrocephalus

Normal pressure hydrocephalus (NPH) is a type of hydrocephalus that occurs in adults, usually older adults (average age >60 years old). NPH is different than other types of hydrocephalus in that it develops slowly over time and would therefore be considered a chronic disease. The drainage of CSF is blocked gradually, and the excess fluid builds up slowly over time. The slow enlargement of the ventricles means that the fluid pressure in the brain may not be as high as in other types of hydrocephalus. However, the enlarged ventricles still press on the brain and can cause the same symptoms. Visualization of the lateral ventricles at any point in the study, especially if it persists, is a typical finding in cases of normal pressure hydrocephalus. This finding, in conjunction with abnormal delay of the tracer in reaching the superior sagittal region, is cause for concern (Fig. 10.17).

CSF Leaks

Cotton swabs can be used to measure abnormal activity in the nose or the ears, which is indicative of a leak. In addition, imaging the site of the suspected leak while the radiopharmaceutical is passing through the suspected area (1–3 hr after injection) may be helpful in localizing the CSF leak. CSF leaks may be intermittent; therefore, negative findings by either cotton swab counting or imaging do not necessarily rule out a leak.

Evaluation of Ventricular Shunts

In many cases, ventricular shunting of the CSF into the circulatory system or abdominal cavity is used to treat cases of normal pressure hydrocephalus. Injection of ^{111}In–pentetate or ^{99m}Tc–pertechnetate directly into the shunt reservoir will clearly demonstrate shunt patency. Persistent radiopharmaceutical uptake in the shunt can indicate partial or complete obstruction of the shunt.

References and Further Reading

Alavi A, Hirsch L, 1991. Studies of central nervous system disorders with single-photon emission computed tomography

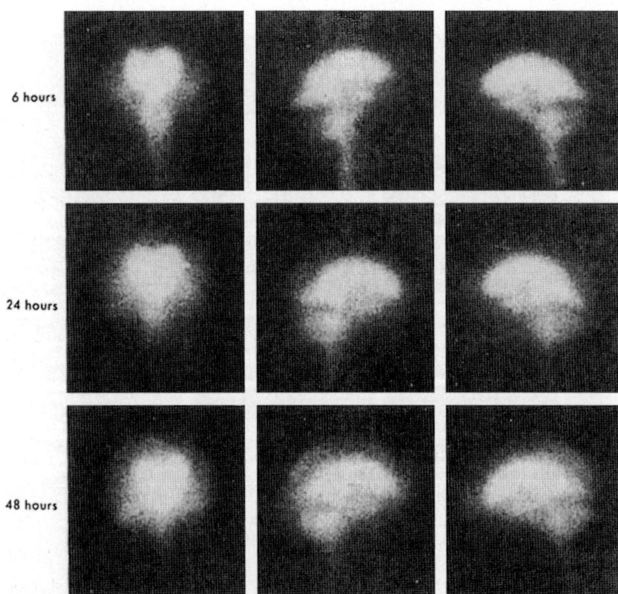

Figure 10.17 Communicating hydrocephalus (normal hydrocephalus) with lateral ventricular reflux on 6-hr images and no significant ventricular clearing on the 24- and 48-hr images. (Reprinted, with permission, from Bernier *et al.*, 1989, p. 294.)

and positron emission tomography: evolution over the past two decades. *Semin Nucl Med.* 21:67.

Bernier DR, Christian PE, Langan JK, Wells LD, eds., 1989. *Nuclear Medicine Technology and Techniques.* 2nd ed. St. Louis, MO: Mosby.

Carter JC, Burt RW, 1992. Acetazolamide intervention for technetium99m-HMPAO SPECT brain imaging. *J Nucl Med Technol.* 20:131–133.

Freeman LM, Johnson PM, eds., 1975. *Clinical Scintillation Imaging.* 2nd ed. New York, NY: Grune and Stratton.

Harkness B, 1992. Computer applications in brain imaging. In: Rowell K, ed. *Clinical Computers in Nuclear Medicine.* Reston, VA: Society of Nuclear Medicine; 51–59.

Holman BL, ed., 1985. *Radionuclide Imaging of the Brain.* New York, NY: Churchill Livingstone.

Holmes RA, Hoffman KA, 1995. Central nervous system. In: Early PJ, Sodee DB. *Principles and Practice of Nuclear Medicine.* 2nd ed. St. Louis, MO: Mosby; 549–578.

Juni JE, Waxman AD, Devous MD, Tikofsky RS, Ichise M, Heertum RV, Carretta RF, Chen CC, 2009. *SNM Procedure Guideline: Procedure Guideline for Brain Perfusion SPECT Using 99mTc Radiopharmaceuticals 3.0.* Reston, VA: Society of Nuclear Medicine.

Karesh SM, Ashburn WL, Dilon WA, Carretta RF, Holmes RA, Hoffman TJ, Valle G, Fuentes R, Singh A, Mountz JM, 1989. *SPECT Brain Imaging with Ceretec: A Clinician's Guide.* Arlington Heights, IL: Amersham.

Klingensmith III WC, Eshima D, Goddard J, eds., 2003. *Nuclear Medicine Procedure Manual.* Englewood, CO: Wick Publishing; 43–46.

Kurtet RW, Lai KK, Tauxe WN, Eidelman BH, Fung JJ, 2000. Tc-99m hexamethylpropylene amine oxime scintigraphy in the diagnosis of brain death and its implications for the harvesting of organs used for transplantation. *Clin Nucl Med.* 24:7–10.

Matin P, 1986. *Clinical Nuclear Medicine Imaging.* New York, NY: Elsevier; 1–47.

Mettler FA, Guiberteau MJ, 1991. *Essentials of Nuclear Medicine Imaging.* 3rd ed. Philadelphia, PA: W.B. Saunders; 55–74.

Park HM, Duncan K, 1994. Nonradioactive pharmaceuticals in nuclear medicine. *J Nucl Med Technol.* 22:240–249.

Perlman SB, Stone CK, 1998. Clinical positron emission tomography. In: Wilson MA, ed. *Textbook of Nuclear Medicine.* Philadelphia, PA: Lippincott-Raven; 331–351.

Shackett P, 2000. *Nuclear Medicine Technology. Procedures and Quick Reference.* Philadelphia, PA: Lippincott Williams & Wilkins; 34–45.

Spieth ME, Ansari AN, Kwada TK, Kimura RL, Siegel ME, 1994. Direct comparison of Tc-99m DTPA and Tc-99m HMPAO for evaluating brain death. *Clin Nucl Med.* 19:867–872.

Tikofsky RS, Tremblath L, Voslar AM, 1993. Radiopharmaceuticals for brain imaging: the technologist's perspective. *J Nucl Med Technol.* 21:57–60.

VanHeertum RL, Tikofsky RS, eds., 1989. *Advances in Cerebral SPECT Imaging.* New York, NY: Trivirum.

Velchik MG, 1990. SPECT: an update and review of clinical indications. *Del Med J.* 62:873–888.

Walker JM, Margouleff D, eds., 1984. *A Clinical Manual of Nuclear Medicine.* Norwalk, CT: Appleton-Century-Crofts; 23–52.

WebMD. eMedicineHealth definition glossary for Normal Pressure Hydrocephalus. http://www.emedicinehealth.com/normal_pressure_hydrocephalus/glossary_em.htm (accessed November 17, 2010).

CHAPTER 11 **Endocrine System**

Ann Steves and Helen Drew

Radionuclide imaging of the endocrine system includes imaging of the thyroid, parathyroid, and adrenal glands. Currently, there are no imaging procedures for the other glands that make up the endocrine system.

Thyroid Imaging

The thyroid gland is located in the anterior neck between the suprasternal notch and the thyroid cartilage (Fig. 11.1). The gland consists of two lobes, each 3–4 cm long from pole to pole. The isthmus (thyroid tissue connecting the right and left lobes of the gland) overlies the trachea. The highly vascular thyroid gland is supplied with blood from the superior and inferior thyroid arteries.

Thyroid imaging, one of the earliest nuclear medicine imaging procedures to be developed, is based on the physiologic process of thyroid hormone production. The thyroid hormones T_3 (triiodothyronine) and T_4 (tetraiodothyronine or thyroxine) are manufactured from iodine absorbed into the blood from the digestive tract. The absorbed blood transports the iodine, in the form of iodide, to the thyroid gland, where it is trapped by the thyroid follicular cells. The process of concentrating iodide in the follicles is referred to as the iodide pump. Through the use of a catalyst present in the thyroid follicles, the iodide is then oxidized to form one or two molecules: monoiodotyrosine (MIT) or diiodotyrosine (DIT). T_3 is formed from the coupling of one MIT molecule and one DIT molecule, whereas T_4 is formed from the combination of two DIT molecules. These hormones are stored in the thyroid gland until they are required by the body for a wide variety of metabolic processes, including growth and development, body temperature regulation, and the metabolism of proteins, lipids, carbohydrates, vitamins, and minerals.

Thyroid hormone production and secretion are controlled by a negative feedback mechanism (Fig. 11.2). Thyroid stimulating hormone (TSH), secreted by the anterior pituitary gland, regulates thyroidal iodide uptake and release of the hormones into the circulation. Low levels of circulating hormone cause more TSH to be produced, thereby stimulating the thyroid gland to produce more T_3 and T_4 for release. Increased levels of circulating hormone signal the anterior pituitary to suppress TSH secretion. The levels of these circulating hormones may also affect the hypothalamus, which secretes thyrotropin-releasing factor (TRF), a hormone that stimulates the anterior pituitary gland to produce TSH.

Radiopharmaceuticals

Table 11.1 compares radiopharmaceuticals commonly used for thyroid imaging and uptake. Because of its significantly higher radiation dose, iodine-131 (^{131}I)–sodium iodide is not recommended for routine imaging.

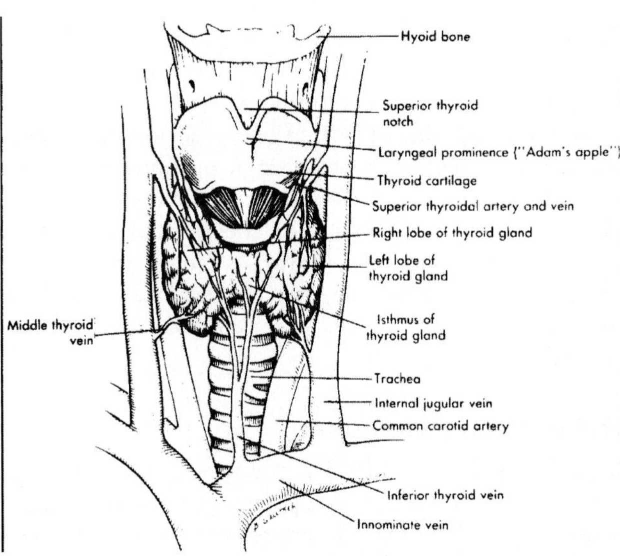

Figure 11.1 Gross anatomy and location of the thyroid gland. (Reprinted, with permission, from McClintic, 1983, p. 500.)

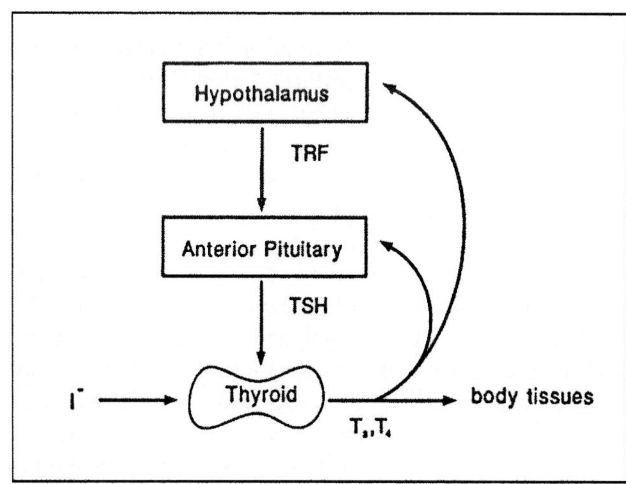

Figure 11.2 Feedback mechanism for controlling thyroid hormone production.

Table 11.1 Thyroid Radiopharmaceuticals

Radiopharmaceutical	$T_{1/2}$	Principal E_γ (keV)	Recommended dosage (mCi)
^{99m}Tc–pertechnetate	6 hr	140	2–10 (imaging)
^{123}I–sodium iodide	13 hr	159	0.1–0.2 (uptake only) 0.2–0.6 (imaging)
^{131}I–sodium iodide	8 days	364	0.004–0.01 (uptake only) 0.05–0.2 (imaging)

Clinical Indications

Thyroid imaging is performed to relate gland structure to function and to evaluate gland size and palpable nodules or masses in the neck. It is also used to identify ectopic thyroid tissue that may be located at the base of the tongue or below the sternum.

Clinical Procedure

Before dose administration, the patient should always be questioned about previous thyroid problems or symptoms, neck surgery, medications, and recent radiographic procedures. A number of medications, iodine-containing foods, and radiographic procedures using iodinated contrast affect radioiodine uptake in the thyroid and can influence both uptake and image results (Table 11.2). A low-iodine diet for 3–10 days before radioiodine administration may be recommended. Certain thyroid medications may need to be discontinued. All female patients of childbearing age should be questioned in this and any other procedure to rule out pregnancy or breast-feeding. Laboratory values for thyroid hormone levels in the blood aid in the interpretation of both the thyroid image and the thyroid uptake.

The radiopharmaceutical is administered orally if radioiodine is used and intravenously if technetium-99m (^{99m}Tc)–pertechnetate is the tracer of choice. Imaging is performed 15–30 min after ^{99m}Tc–pertechnetate administration, 3–4 or 16–24 hr after ^{123}I–sodium iodide, and 6–24 hr after ^{131}I–sodium iodide. The patient is placed in the supine position with the neck hyperextended. Using a scintillation camera with a pinhole collimator, the thyroid is centered in the field of view at a distance from the face of the collimator that will produce an image corresponding to the actual size of the thyroid gland. Images are acquired in the anterior and oblique projections. Images with markers placed on the suprasternal notch or over palpable modules also may be useful. To enhance structural detail, magnified views may be obtained by moving the collimator closer to the surface of the neck. An anterior view of the mediastinum is indicated if ectopic thyroid tissue is suspected. When radioiodine is used as the tracer, a thyroid uptake is usually performed immediately before or after imaging.

Table 11.2 Common Drugs and Chemical Substances Influencing Thyroid Uptake of Iodine

Substance	Duration of effect
Iodine-containing products	
Lugol's solution, SSKI	2–4 weeks
Topical iodine products	2 weeks or longer
Kelp	2–4 weeks
Certain vitamin/mineral supplements	2–4 weeks
Some cough medicines	2–4 weeks
Radiographic contrast media	
Water-soluble intravenous contrast media	2–4 week
Other oral and fat-soluble contrast media	2–4 weeks
Thyroid medications	
Thyroxine	4–6 weeks
Triiodothyronine	2–3 weeks
Antithyroid medications	
Propylthiouracil	2–8 days
Methimazole	2–8 days
Other drugs	
Salicylates	Unknown
Adrenocorticotropic hormone, adrenal steroids	8 days
Competing anions	
Perchlorate	1 week
Pertechnetate	1 week

Image Findings

The normal thyroid gland appears as a butterfly-shaped structure with a uniform, symmetric distribution of activity (Fig. 11.3). The right lobe is often slightly larger than the left, and the isthmus may not be visualized. A pyramidal lobe (a third lobe) is sometimes visualized.

Abnormal findings include gland enlargement and visualization of functioning or nonfunctioning thyroid nodules. Thyroid imaging is not performed to detect nodules but rather to determine whether a nodule concentrates tracer (Fig. 11.4). Whether a nodule is functioning and whether there are single or multiple nodules are important pieces of diagnostic information with implications for management of the thyroid condition. Nonfunctioning nodules, known as "cold" nodules, can represent benign adenoma, cyst, hematoma, and inflammatory conditions, as well as carcinoma. Hot nodules generally are benign.

Technical Considerations

It is important to identify prescribed and over-the-counter medications, food supplements, and other diagnostic tests that may interfere with tracer uptake. Determination of such interferences is best accomplished when the patient is scheduled for thyroid imaging.

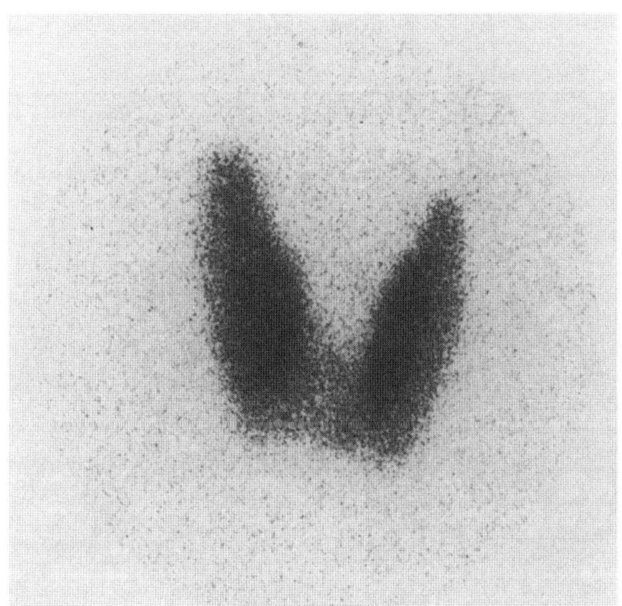

Figure 11.3 Normal thyroid image obtained 24 hr after administration of ^{123}I–sodium iodide. (Courtesy of St. Luke's Episcopal Hospital, Houston, TX.)

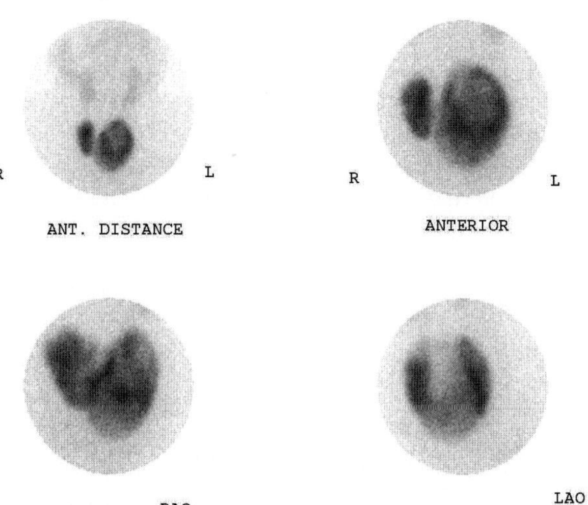

Figure 11.4 Thyroid image demonstrating Graves disease with cold nodule on left. (Courtesy of University of Alabama at Birmingham, Birmingham, AL.)

As with any imaging procedure, movement of the patient during data acquisition will introduce a motion artifact into the diagnostic image. During thyroid imaging, moving the head, swallowing, coughing, or talking should be avoided.

Thyroid Uptake

Thyroid uptake measures the amount of radioactive iodide taken up and retained within the thyroid gland. Different aspects of thyroid metabolism are reflected in the uptake value, depending on how long after tracer administration the uptake is measured. In normal circumstances, thyroid uptake at 2–6 hr after tracer administration reflects iodide trapping and organification within the gland. Uptake values at 24–48 hr are affected by the rate at which iodine is lost from the gland.

Radioiodine uptakes are useful in patients with hyperthyroidism in whom ^{131}I therapy is indicated and in patients with organification defects, which are seen in cases of congenital organification defect and certain types of thyroiditis.

Radiopharmaceuticals

Radioiodine (^{123}I or ^{131}I) is preferred, although it is possible to determine thyroid uptake with ^{99m}Tc–pertechnetate. Radioiodine capsules are easier to handle than radioiodine liquid and minimize the potential for accidental spills and contamination.

Clinical Procedure

Patient preparation is similar to that for radioiodine thyroid imaging. The patient should be instructed not to eat after midnight on the night before the test and to remain fasting for 2 hr after capsule administration to facilitate the intestinal absorption of iodide.

Data are collected with a thyroid uptake probe with a 2-in.-thick sodium iodide crystal and a flat-field collimator connected to a pulse-height analyzer and scaler. The detector should provide a field of at least 10 cm in diameter at the surface of the patient's neck.

If the patient dose capsule is to be used as the standard, the capsule is placed in a neck phantom and counted. The thyroid probe is positioned perpendicular to the capsule, at a distance of 25–30 cm from the face of the collimator to the capsule. The exact distance needs to be determined in each facility. The capsule is counted for 1 min using the appropriate energy setting. Each time an uptake measurement is performed on a patient, a correction factor must be applied to correct for physical decay.

Some facilities use a duplicate capsule as a standard. After being placed in a neck phantom, the standard capsule is counted with the thyroid probe each time an uptake measurement is performed on a patient. The phantom is positioned at the previously calibrated distance from the face of the collimator.

Nonthyroid background measurements are also collected over the thigh. It is important to exclude bladder activity. Therefore, the probe is positioned vertically over one leg, at a distance slightly above the patient's knee.

Some facilities estimate nonthyroid background by placing a lead thyroid shield over the patient's neck to cover the thyroid. The probe is then placed in the uptake position and counts are collected.

Thyroid gland counts are collected with the patient positioned erect or supine with the neck hyperextended. The probe is positioned in front of the neck with the center line of the probe between the thyroid cartilage and the suprasternal notch at the calibrated distance between the face of the collimator and the surface of the neck.

Calculations

Thyroid uptake is calculated using the following equation:

$$\% \text{ uptake} = \frac{N - T}{(S \times D_f) - B} \times 100,$$

where N is patient neck counts per minute, T is patient background counts per minute, S is standard counts per minute, D_f is the decay factor (to account for elapsed time from initial standard count to time uptake measurement is performed), and B is room background counts per minute. A decay factor is not needed if a duplicate capsule is used as a standard. Normal values are 6–18% for a 4-hr uptake and 10–35% for a 24-hr uptake.

Technical Considerations

Medications containing iodine and radiographic procedures using iodinated contrast media will expand the patient's iodide pool, resulting in a low radioiodine uptake. Thyroid medications containing T_4 and antithyroid drugs will suppress the thyroid uptake. Table 11.3 gives a partial list of factors influencing radioiodine uptake.

Because ^{123}I has a low-energy photon of 159 keV, correction for attenuation by soft tissue may be considered when this tracer is used. Patients with extremely large goiters or heavy necks may attenuate the photons, because of variable thyroid depths, thereby causing erroneous results.

Each time an uptake measurement is performed, the patient's prior positioning must be reproduced to ensure constant counting geometry. Standardized distances between the detector and the patient's neck or the neck phantom must be maintained.

To account for residual activity, patients who have received previous radioactive tracers must have a count taken over their thyroid gland to correct for this activity before the tracer is administered. Failure to perform a residual count will result in a falsely increased thyroid uptake value.

Table 11.3 Factors Influencing Thyroidal Iodine Uptake

Increased uptake	Decreased uptake
Iodine deficiency	Suppression by exogenous thyroid hormone
Pregnancy (normal)	Renal failure or severe congestive heart failure
Lithium	Excess iodine (including radiographic contrast agents and iodine-containing drugs)
Rebound after suppression with thyroid hormone	Other drugs including thionamides and glucocorticoids
Rebound after cessation of antithyroid drugs	

Reprinted, with permission, from Drew *et al.* (1987, p. 83).

Radioiodine Whole-Body Imaging

After total thyroidectomy for differentiated thyroid carcinoma, whole-body imaging with radioiodine may be performed (Fig. 11.5). The purpose of this type of imaging is to identify residual functioning thyroid tissue and/or areas of metastases.

^{131}I–sodium iodide is the tracer most commonly used to perform this type of imaging. Dosages of 37–370 megabecquerels (mBq) (1–10 mCi) have been recommended, but the optimum dosage of ^{131}I–sodium iodide is controversial. The β emission of ^{131}I may "stun" thyroid follicular cells, interfering with subsequent ^{131}I uptake when that tracer is used for therapy. For this reason, ^{123}I–sodium iodide (37–74 MBq/1–2 mCi) is now being considered as an alternative to ^{131}I for whole-body imaging. However, the issue of which radioiodine and the dosage to use is still under investigation.

Patient preparation is similar to that for radioiodine thyroid imaging. Sensitivity of whole-body radioiodine

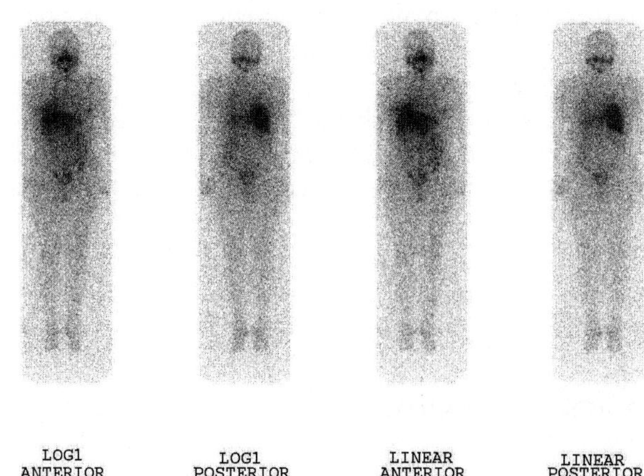

Figure 11.5 Whole-body ^{131}I images 7 days post-therapy. (Courtesy of University of Alabama at Birmingham Hospital, Birmingham, AL.)

imaging can be enhanced by ensuring that the patient has complied with a low-iodine diet and by determining that the serum TSH level is greater than 30–50 milliunits (mU)/L. Pregnancy and lactation should be ruled out in female patients.

Anterior and posterior images of the body to include the head to midfemur are acquired at 24–48 hr after ^{131}I–sodium iodide administration (at 24 hr if ^{123}I is used). Anatomical landmarks should be placed on the images to assist in precise identification of areas of iodine uptake.

Activity may be seen in the salivary glands, thyroid tissue remnants, stomach, esophagus, and thymus, as well as in distant functioning metastases.

Parathyroid Imaging

The four parathyroid glands are located on the posterior aspects of the poles of the thyroid gland. However, their location can be extremely variable (Fig. 11.6). The parathyroid glands produce and secrete parathyroid hormone (PTH), the hormone responsible for regulating the level and distribution of calcium and phosphorus.

Radionuclide imaging of the parathyroid is useful when primary hyperparathyroidism is suspected. This condition results from a tumor in one of the parathyroid glands or from hyperplasia of all four glands, both of which lead to excess secretion of PTH. Excess PTH stimulates removal of large amounts of calcium from the bones, causing weakening and increased fracture risk. The excess calcium level in the blood affects the nervous system function and muscle contraction. The excess calcium may also be deposited in various tissues as calcium phosphate. Death may result in extreme cases.

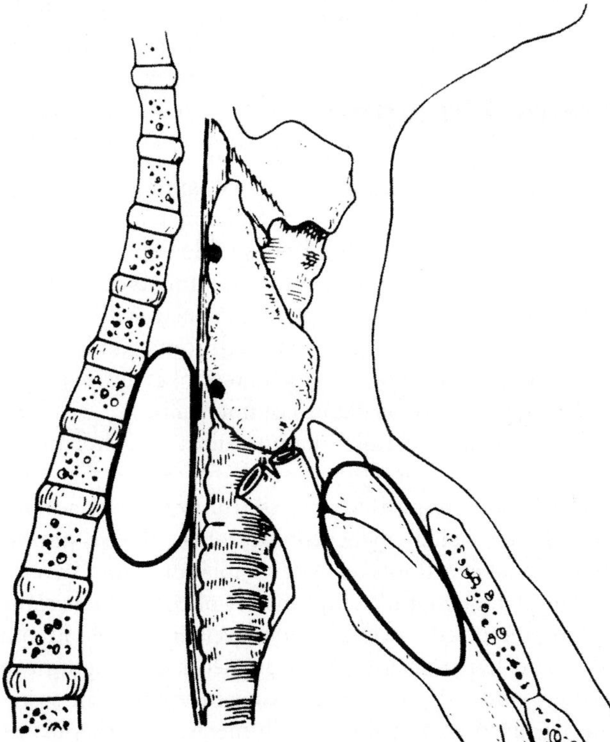

Figure 11.6 Parathyroid glands, represented as solid circles, are located behind the thyroid. Open circles depict common location of ectopic parathyroid glands. (Reprinted, with permission, from Ratliff *et al.*, 1986, p. 35.)

The treatment for primary hyperparathyroidism is surgical removal of the hyperplastic glands or the tumor. Radionuclide imaging is a means of identifying the location of the parathyroid tissue before surgical intervention. Definitive localization of ectopic tissue or tumor is particularly useful. Parathyroid imaging may be accomplished with either the dual-phase technique or a dual-tracer technique.

Clinical Procedure

No special patient preparation is required. The patient is placed in the supine position with the neck hyperextended. Both the neck and the upper mediastinum should be imaged. Because the patient must remain in the same position for an extended period, patient comfort should be optimized. The use of sandbags or some type of restraining device to immobilize the head and neck is recommended. An intravenous line may be placed into an arm vein to permit easy administration of the tracers. Imaging may be performed as a static image acquisition or as single-photon emission computed tomography imaging acquisition.

Dual-Phase Technique

^{99m}Tc–sestamibi (185–925 MBq/5–25 mCi) is administered and localizes in both thyroid and parathyroid tissue. However, the tracer washes out of normal thyroid tissue more rapidly than it does from abnormal parathyroid tissue. Thus, early imaging (10 min after tracer administration) and delayed imaging (1.5–2.5 hr after tracer administration) may demonstrate retention of the tracer in abnormal parathyroid tissue that becomes more obvious on the delayed images (Fig. 11.7).

Dual-Tracer Technique

Two tracers, one that delineates normal thyroid tissue (^{99m}Tc–pertechnetate or ^{123}I–sodium iodide) and one that localizes in both thyroid and abnormal parathyroid tissue (^{99m}Tc–sestamibi or thallium-201 [^{201}Tl]–thallous chloride), are used. Depending on the choice of tracers, there are both advantages and disadvantages as to which is administered first. Downscatter from the higher-energy radionuclide into the lower-energy window, the length of time the patient must remain still, the

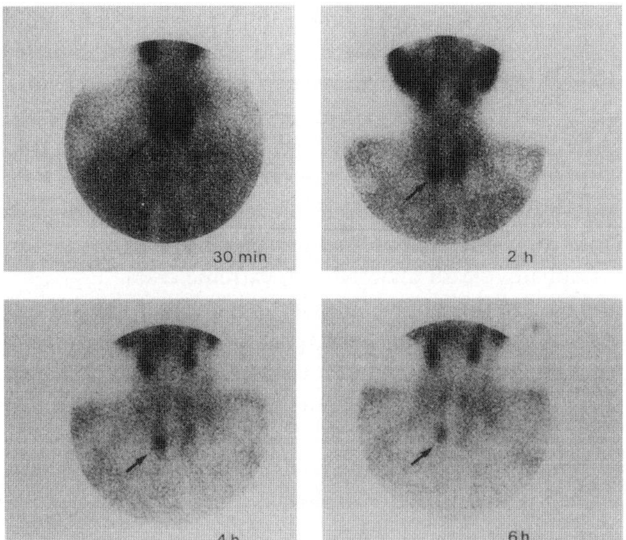

Figure 11.7 Differences in ^{99m}Tc–sestamibi washout from a parathyroid adenoma (arrow) and the surrounding thyroid parenchyma. At 30 min after intravenous injection, slightly increased focal uptake is visualized in the lower right neck (arrow), but the target-to-background ratio is still low. This ratio progressively increases over time and the parathyroid adenoma is well visualized on the 2-, 4-, and 6-hr images. (Reprinted, with permission, from Taillefer and Strashun, 1994.)

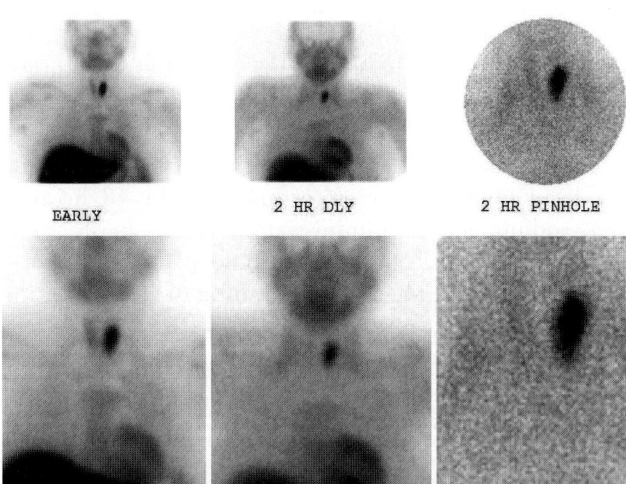

Figure 11.8 Parathyroid images showing adenoma in left lobe using ^{99m}Tc–sestamibi. (Courtesy of University of Alabama at Birmingham Hospital, Birmingham, AL.)

administered activity of each tracer, and the time required for ^{123}I–sodium iodide localization are considerations when choosing the protocol to be used. In all protocols, both images are normalized so that the counts per pixel in the thyroid are the same in both images. Then the ^{99m}Tc–pertechnetate or ^{123}I–sodium iodide image is subtracted from the ^{201}Tl–thallous chloride or ^{99m}Tc–sestamibi image to reveal the area of abnormal parathyroid tissue.

Technical Considerations

Thyroid disease is common in patients with hyperparathyroidism (Fig. 11.8). Such disease may cause nonuniform uptake of both tracers in the thyroid gland and lead to false-positive results when the images are processed with computer subtraction.

The diagnostic quality of the images is dependent on patient cooperation. Movement during data acquisition can have adverse effects. Likewise, image registration, if applicable, must be precise.

When using the dual-tracer technique, ^{99m}Tc–pertechnetate may be administered first to minimize the length of time the patient must remain in one position. After ^{99m}Tc administration, the patient does not need to be positioned until the tracer has concentrated in the thyroid and imaging is ready to begin. This method necessitates correction of the thallium image for ^{99m}Tc downscatter.

There are several advantages to the dual-phase technique. Only one tracer and one intravenous injection are required. Computer subtraction is not required. Also, the radiation dose to the patient may be decreased with the use of a single ^{99m}Tc-labeled agent.

Adrenal Imaging

The adrenal glands are located at the superior poles of the kidneys. They are small glands, weighing only 6–7 g, and consist of an outer cortex and inner medulla. The cortex produces steroid hormones (aldosterone, cortisol, etc.). Cholesterol is a precursor or building block of these hormones. Cholesterol can be radiolabeled with ^{131}I and has been used to image adrenal adenomas and certain other adrenal pathology. Iodocholesterol is an investigational drug and not available commercially.

The adrenal medulla manufactures catecholamines (epinephrine and norepinephrine), hormones that control the body's response to stress. Tumors of the adrenal medulla are called pheochromocytomas. These tumors secrete excessive amounts of catecholamines and may be benign or malignant. Symptoms of pheochromocytoma include increased catecholamine levels in the blood and urine and hypertension. Nuclear medicine imaging can be used to identify sites of excessive catecholamine secretion within the adrenal bed or in metastatic sites outside of this area. The radiopharmaceutical used to image the adrenal medulla is ^{123}I or ^{131}I–methyliodobenzylguanidine (MIBG, also known as iobenguane sulfate). This compound is structurally similar to norepinephrine but does not exert any pharmacologic effect.

Clinical Procedure

In preparation for imaging, the patient should receive Lugol's solution (a concentrated solution of potassium iodide) at least 1 day before tracer administration and for 6–7 days thereafter. The solution saturates the thyroid gland with "cold" iodine, preventing the uptake of any "free" radioiodine (radioiodine not attached to MIBG) that may be present in the tracer and thereby minimizing unnecessary radiation exposure to the thyroid gland.

Approximately 18.5 MBq (0.5 mCi) of ^{131}I–MIBG and approximately 37 MBq (10 mCi) of ^{123}I–MIBG are administered intravenously. Anterior and posterior imaging from the top of the skull to the pelvis is performed at 1, 3, and 7 days after tracer administration for ^{131}I–MIBG and at 24 hr but not later than 48 hr postinjection for ^{123}I–MIBG. The patient should be asked to void immediately before imaging, because free iodine is excreted through the urine.

Image Findings

^{131}I–MIBG and ^{123}I–MIBG uptake is visualized normally in the liver, spleen, and heart. The salivary glands and bladder may also be visualized as a result of uptake of free iodine in the tracer. Areas of abnormal uptake persist over time. Pheochromocytomas may occur in the adrenal bed or in other places in the thorax and abdomen. Metastases from a malignant pheochromocytoma may be visualized in the liver, bone, lymph nodes, heart, lungs, or other sites.

^{131}I–MIBG and ^{123}I–MIBG are used in the detection, localization, staging, and follow-up of neuroendocrine tumors and their metastases, in particular for

- pheochromocytomas,
- neuroblastomas,
- ganglioneuroblastomas,
- ganglioneuromas,
- paragangliomas,
- carcinoid tumors,
- medullary thyroid carcinomas, and
- Merkel cell tumors.

References and Further Reading

Balon HR, Silberstein EB, Meier DA, Charkes ND, Royal HD, Sarkar SD, Donohoe KJ, 2006. *Society of Nuclear Medicine Procedure Guideline for Thyroid Uptake Measurement.* Version 3.0. Reston, VA: Society of Nuclear Medicine (available at http://interactive.snm.org/docs/thyroid%20uptake%20measure%20v3%200.pdf).

Beierwaltes WH, 1991. Endocrine imaging: parathyroid, adrenal cortex and medulla, and other endocrine tumors, II. *J Nucl Med.* 32:1627–1639.

Bombardieri E, Aktolun C, Baum RP, Delaloye AB, Buscombe J, Chatal JF, Maffioli L, Moncayo R, Mortelmans L, Reske SN, 2003. *^{131}I/^{123}I–Metaiodobenzylguanidine (MIBG) Scintigraphy Procedure Guidelines for Tumour Imaging.* Vienna, Austria: European Association of Nuclear Medicine (available at http://www.eanm.org/scientific_info/guidelines/gl_onco_mibg.pdf).

Drew HH, LaFrance ND, Chen JJS, 1987. Thyroid imaging studies. *J Nucl Med Technol.* 15:79–87.

Early PJ, Sodee DB, 1995. *Principles and Practice of Nuclear Medicine.* 2nd ed. St. Louis, MO: Mosby; 617–677.

Ferlin G, Borsato N, Camerani M, Conte N, Zotti D, 1983. New perspectives in localizing large parathyroids by technetium–thallium subtraction scan. *J Nucl Med.* 24:438–441.

Goldsmith SJ, 2004. Endocrine system. In: Christian PE, Bernier DR, Langan JK, eds. *Nuclear Medicine and PET Technology and Techniques.* 5th ed. St. Louis, MO: Mosby; 350–385.

Greenspan BS, Brown ML, Dillehay GL, McBiles M, Sandler MP, Seabold JE, Sisson JC, 2004. *Procedure Guideline for Parathyroid Scintigraphy.* Version 3.0. Reston, VA: Society of Nuclear Medicine (available at http://interactive.snm.org/docs/parathyroid_v3.0.pdf).

McClintic JR, 1983. *Human Anatomy.* St. Louis, MO: Mosby; 500.

O'Doherty MJ, Kettle AG,Wells P, Collins RE, Coakley AJ, 1992. Parathyroid imaging with technetium-99m–sestamibi: preoperative localization and tissue uptake studies. *J Nucl Med.* 33:313–318.

Ratliff B, Soon P, MacFarlane S, Hanelin L, 1986. Parathyroid scanning. *J Nucl Med Technol.* 14: 34–39.

Silberstein EB, Alavi A, Balon HR, Becker D, Charkes ND, Clarke SEM, Divgi CR, Donohoe KJ, Delbeke D, Goldsmith SJ, Meier DA, Sarkar SD, Waxman AD, 2006. *Society of Nuclear Medicine Procedure Guideline for Scintigraphy for Differentiated Papillary and Follicular Thyroid Cancer.* Reston, VA: Society of Nuclear Medicine (available at http://interactive.snm.org/docs/scintigraphy%20for%20differentiated%20thyroid%20cancer%20V3%200%20(9-25-06).pdf).

Taillefer R, Strashun AM, 1994. *Dbuble-Phase ^{99m}Tc–Sestamibi Parathyroid Scintigraphy.* Pocket Lecture Series Vol. 2. Reston, VA: Society of Nuclear Medicine.

CHAPTER 12 **Gastrointestinal System**

Kathleen Murphy, Ann Steves, and Norman Bolus

The gastrointestinal (GI) system structure and function can be assessed using a variety of nuclear medicine procedures. This chapter includes a review of anatomy and physiology and an overview of the clinical indications and technical considerations for nuclear medicine imaging procedures related to the GI system. (Table 12.1 provides a review of the GI system looking at the route of administration and time post-tracer administration in which imaging occurs.)

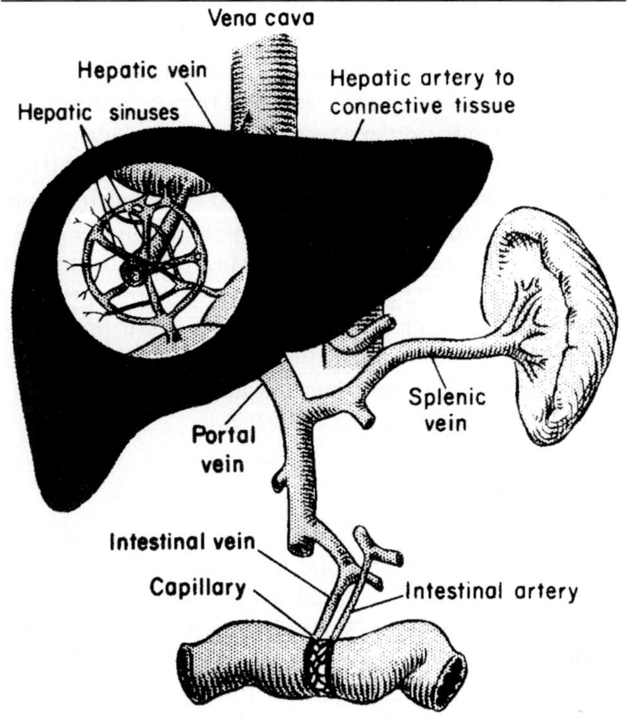

Figure 12.1 Portal and hepatic circulation. (Reprinted, with permission, from Guyton, 1976.)

Liver and Spleen Imaging

Anatomy and Physiology

The liver is the largest solid organ in the body and is located on the right side, underneath the ribs and directly below the diaphragm. Although the shapes of individual livers vary widely, the right lobe is generally larger than the left.

The liver is composed of two cell types, the reticuloendothelial (RE) cells (Kupffer cells) and hepatocytes. The RE cells account for about 15% of the liver's mass. They are responsible for phagocytosis of particulate matter. Approximately 80% of the body's RE cells are in the liver, with the remainder in the spleen, bone marrow, and lymph system. The hepatocytes, the cells that make up most of the liver's mass, perform a variety of functions, including bile formation.

The liver is a highly vascular organ with a dual blood supply (Fig. 12.1). The hepatic artery, a branch of the abdominal aorta, supplies the liver with oxygenated blood. The hepatic portal vein carries blood containing nutrients absorbed from the intestines into the liver for processing.

The spleen is retroperitoneally located in the left upper quadrant of the abdomen. Although it does contain RE cells, it is not considered part of the GI system.

Clinical Indications

1. Determination of the size, configuration, and position of either the liver or the spleen
2. Detection of tumors, hematomas, cysts, abscesses, and trauma
3. Evaluation of functional liver diseases, such as cirrhosis and hepatitis

Radiopharmaceutical

Liver/spleen imaging is performed with technetium-99m (^{99m}Tc)–sulfur colloid. Labeled colloidal particles, averaging 1 μm in size, are engulfed (phagocytosis) by the RE cells in the liver, spleen, and bone marrow. Although the RE cells make up only about 15% of the cells in the liver, they are dispersed homogeneously throughout the liver, allowing for uniform distribution of ^{99m}Tc–sulfur colloid.

Patient History and Preparation

No special patient preparation is required for liver/spleen imaging. A medical history should be obtained and include the following information:

1. Patient diagnosis
2. Pertinent laboratory values: serum bilirubin level, liver enzyme levels (SGOT, SGPT), serum alkaline phosphatase, total serum protein levels (including globulin and albumin), prothrombin time, and urine bilirubin level
3. Previous abdominal surgery

In addition, liver/spleen imaging should be performed before barium or other contrast agents are used for radiographic studies of the GI tract. These agents may cause photon-deficient artifacts to appear on the nuclear medicine images.

Imaging

^{99m}Tc–sulfur colloid (185–370 megabecquerels [MBq]/5–10 mCi) is administered intravenously. If a flow study is indicated, the patient should be positioned under the camera before tracer administration. The flow images are useful in demonstrating the vascularity of any defects that may be visualized on the static images.

After allowing sufficient time for tracer localization within the liver and spleen (usually 10–15 min), static imaging can begin. Standard views include anterior, posterior, right lateral, left lateral, right anterior oblique, left anterior oblique, right posterior oblique, and left posterior oblique projections. An anterior image with a reference marker placed along the right costal margin is also obtained to aid in the assessment of the size and location of the liver. The marker may be placed on the left costal margin for the assessment of splenic size if indicated. Breath-holding views (inspiration and expiration) may be obtained in the anterior position for the assessment of the mobility of the liver. Single-photon emission computed tomography (SPECT) imaging may be performed to better assess the size, location, and depth of liver and/or spleen abnormalities that appear on the planar images. SPECT imaging will also aid the physician in the assessment of abnormalities that may be the result of artifacts or in the detection of lesions that were not identified on planar images.

Image Findings

Approximately 85% of the ^{99m}Tc–sulfur colloid administered is localized in the liver, 10% in the spleen, and the remainder in the bone marrow. The small amount of tracer concentrated in the bone marrow is not normally visualized. The normal liver is usually located above the right costal margin and can have a variety of shapes (Fig. 12.2). One normal variant is a Reidel's lobe, a greatly enlarged right lobe, which may extend down into the pelvis. The left lobe of the liver is relatively thin and anteriorly situated; therefore, it is best visualized on the anterior projection. The normal spleen is located in the left upper quadrant above the left costal margin. Because the spleen lies more posteriorly, splenic size is best determined from the posterior view.

Other surrounding anatomic structures may cause artifacts that are commonly seen on liver/spleen images. The heart, right kidney, porta hepatis, and gallbladder may distort the shape of the liver. SPECT imaging or additional planar views can help distinguish these artifacts from true defects. Certain conditions, such as expansion of the lungs as in emphysema, subphrenic abscess, or an enlarged left hepatic lobe, cause the liver to be displaced below the level of the costal margin.

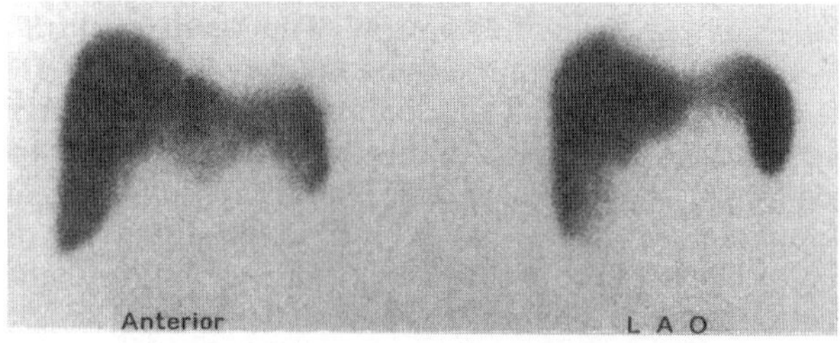

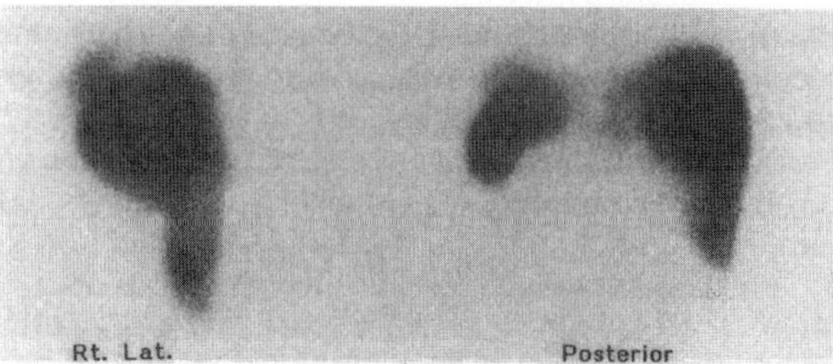

Figure 12.2 Normal liver/spleen images obtained with ^{99m}Tc–sulfur colloid. (Courtesy of St. Luke's Episcopal Hospital, Houston, TX.)

Tumors, cysts, and abscesses appear as single or multiple areas of decreased or absent tracer uptake (Fig. 12.3). Diffuse liver disease, such as cirrhosis and hepatitis, is

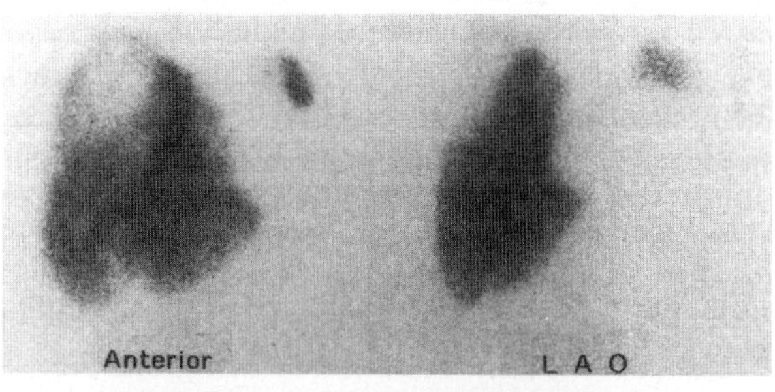

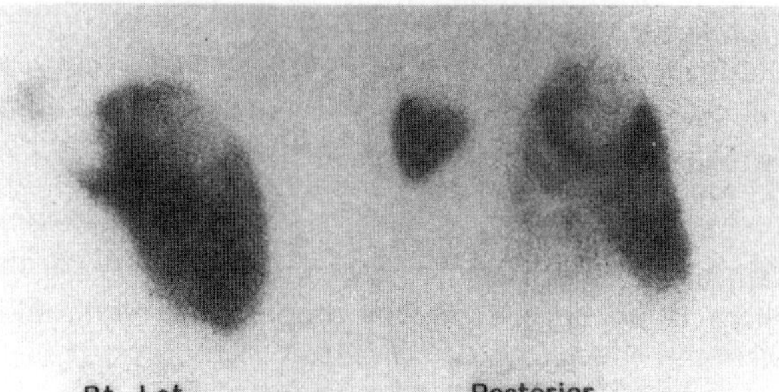

Figure 12.3 Abnormal ^{99m}Tc–sulfur colloid liver/spleen images demonstrate hepatomegaly and multiple areas of space-occupying disease. (Courtesy of St. Luke's Episcopal Hospital, Houston, TX.)

demonstrated by decreased tracer concentration or uneven tracer distribution throughout the liver. In severe cases, colloid shift occurs, resulting in visualization of the bone marrow and markedly increased tracer concentration in the spleen.

Technical Considerations

Imaging too soon after injection of ^{99m}Tc–sulfur colloid may demonstrate cardiac blood pool activity on the images. Allow sufficient time for the tracer to be extracted from the blood by the Kupffer cells.

Attenuation artifacts may appear as a result of residual barium in the GI tract, particularly in the hepatic and splenic flexures, or from female breast tissue overlying the superior portion of the liver's right lobe. Liver/spleen imaging should be performed before radiographic procedures using any contrast agents. Breast shadow artifacts can be eliminated by taping the breast out of the way. Skin folds in obese patients may cause attenuation artifacts that can be alleviated by imaging the patient in an upright position. Respiration may also cause motion artifacts on liver/spleen studies, and imaging the patient in the upright position may decrease the effects of respiration on the images.

Hepatobiliary Imaging

Anatomy and Physiology

The biliary tract begins with the microscopic canaliculi that surround each hepatocyte and carry bile to the right and left hepatic ducts. The common hepatic duct begins below the bifurcation of the right and left hepatic ducts. The cystic duct connects the gallbladder to the biliary tree. The cystic duct and the common hepatic duct join to form the common bile duct. The sphincter of Oddi is a ring of muscle that leads into the duodenum from the common bile duct. If this sphincter is contracted, pressure builds up in the common bile duct and forces the bile up into the cystic duct. The bile then moves into the gallbladder, where it is stored. Bile is released into the duodenum when it is needed to aid in digestion (Fig. 12.4).

Bile is a product of erythrocyte breakdown and hepatocyte metabolism. It is used to emulsify or break down fats (facilitating their digestion), stimulate peristalsis, and enhance absorption of fatty acids. Cholecystokinin (CCK), a hormone produced by the duodenum, stimulates the gallbladder to secrete bile when fatty foods enter the duodenum.

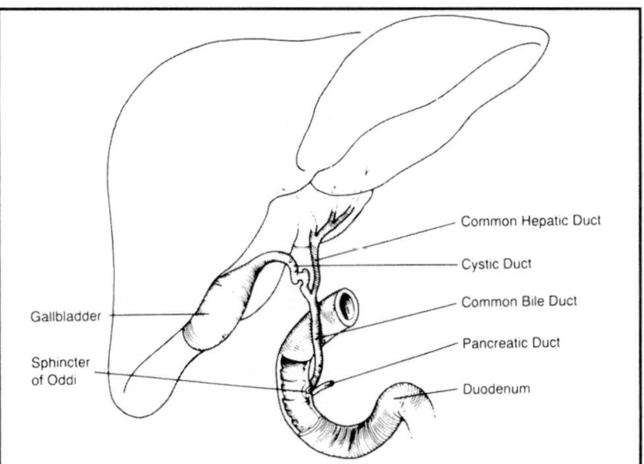

Figure 12.4 Anatomy of the hepatobiliary system.

Clinical Indications

1. Evaluation of patients experiencing upper abdominal pain is needed to rule out cystic duct obstruction (acute cholecystitis).
2. In the case of jaundice, hepatobiliary imaging can help differentiate the cause by ruling out obstruction of the biliary tract.
3. Similarly, such imaging can delineate bile drainage and reflux following surgery.
4. When cold defects are visualized on ^{99m}Tc–sulfur colloid images, subsequent hepatobiliary imaging may identify such defects as normal or abnormal variations of the biliary system.
5. Pediatric applications include the detection of choledochal cysts, biliary atresia, or other congenital abnormalities of the biliary tree.

Radiopharmaceuticals

Mebrofenin, disofenin, and lidofenin, which are ^{99m}Tc-labeled derivatives of iminodiacetic acids (IDA), are the commercially available agents used for hepatobiliary imaging. After intravenous administration, these compounds are carried to the liver, where they are extracted from the blood by hepatocytes. From the hepatocytes, the IDA compounds are transported into the canaliculi along with the bile and follow the path of bile flow.

The amount of hepatic tracer uptake is dependent on several factors, including the chemical structure of the IDA compound, hepatic blood flow, the viability of hepatocytes, and the bilirubin level. Bilirubin, the by-product of hemoglobin breakdown, competes with the uptake of ^{99m}Tc–IDA compounds. For this reason, patients with elevated bilirubin levels may require higher dosages of the tracer than do patients with normal or only slightly elevated bilirubin levels. The adult dosage of ^{99m}Tc–IDA, ranging from 74 to 296 MBq (2–8 mCi), may be determined from the serum bilirubin level.

Patient History and Preparation

Pertinent information from the patient's medical history includes:

1. patient diagnosis and/or clinical indication for the imaging procedure,
2. serum bilirubin level,
3. previous gallbladder surgery or other GI surgery,
4. medications that may affect the transit of the tracer through the biliary tract,
5. time and content of last meal and list of what was eaten.

Certain steps are required in the preparation of the patient to promote bile flow into the gallbladder. If bile flows into the gallbladder, cystic duct obstruction can be ruled out. First, narcotics, sedatives, or other drugs that relax the sphincter of Oddi should be discontinued for 6–12 hr before hepatobiliary imaging. When the sphincter is relaxed, bile flows preferentially into the small intestine rather than the gallbladder. Morphine or other opiates that increase the muscle tone of the sphincter and promote gallbladder filling may be prescribed in certain instances. Second, the patient should fast for 2–4 hr before tracer administration but should not be fasting for more than 24 hr. Again, gallbladder filling is more likely to occur if the duodenum is not stimulated to release CCK by a fatty meal, which will cause the gallbladder to contract, thus expelling the tracer out of the gallbladder.

Imaging

Imaging begins immediately after the tracer is administered intravenously. Images are obtained with a scintillation camera equipped with a low-energy, all-purpose, parallel-hole collimator. The images also may be simultaneously acquired on a computer. The patient is placed in a supine position beneath the detector so that the liver appears in the upper left corner of the field of view. Positioning the patient in this manner permits visualization of the entire biliary tract and the small intestine in a single anterior image. Sequential 5-min images are acquired for 45–60 min.

After the first hour, anterior oblique or right lateral projections may be useful to delineate bowel activity or other structures such as the kidneys. If the gallbladder or biliary ducts are not visualized by 1 hr after tracer administration, delayed images should be obtained at intervals up to 24 hr, as necessary. Likewise, if the gallbladder and common bile duct are visualized but there is no evidence of tracer in the small intestine, delayed views of the abdomen are indicated.

Sincalide (Kinevac)

Sincalide, a synthetic form of CCK, is used in conjunction with hepatobiliary imaging for two purposes. In patients who have fasted for prolonged periods (longer than 24 hr) or who are on hyperalimentation, the gallbladder is full at the beginning of hepatobiliary imaging. Therefore, the radioactive bile produced during imaging will not be able to enter the gallbladder, and cystic duct patency will not be confirmed. Administering 0.01–0.02 μg/kg of sincalide intravenously over 3–5 min before the tracer is injected will cause the gallbladder to contract, leaving it empty in preparation for hepatobiliary imaging. Sincalide should be infused 30–60 min before the tracer is administered.

Sincalide may also be administered near the end of the imaging study (usually 60 min after tracer administration) when the gallbladder is visualized to determine the gallbladder ejection fraction (GBEF). Sincalide has a short serum half-life of only 2.5 min, so it can be given before the administration of the tracer to empty the gallbladder and then administered again at the end of the imaging study to calculate GBEF. Sincalide should not be given after administration of morphine sulfate, because morphine has a serum half-life of 3–6 hr and may counteract the effects of CCK, resulting in a falsely low GBEF.

The gallbladder normally begins to empty approximately 2 min after the administration of sincalide and continues for approximately 11 min. Images are acquired on a computer for approximately 30 min after sincalide infusion at a frame rate of 1–2 frames/min. The normal GBEF value is dependent on the specific technique used (infusion rate, sincalide dosage, and duration of infusion). However, a GBEF of at least 35% is usually considered normal. A GBEF of less than 35% is usually indicative of acalculous cholecystitis.

Sincalide administration is contraindicated in patients with known hypersensitivity or intestinal obstruction. Adverse effects associated with sincalide administration occur frequently and include nausea, abdominal pain, urge to defecate, dizziness, and flushing. These effects usually occur very soon after the infusion and last for only a few minutes. Side effects may be decreased by diluting the sincalide in 10 mL of saline and infusing over 30–45 min. Sincalide may also delay the biliary-to-bowel transit time. Protocols that include the ingestion of a fatty meal have been used when sincalide is not available, but sincalide infusion is more efficient and preferred by most practitioners.

The GBEF is calculated using immediate pre- and postsincalide data. Regions of interest (ROI) are placed around the gallbladder and the liver (background). The liver ROI must not include any ductal activity. The GBEF is calculated using the following formula:

$$\text{GBEF (\%)} = \frac{(\text{max GB counts} - \text{background}) - (\text{min GB counts} - \text{background})}{\text{max GB counts} - \text{background}} \times 100.$$

Morphine Sulfate (Astramorph, Duramorph)

If the gallbladder is not visualized within 40–60 min after tracer administration, morphine sulfate may be administered intravenously as an alternative to delayed imaging. Because acute cholecystitis is usually associated with cystic duct obstruction, visualizing the gallbladder effectively rules out this condition. Morphine causes contraction of the sphincter of Oddi, which, in turn, increases the pressure in the bile ducts. The increased pressure forces tracer through the cystic duct (if it is patent) into the gallbladder. Nonvisualization of the gallbladder after administration of morphine increases the likelihood that the patient has acute cholecystitis. By using morphine, the length of the study is shortened and the specificity of the findings is increased.

A dosage of 0.04–0.1 mg/kg of morphine sulfate is administered intravenously over 2–3 min. Imaging is continued for approximately 30 min after morphine administration. Morphine sulfate administration is contraindicated in patients with respiratory depression, morphine allergy, or acute pancreatitis and in premature neonates. Adverse effects include respiratory depression, dizziness, sedation, nausea, vomiting, sweating, and constipation. Naloxone is a narcotic antagonist and can be given to counteract the adverse effects of morphine, if necessary.

Phenobarbital (Luminal)

Phenobarbital can be used to aid in the differentiation of biliary atresia (blockage of tubes [ducts] from the liver to the gallbladder) from other causes of neonatal jaundice. The patient is pretreated with phenobarbital at a rate of 5 mg/kg/day for 3–5 days before the hepatobiliary study. Phenobarbital enhances the excretion of tracer in patients with patent bile ducts. Nonobstructive causes of neonatal jaundice demonstrate excretion of the tracer into the bowel by 24 hr. The tracer will not be excreted into the bowel in patients with biliary atresia.

Phenobarbital administration is contraindicated in patients who have known allergies to barbiturates and/or respiratory depression. Adverse effects include respiratory depression, drowsiness, hyperexcitability in children, rash, nausea, and vomiting.

Image Findings

Rapid tracer uptake by the hepatocytes is normally seen within several minutes after tracer administration. Visualization of the tracer within the hepatic ducts and gallbladder occurs by 15–30 min. The gallbladder is visualized by 45–60 min, and tracer activity appears in the small intestine by 30 min after injection (Fig. 12.5).

Failure to visualize the gallbladder increases the probability of acute cholecystitis (Fig. 12.6). A rim of increased activity surrounding the gallbladder (known as the rim sign) is indicative of severe, gangrenous, acute cholecystitis. A GBEF of less than 35% may indicate that the patient has acalculous cholecystitis.

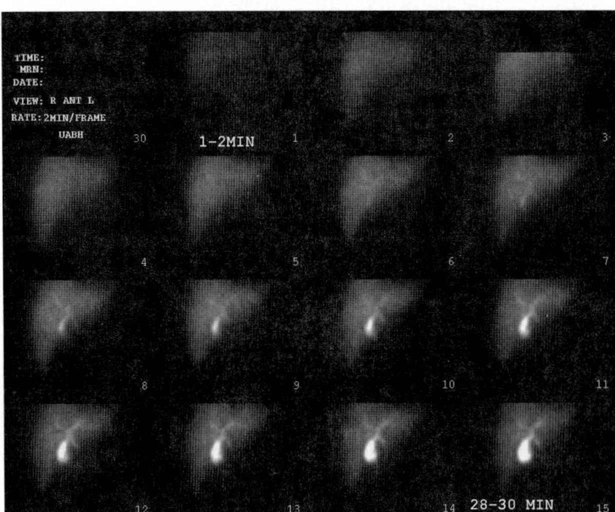

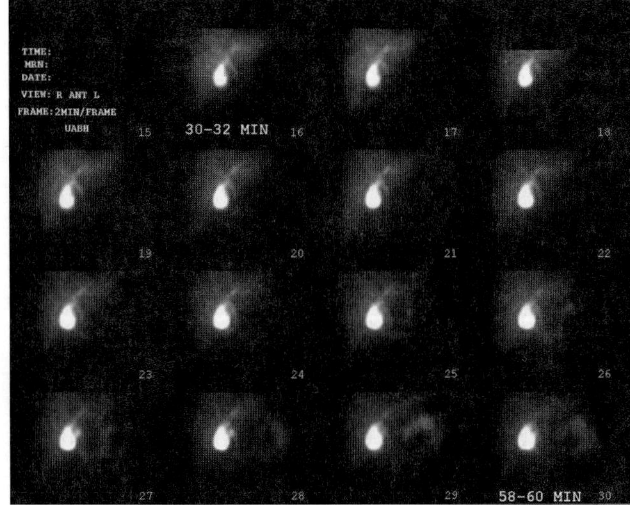

Figure 12.5 Normal hepatobiliary study. Anterior images taken after administration of ^{99m}Tc–mebrofenin demonstrate visualization of common bile duct at 15 min. Gallbladder and small bowel activity are visualized 48 min after tracer administration. (Courtesy of University of Alabama at Birmingham Hospital, Birmingham, AL.)

Nonvisualization of the gallbladder after the administration of morphine or at delayed imaging is indicative of a cystic duct obstruction (acute cholecystitis). Delayed visualization of the gallbladder may be demonstrated in patients with chronic cholecystitis. Nonvisualization of the small intestine or delayed biliary-to-bowel transit time may be the result of a common bile duct obstruction. The presence of bile outside of the normal biliary system may be the result of a bile leak.

Technical Considerations

Prolonged fasting (longer than 24 hr) or hyperalimentation may cause nonvisualization of the gallbladder as a result of the buildup of thick, viscous bile in an atonic gallbladder. In patients with extremely elevated bilirubin levels, clearance of the tracer by the hepatocytes is delayed and tracer is excreted through the kidneys. Lateral and oblique views may assist the physician in identifying kidney uptake.

Detection of Liver Hemangioma

Cavernous hemangiomas are the most common benign tumors of the liver. ^{99m}Tc-labeled red blood cell (RBC) imaging is indicated in patients who present with equivocal findings on computed tomography (CT), ultrasound, or magnetic resonance (MR) imaging. It is important to differentiate these benign tumors from malignant liver carcinomas.

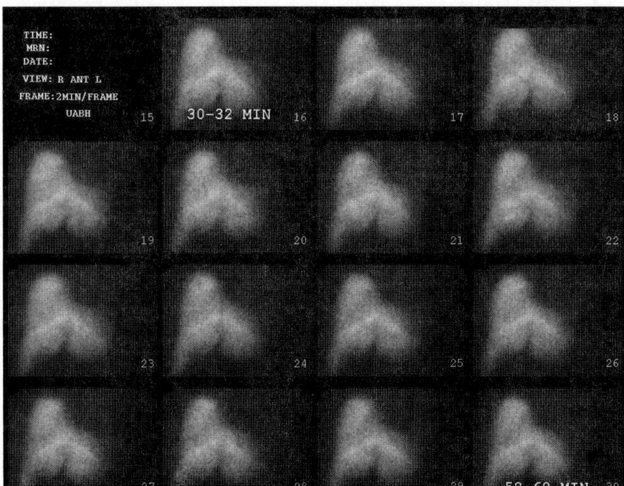

Figure 12.6 Abnormal hepatobiliary study obtained with ^{99m}Tc–mebrofenin. Neither the gallbladder nor the small intestine is visualized on the initial images or on the 2-hr delayed images (not shown). (Courtesy of University of Alabama at Birmingham Hospital, Birmingham, AL.)

Radiopharmaceutical

The RBCs can be labeled using the in vivo, in vitro, or modified in vivo/in vitro method. However, in vitro labeling is preferred because of the high tagging efficiency associated with this method.

Imaging

^{99m}Tc–RBC imaging of the liver is performed in three phases. Labeled RBCs (20–25 mCi/740–925 MBq) are administered, and an optional flow study is performed (1 frame/sec for 60 sec). The positioning for the rapid dynamic study is determined by the physician after reviewing the MR, CT, and/or ultrasound image. The optimum view is chosen to allow visualization of perfusion to the suspected hemangioma. Immediate blood pool images are also optional but, if performed, are acquired in the same view as the flow study, as well as anterior, right lateral, and posterior views. Delayed imaging is acquired at 45–180 min after tracer injection. SPECT imaging is preferred because it is more sensitive than planar imaging in the detection of small hemangiomas.

Image Findings

Hemangiomas usually have decreased or normal perfusion on the flow study but increased uptake on the delayed images (Fig. 12.7). The positive predictive value of ^{99m}Tc-labeled RBC imaging is nearly 100% for hemangioma detection.

Technical Considerations

There is no special patient preparation for this study. However, the presence of contrast material from a CT or radiographic procedure of the abdomen may cause attenuation. The patient should wait several days after having a contrast study before undergoing ^{99m}Tc-labeled RBC liver imaging.

Detection of Meckel's Diverticulum

A Meckel's diverticulum is an outpouching of the intestine, usually located in the distal ileum. It is a remnant of an embryonic duct at the point where the yolk sac is attached to the intestine of the fetus. It is formed when the duct fails to close completely during fetal development. Meckel's diverticulum is found in 2% of the population, but only 25% of these individuals ever display symptoms. Imaging for this abnormality is most commonly performed in children.

The diverticulum may contain gastric mucosa. Just as the gastric mucosa lining of the stomach secretes hydrochloric acid and pepsin, so does the ectopic gastric mucosa in the diverticulum. GI bleeding can result when the secretions of the gastric mucosa cause ulceration of

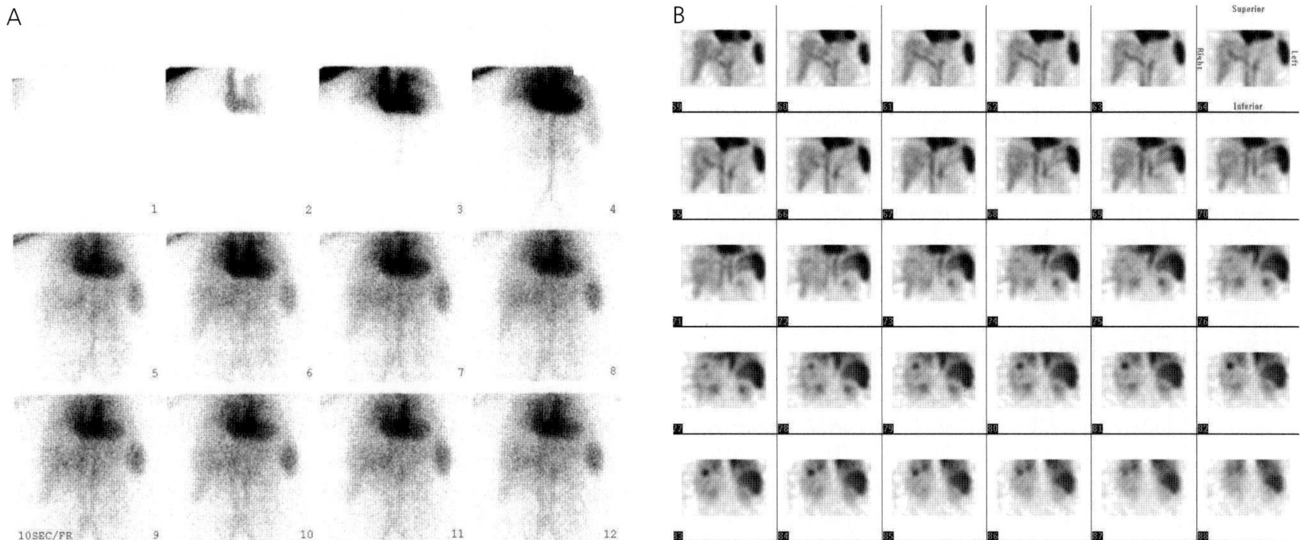

Figure 12.7 (A) Dynamic flow showing positive hemangioma. (B) Positive hemangioma on tomographic sagittal images. (Courtesy of University of Alabama at Birmingham Hospital, Birmingham, AL.)

the adjacent normal intestine. Patients may experience lower abdominal pain as well as GI bleeding. ^{99m}Tc–pertechnetate concentrates in gastric mucosa and has been useful in localizing the Meckel's diverticulum in patients with unexplained GI bleeding.

Patient Preparation

The patient should fast for at least 2 hr and should not receive any laxatives or diagnostic tests (including contrast agents) that might irritate the intestinal tract for at least 3–4 days before imaging. Potassium perchlorate is often administered to children to prevent thyroid uptake of ^{99m}Tc–pertechnetate, but it should not be used in this instance because it also blocks gastric mucosa secretions and may cause false-negative results.

Administration of certain drugs may enhance visualization of the Meckel's diverticulum. Pentagastrin (Peptavlon) stimulates gastric secretion, thereby increasing pertechnetate secretion in the stomach and diverticulum. It is administered subcutaneously 15–20 min before the tracer. The dosage is 6 µg/kg, and it should be used cautiously in patients with pancreatic or hepatobiliary diseases. Hypersensitivity to pentagastrin is a contraindication. Adverse effects are usually related to the GI tract and include abdominal pain, nausea, vomiting, and the urge to defecate. Other side effects include tachycardia, flushing, dizziness, headache, and drowsiness. An allergic reaction may occur if the patient has an unknown hypersensitivity to pentagastrin.

Alternatively, cimetidine (Tagamet) may be administered, because it helps retain ^{99m}Tc–pertechnetate in the gastric mucosa. Cimetidine is usually given orally but may be administered intravenously 1 hr before imaging. The oral administration of cimetidine is carried out over 2 days before imaging. The dosages are: adults, 300 mg four times a day; children, 20 mg/kg/day; and neonates, 10–20 mg/kg/day. Few adverse effects are associated with the administration of cimetidine, but these may include dizziness, confusion, bradycardia, and diarrhea.

Glucagon relaxes the smooth muscle of the GI tract, thus slowing down peristalsis and allowing the pertechnetate to remain stationary for a longer period of time. Fifty micrograms per kilogram are administered intravenously 10 min after injection of ^{99m}Tc–pertechnetate. The adverse effects are few but may include nausea and vomiting, as well as an allergic response in patients with hypersensitivity to glucagon. Pentagastrin and glucagon may be used in the same patient to increase the uptake of pertechnetate while slowing down the movement of the tracer in the GI tract.

Imaging

The patient is placed supine beneath the scintillation camera so that the area between the xiphoid and symphysis pubis is centered in the field of view. After intravenous administration of ^{99m}Tc–pertechnetate, static images are acquired every 30–60 sec for 30–60 min. Performance of a flow study (1–5 sec/frame for 1 min) is optional. Precise localization of a site of increased activity can be accomplished with additional views (e.g., obliques, laterals, posterior, postvoid).

Image Findings

A Meckel's diverticulum containing functioning gastric mucosa should be visualized by 10–15 min after injection, at the same time that tracer activity appears in the

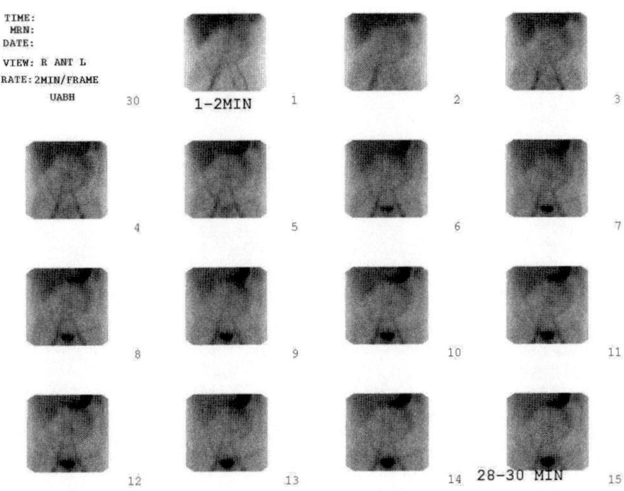

Figure 12.8 Negative Meckel's scan showing dynamic flow and bifurcation of iliac arteries and bladder tracer concentration. (Courtesy of University of Alabama at Birmingham Hospital, Birmingham, AL.)

stomach (see Fig. 12.9 and for comparison, a negative scan is shown in Fig. 12.8). It is usually seen in the right lower quadrant but can appear anywhere in the abdomen.

Technical Considerations

Failure to image the entire abdominal area can result in a false-negative examination. False-negative results also can be caused by insufficient gastric mucosa in the diverticulum to permit detection or by the removal of pertechnetate by bowel secretions. False-positive results are also possible and are most often caused by other pathologies.

Localization of Gastrointestinal Bleeding

Detection and localization of the site of GI bleeding can be accomplished with ^{99m}Tc–sulfur colloid or ^{99m}Tc-labeled RBCs. Sulfur colloid is best used in cases of active bleeding, because it leaves the blood pool rapidly and may be cleared before the next bleeding episode. However, bleeding in the right upper quadrant may be obscured by sulfur colloid uptake in the liver. Labeled RBCs are the better choice when the bleeding is intermittent, because the tracer remains in the blood pool for a long period and allows delayed imaging.

Imaging

No special patient preparation is required. The patient is placed under the scintillation camera in the supine position with the abdomen centered in the field of view.

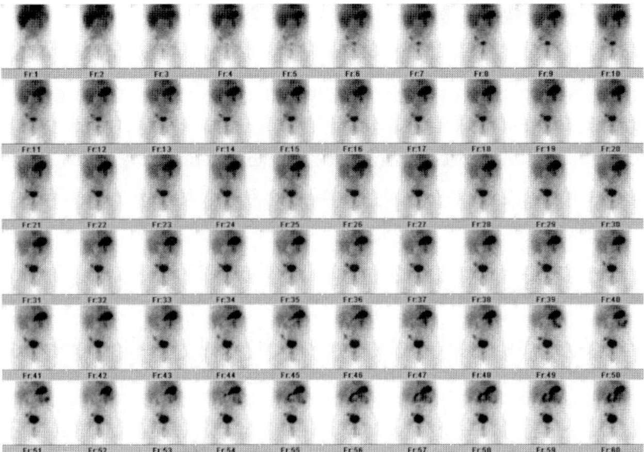

Figure 12.9 Positive Meckel's diverticulum study of a young child. Note the small area of increasing tracer concentration medially located between the stomach and the bladder. (Courtesy of The Children's Hospital of Alabama, Birmingham, AL.)

Rapid sequential images are acquired as the tracer is administered. After the dynamic study, short static images are obtained at intervals (every 5 min or more frequently) for up to 60–90 min after injection of the tracer. Dynamic images may be acquired at 10–60 sec/frame instead of the static images. If no areas of tracer accumulation are visualized and ^{99m}Tc-labeled RBCs have been used, delayed images may be obtained at intervals. The dynamic images should be displayed in cine format for the physician to review.

Image Findings

In ^{99m}Tc-labeled RBC imaging, the liver, spleen, abdominal vessels, kidneys, bladder, genital organs, and stomach are normally visualized. Progressive tracer accumulation in other areas indicates a bleeding site (Fig. 12.10). If ^{99m}Tc–sulfur colloid is the tracer, an area of active bleeding is demonstrated within the first 5 min of imaging and may become more intense as background activity decreases.

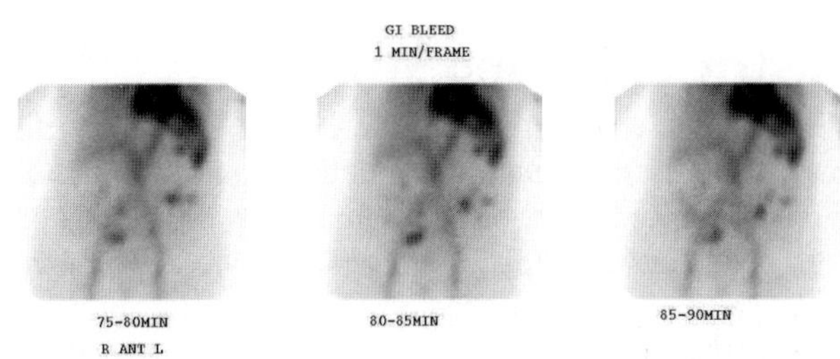

Figure 12.10 Positive gastrointestinal bleeding study obtained with ^{99m}Tc–RBCs. (Courtesy of University of Alabama at Birmingham Hospital, Birmingham, AL.)

Gastroesophageal Reflux

In adults, recurring or continual reflux of gastric or duodenal contents into the esophagus can lead to esophagitis and dysphagia. In infants, chronic reflux may cause failure to thrive and aspiration pneumonia. Gastroesophageal scintigraphy is a sensitive method for detecting reflux.

Patient Preparation

The patient should fast for several hours before imaging. For adults, ^{99m}Tc–sulfur colloid is mixed with 150 mL of orange juice and 150 mL of dilute hydrochloric acid and administered orally. For infants, the tracer is mixed with infant formula and administered through a nasogastric tube or orally through a baby bottle. It is important that the entire volume be consumed.

Imaging

After tracer administration, the patient is placed in a supine position under the scintillation camera. The stomach is positioned low in the field of view to ensure that the esophagus and lung fields are included. Serial images are obtained as varying amounts of pressure are applied to the abdomen using an abdominal binder. Delayed images of the lung fields up to 24 hr after tracer administration are useful for detecting intermittent reflux, which may lead to aspiration of the tracer into the lungs.

Image Findings

A normal study demonstrates no esophageal reflux. The stomach is visualized, but no radioactivity is observed in the esophagus. Esophageal reflux is confirmed by the presence of activity in the esophagus or in the lungs (Fig. 12.11).

Technical Considerations

The patient may experience emesis. The technologist should take steps to minimize possible radioactive contamination before the procedure begins.

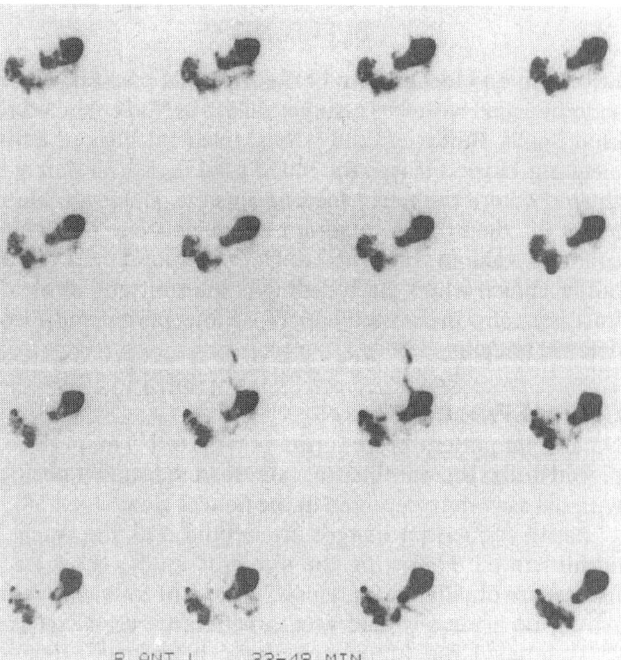

Figure 12.11 Serial images of gastroesophageal reflux study in an infant demonstrate intermittent reflux (second and third images in third row) into the esophagus approximately 42 min after tracer injection into the stomach. (Courtesy of the Children's Hospital of Alabama, Birmingham, AL.)

Gastric Emptying Study

Abnormal gastric emptying rates can be caused by diseases or surgical procedures. Patients experience nausea, vomiting, weight loss, or abdominal fullness and distention. In 2009, the Society of Nuclear Medicine introduced a new standardized gastric-emptying protocol because the procedure was performed in a variety of different ways. The following is pertinent summary information for this standard protocol.

Patient Preparation

The patient should take nothing by mouth for a minimum of 4 hr before the study. It is preferable for the patient to take nothing by mouth starting at midnight and then to be given the radiolabeled meal in the morning. The patient should be advised of the logistical demands of the procedure (e.g., the meal to be used, the time required for eating the meal [less than 10 min] and for imaging, the number of images required, and what the patient is allowed to do between images). Instructions for diabetic patients include that insulin-dependent diabetic patients should bring their glucose monitors and insulin with them. The serum glucose level at the time of meal ingestion should be recorded and included in the final report. Diabetic patients should have their diabetes under good control, with the blood sugar ideally less than 200 mg/dL. Diabetic patients should monitor their glucose level and adjust their morning dose of insulin as needed for the prescribed meal. Premenopausal women should ideally be studied on days 1–10 of their menstrual cycle, if possible, to avoid the effects of hormonal variation on gastrointestinal motility. Prokinetic agents such as metoclopramide, tegaserod, domperidone, and erythromycin are generally stopped 2 days before the test unless the test is done to assess the efficacy of these drugs. Medications that delay gastric emptying, such as opiates or antispasmodic agents, should generally also be stopped 2 days before testing. Some other medications that may have an effect on the rate of gastric emptying include atropine, nifedipine, progesterone, octreotide, theophylline, benzodiazepine, and phentolamine.

Standard Meal Preparation and Imaging

The recommended meal is a standard meal consisting of 118 mL (4 oz.) of liquid egg whites (e.g., Eggbeaters, ConAgra Foods, or an equivalent of generic liquid egg white), two slices of toasted white bread, 30 g of jam or jelly, and 120 mL of water. The meal preparation is to mix 18.5–37 MBq (0.5–1 mCi) of ^{99m}Tc sulfur colloid into the liquid egg whites. Cook the eggs in a microwave or on a hot nonstick skillet (see Ziessman *et al.*, 2007, for more information on preparation techniques). Stir the eggs once or twice during cooking and cook until firm—to the consistency of an omelet. Toast the bread and spread the jelly on the toasted bread. The meal may be eaten as a sandwich to decrease the time required for ingestion; if preferred, the eggs and toast may be eaten separately.

Immediately after eating, the patient is positioned supine under the scintillation camera with the stomach in the middle of the field of view (optimally within 10 min). Anterior and posterior planar images (or a single left anterior oblique image) with the distal esophagus, stomach, and proximal small bowel in the field of view should be obtained for 1 min immediately after ingestion of the meal. Repeated images are obtained in the same projection(s) for 1 min at hourly intervals up to 4 hr on the same camera as was used for the initial images. If dynamic imaging cannot be performed, static images can be acquired at 15-min intervals, but this method does not allow for the accurate calculation of an emptying half-time from a time–activity curve. Data are stored in a computer for processing a gastric retention/emptying time. The images themselves are not considered diagnostic (Figs. 12.12 and 12.13).

Processing

An ROI is drawn around the activity in the entire stomach in anterior and posterior views (or the left anterior oblique view, if acquired). The ROI should include any visualized activity in the fundic (proximal) and antral (distal) regions of the stomach, with care to adjust the ROI to avoid activity from adjacent small bowel, if possible. A marker placed on the patient in a fixed position such as the iliac crest may be helpful for ensuring reproducibility in gastric positioning and ROI placement. All data must be corrected for radioactive decay. The final measurement of gastric emptying is based on the percentage of gastric retention at specific times after meal ingestion (e.g., at 2, 3, and 4 hr). A time–activity curve obtained from the geometric mean of gastric counts displayed for all time points may be helpful.

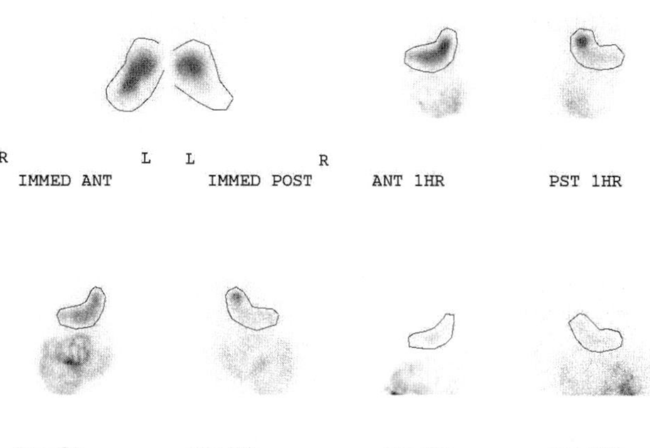

Figure 12.12 Normal gastric emptying scan with ROIs drawn for quantification. (Courtesy of University of Alabama at Birmingham Hospital, Birmingham, AL.)

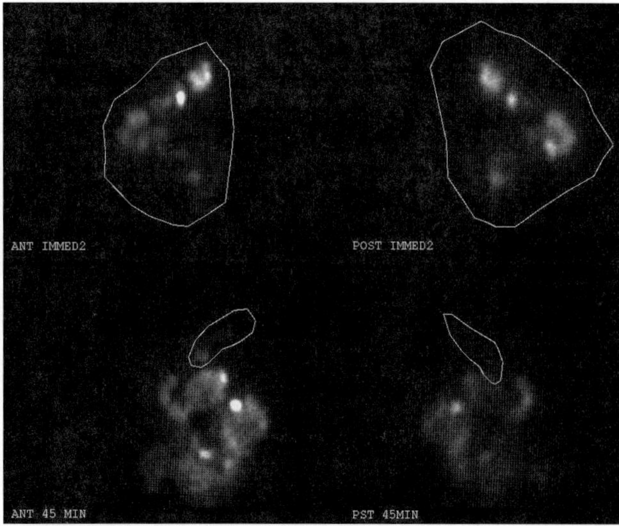

Figure 12.13 Gastric emptying showing rapid clearance. (Courtesy of University of Alabama at Birmingham Hospital, Birmingham, AL.)

Salivary Gland Imaging

There are three pairs of salivary glands: parotids, submandibular, and sublingual. These excretory glands secrete saliva in the oral cavity to aid in the digestion of food.

Clinical Indications

1. To assess salivary gland function
2. To evaluate palpable masses

3. To evaluate xerostomia (dry mouth)
4. To rule out an obstruction

Imaging

There is no special patient preparation. After interviewing the patient, the physician will determine whether a flow study is needed. The patient's neck must be hyperextended to prevent overlap of the thyroid and the salivary glands. Anterior images are acquired at 5-min intervals after the injection of 370 MBq (10 mCi) of ^{99m}Tc–pertechnetate. At 30 min after injection, right and left lateral images are obtained. A marker image should be acquired if the patient has a palpable mass. If an obstruction is suspected after the initial set of images, the patient may be asked to suck on a lemon drop to stimulate the secretion of saliva from the glands. Anterior and right and left lateral images are then obtained at 10 min poststimulation.

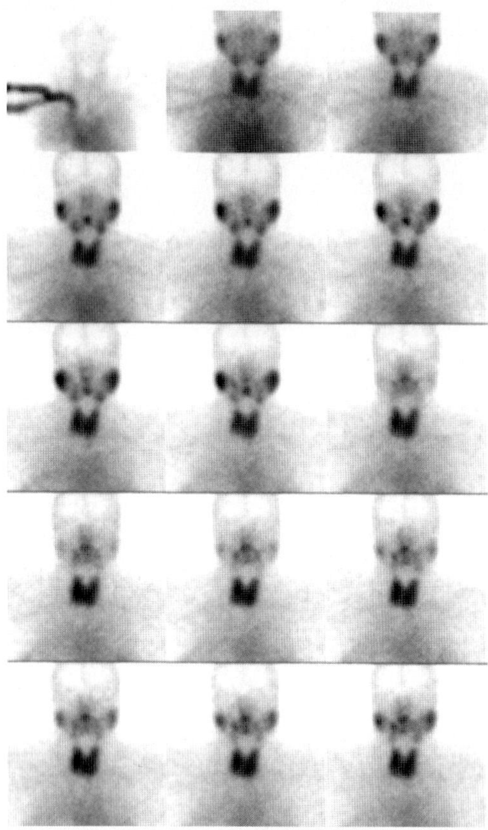

Figure 12.14 Reframed dynamic images (1 min per frame) show parotid and submandibular glands. Washout after lemon juice is seen halfway through study (third frame of third row). (Reprinted, with permission, from Loutfi *et al.*, 2003.)

Image Findings

Normal salivary glands will appear with smooth margins and uniform distribution of the tracer (Fig. 12.14). Metastatic disease will appear as areas of decreased uptake, whereas Warthin's tumor will demonstrate increased uptake. Benign tumors, cysts, and other pathologies may appear as cold defects. Sjögren syndrome is an autoimmune disorder that involves insufficient moisture production in the lacrimal and salivary glands. The characteristic appearance of Sjögren syndrome on a radionuclide salivary gland study includes asymmetrical arrival of the tracer or delayed uptake in the salivary glands as compared with the thyroid. There is bilateral decreased uptake on the delayed images and an absent or suppressed response poststimulation.

LeVeen Shunt Patency

The LeVeen shunt is used to control ascites by draining the fluid in the peritoneal cavity through a tube implanted through the internal jugular vein into the superior vena cava. A patency study is performed to ensure that the tube is functioning and that it is not blocked.

Imaging

No special patient preparation is required. The patient is placed in a supine position under the scintillation camera with the shunt tube in the field of view. The tube is palpable in the thoracic wall and neck. ^{99m}Tc–sulfur colloid or ^{99m}Tc–macroaggregated albumin (37–74 MBq/1–2 mCi) is introduced into the peritoneal space with a needle. Serial imaging begins when the radioactivity appears in the lower portion of the tube. Liver/spleen or lung imaging is performed 1 hr after tracer administration. If the tube is not visualized, delayed views are performed as necessary.

Image Findings

A patent shunt is demonstrated by early visualization of the tube. Liver/spleen or lung visualization occurs within 20 min of tracer administration (Figs. 12.15, 12.16). Lack of tube visualization and delayed tracer concentration in the liver/spleen or lung indicate shunt malfunction.

Carbon-14 Urea Breath Test

Clinical Indications

- Initial diagnosis of non-NSAID-induced gastric ulcers (nonsteroidal anti-inflammatory drugs, e.g., ibuprofen, naproxen, indomethacin, piroxicam)
- Documentation of eradication of *Helicobacter pylori* treatment for duodenal ulcers.

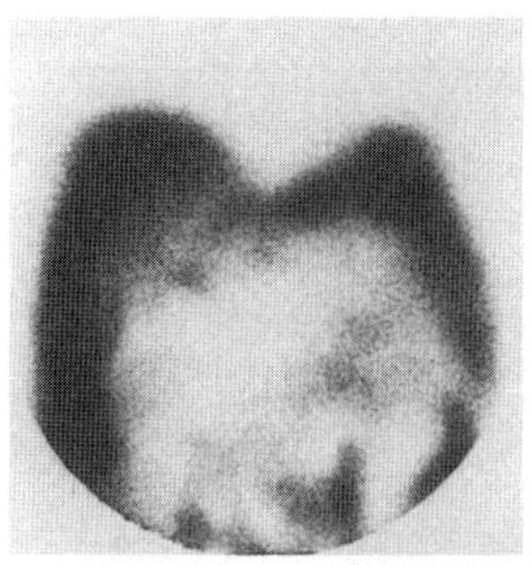
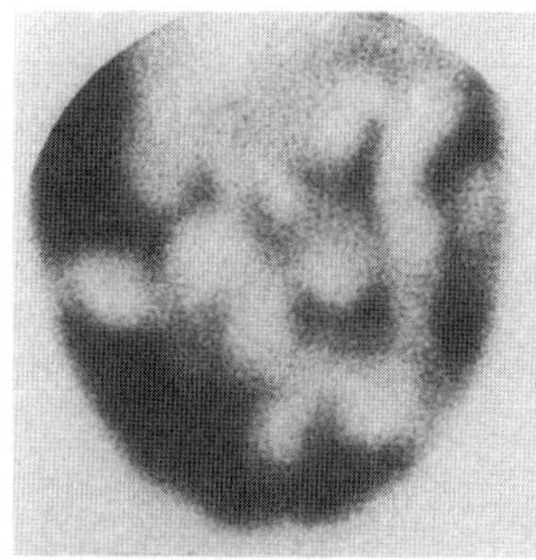

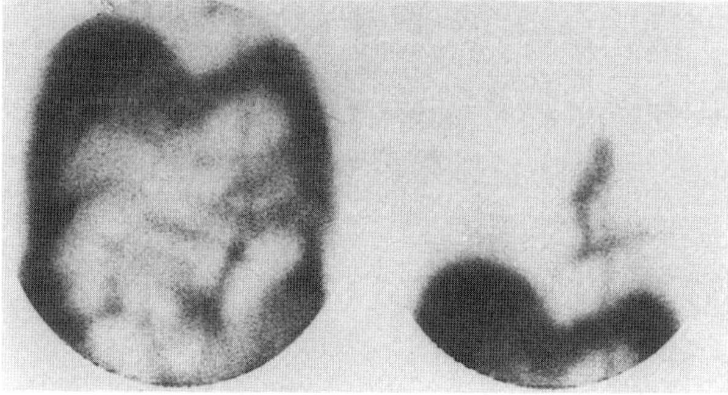

Figure 12.15 LeVeen shunt study performed by intraperitoneal administration of ^{99m}Tc–sulfur colloid. Delayed abdominal images demonstrate visualization of the shunt tubing along the left midclavicular line. (Courtesy of St. Luke's Episcopal Hospital, Houston, TX.)

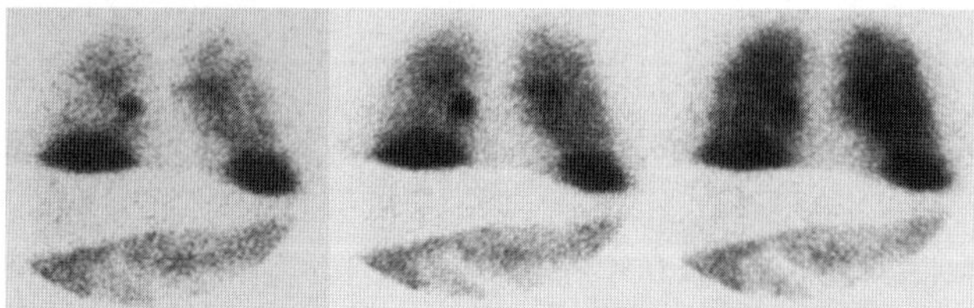

Figure 12.16 Normal LeVeen shunt study. Images at 10, 20, and 30 min demonstrate rapid arrival of ^{99m}Tc–MAA in lungs with increasing activity over time, confirming patency of shunt. Activity inferior to lungs represents injected activity in peritoneal cavity (MacDonald and Burrell, 2008).

Principle

The urea breath test is based on the detection of urase, an enzyme produced by *H. pylori*. Since urase is not present in normal tissue and other urase-producing bacteria do not colonize the stomach, the detection of urase in the stomach means that there is *H. pylori* infection. The organism is usually present in the gastric antrum and lives beneath the mucus layer. One of its special characteristics is its ability to produce urease, an enzyme that is not normally found in the human stomach.

The procedure is as follows:

1. the patient presents following an overnight fast and is given 35 kBq (~1 μCi) ^{14}C urea (oral pill),
2. a single breath sample with a known amount of CO_2 is taken 10–15 min later and measured in a liquid scintillation counter (or sent off to be read),
3. uninfected subjects exhale ~<150 dpm.

^{14}C urea is radioactive but the ingested urea is rapidly excreted and the radiation dosage from this test is very low (equal to one day's background radiation).

Results

- Negative: <50 dpm net counts
- Indeterminate: 50–199 dpm net counts
- Positive: >199 dpm net counts or anything four times above background or greater

References and Further Reading

Balon HR, Brill DR, Donohoe KJ, Ganske MA, Machac J, Parker JA, Royal HD, Shulkin BL, Wittry MD, 2001. Guidelines and Communications Committee, Commission on Health Care Policy and Practice. *Society of Nuclear Medicine Procedure Guidelines Manual 2001–2002.* Reston, VA: Society of Nuclear Medicine; 33–60.

Bernier DR, Christian PE, Langan JK, 1997. *Nuclear Medicine Technology and Techniques.* 4th ed. St. Louis, MO: Mosby; 355–388.

Chester M, Glowniak J, 1992. Hepatobiliary imaging update. *J Nucl Med Technol.* 20:3–7.

Christian PE, Datz FL, Moore JG, 1987. Technical considerations in radionuclide gastric emptying studies. *J Nucl Med Technol.* 15:200–207.

Donohoe, KJ, Maurer AH, Ziessman HA, Urbain JC, Royal HD, Martin-Comin J, 2009. *Procedure Guideline for Adult Solid-Meal Gastric Emptying Study 3.0.* Reston, VA: Society of Nuclear Medicine.

Gilbert SA, Brown PH, Krishnamurthy GT, 1987. Quantitative nuclear hepatology. *J Nucl Med Technol.* 15:38–43.

Guyton AC, 1976. *Textbook of Medical Physiology.* 5th ed. Philadelphia, PA: WB Saunders; 375.

Loutfi I, Nair MK, Ebrahim AK, 2003. Salivary gland scintigraphy: the use of semiquantitative analysis for uptake and clearance. *J Nucl Med Technol.* 31(2):83.

MacDonald A, Burrell S, 2008. Infrequently performed studies in nuclear medicine, 1. *J Nucl Med Technol.* 36(3):135.

Nowak TJ, Handford AG, 1999. *Essentials of Pathophysiology: Concepts and Applications for Health Care Professionals.* Boston, MA: McGraw-Hill; 323–377.

Park HM, Duncan K, 1994. Nonradioactive pharmaceuticals in nuclear medicine. *J Nucl Med Technol.* 22:240–249.

Shackett P, 2000. *Nuclear Medicine Technology: Procedures and Quick Reference.* Philadelphia, PA: Lippincott Williams & Wilkins; 46–50, 109–113, 119–153, 178–182, 236–239.

Shier D, Butler J, Lewis R, 2003. *Hole's Essentials of Human Anatomy and Physiology.* 8th ed. New York, NY: McGraw-Hill; 391–432.

Sodee DB, Velchik MG, Noto RB, *et al.*, 1995. Gastrointestinal system. In: Early PJ, Sodee DB. *Principles and Practice of*

Table 12.1 GI Section Procedure Review Table

Nuclear medicine examination	Radiopharmaceutical (generic name)	Route of administration	Imaging time post-tracer administration
Liver imaging	4–6 mCi ^{99m}Tc–sulfur colloid (SC)	IV	10–15 min
Hepatobiliary imaging	1–5 mCi of ^{99m}Tc–mebrofenin or disofenin/10 mCi if bilirubin levels high	IV	Flow 60 min or longer; depends on findings
Meckel's diverticulum imaging	10–15 mCi ^{99m}Tc–pertechnetate	IV	Dynamic 30–60 sec per frame for 30–60 min
GI bleeding imaging	20–50 mCi ^{99m}Tc-labeled RBCs	IV	Flow: dynamic out to ~60 min or longer; depends on findings
Hemangioma imaging	20–50 mCi ^{99m}Tc-labeled RBCs	IV	Flow: dynamic, static, delayed out to 180 min or longer
Gastroesophageal reflux imaging	300 μCi–2 mCi ^{99m}Tc–SC	Orally with liquid or semisolid (recommended: acidified orange juice + abdominal binder)	Serial images for 1 hr post ingestion; 24-hr delay of lungs if possible
Gastric emptying	200 μCi–1 mCi ^{99m}Tc–SC mixed with std meal	Orally with liquid and/or solid	ASAP–90-min serial images of 30–60 sec each
LeVeen shunt patency	1–2 mCi of either ^{99m}Tc–SC or MAA	Intraperitoneal	15–20 min or longer
Schilling test	^{57}Co–cyanocobalamin (vitamin B_{12})	Orally; intrinsic factor given IM	None
^{14}C–urea breath test	1 μCi ^{14}C–urea capsule	Orally with 30 mL warm water	None

Nuclear Medicine. 2nd ed. St. Louis, MO: Mosby; 476–534.

Spencer RP, 1995. The spleen. In: Early PJ, Sodee DB. *Principles and Practice of Nuclear Medicine.* 2nd ed. St. Louis, MO: Mosby; 535–548.

Thrall JH, Ziessman HA, 2001. *Nuclear Medicine: The Requisites.* St. Louis, MO: Mosby; 265–293.

Vitti RA, Malmud LS, 1997. Gastrointestinal system. In: Bernier DR, Christian PE, Langan JK, eds. *Nuclear Medicine Technology and Techniques.* 4th ed. St. Louis, MO: Mosby; 355–388.

Weiss SC, Conway JJ, 1997. Pediatrics. In: Bernier DR, Christian PE, Langan JK, eds. *Nuclear Medicine Technology and Techniques.* 4th ed. St. Louis, MO: Mosby; 468–489.

Ziessman HA, Goetze S, Bonta D, Ravich W, 2007. Experience with a new standardized 4-hr gastric emptying protocol. *J Nucl Med.* 48:568–572.

CHAPTER 13 Genitourinary System

Kathleen Murphy, Melanie Stepherson, Ann Steves, and Norman Bolus

Nuclear medicine imaging provides information about the function and the structure of the organs in the genitourinary system. In particular, assessment of renal function is a common indication for patients arriving in the nuclear medicine department. This chapter contains an overview of genitourinary (GU) procedures performed in the nuclear medicine department. (Table 13.1 gives a review of the GU system looking at the route of administration and time post-tracer administration in which imaging occurs.)

Renal Imaging

Renal imaging is a reliable method of evaluating the structure, location, and function of the kidneys. This can be easily accomplished without danger of allergic reaction and with little or no patient discomfort.

Anatomy and Physiology

The kidneys regulate the volume and composition of the body's extracellular fluid through their excretory function. The kidneys are retroperitoneal organs located between the 12th thoracic and 4th lumbar vertebrae (Fig. 13.1). The right kidney is positioned slightly lower than the left because of the presence of the liver superiorly. The ureters and the blood vessels attach at the hilus, an indentation on the medial border of the kidneys. The kidneys receive blood from the right and left renal arteries, which branch directly off the descending aorta.

Each kidney consists of an outer renal cortex and an inner renal medulla (Fig. 13.2). The cortex contains the majority of the nephrons, which are the microscopic functional units of the kidney. Each kidney contains more than one million nephrons. The nephron consists of a renal corpuscle and its attached tubule (Fig. 13.3). Each corpuscle is composed of a glomerulus surrounded

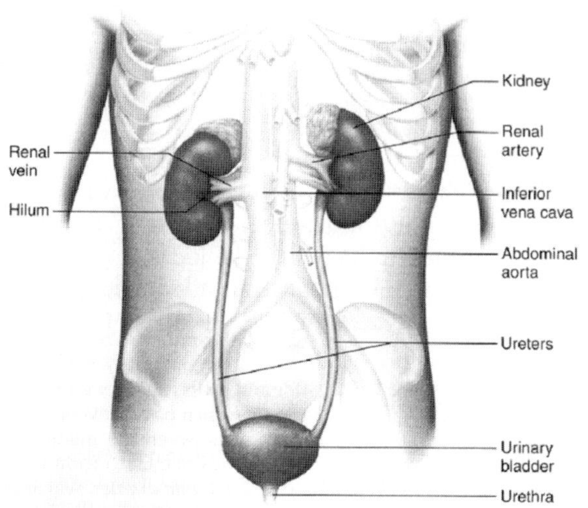

Figure 13.1 The urinary system. (Reprinted, with permission, from Shier *et al.*, 2003, p. 461.)

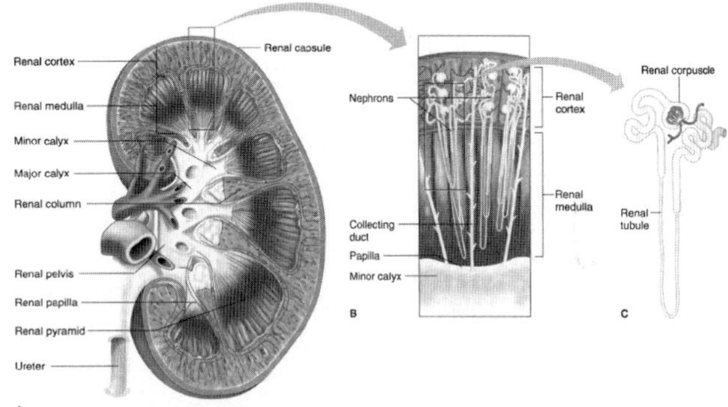

Figure 13.2 Cross-section of a kidney. (Reprinted, with permission, from Shier *et al.*, 2003, p. 462.)

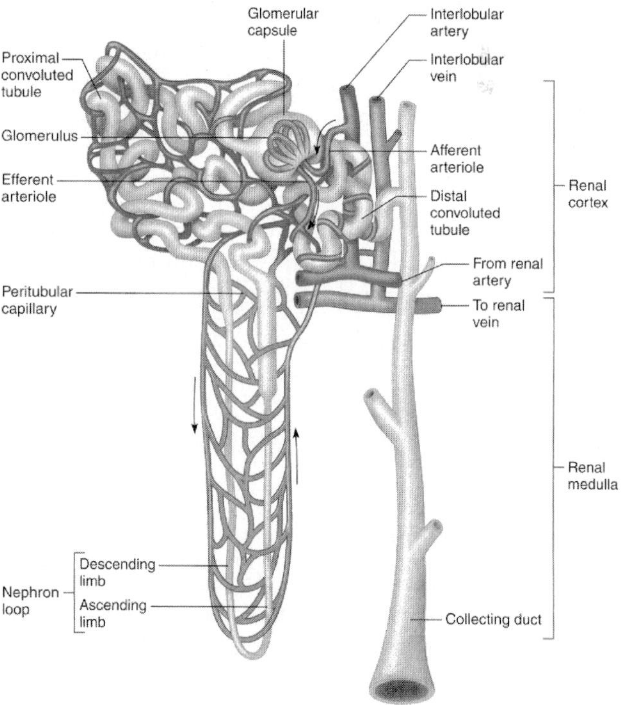

Figure 13.3 The nephron. (Reprinted, with permission, from Shier *et al.*, 2003, p. 465.)

by Bowman's capsule. The glomerulus receives blood from the afferent arteriole, which also helps regulate blood pressure through the juxtaglomerular apparatus. The tubules consist of the proximal convoluted tubule, the loop of Henle, and a distal convoluted tubule. The renal medulla contains the renal pyramids, which empty urine into the minor and major calyces of the renal pelvis.

Three processes are involved in urine formation: glomerular filtration, tubular reabsorption, and tubular secretion. Glomerular filtration involves the filtration of water and solutes out of the glomeruli and into Bowman's capsule. The glomerular filtration rate (GFR) is the volume of plasma filtrate produced in 1 min by the renal glomeruli of both kidneys. Tubular reabsorption occurs in the walls of the renal tubules and collecting system, where most of the water and other physiologically important substances are reabsorbed into the blood. Tubular secretion also occurs in the tubular cells and involves the secretion of certain substances out of the blood and into the filtrate.

The urine passes into the renal calyces, the renal pelvis, and into the ureters. Peristalsis forces urine down the ureters and into the bladder. The urine travels out of the body through the urethra, exiting via the urinary meatus.

Clinical Indications

Renal imaging is most often used to determine renal function rather than morphology. Functional imaging is indicated in evaluation of:

1. relative blood flow and renal function,
2. obstructive uropathy,
3. renal transplant function,
4. renal function of potential kidney donors,
5. renovascular hypertension.

Renal morphology usually is better demonstrated with other imaging modalities, such as ultrasound or radiography. However, static renal imaging may be useful in:

1. evaluation of renal trauma,
2. demonstration of congenital abnormalities, tumors, and cysts,
3. evaluation of patients who are allergic to radiographic contrast media.

Contraindications

A false-positive study may result if a patient is experiencing transient contrast-induced acute tubular necrosis after undergoing a renal arteriogram. This can be avoided by waiting several days after the arteriogram before performing the radionuclide renal study. Probenecid and other drugs that block tubular secretion may interfere with the uptake of renal radiopharmaceuticals.

Radiopharmaceuticals

The choice of radiopharmaceutical depends on the reason for renal imaging. Renal radiopharmaceuticals are localized in the kidneys by glomerular filtration, tubular secretion, tubular binding, or a combination of these processes.

Technetium-99m (^{99m}Tc)–Pentetate (DTPA)

Pentetate is cleared by glomerular filtration with minimal binding to the renal parenchyma. Because of its rapid clearance rate, it is useful in demonstrating glomerular filtration capabilities as well as relative blood flow to each kidney.

^{99m}Tc–Mertiatide (MAG3)

Mertiatide is excreted by the kidneys via tubular secretion. It has a high first-pass extraction fraction and rapid plasma clearance. This agent can be used to assess effective renal plasma flow (ERPF).

^{99m}Tc–Succimer (DMSA)

Succimer binds to the tubules in the renal cortex. Approximately 50% is bound within 2 hr of administration. Because this tracer remains fixed in the renal parenchyma for a relatively long period of time, it is most useful for imaging space-occupying lesions (cysts or tumors) or gross renal anatomy.

Patient History and Preparation

Before the start of the study, fully explain the procedure to the patient to elicit full cooperation. A medical history should be obtained that includes:

1. Patient's diagnosis.
2. Pertinent laboratory values: Laboratory analysis of blood chemistry is useful in determining renal function. Creatinine, urea, and nitrogen are metabolic waste products that the kidneys normally remove from the circulation. Elevated blood urea nitrogen and creatinine levels may indicate poor renal function.
3. Previous abdominal surgery, particularly to the kidneys.
4. Patient's blood pressure to determine whether renovascular hypertension is a consideration.

Renal Perfusion Imaging

Acquisition

Renal blood flow imaging can be performed with a number of ^{99m}Tc-labeled agents. The procedure is conducted as follows:

1. position the patient supine with the kidneys centered over the detector to obtain a posterior projection,
2. administer 370–555 megabecquerels (MBq) (10–15 mCi) of the tracer intravenously using a bolus injection technique,
3. obtain sequential images every 2 sec for 30–60 sec,
4. obtain a blood pool image immediately after the flow acquisition, as necessary.

Normal Findings

Soon after its arrival in the aorta, the radiopharmaceutical bolus perfuses each kidney in a vascular blush. The activity should arrive in each renal area at approximately the same time and with equal intensity (Fig. 13.4). Subsequent concentration levels and disappearance of the tracer depend on the agent used. A gradual increase will be seen in the concentration of pentetate as a result of glomerular filtration. Activity will then be seen in the renal collecting system, ureters, and bladder. ^{99m}Tc–mertiatide is taken up promptly in the kidneys, followed by excretion into the collecting system and bladder. With succimer, activity accumulates gradually, outlining the tubular cells. A minute amount of the agent is excreted in the urine, and, therefore, the collecting systems will not concentrate the radiopharmaceutical.

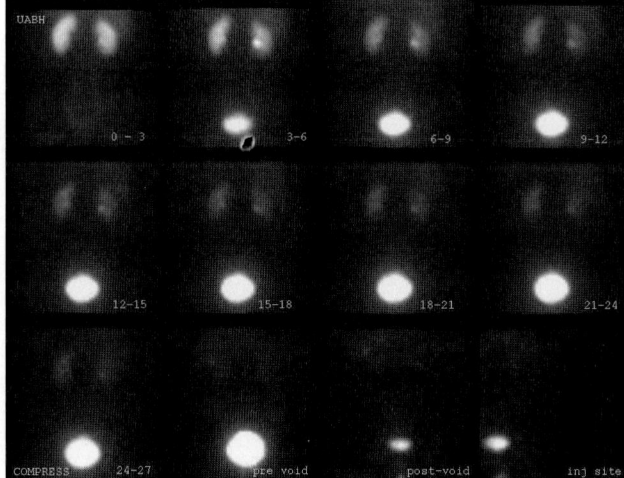

Figure 13.4 Normal ^{99m}Tc–mertiatide study. (Courtesy of University of Alabama at Birmingham Hospital Birmingham, AL.)

Abnormal Findings

Vascular tumors and arteriovenous malformations (AVMs) are seen as areas of increased activity during the flow sequence. Areas of relative decreased activity resulting from cysts or avascular tumors may also be seen in the flow sequence.

Technical Considerations

Positioning errors are a common pitfall. They may be minimized by the following actions:

1. Place the iliac crests in the lower one-third of the field of view to ensure that both kidneys are included.
2. Position the detector over the right or left iliac fossa when performing a flow study on a patient who has undergone a renal transplant. The aortic bifurcation, iliac artery, and urinary bladder should be included in the field of view. For an accurate flow study, it is also important that the tracer be given as a compact bolus and is not infiltrated.

Renal Function Imaging (Renogram)

Acquisition

Renal function imaging is performed with ^{99m}Tc–mertiatide or ^{99m}Tc–pentetate. Along with a set of sequential images, a time–activity curve (renogram) is generated to demonstrate renal function. It is important that the patient be well hydrated before the study begins. Also, the patient should void immediately before the study. Data are acquired as follows:

1. Position the patient prone or supine to obtain a posterior projection over the kidneys. In the case of a renal transplant, the patient should be placed supine with the detector over the iliac fossa, where the kidney is located.
2. Administer the tracer intravenously.
3. A dynamic flow study (see section on renal perfusion imaging) is acquired. Sequential 30- to 60-sec images are obtained immediately after the flow for a total of 20–30 min. All images are saved in a computer for later processing.
4. Administration of furosemide (Lasix) may be indicated to rule out ureteral obstruction if tracer activity does not clear from the renal pelvis or ureteropelvic junction after the initial acquisition is completed (see section on diuresis renography).

Normal Findings

Normal kidneys show prompt tracer uptake with peak uptake at 3–5 min. The kidney activity then gradually decreases as the tracer is excreted. Renal pelvis and bladder activity is usually seen by 3–6 min.

The computer-generated time–activity curves represent three phases: vascular, secretory, and excretory (Fig. 13.5). The vascular phase reflects the arrival of the bolus of activity in the renal area. In the secretory phase, the tracer is concentrated in the kidneys. The peak transit time, usually 3–5 min after injection, is the time at which the tracer reaches its maximum concentration in the kidneys. The excretory phase follows, with a fairly rapid drop in the activity curve as the tracer is excreted from the kidney into the bladder.

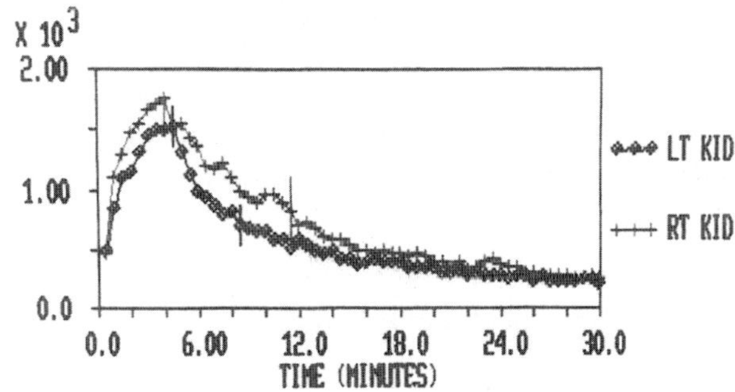

Figure 13.5 Normal renogram curves for left and right kidneys. (Courtesy of the Department of Veterans Affairs Medical Center, Buffalo, NY.)

Abnormal Findings

Abnormalities of the renogram are usually reflected in the second and third phases of the curve (Fig. 13.6). An activity curve that exhibits an adequate upslope but no subsequent fall in activity is usually the result of an obstruction and indicates that the renal tubules take up the material but cannot excrete the activity. A curve that displays a below-normal level of activity throughout the renogram indicates poor renal function. Serial images corresponding to the curve provide additional visual demonstration of the abnormalities.

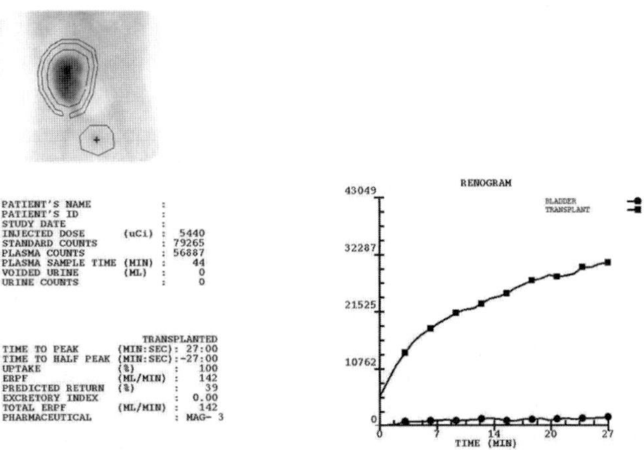

Figure 13.6 Transplant renogram showing obstruction. (Courtesy of University of Alabama at Birmingham Hospital, Birmingham, AL.)

Technical Considerations

Be sure to ascertain the patient's state of hydration, because a dehydrated patient may exhibit delayed transit time.

Diuresis Renography

If, at the conclusion of renal function imaging, tracer is retained in the renal pelvis or calyces, the administration of a diuretic to rule out a urinary tract obstruction may be indicated. Furosemide is administered intravenously to increase urine production. If there is no obstruction, increased urine flow will promptly wash out the residual tracer activity (Fig. 13.7).

The patient should be well hydrated, as required for functional imaging, and the bladder should be emptied before furosemide is administered. Patients who are unable to void voluntarily should be catheterized. Increased bladder pressure may diminish the effect of the diuretic. Furosemide is contraindicated in anuric and/or dehydrated patients. Extreme care must be taken when using furosemide in patients who have just undergone urologic surgery, because the increased rate of urine flow may tear new sutures.

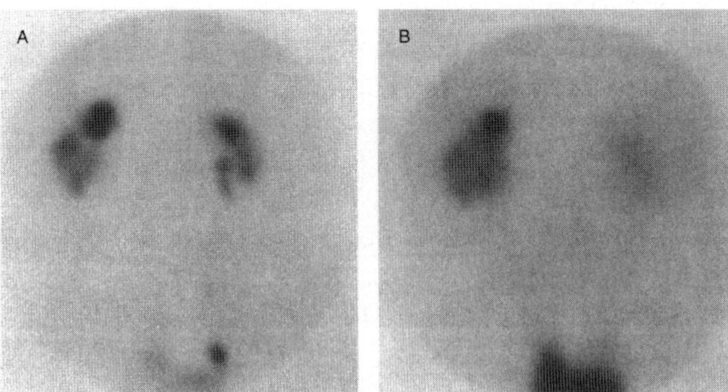

Figure 13.7 (A) Approximately 12 min after administration of ^{99m}Tc–pentetate, tracer activity remains in the pelvis and calyces of the right kidney and in the calyces of the upper pole of the left kidney. (B) After intravenous administration of furosemide, activity drains from the right kidney but remains in the upper pole of the left kidney. (Courtesy of the Department of Veterans Affairs Medical Center, Buffalo, NY.)

Data acquisition is the same as for the renal function study. Furosemide dosages range from 20–40 mg for adults and 0.5–1 mg/kg for pediatric patients. The diuretic is injected slowly over 1–2 min while images are acquired and should have an effect within 30–60 sec. Imaging is continued for approximately 20 min.

Quantitative Renal Studies

Quantitative techniques provide numerical values that indicate the level of tubular and glomerular function. In addition to the renogram curve and serial images, such values are useful in monitoring the course of patients with many different types of renal pathology. Quantitative studies are based on either a blood sampling technique to estimate tracer clearance from the blood or a camera method to determine the amount of tracer accumulated in the kidneys. The advantage of radionuclide techniques over chemical measurements, such as creatinine clearance, is that the function of each kidney (differential function) can be determined.

Effective Renal Plasma Flow

ERPF is a measure of renal tubular function and is performed after the administration of ^{99m}Tc–mertiatide. Renal plasma flow was first measured using a nonradioactive substance, *p*-aminohippuric acid (PAH). The term "effective" is used to describe the measurement of renal plasma flow with mertiatide, because its urinary clearance is slightly different than that of PAH. Several methods have been developed to estimate ERPF. Some require imaging and computer data processing, whereas others also require the collection of blood and urine samples. A normal ERPF value is 500–600 mL/min. However, normal values vary with the patient's age and gender.

Glomerular Filtration Rate

^{99m}Tc–pentetate is commonly used to determine GFR because its renal uptake is proportional to GFR. Measurement of the renal activity before the tracer is excreted into the ureters provides an estimate of the differential GFR of both kidneys. Several methods, using either a single blood sample or imaging with computer data processing, have been developed to determine GFR. A normal GFR value is 125 mL/min. However, the normal value varies with the patient's age and gender.

Renal Imaging with ACE Inhibitors

Renal artery stenosis (RAS) causes a decrease in the kidney's perfusion pressure, which results in a decrease in the afferent arteriole's pressure. This leads to a decline of filtration pressure and decreased GFR. The kidneys are able to compensate for RAS, because the decreased pressure in the afferent arteriole stimulates the juxtaglomerular apparatus to release renin. Renin converts angiotensinogen to angiotensin I. Angiotensin-converting enzyme (ACE) converts angiotensin I to angiotensin II, which causes vasoconstriction of the efferent arteriole, maintains the proper filtration pressure, and restores the GFR.

ACE inhibitors can be administered to assist in the diagnosis of renovascular hypertension resulting from RAS. The kidneys' compensatory mechanisms may cause baseline renograms to appear normal. The administration of ACE inhibitors blocks the conversion of angiotensin I to angiotensin II, resulting in decreased efferent glomerular arteriole vasoconstriction, decreased filtration pressure, and abnormally low GFR. The perfusion to the affected kidney remains the same or increases because of the decreased vascular resistance. After the administration of an ACE inhibitor, renal perfusion may present as normal initial uptake. The initial uptake of GFR agents (^{99m}Tc–pentetate) may be markedly decreased, but decreased GFR results in prolonged retention of either type of renal radiopharmaceutical. A patient who has an abnormal renogram after the administration of an ACE inhibitor has a high likelihood of having renovascular hypertension resulting from RAS.

Patients should discontinue ACE inhibitor therapy for 3–7 days before the study, remain well hydrated (7 mL/kg), and void before the procedure. Baseline sitting and standing blood pressures and heart rate should be recorded before the administration of the ACE inhibitor. The blood pressure and pulse should be monitored every 10–15 min during the infusion. The patient is not released until his or her standing blood pressure returns to at least 70% of the baseline reading. Diuretic medications may enhance the hypotensive effect associated with ACE inhibitor administration. Therefore, patients should discontinue any diuretic medications for several days before the study.

The two most commonly used ACE inhibitors are captopril (Capoten) and enalaprilat (Vasotec IV). The usual dosage of captopril is 25–50 mg orally (the tablets may be crushed and dissolved in 150–200 mL of water to enhance absorption). Adverse effects of captopril include orthostatic hypotension, dizziness, tachycardia, chest pain, rash, and loss of taste. The radiopharmaceutical is administered at 60 min after captopril administration, because this is when peak blood levels of captopril occur after oral ingestion.

The recommended dosage of enalaprilat is 40 μg/kg in 10 mL of normal saline. It is administered via a slow intravenous push over 3–5 min to avoid adverse effects. The establishment of an intravenous line is recommended because of the increased risk of hypotension. A drop in blood pressure is usually observed at 10–15 min, so the renal tracer is injected at least 15 min after the administration of enalaprilat is complete. Adverse effects of enalaprilat include orthostatic hypotension, dizziness, chest pain, headache, dry cough, electrolyte disturbances, fatigue, abdominal pain, vomiting, and diarrhea.

Static Renal Imaging

Acquisition

Delayed static imaging is performed with ^{99m}Tc–succimer (37–222 MBq/1–6 mCi). Static imaging permits the visualization of the renal cortical outline and size, shape, and contour of the kidneys. This is extremely useful in providing an accurate quantification of viable renal parenchyma. Image acquisition begins 2–3 hr after the flow study. The patient is positioned for a posterior projection. Left and right posterior oblique images are obtained as required.

Normal Findings

Normal static images show a smooth renal contour. Both kidneys should have equal amounts of tracer accumulation and uniform tracer distribution (Fig. 13.8).

Abnormal Findings

Abnormal findings include congenital abnormalities, such as horseshoe kidney, ectopic kidneys, and the absence of a kidney. Horseshoe kidneys are located anteriorly in the pelvis and are the result of the failure of the kidneys to separate during fetal development.

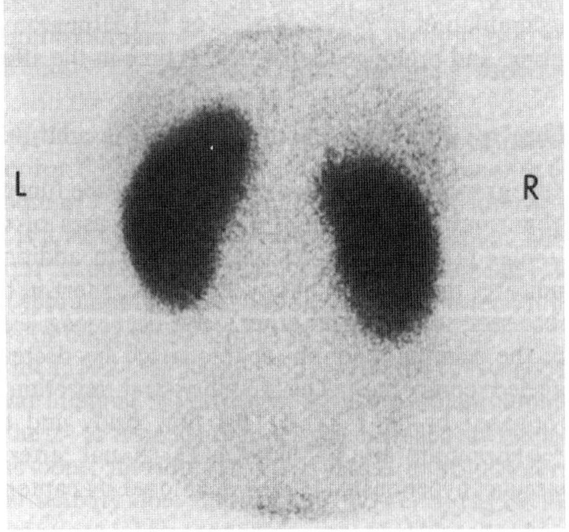

Figure 13.8 Normal ^{99m}Tc–succimer study. (Reprinted, with permission, from Saha, 1998.)

Congenital malformations, such as fetal lobulations and horseshoe kidneys, are easily identified on the images as areas of activity outside the normal renal outline. Areas of increased or decreased activity may represent cysts, neoplasms, infarcts, or renal trauma.

Technical Considerations

If the patient is in severe renal failure, images obtained with succimer may be delayed up to 24 hr to improve visualization of the kidneys. Horseshoe kidneys and pelvic kidneys are located more anteriorly from the normal renal position. If these anomalies are a consideration, an anterior projection may be helpful.

Radionuclide Cystography

Radionuclide cystography is performed for the evaluation of vesicoureteral reflux and is most commonly performed in children. Vesicoureteral reflux may be the result of a congenital malformation of the joining of the ureters to the bladder and results in the flow of urine from the bladder back up into the ureters. This condition is often responsible for recurrent urinary tract infections, which may damage the kidneys.

Acquisition

Two methods are used to perform radionuclide cystography. The indirect method involves intravenous administration of a functional renal agent, such as ^{99m}Tc–pentetate or ^{99m}Tc–mertiatide. After the agent is cleared from the kidneys into the bladder, the patient is asked to void while being imaged. Reflux that occurs during voiding can then be observed.

The more commonly used direct method is performed as follows:

1. Have patient void before the study begins.
2. Catheterize the patient.
3. Connect the catheter to a bottle of normal saline to which 37 MBq (1 mCi) ^{99m}Tc–pertechnetate has been added.
4. Position the patient supine on the imaging table with the upper portion of the bladder in the lower part of the field of view.
5. Obtain multiple sequential images as the bladder is filled with the radioactive saline solution.
6. Discontinue saline infusion when bladder capacity is reached. Obtain a posterior prevoid image that includes the entire bladder and upper urinary tracts.
7. Obtain voiding images with the patient in the seated position and the camera against the patient's back. Remove the catheter and encourage the patient to void into a bed pan or urinal.

8. Obtain a postvoid image that includes the entire bladder and upper urinary tracts.

Image Findings

A normal exam will show increasing activity in the bladder without reflux into the ureters. An abnormal exam will show ureteral reflux, especially during urination (Fig. 13.9). Reflux usually increases as the study progresses, although transient reflux may occur. Certain quantitative information, such as the reflux bladder volume and the volume of reflux into the kidney, can also be calculated.

Technical Considerations

1. Equipment and the surrounding area should be covered with absorbent paper to prevent contamination with radioactive urine.
2. It is important to establish adequate bladder filling before the voiding portion of the exam. An increase in patient discomfort, leakage of urine around the catheter, or cessation of flow from the saline infusion bottle may all indicate sufficient bladder filling. Bladder capacities vary according to age and condition of the bladder.
3. If quantitative results are desired, note that any loss of urine will cause inaccuracies in the calculations.
4. Depending on their age, children may not cooperate when asked to void.
5. Catheterization should be performed by someone who is well trained in the technique to ensure correct placement and to avoid physical or psychological trauma to the child.

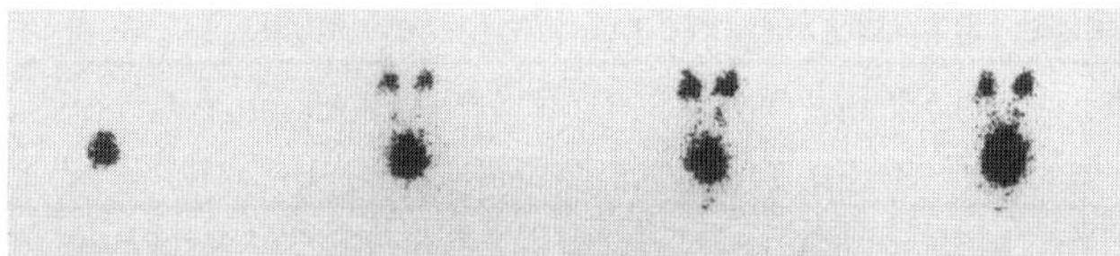

Figure 13.9 Positive radionuclide cystogram shows increase in bilateral vesicoureteral reflux as the bladder is filled. (Courtesy of The Children's Hospital of Alabama, Birmingham, AL.)

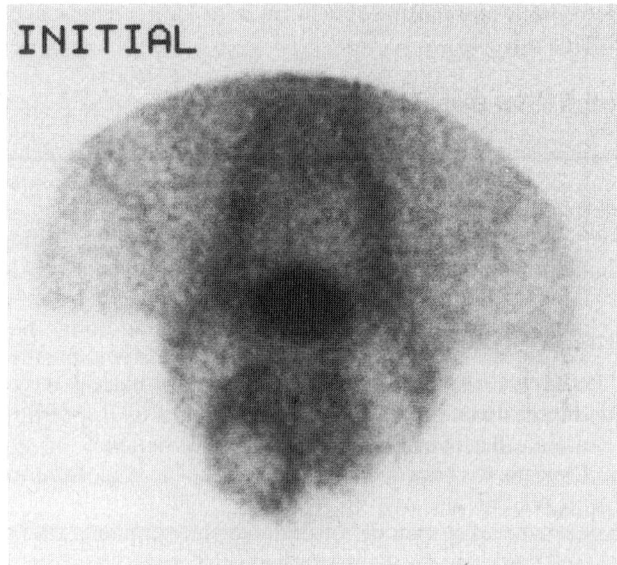

Figure 13.10 Testicular torsion. Scrotal image obtained with ^{99m}Tc–pertechnetate shows decreased activity in the right testicle surrounded by an intense halo of activity. (Courtesy of The Children's Hospital of Alabama, Birmingham, AL.)

Testicular Imaging

Testicular imaging is most often performed to differentiate acute torsion (twisting) of the spermatic cord and epididymitis (inflammation of the epididymis). Torsion of the spermatic cord is often spontaneous and occurs most commonly in young men, with an acute onset of pain. The distinction is important, because torsion requires immediate surgical intervention to prevent necrosis of the affected testicle. Epididymitis is treated with antibiotics.

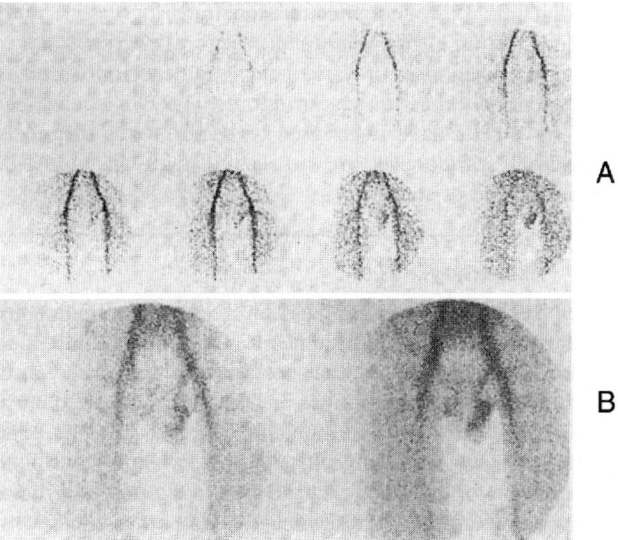

Figure 13.11 Acute epididymitis. Increased perfusion and uptake in the left scrotum. (Reprinted, with permission, from Thrall and Ziessman, 2001, p. 361.)

Acquisition

With the patient in the supine position, the penis is taped to the pubic symphysis. The scrotal sac is supported on towels or a sling to permit close placement to the anteriorly placed camera. The testes should be positioned as symmetrically as possible. With the scrotum positioned in the lower center of the field of view, dynamic images are obtained at 2- to 3-sec intervals after the intravenous injection of 185–555 MBq (5–15 mCi)

Table 13.1 GU Section Procedure Review Table

Nuclear medicine examination	Radiopharmaceutical (generic name)	Route of administration	Imaging time post-tracer administration
Renal tubular binding	2–6 mCi ^{99m}Tc–succimer (DMSA)	IV	2–3 hr
Captopril renography	5–10 mCi ^{99m}Tc–mertiatide; low-dose:high dose is 1 mCi then 10 mCi	IV	Flow-serial images for ~30 min
ERPF	5–10 mCi ^{99m}Tc–mertiatide (MAG_3)	IV	Flow-serial images for ~30 min
GFR	5–15 mCi ^{99m}Tc–pentetate (DTPA)	IV	Flow-serial images for ~30 min
Testicular imaging images may be needed	5–20 mCi ^{99m}Tc–pertechnetate	IV	Flow followed by static images; delay
Radionuclide indirect cystography	3–10 mCi ^{99m}Tc–pentetate or ^{99m}Tc–mertiatide	IV	Flow image while voiding
Radionuclide direct cystography	1 mCi ^{99m}Tc–SC or pertechnetate	Instill via urinary catheter	Flow during filling and voiding

of ^{99m}Tc–pertechnetate. After dynamic imaging, immediate static images are acquired.

Image Findings

The normal flow study demonstrates symmetrical activity distribution. Scrotal perfusion, if seen at all, is of minimal intensity. The static images will show the scrotum and contents to have homogeneous areas of activity of similar intensity to that of the thigh.

Acute torsion will be seen on the dynamic images as normal or absent perfusion of the affected side. The static images will demonstrate an area of absent or decreased activity when compared with that of the opposite testicle or the thigh (Fig. 13.10). Epididymitis is indicated by increased blood flow to the affected side. The static images will also show increased activity (Fig. 13.11).

References and Further Reading

Alazraki NP, Mishkin FS, 1988. *Fundamentals of Nuclear Medicine.* 2nd ed. Reston, VA: Society of Nuclear Medicine; 102–111.

Balon HR, Brill DR, Donohoe KJ, Ganske MA, Machac J, Parker JA, Royal HD, Shulkin BL, Wittry MD, 2001. Society of Nuclear Medicine Guidelines and Communications Committee, Commission on Health Care Policy and Practice. *Society of Nuclear Medicine Procedure Guidelines Manual 2001–2002.* Reston, VA: Society of Nuclear Medicine; 81–86.

Beschi RJ, Dubovsky E, Kontzen FN, 1994. Genitourinary system. In: Bernier DR, Christian PE, Langan JK, eds. *Nuclear Medicine Technology and Techniques.* 3rd ed. St. Louis, MO: Mosby; 335–360.

Datz FL, 1988. *Handbooks in Radiology: Nuclear Medicine.* Chicago, IL: Yearbook Medical Publishers; 185–219.

Nowak TJ, Handford AG, 1999. *Essentials of Pathophysiology: Concepts and Applications for Health Care Professionals.* Boston, MA: McGraw-Hill; 378–403.

Park HM, Duncan K, 1994. Nonradioactive pharmaceuticals in nuclear medicine. *J Nucl Med Technol.* 22:240–249.

Rowell KL, ed. 1992. *Clinical Computers in Nuclear Medicine.* Reston, VA: Society of Nuclear Medicine; 39–50.

Rowell KL, Stutzman ME, Scott JW, 1987. Quantitation of renal function. *J Nucl Med Technol.* 15:146–152.

Royal HD, 1997. Genitourinary system. In: Bernier DR, Christian PE, Langan JK, eds. *Nuclear Medicine Technology and Techniques.* 4th ed. St. Louis, MO: Mosby; 389–406.

Saha G, 1998. *Fundamentals of Nuclear Pharmacy.* 4th ed. New York, NY: Springer-Verlag; 279.

Sfakianakis GN, Georgiou M, Cavagnaro F, Strauss J, Bourgoignie J, 1992. Fast protocols for obstruction (diuretic renography) and for renovascular hypertension (ACE inhibition). *J Nucl Med Technol.* 20:193–206.

Shackett P, 2000. *Nuclear Medicine Technology: Procedures and Quick Reference.* Philadelphia, PA: Lippincott Williams & Wilkins; 217–235, 258–261.

Shier D, Butler J, Lewis R, 2003. *Hole's Essentials of Human Anatomy and Physiology.* 8th ed. New York, NY: McGraw-Hill; 459–479.

Sodee DB, 1995. Special imaging procedures. In: Early PJ, Sodee DB. *Principles and Practice of Nuclear Medicine.* 2nd ed. St. Louis, MO: Mosby; 802–804.

Solomon EP, Phillips GA, 1987. *Understanding Human Anatomy and Physiology.* Philadelphia, PA: W.B. Saunders Company.

Taylor A, Ziffer J, 1995. Urinary tract. In: Early PJ, Sodee DB, eds. *Principles and Practice of Nuclear Medicine.* 2nd ed. St. Louis, MO: Mosby; 579–616.

Thrall JH, Ziessman HA, 2001. *Nuclear Medicine: The Requisites.* 2nd ed. St. Louis, MO: Mosby; 322–362.

Vogel JM, Martin P, 1986. Genitourinary tract scintigraphy. In: Matin P, ed. *Clinical Nuclear Medicine Imaging.* New York, NY: Medical Examination Publishing; 117–140.

Weiss SC, Conway JJ, 1987. Radionuclide cystography. *J Nucl Med Technol.* 15:66–74.

CHAPTER 14 **Respiratory System**

Ann Steves and Norman Bolus

The anatomic relationship of the lungs to other structures in the thoracic cavity is shown in Figure 14.1. The major airways, the bronchi, divide into successively smaller branches, called bronchioles, and terminate with the alveoli (Fig. 14.2). In the alveoli, carbon dioxide and oxygen are exchanged. Each alveolus is surrounded by approximately 1000 capillaries of the pulmonary circulation.

Respiration is the transport of oxygen and carbon dioxide to and from the cells of the body. Four processes are involved in respiration: (a) ventilation, the flow of air into and out of the lungs; (b) gas exchange, the diffusion of oxygen and carbon dioxide between the alveoli and the blood; (c) gas transport, the movement of oxygen and carbon dioxide to and from the cells through the circulation; and (d) regulation of ventilation. In the healthy lung, ventilation and perfusion (blood flow) are matched for efficient and complete exchange of oxygen and carbon dioxide. Pulmonary disease upsets this balance.

The most common clinical indication for lung imaging is evaluation of pulmonary emboli (PE), including initial screening to rule out PE or follow-up imaging to evaluate response to therapy. Diagnosing a PE is the primary use of radionuclide lung imaging. The technique is used less frequently for preoperative evaluations and evaluations of lung transplant and right-to-left cardiac shunts.

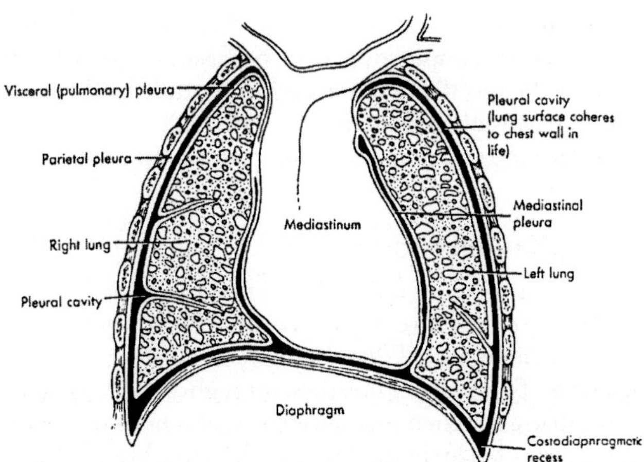

Figure 14.1 Mediastinum (heart, its great vessels, trachea, and bronchi have been removed). (Reprinted, with permission, from McClintic, 1983, p. 412.)

Perfusion Imaging

Perfusion imaging is used to demonstrate blood flow to the lungs. Technetium-99m (^{99m}Tc)–macroaggregated albumin (MAA) particles are injected intravenously and are trapped in the vasculature of the lungs. The majority of these particles are 10–90 μm in diameter and, thus, will block arterioles of this size within the lung. Areas of the lung in which perfusion is decreased or absent will receive little or no tracer. The number of arterioles that are blocked with tracer depends on the number of particles injected. An adult patient should receive 200,000–700,000 tracer particles, which will occlude less than 1% of the lung arterioles but provide uniform tracer distribution. Patients with pulmonary hypertension or right-to-left cardiac shunts should receive fewer particles (100,000–200,000 particles is the recommended dosage in these instances). Likewise, the number of particles should be reduced for pediatric patients (the number of particles is dependent on the age of the child).

Clinical Procedure

Relevant medical history includes the following:

1. Factors predisposing the patient to PE: recent surgery, cancer, chronic obstructive pulmonary

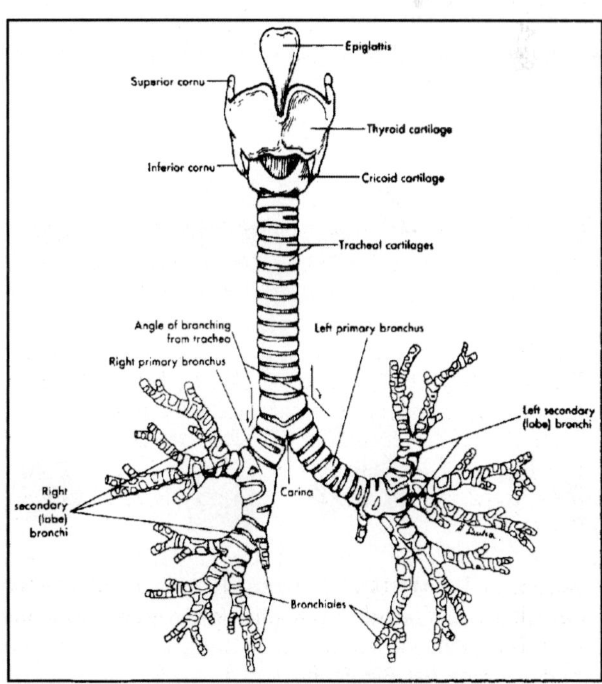

Figure 14.2 Larynx, trachea, and bronchi. (Reprinted, with permission, from McClintic, 1983, p. 411.)

disease, immobility, obesity, or prior history of PE (including previous anticoagulant or thrombolytic therapy).
2. Symptoms of PE: shortness of breath, chest pain, fever, cough, syncope, tachycardia, jugular venous distension, or hemoptysis. These signs and symptoms are not specific to PE and can occur in a variety of conditions.
3. Other clinical history: right-to-left cardiac shunt, pulmonary hypertension, medications.
4. Recent chest radiograph findings: chest radiograph findings are needed for interpretation of the lung images. Because the symptoms of PE are common to many other conditions, it is necessary to rule out other pathology that may mimic PE or obscure its diagnosis. The chest radiograph should be obtained within 24 hr of imaging or within 1 hr for patients whose signs and symptoms have changed.
5. Results of diagnostic tests for deep vein thrombosis (DVT).

Imaging

The patient should be placed in the supine position for injection of the radiopharmaceutical. When the patient is supine, the effect of gravity, which hinders blood flow to the lung apices, is minimized, allowing uniform tracer distribution throughout the lung. ^{99m}Tc–MAA (1–4 mCi/37–148 megabecquerels [MBq]) is administered intravenously.

Imaging can begin immediately after tracer administration. Static images are acquired for the following anatomic views: anterior, posterior, laterals, and posterior or anterior obliques (see Fig. 14.3 for all eight views associated with imaging the lungs).

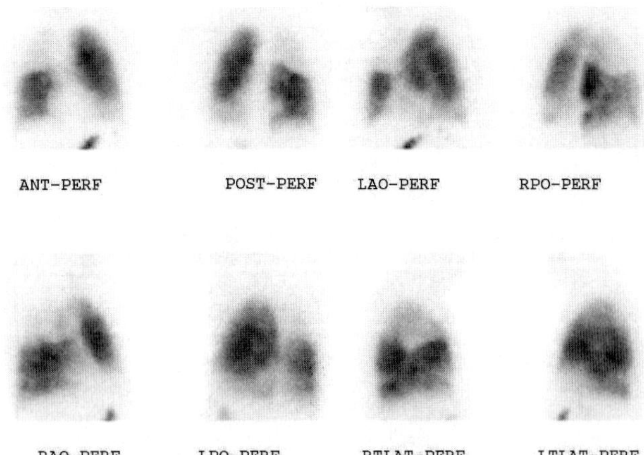

Figure 14.3 Low-probability lung perfusion scan showing all eight views of the lungs. (Courtesy of University of Alabama at Birmingham Hospital, Birmingham, AL.)

Image Findings

The radiopharmaceutical is normally distributed evenly throughout the lungs. Because the lung apices are thinner than the lower portions of the lungs, tracer distribution may appear to be somewhat decreased at the apices. The cardiac impression may be seen on the anterior and left lateral views. Decreased areas of tracer uptake indicate a disruption of blood flow, which can be the result of a variety of conditions.

Technical Considerations

Common technical errors associated with perfusion imaging include the following:

1. Extravasation of the tracer at the injection site, which may cause an insufficient number of particles to be delivered to the lungs, resulting in nonuniformities not related to pathology in the lungs.
2. Small blood clots in the syringe, formed when blood is withdrawn into the syringe and allowed to stand for a period of time. When these clots are injected into the patient, they may result in hot spots on the images (again, not related to pathology).
3. Failure to remove attenuating objects, such as jewelry and electrocardiographic leads, which results in cold-spot artifacts on images.
4. Tracer administration with the patient in an upright position, which causes decreased tracer concentration in the lung apices.

Ventilation Imaging

Ventilation imaging demonstrates the flow of air into and out of the lungs. Whereas perfusion imaging is very sensitive for detecting changes in blood flow, it is unable to specify the cause of the change. Ventilation imaging, performed in conjunction with perfusion imaging, can increase the specificity of the perfusion study by differentiating perfusion defects that are the result of a PE from those that are associated with obstructive lung disease.

Radiopharmaceuticals

Ventilation imaging may be performed with xenon-133 (^{133}Xe), a radioactive inert gas, or with an aerosol of ^{99m}Tc–pentetate (DTPA). Both are administered by inhalation. The patient breathes through a face mask or mouthpiece attached to a spirometry system to inhale radioxenon, or a nebulizer to inhale aerosolized ^{99m}Tc–pentetate.

Clinical Procedure

Relevant medical history includes the same items obtained for perfusion imaging. The procedure should be reviewed thoroughly with the patient to elicit full cooperation. The administration apparatus should be placed on the patient for a practice run before the tracer is inhaled. If radioactive gas is used as the tracer, the patient should be positioned before administration. The patient may be placed in a supine or upright position, whichever is more comfortable.

Imaging

^{133}Xe

The standard view is the posterior, because more lung area is exposed in this projection. Other views, however, may be appropriate when a specific segment of the lung is of interest and would be better visualized with a different projection. The following images are obtained: single breath, acquired during initial inhalation of the gas; wash-in or equilibrium, collected while the xenon distributes throughout the aerated portions of the lungs; and washout, taken while the radioactivity is cleared from the lungs. The length of time for which equilibrium and washout images are obtained varies from department to department.

^{99m}Tc–Pentetate Aerosol

The tracer is injected into a nebulizer to generate the aerosol particles. ^{99m}Tc–pentetate (925–1295 MBq/25–35 mCi) placed in the nebulizer will deliver 18.5–37 MBq (0.5–1 mCi) of activity to the patient. After a single 5-min inhalation of the aerosolized tracer, multiple projections matching those of the perfusion study can be obtained. Single-breath or washout images are not possible.

Image Findings

Radioxenon is normally distributed uniformly throughout both lungs, with no retention of tracer during the washout phase. Retention of the xenon after 2–3 min of the washout phase may indicate obstructive lung disease.

Normal aerosol images demonstrate symmetric deposition of the tracer from the apex to the base of both lungs. Segments of the lungs that are not ventilated will show decreased or absent tracer activity (Fig 14.4).

Technical Considerations

In performing ventilation imaging, the following technical points should be considered. Certain patients may not be able to tolerate an oxygen mask, mouthpiece, or nose clips. They may attempt to remove the apparatus during the procedure, allowing xenon to escape into the room. Patients who have difficulty holding a mouthpiece tightly may cause the same problem. Trapping equipment is necessary to contain xenon exhaled by the patient to prevent unnecessary radiation exposure to personnel. The equipment should be checked periodically to ensure that there are no leaks in the closed system and that the charcoal filter has not become saturated with xenon, thereby decreasing its trapping effectiveness.

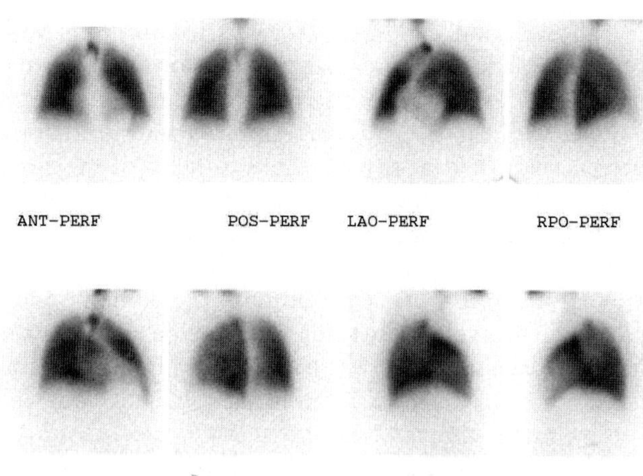

Figure 14.4 Normal ventilation images obtained with aerosol DTPA. (Courtesy of University of Alabama at Birmingham Hospital, Birmingham, AL.)

A room in which xenon ventilation imaging is performed should be equipped with a ventilation system that maintains negative pressure within the room. The system should be activated when xenon is in use to contain the gas inside the room should a leak occur.

When performing aerosol imaging, it is important to maintain the correct oxygen flow rate through the nebulizer. Improper flow rate may affect particle size. Particles that are too large will lodge in the central airways instead of being carried throughout the lungs. Also, significant contamination of the patient's nose and mouth, upper chest, and the floor under the nebulizer may occur during the performance of aerosol studies. Some studies have shown that allowing the patient to practice breathing from the nebulizer before introduction of the tracer and coaching the patient throughout the study decrease the amount of contamination.

Combined Ventilation/Perfusion Imaging

If perfusion imaging is performed first and the results are normal, ventilation imaging may not be necessary. This may be a particularly useful technique if a lung V/Q is requested on a pregnant patient as a way to decrease overall radiation exposure. However, performing both ventilation and perfusion examinations on the same patient at the same time permits the physician to determine whether perfusion defects are associated with ventilation defects, which may increase the specificity of the findings. In cases in which both examinations are required, the following procedures are recommended.

When ^{99m}Tc–pentetate and ^{99m}Tc–MAA imaging are performed together, the aerosol study should be completed first, because less activity will be delivered to the lungs. The count rate of the perfusion study should be at least four times greater than that obtained from the aerosol study. This can be achieved if a smaller amount of ^{99m}Tc–pentetate (e.g., 1 mCi) is administered.

When ^{133}Xe and ^{99m}Tc–MAA imaging are performed together, completing the xenon ventilation first is the better option from a technical point of view. If the perfusion images are performed first, a ^{99m}Tc background image must be obtained in the ^{133}Xe photopeak window.

Lung Quantitation

Quantitation of blood flow to the lungs may be used to assess the status of patients before lung resection or to monitor resolution of PEs. Normally, 55% of the pulmonary arterial blood flow is to the right lung and 45% to the left. By drawing one or more regions of interest around each lung in the posterior view of a perfusion image, one can determine the percentage of tracer uptake in each lung. Other calculations may also relate the percentage tracer uptake and the results of the patient's pulmonary function test to predict the expiratory volume of each lung after surgery (Fig. 14.5).

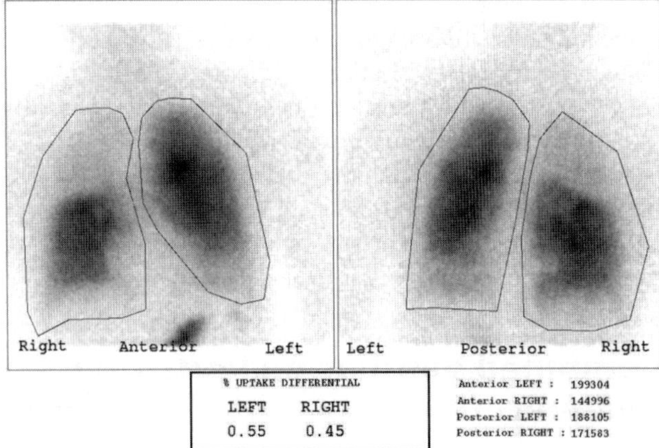

Figure 14.5 Example of lung quantification with percentage uptake of right vs. left lung. (Courtesy of University of Alabama at Birmingham Hospital, Birmingham, AL.)

Radionuclide Venography

Radionuclide venography performed with ^{99m}Tc–MAA or ^{99m}Tc–RBCs is used to image acute DVT in the lower extremities. DVT of the lower extremities may lead to a PE. Immobility, surgery, certain medications, obesity, cancer, congestive heart failure, and recent myocardial infarction predispose patients to developing thrombophlebitis and DVT.

Relevant history includes:

1. location/duration of edema, warmth, redness, or pain in the lower extremities,
2. prior history of DVT,
3. presence of factors that increase the risk of DVT,
4. presence of arthritis, cellulitis, or varicose veins,
5. results of other diagnostic tests, specifically, ultrasound of the lower extremities and D-dimer assay (a by-product of blood clot degradation).

No special patient preparation is required. Approximately 222 MBq (6 mCi) of ^{99m}Tc–MAA or approximately 740–1,110 MBq (20–30 mCi) of ^{99m}Tc–RBCs are injected intravenously. Imaging of the anterior and posterior pelvis, thighs, knees, and calves is performed at 10 min and 60–90 min after injection. Areas of increased concentration are indicators of possible DVT. Increased tracer uptake may also occur in recent surgical sites and in collateral and superficial veins.

References and Further Reading

Alazraki NP, Mishkin FS, 1988. *Fundamentals of Nuclear Medicine.* 2nd ed. Reston, VA: Society of Nuclear Medicine; 68–72.

Caretta RF, Vande Streek P, Weiland FL, 1999. Optimizing images of acute deep-vein thrombosis using technetium-99m apcitide. *J Nucl Med Technol.* 27:271–275.

Crawford ES, Quain BC, Zaken AM, 1992. Air and surface contamination resulting from lung ventilation aerosol procedures. *J Nucl Med Technol.* 20:151–154.

Gilworth DL, Donovan BC, Morrison R, Ryan K, Reagan K, Goldhaber SZ, 1988. Patient management of pulmonary embolism. *J Nucl Med Technol.* 16:33–36.

Hanson PC, 1987. Ventilation scintigraphy. *J Nucl Med Technol.* 15:193–197.

Ikehira H, Kinjo M, Yamamoto Y, Makino H, Furuichi Y, Nakamura H, Aoki T, 1999. Hot spots observed on pulmonary perfusion imaging: a case report. *J Nucl Med Technol.* 27:301–302.

McClintic JR, 1983. *Human Anatomy.* St. Louis, MO: Mosby.

McGraw RS, Culver CM, Juni JE, Schane SC, Nagle CE, 1992. Lung ventilation studies: surface contamination associated with technetium-99m-DTPA aerosol. *J Nucl Med Technol.* 20:228–230.

Mettler FA, Guiberteau MJ, 1991. *Essentials of Nuclear Medicine Imaging.* 3rd ed. Philadelphia, PA: WB Saunders; 141–176.

Palla A, Tumeh SS, Giuntini C, 1995. Lung. In: Early PJ, Sodee DB, eds. *Principles and Practice of Nuclear Medicine.* 2nd ed. St. Louis, MO: Mosby; 443–475.

Parker JA, Coleman RE, Hilson AJW, Royal HD, Siegel BA, Sostman HD, 2004. Procedure guideline for lung scintigraphy 3.0. *Society of Nuclear Medicine Procedure Guidelines.* Reston, VA: Society of Nuclear Medicine.

Phegley DJ, Secker-Walker RH, 1997. Respiratory system. In: Bernier DR, Christian PE, Langan JK, eds. *Nuclear Medicine Technology and Techniques.* 4th ed. St. Louis, MO: Mosby; 303–322.

Schuster K, Peterson J, Sirr S, Stuart DD, 1987. Quality control in the production of radioaerosols [letter]. *J Nucl Med Technol.* 15:97.

Wagner HN Jr., 1995. Regional ventilation and perfusion. In: Wagner HN Jr., Szabo Z, Buchanan JW, eds. *Principles of Nuclear Medicine.* 2nd ed. Philadelphia, PA: WB Saunders; 893–894.

Williams DA, Carlson C, McEnerney K, Hope E, Hoh CK, 1998. Technetium-99m DTPA aerosol contamination in lung ventilation studies. *J Nucl Med Technol.* 26:43–44.

CHAPTER 15 **Skeletal System**

Ann Steves and Norman Bolus

Bone imaging is one of the most commonly ordered procedures in nuclear medicine. Standard clinical indications for performing bone imaging include the following:

1. Staging of malignant disease: screening of patients with primary tumors (e.g., breast, lung, prostate carcinoma) known to metastasize readily to bone, evaluation of response to therapy, localization of biopsy sites
2. Evaluation of primary bone neoplasms (e.g., Ewing sarcoma, osteogenic sarcoma): detection of sites in other bones, detection of soft-tissue metastases
3. Diagnosis of skeletal inflammatory disease (e.g., osteomyelitis)
4. Evaluation of skeletal pain of unknown cause
5. Determination of bone viability when blood supply to the area is in question
6. Detection of occult fractures (e.g., sports injury) not demonstrated radiographically

All of these indications are important reasons for performing bone imaging. However, staging and assessment of treatment for malignant disease is the most frequent.

Technetium-99m (^{99m}Tc)–medronate (MDP) and ^{99m}Tc–oxidronate (HDP) are currently the two radiopharmaceuticals of choice. Medronate has been shown to have a faster blood clearance than other labeled phosphate compounds, and oxidronate has greater bone uptake. Approximately 50% of the administered tracer is concentrated in bony tissue. The other 50% is excreted from the body through the kidneys.

Localization of these tracers in the bone is dependent on blood flow and the rate of bone production or remodeling. Blood flow is required to carry the radiopharmaceutical to the bone, where an exchange between ions in the bone crystal and the tracer takes place. Hydroxyapatite, with a chemical makeup of $Ca_{10}(PO_4)(OH)_2$, is the inorganic compound forming crystal structures within bone. Although the mechanism is not completely understood, it is believed that the phosphorus groups of the tracer exchange onto the calcium of the hydroxyapatite crystal.

Throughout life, bone is constantly being destroyed and replaced with new bone, a process called bone remodeling. Hence, bone tracers are concentrated to some extent in even normal skeletal tissue. Any process that increases osteoblastic (bone formation) activity causes increased tracer uptake. Conversely, areas of osteolytic (bone destruction) activity are visualized as areas of decreased tracer activity.

A thorough knowledge of the gross anatomy of the skeletal system is essential for the technologist. Figures 15.1 and 15.2 illustrate the more important skeletal structures visualized during bone imaging, but the reader is encouraged to review other more comprehensive anatomy texts.

Clinical Procedure

Patient History

Relevant medical history should include patient's diagnosis, if known; recent injuries and/or surgeries; previous injuries to bones; medications (certain medications may

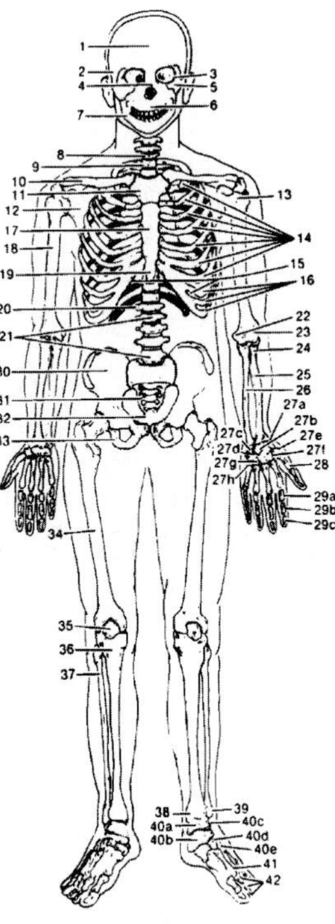

1. Frontal bone
2. Temporal bone
3. Orbit
4. Nasal bone
5. Zygomatic bone
6. Maxilla
7. Mandible
8. Seventh cervical vertebra
9. Thoracic vertebra I
10. Clavicle
11. Manubrium of sternum
12. Scapula
13. Head of humerus
14. True ribs
15. Kidneys
16. False ribs
17. Body of sternum
18. Humerus
19. Xiphoid process
20. Transverse process
21. Lumbar vertebrae
22. Medial condyle of humerus
23. Lateral epicondyle of humerus
24. Capitulum of radius
25. Radius
26. Ulna
27. Carpal bones
    a. Scaphoid bone of hand
    b. Lunate bone
    c. Triangular bone
    d. Pisiform bone
    e. Trapezium
    f. Trapezoid
    g. Capitate bone
    h. Hamate bone
28. Metacarpal bones
29. Phalanges
    a. Proximal phalanx
    b. Middle phalanx
    c. Distal phalanx
30. Iliac bone
31. Sacrum
32. Bladder
33. Ischium
34. Femur
35. Patella
36. Tibia
37. Fibula
38. Medial malleolus
39. Lateral malleolus
40. Tarsal bones
    a. Talus
    b. Navicular bone
    c. Calcaneus
    d. Cuneiform bones
41. Metatarsal bones
42. Phalanges of toes

Figure 15.1 Anterior skeleton. (Reprinted, with permission, from Early, 1985, p. 571.)

alter tracer distribution); location, duration, and frequency of pain (if patient is experiencing pain); serum alkaline phosphatase level (alkaline phosphatase is an enzyme involved in the calcification of bone and the serum level may be elevated in certain diseases of bone); prostate-specific antigen level in patients with prostate cancer; and therapy that may affect results (e.g., radiation therapy, chemotherapy, iron therapy).

Patient Preparation

1. Explain the reason for the delay between tracer administration and imaging.
2. Administer 740–1110 megabecquerels (MBq) (20–30 mCi) ^{99m}Tc-labeled phosphate compound intravenously. If a flow study is requested, position patient under the scintillation camera before tracer administration.

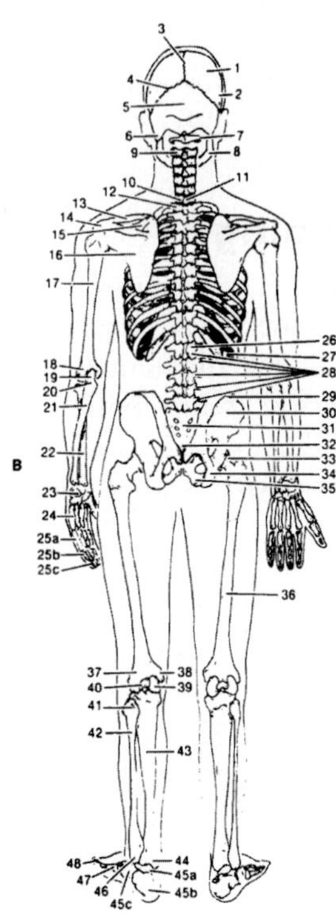

1. Parietal bone
2. Temporal bone
3. Sagittal suture
4. Lambdoidal suture
5. Occipital bone
6. Mastoid process
7. Atlas
8. Mandible
9. Axis or second cervical vertebra
10. Seventh cervical vertebra
11. Spinous process
12. Thoracic vertebra I
13. Clavicle
14. Acromion
15. Spine of scapula
16. Scapula
17. Humerus
18. Lateral epicondyle of humer
19. Olecranon
20. Head of radius
21. Ulna
22. Radius
23. Carpal bones
24. Metacarpal bones
25. Phalanges
    a. Proximal phalanx
    b. Middle phalanx
    c. Distal phalanx
26. Transverse process
27. Kidneys
28. Lumbar vertebrae
29. Iliac crest
30. Upper part of ilium
31. Sacrum
32. Bladder
33. Head of femur
34. Ischium
35. Pubic bone
36. Femur
37. Lateral epicondyle of femur
38. Medial epicondyle of femur
39. Medial condyle of femur
40. Lateral condyle of femur
41. Head of fibula
42. Fibula
43. Tibia
44. Medial malleolus
45. Tarsal bones
    a. Talus
    b. Calcaneus
    c. Cuboid bone
46. Lateral malleolus
47. Metatarsal bones
48. Phalanges of toes

Figure 15.2 Posterior skeleton. (Reprinted, with permission, from Early, 1985, p. 572.)

3. Unless contraindicated, encourage the patient to drink two or more 8-ounce glasses of water and to void frequently during the delay before imaging. Hydration of the patient helps clear the tracer from the body. Frequent voiding decreases the bladder's exposure to radiation.
4. The patient should void immediately before imaging. A large amount of radioactive urine in the bladder can obscure bony structures of the pelvis.

Imaging

1. Imaging can begin 2 hr after tracer administration.
2. Ascertain that patient has voided before proceeding with imaging.
3. Set camera controls (photopeak energy, percentage window, etc.).
4. Place the patient in a supine or prone position, whichever is better tolerated. The patient–detector distance should be minimized for each view.
5. Use the spot-image technique, whole-body technique, or single-photon emission computed tomography (SPECT) imaging to acquire data.

Spot-Image Technique

Depending on the size of the field of view, 10–30 separate spot images may be required to image the entire skeleton. A medium- or high-resolution, parallel-hole, or diverging-hole collimator can be used. An anterior or posterior view of the chest is imaged for a preset number of counts.

Adequate counting statistics must be achieved; 500,000–1,000,000 counts are recommended. All subsequent images are collected for the same time interval. Because all images are collected for the same length of time, the film density in one image can be compared with that of another. For each image, the distance between the patient and the surface of the detector should be minimized to obtain the best possible spatial resolution.

Whole-Body Technique

A miniaturized image of the total skeleton is attained with a device that moves either the camera detector or the patient through the scintillation camera's field of view. Depending on the size of the field of view and the type of collimator used, one to three passes are required to cover the width of the patient's body. A high-resolution, low-energy all purpose (LEAP) parallel-hole or special type of diverging collimator specifically designed for this application can be used. The speed at which the detector travels over the patient depends on the count rate obtained from the anterior or posterior chest. The same scanning speed is used for both anterior and posterior images. Each view of the total-body scan should contain more than 1.5 million counts. Again, the detector should be as close to the patient as possible for optimum spatial resolution.

SPECT Imaging

The use of SPECT for bone imaging is a specialized type of spot imaging. SPECT is not appropriate for total-body imaging but can be very useful for imaging limited areas of the skeleton where bony structures are superimposed on one another. These areas include the knees, hips, lumbar spine, and facial bones. Abnormalities not seen on planar imaging are frequently demonstrated with SPECT imaging. A low-energy, all-purpose, parallel-hole collimator is recommended. The detector–patient distance should be minimized. This distance will vary, depending on the area of the body being imaged, because the detector must be able to travel around the patient, unimpeded, for 360°.

Image Findings

Normal Tracer Distribution

The radiopharmaceutical is normally taken up symmetrically throughout the skeleton (Fig. 15.3). Areas of normally increased activity include the sacroiliac joints, anterior iliac crests, sternum, nasopharyngeal area, shoulder joints, and spine. In children, increased tracer concentration at epiphyseal plates of the long bones and costochondral junctions is the result of increased bone production (Fig. 15.4). Conversely, overall skeletal uptake in the elderly is lower than in younger people. Activity in the kidneys is usually less than bone activity but can vary and may even indicate certain types of renal disease. Tracer accumulation can also occur in normal female breast tissue, as well as in certain diseases of the breast.

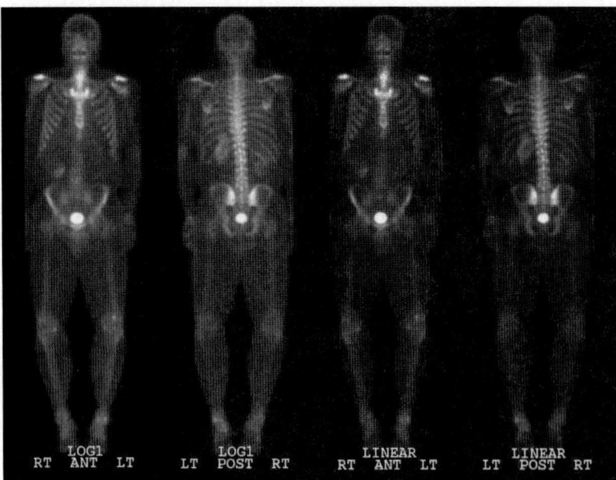

Figure 15.3 Normal adult bone image obtained with ^{99m}Tc–medronate also showing a right renal mass. (Courtesy of University of Alabama at Birmingham Hospital, Birmingham, AL.)

Abnormal Tracer Distribution

Abnormal tracer distribution can include areas of increased tracer accumulation within the skeleton itself or outside in soft tissue. Increased blood flow and/or bone production are responsible for increased tracer concentration and can occur in neoplastic disease, both primary and metastatic; bone trauma; inflammatory processes (e.g., osteomyelitis); metabolic bone disease (e.g., Paget's disease); and arthritic changes.

Extraosseous activity is sometimes seen in renal abnormalities, soft-tissue inflammation (e.g., surgical sites), neoplastic masses, female breasts, and acute myocardial infarction.

Photopenic areas (areas of decreased tracer accumulation) are usually related to diminished blood flow to the area or to complete destruction or replacement of normal bone tissue. The following conditions may result in photopenic areas on images: radiation injury as a result of therapy, bone cyst, disuse atrophy of an extremity, avascular necrosis, and artifacts (e.g., pacemaker, prosthesis).

Multiphase Bone Imaging

When an inflammatory process, such as osteomyelitis, is suspected, dynamic or multiple-phase bone imaging may be helpful to the physician in making a differential diagnosis. In this technique, the patient is first positioned under the gamma camera with the affected area in the field of view. The standard tracer dosage is administered as a bolus injection while dynamic images to assess blood flow are acquired, beginning at the time of injection and continuing for about 1 min (first phase, Fig. 15.5). Immediate static images of the blood pool are then acquired within 10 min of tracer administration (second phase, Fig. 15.6), followed by delayed images at 2–4 hr (third

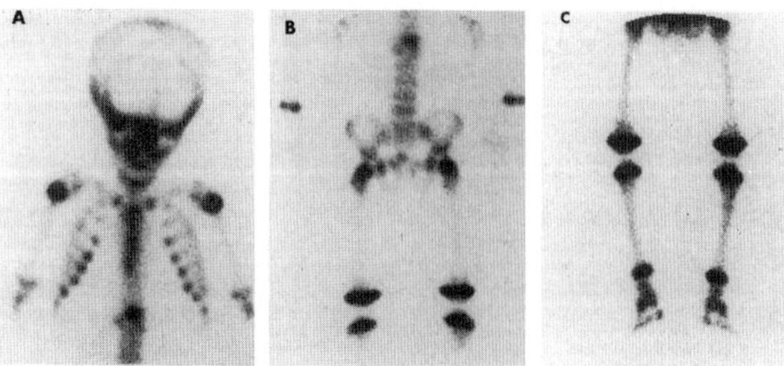

Figure 15.4 Total-body pediatric image. Note areas of normally increased tracer accumulation in children in the epiphyseal plates and costochondral junctions. (Courtesy of The Children's Hospital of Alabama, Birmingham, AL.)

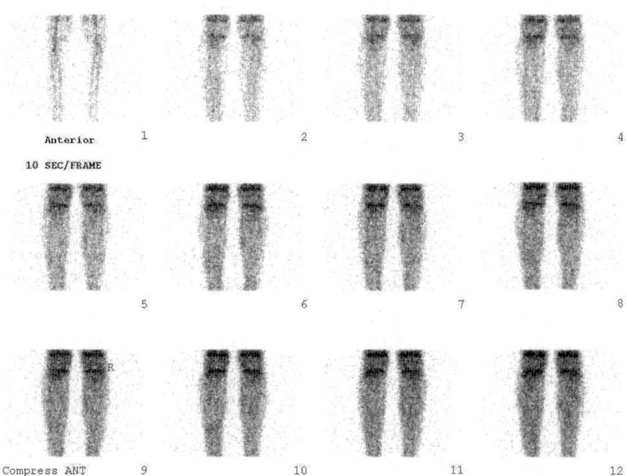

Figure 15.5 First-phase pediatric stress fracture flow study. (Courtesy of University of Alabama at Birmingham Hospital, Birmingham, AL.)

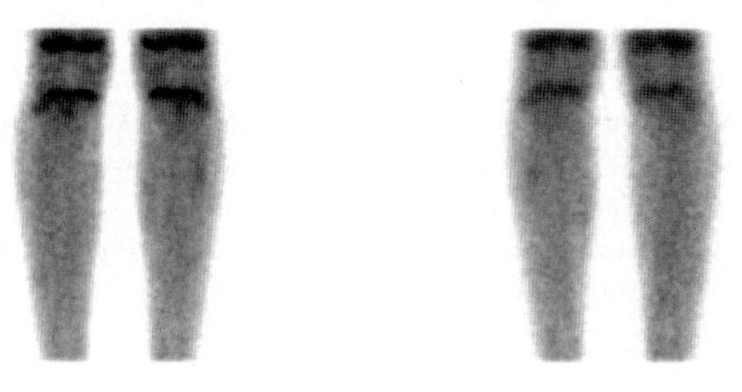

Figure 15.6 Second-phase pediatric stress fracture, immediate static images. (Courtesy of University of Alabama at Birmingham Hospital, Birmingham, AL.)

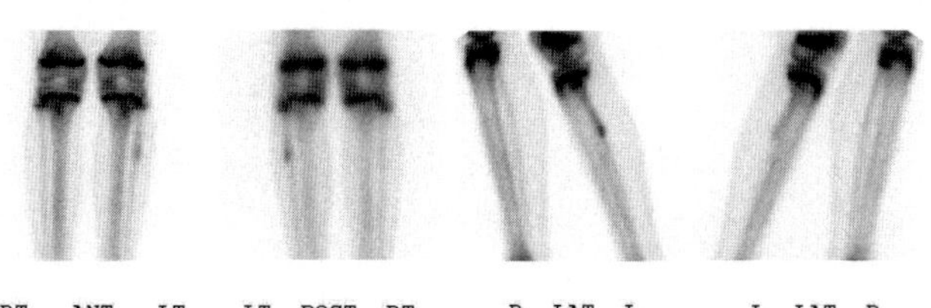

Figure 15.7 Third-phase pediatric stress fracture upper left tibia. (Courtesy of University of Alabama at Birmingham Hospital, Birmingham, AL.)

phase, Fig. 15.7). Additional delayed images may be necessary at 24 hr after injection (sometimes referred to as fourth phase).

Both cellulitis and osteomyelitis demonstrate increased activity on the early images. With osteomyelitis, however, the tracer concentration persists throughout the delayed images.

Technical Considerations

Although bone imaging is one of the simplest and most frequently performed nuclear medicine imaging procedures, technical errors sometimes occur. These errors, discussed here, result in a variety of image artifacts.

Extravasation of the tracer at the injection site may be construed as pathology or obscure bony pathology underlying the area of infiltration. Additional images of the affected area may be helpful in confirming the cause of the increased accumulation and in ruling out skeletal disease. Considerations should be made to do oblique or lateral views to determine depth if not doing SPECT imaging. Furthermore, there may appear to be overall decreased activity concentration in the bones if a significant amount of the tracer is not administered intravenously. Imaging times may be extended in such instances to achieve adequate counting statistics.

Because the tracer is excreted from the body through the urinary tract, radioactive urine contamination is possible with young children or incontinent patients. Equipment should be protected, and the patient should be checked for contaminated garments or linens before imaging begins.

It is important that patients void immediately before imaging the pelvis. Excess activity in the bladder can obscure pelvic structures. Images of the pelvis should be obtained first if the spot-view technique is being used. Separate spot images of the pelvis may be necessary when whole-body imaging is performed.

Any attenuating materials, such as jewelry, belt buckles, various body piercings, removable prostheses, pocket contents, or metallic electrocardiographic leads, could cause a photopenic area on the image. The patient should remove these attenuating materials before imaging.

Close attention to precise patient positioning is essential. Contralateral sides of bony structures (e.g., iliac crests, shoulder joints) must be positioned at the same angle and at the same distance from the detector. Failure to do so may cause one side to appear to have a greater tracer concentration than the other. Asymmetry of contralateral sides may be falsely interpreted as an abnormality. It is equally important to include all areas of interest on the bone images. A problem sometimes arises when certain parts of the skeleton, usually the arms, cannot be positioned within the field of view during whole-body imaging. Greater care should be taken to include the entire skeleton in the field of view, or additional spot images of the excluded parts of the skeleton should be obtained to avoid missing any abnormalities.

When imaging pathology associated with the extremities, such as a hand or foot, care should be taken to image both in the same frame if possible. Sometimes this is done by putting the extremities (feet or hands) both directly on the camera head. In such situations, often an external marker is used to identify left from right. If used, the marker should be used on the side that does not have pathology so that there is no concern of the marker interfering with the view of the pathology.

An unexpected pattern of tracer distribution may indicate improper preparation of the radiopharmaceutical and can degrade the quality of bone images. Excess free pertechnetate appears as tracer concentration in the thyroid, salivary glands, and stomach. Liver uptake or increased soft-tissue and kidney uptake can also be indicators of radiopharmaceutical problems. Adequate and timely radiopharmaceutical quality control is necessary to identify formulation problems before the preparation is administered to patients (see Chapter 3).

^{18}F–Sodium Fluoride (NaF)

^{18}F–Sodium fluoride (NaF) positron emitting tomography (PET) imaging is used to provide physiologic information about bone. ^{18}F-NaF bone scans are very sensitive to bone metastatic disease for both osteoblastic and osteolytic cancers. With ^{18}F-NaF, bone metastases are seen at sites of high bone turnover and remoldeling, and it is therefore used to detect and follow up on bone metastases.

References and Further Reading

Anaheim Nuclear CT/PET Imaging Center. Retrieved from http://anaheimctpet.com/bonescans.html March 9, 2011.

Christian PE, Coleman RE, 1997. Skeletal system. In: Bernier DR, Christian PE, Langan JK, eds. *Nuclear Medicine Technology and Techniques.* 4th ed. St. Louis, MO: Mosby; 407–432.

Collier BD, Sodee DB, Robinson RG, 1995. Bone. In: Early PJ, Sodee DB, eds. *Principles and Practice of Nuclear Medicine.* 2nd ed. St. Louis, MO: Mosby; 339–369.

Donohoe KJ, Brown ML, Collier BD, Carretta RF, Henkin RE, O'Mara RE, Royal HD, 2003. Society of Nuclear Medicine Procedure Guideline for Bone Scintigraphy 3.0. In: *Society of Nuclear Medicine Procedure Guidelines.* Reston, VA: Society of Nuclear Medicine.

Early PJ, Sodee DB, 1985. *Principles and Practice of Nuclear Medicine.* 2nd ed. St. Louis, MO: Mosby.

English RJ, 1995. *SPECT: A Primer.* 3rd ed. Reston, VA: Society of Nuclear Medicine; 123–126, 168–171, 177–178.

Hladik WB III, Saha GB, Study KT, eds., 1987. *Essentials of Nuclear Medicine Science.* Baltimore, MD: Williams and Wilkins.

Nagle CE, Morayati SJ, Carichner S, Winkes B, Cassisi R, McGraw R, Schane E, 1988. The whole-body bone scan?: case report. *J Nucl Med Technol.* 16:15–16.

Thrall JH, Ziessman HA, 1995. *Nuclear medicine: The Requisites.* St. Louis, MO: Mosby; 93–128.

CHAPTER 16 **Infection/Inflammation Imaging**

Ann Steves

Gallium-67 (^{67}Ga)–citrate, which is recommended for chronic cases, and white blood cells labeled with indium-111 (^{111}In) or technetium-99m (^{99m}Tc), which are recommended for acute cases, are tracers used to visualize areas of inflammation and infection.

Gallium Imaging

^{67}Ga–citrate has been used to image both neoplastic and inflammatory diseases. Although a variety of processes have been suggested, the exact mechanism by which gallium concentrates in tumor or infection sites is not known. In the case of inflammatory processes, common clinical indications for gallium imaging include the following:

1. localization of sources of fever of unknown origin,
2. diagnosis of osteomyelitis,
3. detection of lung infections in immunocompromised patients,
4. evaluation and monitoring of inflammatory processes, such as sarcoidosis.

Clinical Procedure

No special preparation is needed before administration of ^{67}Ga–citrate. Knowledge of the clinical indication for a specific study will assist the technologist in determining the areas of interest to be imaged. The amount of ^{67}Ga–citrate administered ranges from 148 to 222 megabecquerels (MBq) (4–6 mCi), depending on the pathology being imaged. In very large patients, up to 333 MBq (9 mCi) may be administered.

Imaging is performed 4–72 hr after intravenous injection of the tracer. Earlier imaging times are indicated when imaging the abdomen, so that bowel activity will be at a minimum. Planar or tomographic techniques may be performed.

^{67}Ga has a range of photon energies (93, 184, 296, and 388 keV), so an appropriate choice of collimator is critical to minimize scatter and septal penetration and to obtain optimal resolution. Depending on the individual collimator rating, a medium- or high-energy parallel-hole collimator typically is used. If the scintillation camera can be set to accept multiple photopeaks, acquiring photons of two or three energies (93 and 184 keV or 93, 184, and 296 keV, respectively) decreases imaging time.

Image Findings

The normal distribution of ^{67}Ga–citrate includes tracer uptake in the nasopharynx, lacrimal glands, salivary glands, bony thorax (ribs, sternum, clavicle, scapulae), external genitalia, liver, kidney (up to 48 hr after injection), colon contents, and pelvis (lumbar spine, sacrum, ileum, ischium) and, in children, in active epiphyses of long bones.

Liver uptake is intense, and the liver is the most prominent structure seen in a normal gallium image

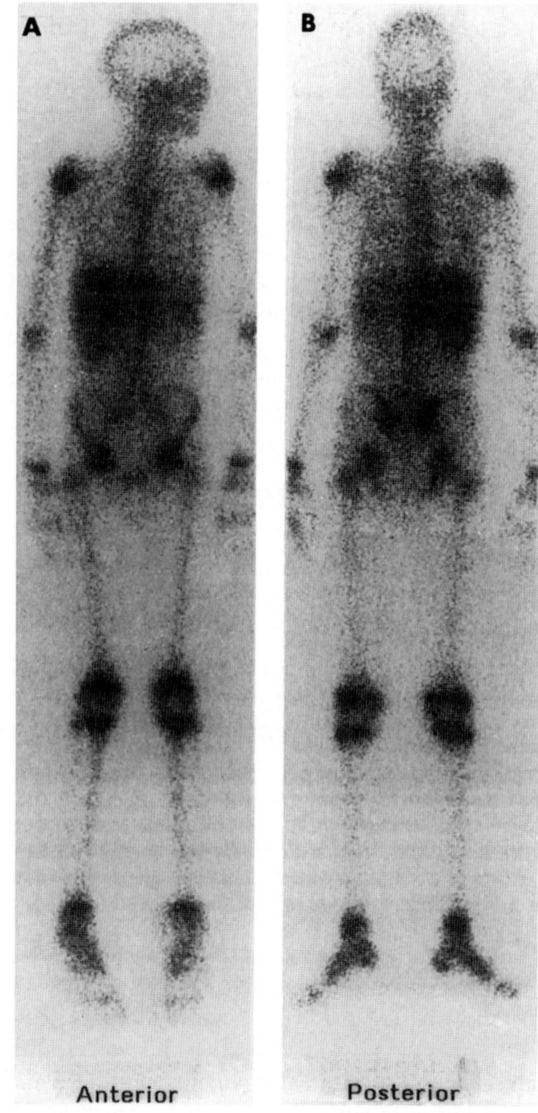

Figure 16.1 Normal ^{67}Ga images obtained 72 hr after tracer administration. (Courtesy of St. Luke's Episcopal Hospital, Houston, TX.)

(Fig. 16.1). Because the kidneys excrete 20–30% of the administered dose during the first 24 hr, renal activity is normally visualized up to 48 hr after tracer administration. After 48 hr, persistent renal activity is indicative of disease.

Changes in biodistribution may result from blood transfusions, chemotherapy, or iron therapy. These changes cause increased gallium concentration throughout the skeleton. Recent trauma may result in areas of increased uptake. Decreased gallium uptake may be noted when gadolinium for magnetic resonance imaging has been administered within 24 hr before gallium administration.

Technical Considerations

Because gallium is excreted initially through the kidneys, patients who are being imaged earlier than 48 hr should be asked to void before the pelvis is imaged. Gallium is also excreted through the gastrointestinal tract. Images of patients taken later than 48 hr after injection will usually show a concentration of ^{67}Ga within the intestinal contents, particularly within the large bowel. Areas of increased tracer concentration within the bowel may be mistaken for disease. Laxatives or enemas may be prescribed to help bowel clearance. This will also decrease the radiation dose to the bowel wall. Bowel preparations are contraindicated in patients who are acutely ill or unable to eat solid food. Radiographic examinations of the gastrointestinal tract performed with barium should be scheduled after gallium imaging.

^{111}In-Labeled Leukocyte Imaging

Leukocytes, which are white blood cells, accumulate in areas of infection. Labeling these cells with a radiotracer permits detection of infection sites using nuclear medicine imaging techniques.

Unlike ^{67}Ga–citrate, ^{111}In-labeled leukocytes do not normally accumulate in the bowel. For this reason, labeled leukocytes are the tracer of choice when imaging the abdomen. Common clinical indications for using ^{111}In-labeled leukocytes include the following:

1. detection of sources of fever of unknown origin,
2. detection of sites of inflammatory bowel disease,
3. detection of osteomyelitis.

Leukocyte Labeling

White cells are isolated from a sample of the patient's blood. ^{111}In–oxine is added to the leukocytes. It diffuses into the cells and binds to components within them. The labeling procedure takes approximately 2 hr (Fig. 16.2). Strict aseptic technique must be maintained, because the labeled cells will be reinjected into the patient. Depending on the method used to tag the cells, a white cell labeling efficiency of 70–90% can usually be achieved. Patients who are taking steroids, aspirin, or antibiotics will exhibit lower labeling efficiencies, because these medications affect the labeling process. Utmost measures should be taken to ensure that the donor patients receive their own blood back.

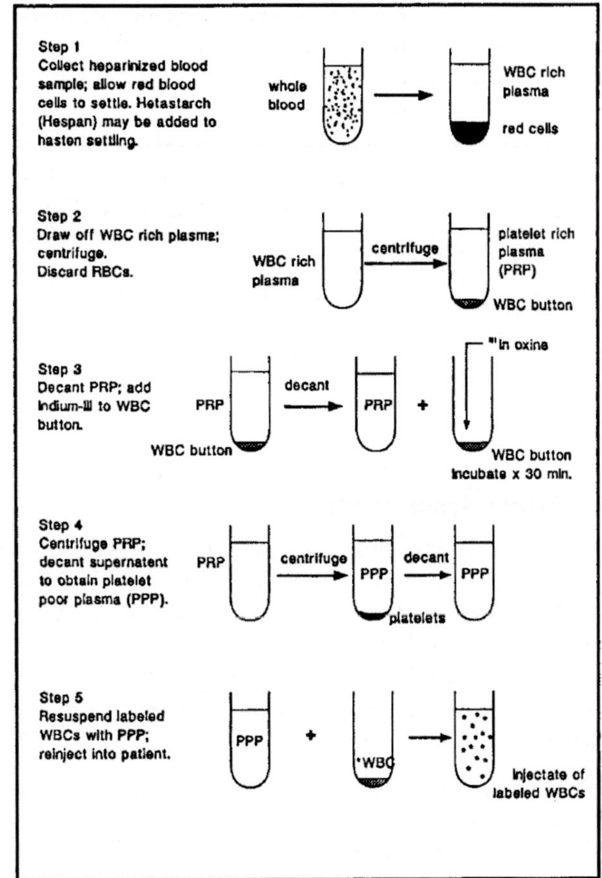

Figure 16.2 Leukocyte-labeling technique.

During the labeling procedure, it is important to separate the white blood cells from the red blood cells and platelets. If platelets are tagged along with the leukocytes, a false-positive image may result, because platelets concentrate in sites of thrombosis rather than in areas of infection. Use of the proper centrifuge speed when separating the various types of cells minimizes platelet labeling.

Patients with extremely low white cell counts may not be able to provide sufficient white cells for labeling. In such cases, donor cells may be tagged.

Imaging

Radiolabeled leukocytes should be administered within 1–2 hr of cell labeling to ensure maximum cell viability. Imaging is performed at 1–4 or 16–30 hr after the labeled leukocytes are administered to the patient. If the infection site is unknown, anterior and posterior views of the head, abdomen, pelvis, and chest, as well as views of the extremities, should be obtained.

^{111}In emits two γ photons with energies of 173 and 247 keV, respectively. Therefore, a medium- or high-energy parallel-hole collimator should be used. Acquisition of photons from both photopeaks decreases imaging time.

In the case of osteomyelitis, simultaneous ^{111}In-labeled leukocyte/^{99m}Tc–medronate bone images may be obtained using two or three different photopeak windows to differentiate the 140-keV ^{99m}Tc photons from the ^{111}In photons.

Image Findings

A normal image demonstrates tracer activity in the spleen, liver, and bone marrow. The most intense activity occurs in the spleen, with less activity in the liver and an even smaller amount of activity in the bone marrow. Any other areas of tracer uptake represent infection (Fig. 16.3).

Technical Considerations

Damage to the labeled leukocytes can be avoided by injecting them into the patient slowly through a large-gauge needle. Extravasation of the labeled cells compromises image quality and may result in a false-negative image if insufficient leukocytes are administered intravenously.

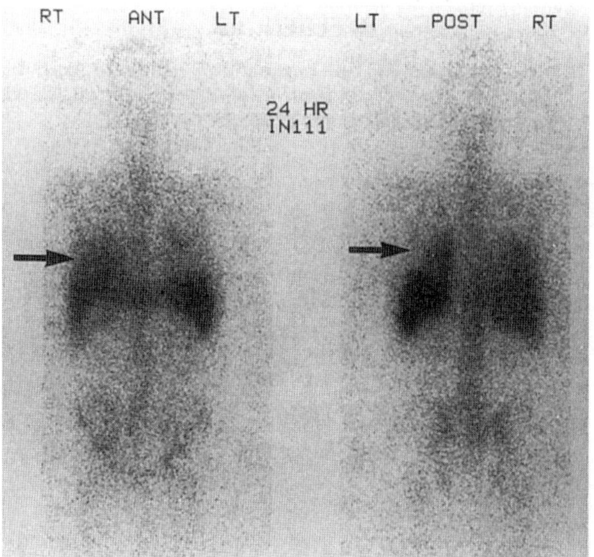

Figure 16.3 Infection in lower lobes of both lungs is visualized on ^{111}In-labeled leukocyte images. (Courtesy of Baptist Memorial Hospital East, Memphis, TN.)

^{99m}Tc-Labeled Leukocyte Imaging

There are many advantages to using ^{99m}Tc as the radioactive tag. Today's gamma cameras are designed to work best with ^{99m}Tc's photon energy. More radioactivity may be administered, which results in shorter acquisition times, better-quality images, and lower absorbed radiation dose to the patient.

Clinical indications for using ^{99m}Tc-labeled leukocytes are similar to those for ^{111}In-labeled leukocytes. However, ^{99m}Tc-labeled leukocytes may be more sensitive in the detection of inflammation or ischemia in the small bowel and the detection of acute osteomyelitis.

Leukocyte Labeling

Leukocytes may be labeled with ^{99m}Tc using ^{99m}Tc–exametazime (HMPAO). Exametazime is available as a radiopharmaceutical kit that is reconstituted with ^{99m}Tc–pertechnetate. The radiolabeled exametazime is then added to white cells isolated from a sample of the patient's whole blood. The procedure is very similar to the ^{111}In labeling process shown in Figure 16.2, except that ^{99m}Tc–exametazime is added to the white cells suspended in plasma in place of ^{111}In–oxine. When ^{99m}Tc–exametazime is prepared for white cell labeling, the stabilizer (methylene blue) supplied in the radiopharmaceutical kit is *not* added to the preparation.

Imaging

The imaging protocol is similar to that for ^{111}In–white blood cell imaging. However, early imaging of the pelvis and abdomen is critical, because bowel activity appears very early after administration of ^{99m}Tc-labeled leukocytes. A low-energy, all-purpose, or high-resolution parallel-hole collimator or pinhole collimator should be used. Single-photon emission computed tomography imaging is also possible with ^{99m}Tc–leukocytes. Relevant areas of the body are imaged depending on the clinical indication for the examination.

Image Findings

The normal biodistribution of ^{99m}Tc-labeled leukocytes is different from that of ^{111}In-labeled leukocytes. Because of slow blood clearance of ^{99m}Tc-labeled leukocytes, activity in the heart, lungs, and great vessels may be visualized on delayed images. Bowel activity in adults increases over time. The spleen, liver, bone marrow, kidneys, bowel, bladder, and major blood vessels will normally be visualized. The patient should empty his or her bladder before imaging.

Areas of abnormal tracer bowel localization may be seen very early (15–30 min after injection) and increase over time. Lung activity that persists longer than 4 hr may indicate pathology (Fig. 16.4).

Technical Considerations

Both early and delayed images are important for accurate interpretation. Technical considerations similar to those described for ^{111}In-labeled leukocyte imaging apply.

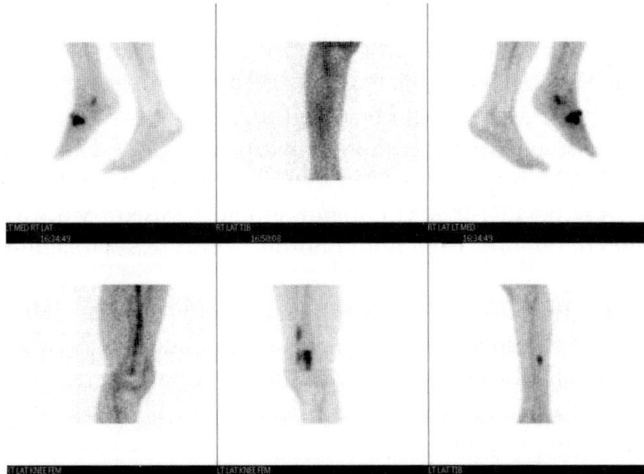

Figure 16.4 White blood cell scan showing an infection in the foot and leg. (Courtesy of University of Alabama at Birmingham Hospital, Birmingham, AL.)

References and Further Reading

Alazraki NP, 1995. Gallium-67 imaging in infection. In: Early PJ, Sodee DB. *Principles and Practice of Nuclear Medicine.* 2nd ed. St. Louis, MO: Mosby; 702–713.

Baker WJ, Datz FL, 1984. Preparation and clinical utility of ^{111}In-labeled leukocytes. *J Nucl Med Technol.* 12:131–136.

Ceretec (^{99m}Tc–exametazime injection), 1995. Package insert. Arlington Heights, IL: Amersham Healthcare.

Kao CH, Wang YL, Wang SJ, 1992. Elution analysis and normal biodistribution of technetium-99m–HMPAO-labeled white blood cells. *J Nucl Med Technol.* 20:224–227.

Kipper MS, Williams RJ, 1983. Indium-111-white blood cell imaging. *Clin Nucl Med.* 8:449–455.

Palestro CJ, Brown ML, Forstrom LA, Greenspan BS, McAfee JG, Royal HD, Schauwecker DS, Seabold JE, Signore AS, 2004. Society of Nuclear Medicine procedure guideline for ^{99m}Tc–exametazime (HMPAO) labeled leukocyte scintigraphy for suspected infection/inflammation 3.0. In: *Society of Nuclear Medicine Procedure Guidelines* Reston, VA: Society of Nuclear Medicine.

Palestro CJ, Brown ML, Forstrom LA, Greenspan BS, McAfee JG, Royal HD, Schauwecker DS, Seabold JE, Signore AS, 2004. Society of Nuclear Medicine procedure guideline for In-111 leukocyte scintigraphy for suspected infection/inflammation 3.0. In: *Society of Nuclear Medicine Procedure Guidelines.* Reston, VA: Society of Nuclear Medicine.

Palestro CJ, Brown ML, Forstrom LA, Greenspan BS, McAfee JG, Royal HD, Schauwecker DS, Seabold JE, Signore AS, 2004. Society of Nuclear Medicine procedure guideline for gallium scintigraphy in inflammation 3.0. In: *Society of Nuclear Medicine Procedure Guidelines.* Reston, VA: Society of Nuclear Medicine.

Preston DF, 1997. Inflammatory process and tumor imaging. In: Bernier DR, Christian PE, Langan JK, eds. *Nucl Med Technol Techn.* 4th ed. St. Louis, MO: Mosby; 451–467.

Preston DF, 1995. Indium-111 label in inflammation and neoplasm imaging. In: Early PJ, Sodee DB. *Principles and Practice of Nuclear Medicine.* 2nd ed. St. Louis, MO: Mosby; 714–724.

Steffel FG, Rao SA, 1987. Rapid and simple methods for labeling white blood cells and platelets with indium-111–oxine. *I Nucl Med Technol.* 15:61–65.

CHAPTER 17 **Nuclear Oncology**

Ann Steves and Norman Bolus

Cancer is the second leading cause of death in the United States, behind heart disease. Accurate staging, assessment of therapy, and early detection of disease recurrence are essential to obtaining the best outcomes for patients. Radioimmunoscintigraphy, positron emission tomography, and other types of radionuclide imaging offer many options for assisting oncologists in treating patients and make nuclear medicine technologists important members of the team that treat patients with cancer.

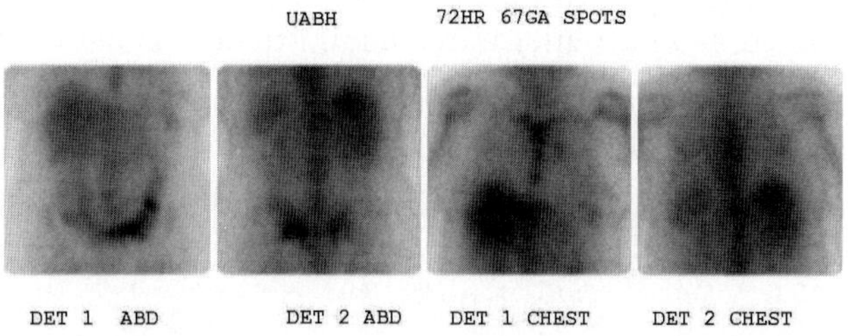

Figure 17.1 Lymphoma determination on a ^{67}Ga scan. (Courtesy of University of Alabama at Birmingham Hospital, Birmingham, AL.)

Gallium Imaging

Gallium-67 (^{67}Ga)–citrate is most commonly used in imaging lymphoma to assess the extent of the disease, detect its progression, and monitor the patient's response to treatment. Other tumors, such as lung cancer and multiple myeloma, also concentrate this tracer. Patient preparation for gallium imaging may include oral laxatives or enemas, but the usefulness of these bowel preparations to clear activity from the bowel is still being debated. Relevant medical history includes recent surgery, chemotherapy, or diagnostic tests; any drugs that may change the biodistribution of ^{67}Ga–citrate, such as iron therapy or gadolinium magnetic resonance contrast agents; areas of recent trauma or infection; and the results of other imaging tests.

For adults, the suggested dosage of ^{67}Ga–citrate is 185–370 megabecquerels (MBq) (5–10 mCi). Imaging takes place 48–72 hr after intravenous administration of the tracer. The reader is referred to Chapter 16 for information about the biodistribution of ^{67}Ga–citrate and other technical considerations. Anterior and posterior images of the head, chest, and abdomen are obtained using either the spot view or whole-body technique. Special views and single-photon emission computed tomography (SPECT) imaging may be performed as indicated. Delayed imaging beyond 72 hr is sometimes necessary (Fig. 17.1).

Indium-111 (^{111}In)–Capromab Pendetide

^{111}In–capromab pendetide (ProstaScint) is a monoclonal antibody that is directed against prostate-specific membrane antigen (PSMA), an antigen that is secreted to a greater extent by malignant prostate cells than nonmalignant cells. The antibody is tagged with ^{111}In and injected into the patient to identify metastases from the primary prostate cancer. Because understaging the extent of disease occurs frequently in prostate cancer, ^{111}In–capromab pendetide may be used in patients who have been newly diagnosed to more accurately stage the disease before surgery. After surgery or radiation therapy, it is used to detect recurrence or residual cancer in patients with rising PSA levels but no other evidence of disease.

Relevant patient history includes previous therapy and surgery, recent laboratory results including PSA levels and human antimurine antibody (HAMA) titer, results of other imaging examinations, and prior history of allergies or allergic reactions. Because monoclonal antibodies are produced from mouse spleen cells, the patient's immune system may identify the monoclonal antibody as a foreign protein. The patient's immune system then begins to produce antibodies against the monoclonal antibody, a process called a HAMA response. A HAMA response increases the possibility of an allergic response to a second administration of monoclonal antibody and decreases the likelihood of a second successful imaging procedure. For this reason, patients receiving a second administration of radiolabeled monoclonal antibodies may be tested for this antibody before tracer administration.

Patient preparation includes laxatives beginning the day before imaging. Some sources recommend continuing laxatives for 4–5 days until imaging is completed. Likewise, some sources recommend bladder catheterization and bladder irrigation before imaging to remove all residual radioactive urine from the field of view. Patients should also be encouraged to increase fluid intake for the duration of the examination.

After intravenous administration of approximately 185 MBq (5 mCi) of ^{111}In–capromab pendetide, an early image of the abdomen and pelvis is obtained at 30 min to 4 hr to delineate the blood pool for use during interpretation. Alternatively, a SPECT blood pool image using technetium-99m (^{99m}Tc)-labeled red blood cells may be obtained simultaneously with the ^{111}In images on day 4 or 5. Anterior and posterior spot views or whole-body imaging to include the skull to midfemur are performed 4–5 days after tracer administration, along with SPECT images of the abdomen and pelvis (Fig. 17.2).

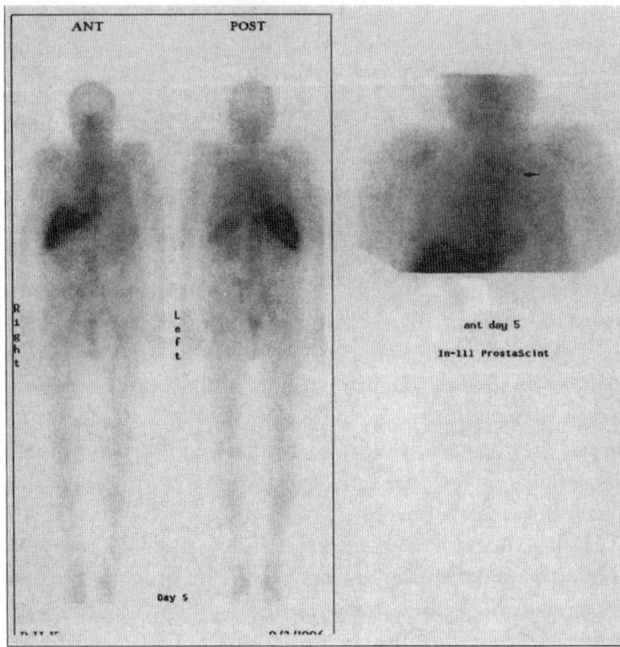

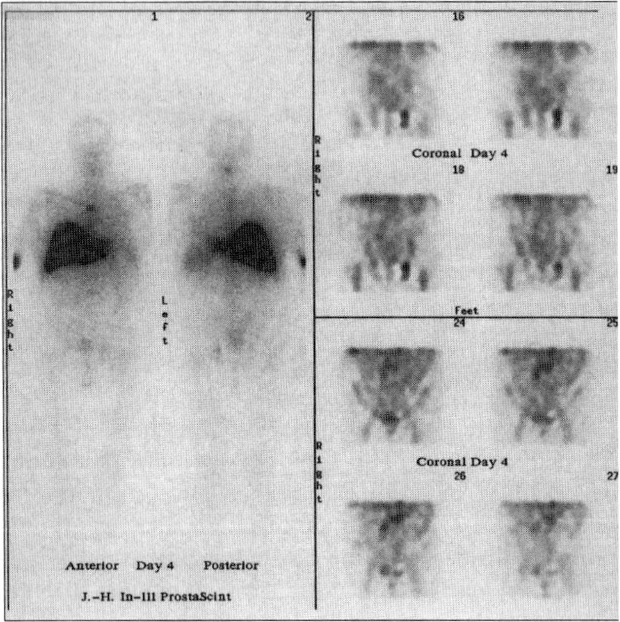

Figure 17.2 A patient with abnormal uptake in the regions of the posterior cervical spine and manubrium. Coronal SPECT views show periaortic and left obturator areas of uptake. Infiltration is noted in the right antecubital injection site. (Reprinted, with permission, from Williams *et al.*, 1997, p. 214.)

Normal biodistribution of ^{111}In–capromab pendetide includes activity in the blood pool and blood-filled structures (liver, spleen, and penis), bone marrow, and large bowel.

^{111}In–Pentetreotide

^{111}In–pentetreotide (OctreoScan) is a form of octreotide. Octreotide is an analog of the hormone somatostatin. ^{111}In–pentetreotide binds to somatostatin receptors on the surface of cells, concentrating in tumors with a high density of receptor sites. It is a peptide, which is the portion of an amino acid molecule that naturally binds to receptors on the cell surface.

Somatostatin is a hormone concentrated in the hypothalamus, cerebral cortex, brain stem, gastrointestinal tract, and pancreas. Its functions include neurotransmission and inhibition of the release of growth hormone, insulin, glucagon, and gastrin and hormone production by certain types of tumors. Receptor sites for somatostatin are located in the anterior pituitary gland, pancreatic islet cells, lymphocytes, and certain types of tumors (brain, breast, and lung cancer and lymphoma).

^{111}In–pentetreotide is approved for localizing primary and metastatic tumors originating from neuroendocrine cells, cells that contain somatostatin receptor sites. This includes many types of tumors, such as pituitary and endocrine tumors, paraganglioma, medullary thyroid carcinoma, carcinoids, and small-cell lung cancer.

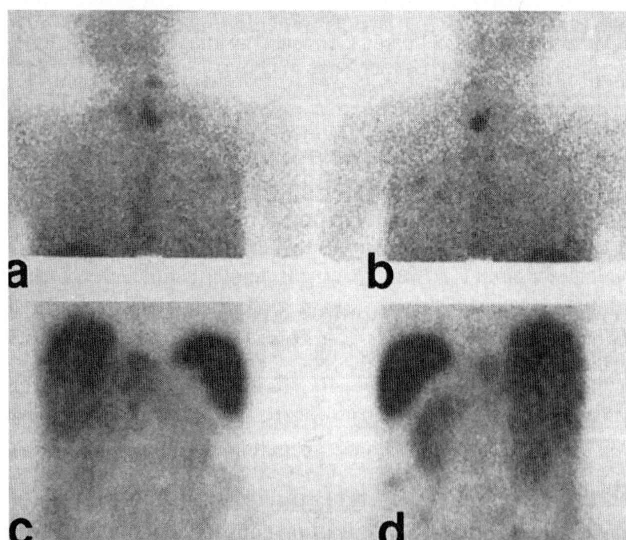

Figure 17.3 ^{111}In–pentetreotide images. (a) Anterior view. (b) Posterior view of the chest. (c) Anterior and (d) posterior view of the abdomen of patient with known liver metastases. Somatostatin receptor scintigraphy discovered bone metastases. (Reprinted, with permission, from Lebtahi *et al.*, 1997.)

Relevant patient history includes type of primary tumor; results of other imaging studies and tumor marker assays; recent surgery, chemotherapy, radiation therapy, and octreotide therapy; and history of cholecystectomy. The patient should be well hydrated for at least 24 hr after tracer administration. It is recommended that a mild laxative be given to the patient 24 hr before tracer administration and continue for 48 hr afterward to remove any radioactivity in the gastrointestinal tract. The patient should void immediately before imaging, because the tracer is eliminated from the body primarily through the genitourinary system. Imaging can begin 24–48 hr after the administration of 222 MBq (6 mCi) of activity. Because the purpose of the procedure is to visualize the unknown primary site of the cancer or to demonstrate the extent of the disease, anterior and posterior whole-body imaging should be performed (Fig. 17.3). SPECT imaging may be performed as indicated by the clinical history. Four-hour images may be performed before activity appears in the gastrointestinal tract.

Normal distribution of ^{111}In–pentetreotide includes tracer uptake in the pituitary and thyroid glands, liver, spleen, kidneys, bladder, and sometimes the gallbladder. Intestinal activity typically does not appear until 24 hr after tracer administration.

Fewer than 1% of patients in clinical trials with this agent have experienced any adverse effects. These effects were transient and mild, because this agent is a peptide, not an antibody, and no HAMA effect occurs. Patients with suspected insulinomas are at risk for developing severe hypoglycemia. An intravenous infusion of glucose should be available for these patients. ^{111}In–pentetreotide should not be administered into intravenous lines or administered with total parenteral nutrition solutions.

^{99m}Tc–Depreotide

^{99m}Tc–depreotide (NeoTect) is a synthetic peptide that binds to somatostatin receptors found in normal tissue and in many malignant tumors. It may not be commercially available for nuclear medicine in the United States. However, it is used to evaluate certain lung nodules identified on a chest X ray or CT to determine which should be biopsied to rule out lung cancer. If a single pulmonary nodule concentrates ^{99m}Tc–depreotide, there is a greater chance that the nodule is malignant.

Relevant history includes the results of the chest X ray or CT, other lung conditions, recent surgery, and any allergies or previous allergic reactions. The only preparation is that the patient should be well hydrated before tracer administration and for the first few hours afterward. Anterior and posterior planar projections of the chest or chest SPECT are obtained 2–4 hr after intravenous administration of 555–740 MBq (15–20 mCi) of ^{99m}Tc–depreotide. The tracer should not be administered with total parenteral solutions or through those intravenous lines. Normal biodistribution includes the kidneys, liver, spleen, and bone marrow. On SPECT images the ends of the ribs, sternum, and spine may appear to have more tracer uptake than normal lung tissue.

^{99m}Tc–Arcitumomab

^{99m}Tc–arcitumomab (CEA-Scan) is a fragment of an antibody that is expressed against carcinoembryonic antigen (CEA), an antigen that is secreted by most colorectal cancers and up to 75% of adenocarcinomas. The principle behind CEA imaging is that the labeled antibody fragment will bind to the CEA on the tumor, demonstrating small areas of metastases that are not easily visualized with other types of imaging modalities. ^{99m}Tc–arcitumomab is used for two main reasons in patients with colorectal cancer: (1) to monitor patients who have rising CEA levels but who do not have clinical symptoms of cancer recurrence and (2) to identify which patients may benefit the most from surgical resection of the primary tumor. In the latter group of patients, a surgical cure may be possible if the tumor has not spread. Extensive spread of the disease negates the appropriateness of surgery.

Relevant patient history includes information about the primary tumor, previous surgery, location of colostomy site, results of other medical imaging examinations, and CEA and liver enzyme levels. The patient should be well hydrated before tracer administration to enhance tracer clearance. Imaging may be performed 2–5 hr after intravenous administration of 925–1110 MBq (25–30 mCi) of ^{99m}Tc–arcitumomab, although imaging times closer to 5 hr permit better blood clearance, with the potential for better tumor visualization. Anterior and posterior planar images of the head, chest, abdomen, and pelvis are obtained along with SPECT imaging of the chest and pelvis. The patient's bladder should be emptied immediately before pelvic imaging to prevent masking of disease close to the bladder. Catheterization of the patient may be indicated. The colostomy bag should also be changed before imaging, and the location of the colostomy site should be noted on an additional image of the abdomen. Delayed imaging of the chest or abdomen at 18–24 hr may be necessary to better delineate tumor uptake.

Normal biodistribution of ^{99m}Tc–arcitumomab includes tracer uptake in the heart, lungs, major blood vessels, liver, spleen, kidneys, bowel, and bladder (Fig. 17.4). Uptake at the colostomy site may be faint or as intense as that in the blood pool.

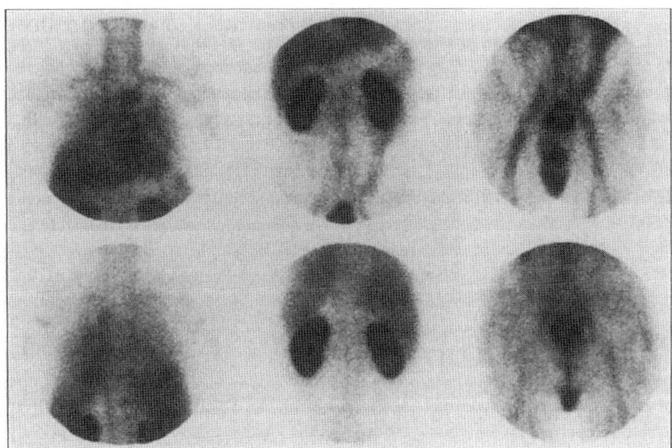

Figure 17.4 Normal biodistribution of ^{99m}Tc–CEA-Scan at 4 hr after injection. Top row shows anterior planar images of the chest, abdomen, and pelvis. Bottom row shows posterior planar images of the chest, abdomen, and pelvis. (Reprinted, with permission, from Erb and Nabi, 2000.)

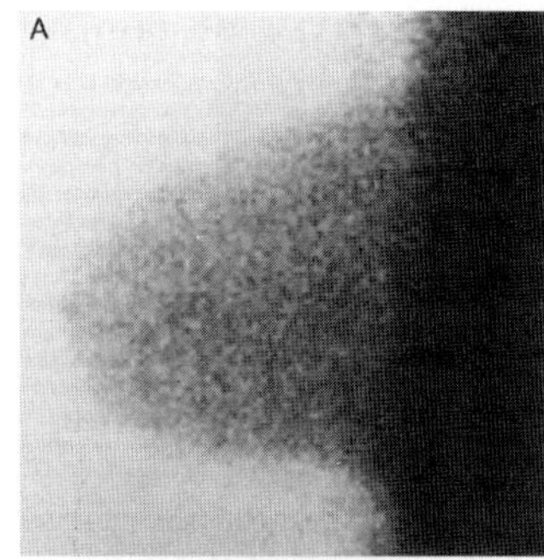

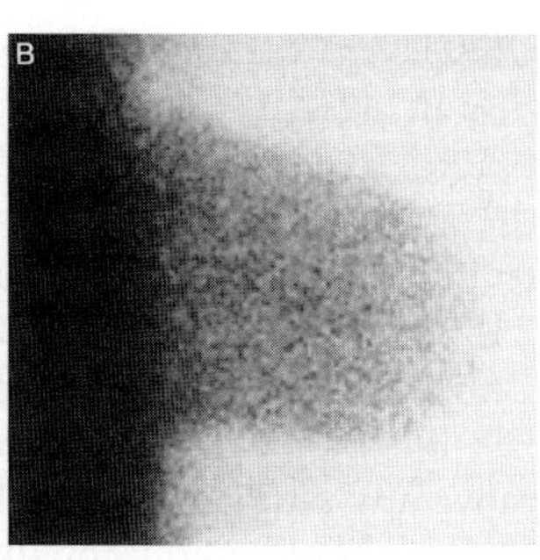

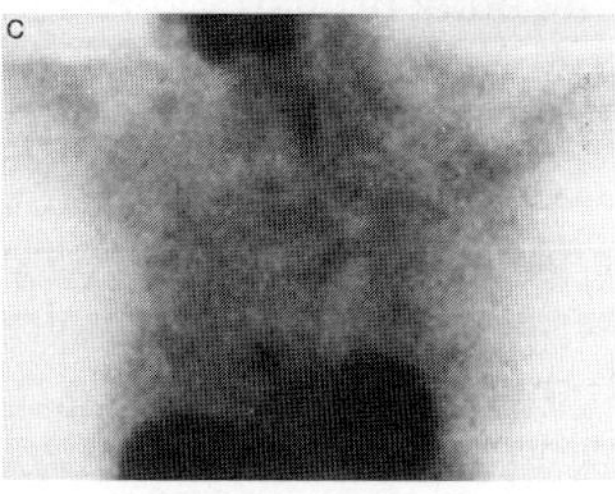

Figure 17.5 Left (A) and right (B) lateral prone and anterior upright (C) scintimammography images of a 52-year-old female with negative mammography and a normal breast physical examination show no area of increased ^{99m}Tc–sestamibi uptake in the breast. The breast contours and anterior chest wall are clearly seen in the lateral images, and there is good visualization of the axillae in the anterior image. (Reprinted, with permission, from Diggles *et al.*, 1994.)

Scintimammography

Radionuclide breast imaging is performed in cases of an indeterminate X-ray mammogram, dense breast tissue, and suspected recurrence of breast cancer after surgery or radiation therapy and as an aid in treatment planning for breast cancer. ^{99m}Tc–sestamibi is taken up into breast tumors as a result of the increased blood flow and metabolic rate of the neoplastic cells.

No special preparation of the patient is required. Pertinent medical history includes the results of prior X-ray mammograms, prior breast surgery or other therapy, lactation and pregnancy status of the patient, date of the last menstrual period, and any physical signs or symptoms the patient is experiencing. Scintimammography should not be performed within 2 weeks of a needle aspiration or within 4–6 weeks of a breast biopsy.

^{99m}Tc–sestamibi (740–1110 MBq/20–30 mCi) is administered intravenously in the arm contralateral to the involved breast. If abnormalities are suspected in both breasts, the tracer should be administered into a vein in the foot. Imaging begins 5–10 min after the tracer is injected. Planar views of the anterior chest and axillae and lateral views of each breast are acquired. The lateral views are acquired with the patient in the prone position with the breast suspended; the contralateral breast is compressed under the patient against the table. The anterior view may be acquired with the patient upright or supine. If nodules can be palpated, additional images with markers placed over the areas of abnormality may be helpful. The markers should be placed after the patient has been positioned for imaging. Tables specially designed for breast imaging may be helpful in correctly positioning the patient and increasing patient comfort. Specialized cameras as well are available specifically for scintimammography including positron emission mammography (PEM). Normal biodistribution of ^{99m}Tc–sestamibi includes uptake in the salivary and thyroid glands, myocardium, liver, gallbladder, intestines, skeletal muscles, kidneys, and bladder (Fig. 17.5).

Lymphoscintigraphy

Lymphoscintigraphy is a method by which the lymph drainage pattern can be mapped or a sentinel lymph node (SLN) can be identified by injecting radioactive particles within or under the skin. This technique is most commonly performed in patients with melanoma or breast cancer to identify the SLN, the node nearest to a tumor. If an SLN can be identified and excised, a sample of the node is viewed under a microscope to determine whether malignant cells from the tumor have spread into the lymph system that will carry them to distant parts of the body. If the SLN is negative for malignant cells, extensive surgery to dissect the lymph nodes is not necessary.

Lymphoscintigraphy is often performed several hours before surgery, so coordination with surgical staff may be necessary to ensure that the patient is properly prepared for surgery. No special preparation is needed for the nuclear medicine examination. Relevant patient history includes information about the site and type of cancer and the results of other imaging examinations. Tracer uptake into the lymphatics is dependent, in part, on the particle size of the tracer. ^{99m}Tc–sulfur colloid is filtered through a 0.22-μm filter to obtain a preparation with smaller particles. Two to six injections around the lesion, totaling approximately 37 MBq (1 mCi), are introduced into the dermis. The injection sites may be numbed with a local anesthetic before injection of the tracer. Imaging begins immediately. If no lymph nodes are observed, imaging is repeated at 45 min to 1 hr and at 30- to 45-min intervals until a lymph node is observed. Other imaging protocols may be preferred. To assist in pinpointing the location of a lymph node, performing a transmission scan of the area in question to produce a silhouette of the body or outlining the body with intravenous tubing containing ^{99m}Tc is helpful (Fig. 17.6).

Contamination of the imaging site may occur if the tracer leaks out of the injection site. Technologists should be alert to this possibility, because the contamination may be misinterpreted as a lymph node.

Tumor Imaging Using ^{18}F-Fluorodeoxyglucose

^{18}F-Fluorodeoxyglucose (^{18}F-FDG) is a positron-emitting radiopharmaceutical used for metabolic imaging and the tracer most commonly used for positron emission tomography (PET) imaging. Malignant cells take up ^{18}F-FDG to a greater extent than do nonmalignant cells, making this tracer clinically useful for differentiating between benign and malignant disease, staging malignancies, detecting the recurrence of cancer, and monitoring a patient's response to therapy.

Although ^{18}F-FDG has been used to image many types of cancer, the Centers for Medicare and Medicaid Services have approved reimbursement for specific clinical indications involving certain cancers.

Relevant patient history includes recent surgery, chemotherapy, radiation therapy, results of other imaging examinations, diabetes status, and the patient's ability to cooperate by lying still for several hours and lying with arms overhead. Patient preparation includes fasting for at least 4 hr to minimize ^{18}F-FDG uptake in certain organs, such as the heart. A laxative may be prescribed the night before imaging. Because tumor uptake is reduced if the patient is hyperglycemic, the blood glucose level may be checked with a glucometer before the tracer is administered. ^{18}F-FDG (185–740 MBq/5–20 mCi) is administered intravenously. During the waiting period before imaging, the patient should rest quietly as excessive movement can cause tracer uptake in muscles that may be misinterpreted as disease. Likewise, the patient may receive a mild sedative to help relax and avoid muscle uptake related to tension. Imaging begins 30–60 min later. Imaging protocols vary widely, depending on the type of imaging instrumentation available and the area of the body to be imaged. Both emission (delineating the distribution of ^{18}F-FDG) and transmission (needed for attenuation correction) images are acquired. Image processing varies, depending on the type of equipment and software. Images are displayed in the three tomographic planes and may include both attenuation-corrected and uncorrected images.

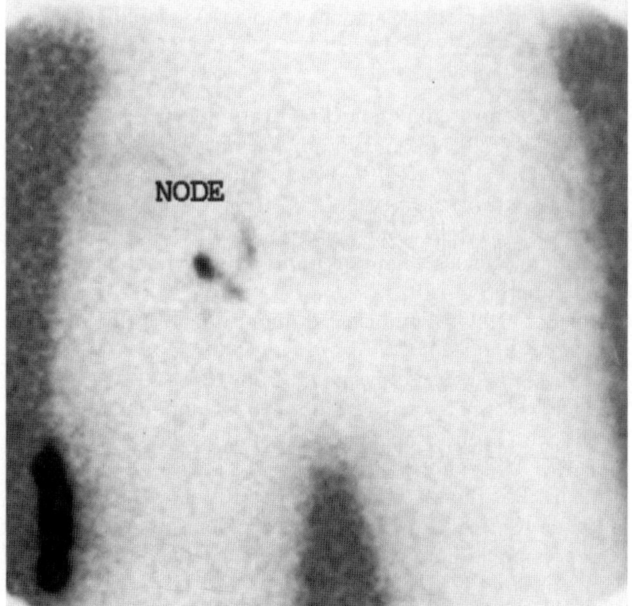

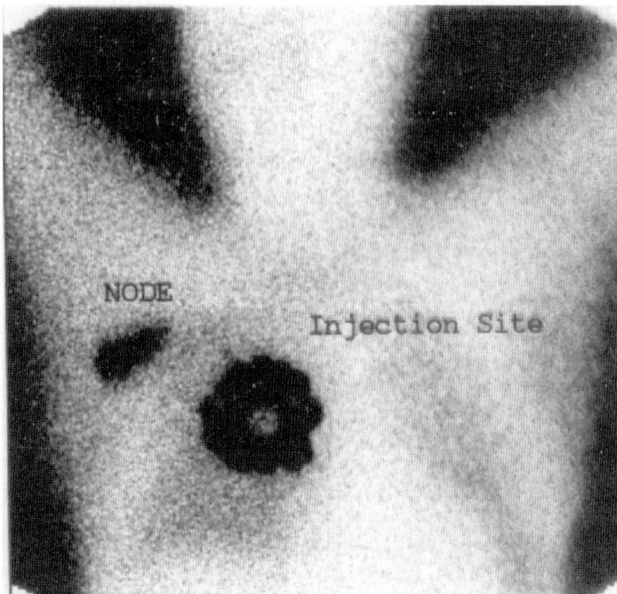

Figure 17.6 (Left) Sentinel node study of melanoma on outer aspect of right thigh demonstrating sentinel node in right groin. (Right) Sentinel node study of breast carcinoma demonstrating sentinel node in right axilla. (Courtesy of University of Alabama Hospital, Birmingham, AL.)

Normal ^{18}F-FDG tracer uptake is visualized in the brain, myocardium, liver, spleen, stomach, intestines, kidneys, and bladder. Areas of increased uptake can also be seen in areas of healing wounds, infections, and granulomatous tissue, as well as in malignancies (Fig. 17.7). Certain patients may require bladder catheterization or diuretics to eliminate urinary tract activity that interferes with image interpretation.

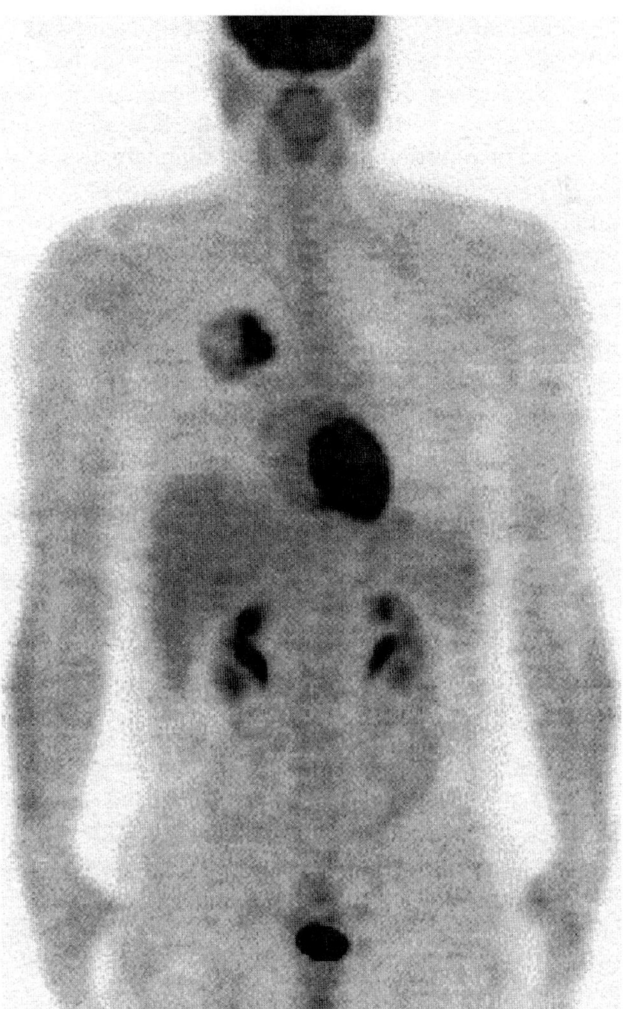

Figure 17.7 PET image demonstrating tumor in right lung. (Courtesy of Regional Metabolic Imaging, Birmingham, AL.)

References and Further Reading

Balon HR, Goldsmith SJ, Siegel BA, Silberstein EB, Donohoe KJ, Krenning EP, Lang O, 2001. Society of Nuclear Medicine procedure guideline for somatostatin receptor scintigraphy with In-111 pentetreotide 1.0. In: *Society of Nuclear Medicine Procedure Guidelines Manual 2001–2002.* Reston, VA: Society of Nuclear Medicine; 127–131.

Bartold SP, Donohoe KJ, Haynie TP, Henkin RE, Silberstein EB, Lang O, 2001. Society of Nuclear Medicine procedure guideline for gallium scintigraphy in the evaluation of malignant disease 3.0. In: *Society of Nuclear Medicine Procedure Guidelines Manual 2001–2002.* Reston, VA: Society of Nuclear Medicine; 121–125.

Diggles L, Mena I, Khalkhali I, 1994. Technical aspects of prone dependent breast scintimammography. *J Nucl Med Technol.* 22:165–170.

Dunnwald LK, Mankoff DA, Byrd DR, Anderson BO, Moe RE, Yeung RS, Eary JF, 1999. Technical aspects of sentinel node lymphoscintigraphy for breast cancer. *J Nucl Med Technol.* 27:106–111.

Erb DA, Nabi HA, 2000. Clinical and technical considerations for imaging colorectal cancers with technetium-99m-labelel antiCEA Fab' fragment. *J Nucl Med Technol.* 28:12–18.

Khalkhali I, Caravaglia G, Abdel-Nabi HH, Peller PJ, Tallefer R, Vande Streek PR, Van de Wiele C, 2004. Society of Nuclear Medicine procedure guideline for breast scintigraphy 2.0. *Society of Nuclear Medicine Procedure Guideline* Reston, VA: Society of Nuclear Medicine.

Lebtahi R, Cadiot G, Sarda L, Daou D, Faraggi M, Petegnief Y, Mignon M, Le Guludec D, 1997. Clinical impact of somatostatin receptor scintigraphy in the management of patients with neuroendocrine gastroenteropancreatic tumors. *J Nucl Med.* 38:853–858.

Mar MV, Gee-Johnson S, Kim EE, Podoloff DA, 2002. Whole-body lymphoscintigraphy using transmission scans. *J Nucl Med Technol.* 30:12–17.

Nabi HA, Zubeldia JM, 2002. Clinical applications of ^{18}F-FDG in oncology. *J Nucl Med Technol.* 30:3–9.

Neotect Technical User's Guide, 2002. Wayne, NJ: Berlex Laboratories.

Peller PJ, Khedkar NY, Martinez CJ, 1996. Breast tumor scintigraphy. *J Nucl Med Technol.* 24:198–203.

Preston DF, 1997. Inflammatory process and tumor imaging. In: Bernier DR, Christian PE, Langan JK, eds. *Nuclear Medicine Technology and Techniques.* 4th ed. St. Louis, MO: Mosby; 451–458, 461–467.

Schelbert HR, Hoh CK, Royal HD, Brown M, Dahlbom MN, Dehdashti F, Wahl RL, 2001. Society of Nuclear Medicine procedure guideline for tumor imaging using F-18 FDG 2.0. In: *Society of Nuclear Medicine Procedure Guidelines Manual 2001–2002.* Reston, VA: Society of Nuclear Medicine; 133–137.

Serafini AN, 1993. From monoclonal antibodies to peptides and molecular recognition units: an overview. *J Nucl Med.* 34(suppl):533–536.

Wahl RL, 1995. Radiolabeled monoclonal antibodies. In: Early PJ, Sodee DB. *Principles and Practice of Nuclear Medicine.* 2nd ed. St. Louis, MO: Mosby; 678–701.

Warner J, Hovey S, Crawford ES, 2002. Contamination problem with sentinel node localization procedure: a case study. *J Nucl Med Technol.* 30:18–20.

Williams BS, Hinkle GH, Lamatrice RA, Fry JP, Loesch JA, Olsen JO, 1997. Technical considerations for acquiring and processing indium-111 capromab pendetide images. *J Nucl Med Technol.* 25:205–216.

Williams BS, Hinkle GH, Douthit RA, Fry JP, Pozderac RV, Olsen JO, 1999. Lymphoscintigraphy and intraoperative lymphatic mapping of sentinel nodes in melanoma patients. *J Nucl Med Technol.* 27:309–317.

CHAPTER 18 Hematopoietic System

Helen Drew and Norman Bolus

In several nuclear medicine procedures, the patient receives radioactive material but is not imaged. Instead, the amount of radioactivity concentrated in a particular organ is quantified using an external counting device, usually an uptake probe (however, some protocols enable us to conduct these types of studies with a gamma camera). Alternatively, a blood or urine sample is collected from the patient and counted in a scintillation well counter. Diagnostic procedures such as these are referred to as in vivo nonimaging techniques.

Hematologic Studies

Circulating blood is a complex mixture made up of the plasma compartment and the cellular compartment. Plasma is a watery fluid containing various ions and inorganic and organic molecules, such as sodium (Na^+), potassium (K^+), chloride ion (Cl^-), magnesium (Mg^{2+}), bicarbonate (HCO_3^-), calcium (Ca^{2+}), and sugar. Plasma proteins, such as albumin, immunoglobulins, transport proteins, lipoproteins, and clotting proteins, make up the solid portion and exert an osmotic force, which decreases the amount of fluid lost through the capillary pores.

When blood is collected with an anticoagulant (a substance that prevents normal clotting), the whole blood separates into plasma and cellular components. If the blood is collected without an anticoagulant, the clot formed contains most of the cells and the coagulation proteins, leaving behind a straw-colored fluid called serum.

Red blood cells (or erythrocytes) make up the largest volume of the cellular compartment, about $5 \times 10^6/\mu L$ of blood. Red cells are biconcave disks and measure 6–8 μm in diameter. The primary function of the red cell is to transport oxygen to the body's tissues and carry carbon dioxide, the by-product of metabolism, back to the lungs for elimination from the body.

Red cells are produced from a bone marrow stem cell, which is initially a pro-erythroblast with the ability to synthesize hemoglobin. The cell matures into a normoblast and, after extruding its nucleus, becomes a reticulocyte. At this stage, the reticulocyte enters the peripheral circulation. The level of tissue oxygenation regulates red cell production. Tissue hypoxia stimulates erythropoietin production from the kidneys, which in turn stimulates bone marrow red cell production. Therefore, obese patients or those with conditions such as cardiac failure or severe lung disease, which cause tissue hypoxia, exhibit increased red cell production. Red blood cells have a normal life span of 120 days. Old red cells are destroyed primarily by the spleen.

Included in the cellular compartment but not easily measured are leukocytes and platelets. Leukocytes constitute a major defense system within our bodies and can be divided into granulocytes, lymphocytes, and monocytes. These cells are present in a volume of $5 \times 10^3/\mu L$ blood. The primary function of platelets is blood coagulation and clot retraction. Platelets also participate in hemostasis and in maintaining integrity of blood vessel walls by aggregating and sealing wall defects. Platelets are present in a volume of $3.5 \times 10^5/\mu L$ blood. Each of these cell types—red blood cells, leukocytes, and platelets—have different pathways within the open circulatory system.

A common method used to ascertain whether a patient has a normal number of red cells is to perform a standard laboratory test to determine the hematocrit. This is done by placing a well-mixed sample of anticoagulated blood into a capillary tube and centrifuging the tube for an appropriate period of time and gravitational force. By definition, a hematocrit is the volume of packed red cells expressed as a percentage of the total volume (Fig. 18.1). When hematocrits are performed on normal blood, red cells make up the majority of the volume of packed cells. The grayish layer just above the packed red cells is made up of white cells. Just above that layer is a minute, cream-colored layer representing platelets. Readings of venous hematocrits, performed on individuals with normal blood, show red cell volumes of 35–48%.

A simple hematocrit reading can sometimes yield misleading results when estimating red cell volume or plasma volume. If the patient is dehydrated and has a decreased plasma volume, the hematocrit will be falsely elevated. If the patient has an increased plasma volume, the hematocrit will be falsely low. Direct measurement of red cell volume and plasma volume is the only method for determining these values accurately.

Total Blood Volume Determination

Determining total red cell volume (TRCV) and total plasma volume (TPV) through use of radiolabeled blood components is an accepted method performed by the nuclear medicine laboratory. Estimations of total blood volume (TBV) are clinically useful in the diagnosis and management of polycythemia or when changes in the venous hematocrit fail to reflect accurately changes in

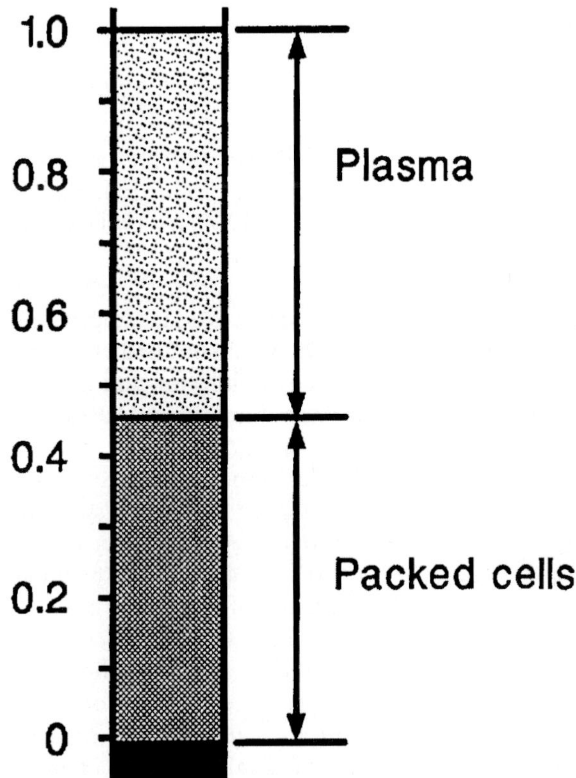

Figure 18.1 Hematocrit determination.

TRCV or TPV. When the venous hematocrit is increased, TRCV measurements distinguish absolute increases in red cell volume from decreases in plasma volume. In cases of gross splenomegaly, red cells pool in the spleen, and increases in the plasma volume may give misleading venous hematocrit readings.

TBV measurements are calculated using the isotope dilution principle equation

$$V = \frac{Q}{C},$$

where V represents the volume, Q represents the dose administered in counts per minute (cpm), and C represents the concentration of dose after dilution in counts per minute. The larger the volume into which the label is mixed, the lower the counts in the sample withdrawn, and, conversely, the smaller the volume, the higher the counts in the sample. The isotope dilution principle is true only when working with a closed system in which no radiopharmaceutical is allowed to leak out of the system being measured. In addition, the volume of the unknown must not change significantly during the measurement. In most cases, red cell volume measurements are performed in a closed system using radiolabeled red blood cells.

Plasma Volume Determination

Plasma volume measurements are performed using radiolabeled albumin. Albumin does not remain within the intravascular space but diffuses rapidly into the extravascular compartments. Because this vascular space is now an open system, use of the closed-system isotope dilution principle for calculations would cause errors in the plasma volume result. If the injected radiopharmaceutical leaves the open system at a slower rate than the uniform mixing rate within that system and samples are taken only after mixing has been completed, the volume can be obtained by an extrapolation procedure.

Plasma Volume Technique

Materials

The patient is administered 370 kilobecquerels (kBq) (10 microcuries [μCi]) iodine-125 (^{125}I)–human serum albumin (HSA) contained in a volume of 1.5 mL. No more than 2% of the radioactivity can be in the free form. The free form is removed from the intravascular space more rapidly than the labeled albumin, which causes overestimation of the plasma volume. Technetium-99m (^{99m}Tc)–HSA can also be used, but labeling efficiency at time of injection must be performed and must be at least 98% bound. All equipment for collecting blood samples and injecting the radiopharmaceutical must be prepared in advance. This equipment includes gloves, 23-gauge needles, syringes, and labeled heparinized blood collection tubes.

Patient Preparation

The patient should be supine and at rest for at least 15–20 min before starting the study. Plasma volume decreases when a person is standing, because venous pressure increases in the legs, and water moves from the intravascular to the extracellular nonvascular space.

Tracer Administration/Sample Collection

Before tracer administration, collect a background heparinized blood sample. Inject the radiolabeled albumin intravascularly, taking care to avoid infiltration of the tracer. The exact volume injected must be known for the calculations; therefore, weighing the syringe on an analytical balance before and after injection is recommended. The difference between the preinjection and postinjection syringe weights is equivalent to the volume injected. Record the exact time of injection. Do not rinse the syringe with blood. Three 10-mL heparinized blood samples are collected at exactly 10, 20, and 30 min after injection from a venous site other than the injection site.

Sample Handling

Centrifuge the samples and pipette 1-mL aliquots of plasma into labeled counting tubes. Prepare a standard by diluting a duplicate dosage (10 μCi ^{125}I–HSA in 1.5 mL) into a 500-mL volumetric flask. Again, the exact volume must be known, so the syringe should be weighed. Do not rinse the standard syringe in the water. Bring the volume in the flask up to the line using distilled water. Mix well by inverting and shaking the flask. Pipette duplicate 1-mL aliquots of the standard into labeled counting tubes.

Counting

Adjust the pulse-height analyzer of the scintillation spectrometer to count ^{125}I. Count each 1-mL sample for a time period that is long enough to assure a counting error of no more than 1%. After counting, adjust all samples to net counts per minute by subtracting patient background from the patient samples and room background from the standard samples.

Calculations

The net counts per minute of each postinjection sample are plotted against time on semilogarithmic graph paper. The best straight line is drawn through these points (Fig. 18.2). The zero-time activity is estimated by extrapolation; this value is used to calculate the TPV using the equation:

$$\text{TPV} = \frac{\text{volume injected} \times \text{net standard activity}}{\text{net patient activity at time zero}}.$$

Sources of Error

If the radiopharmaceutical is infiltrated, an erroneously high result will be obtained. If the patient contains a radiotracer from a previous diagnostic test and the count rate of the postinjection samples is not corrected for this contamination, an erroneously low result will be obtained. Inaccurate measurement of the injected volume and the standard volume can cause errors in the results.

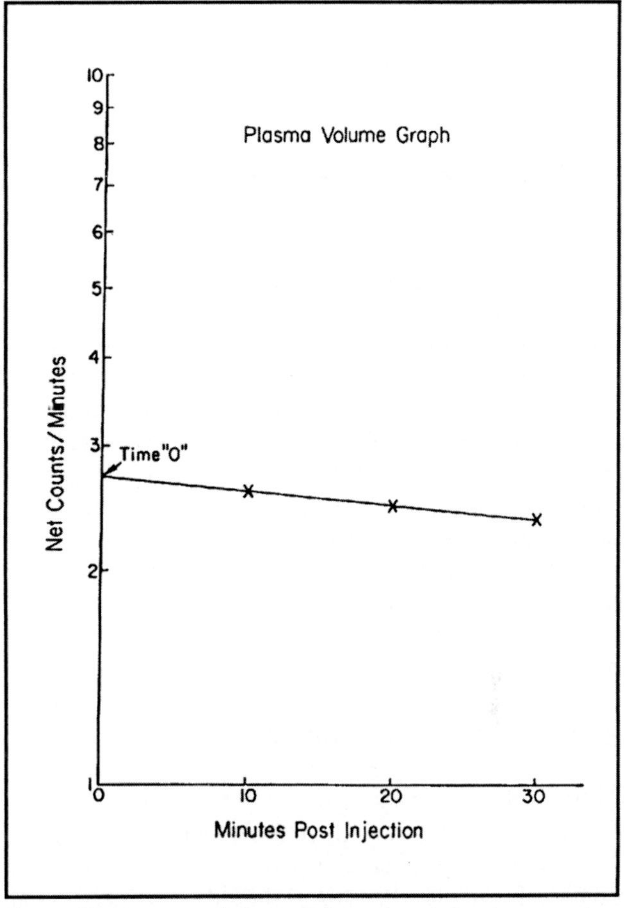

Figure 18.2 Extrapolation graph used to determine zero-time activity to calculate plasma volume.

Red Cell Volume Determination

Radiolabeling of red blood cells for red cell volume measurement is referred to as random labeling. The radionuclide labels erythrocytes circulating in the peripheral blood. This process labels all cells in the sample, from the youngest to the oldest erythrocytes or erythrocytes of random age.

The most commonly used radionuclides for random red cell labeling are ^{99m}Tc–pertechnetate and chromium-51 (^{51}Cr)–sodium chromate. Because of the high rate of elution of ^{99m}Tc–pertechnetate from the labeled red cells, this tracer is not recommended for red cell volume determinations.

Ascorbic Acid Method for Labeling Red Cells

Ten milliliters of whole venous blood are collected from the patient into a 20-mL syringe containing 2 mL of the anticoagulant acid–citrate–dextrose (ACD) solution. Heparin and ethylenediaminetetraacetic acid (EDTA) are not satisfactory anticoagulants for use in this labeling procedure. After inverting to mix, transfer blood into a sterile vial. Add 1.11 MBq (30 μCi) ^{51}Cr to the vial. Gently mix and incubate for 30 min at room temperature. During this time, 80–95% of the chromate ion is transported across the red cell membrane and binds to the beta chain of the hemoglobulin molecule. The hexavalent chromate ion is reduced to a trivalent chromic ion. Fifty milligrams (mg) of ascorbic acid are then added to reduce the free chromate to chromic ion. This prevents extracellular chromate from labeling circulating red cells after reinjection of the labeled red cell mixture. The reinjection mixture will contain both red cell-bound and -free ^{51}Cr.

Wash Method for Labeling Red Cells

Ten milliliters of whole venous blood are collected from the patient into a 20-mL syringe containing 2 mL ACD anticoagulant. After mixing, transfer blood into a sterile vial. Centrifuge this mixture at 1000–1500 *g* for 5–10 min. Remove and discard the supernatant plasma, taking care not to remove any red cells. Add 1.11 MBq (30 μCi) ^{51}Cr to the packed red cells and mix gently. Allow this mixture to stand for 30 min at room temperature. Wash the labeled red cells in 4–5 mL isotonic saline, then centrifuge at 1000 *g* for 5–10 min. Remove the supernatant saline, resuspend the labeled red cells in saline, and recentrifuge. After the last centrifugation, resuspend the red cells in saline to the original volume. This method removes all of the free chromate ion so that the reinjection mixture contains only red cell-bound ^{51}Cr.

Red Cell Volume Technique

Materials

Use red cells labeled with 370–740 kBq (10–20 μCi) ^{51}Cr–sodium chromate. The exact volume must be known. Therefore, the syringe should be weighed on an analytical balance before and after injection. Equipment for collecting blood samples and injecting the radiopharmaceutical must be prepared in advance. This includes gloves, 20-gauge needles, and heparinized blood collection tubes.

Patient Preparation

Patients should be supine and at rest for 15–20 min before the start of the study. A patient background sample must be collected.

Tracer Administration/Sample Collection

Inject intravenously 5 mL ^{51}Cr-labeled red cells, taking care not to infiltrate any of the tracer. Record the exact time of injection. Do not rinse the syringe with the patient's blood. After waiting a sufficient length of time (usually 10–20 min) to ensure complete mixing of the labeled red cells within the circulation, withdraw 10 mL blood into a heparinized tube from a vein other than the one used for tracer injection. In seriously ill patients, a delay of up to 30 min for complete mixing may be necessary. For this reason, it is recommended that the postinjection sample be drawn at 30 min.

In certain disease states, such as severe polycythemia and splenomegaly, complete mixing of the labeled red cells may be greatly delayed. In such instances, serial postinjection samples at 30, 60, and 90 min should be collected.

Sample Handling

Perform a microhematocrit determination on the stock-labeled red cell mixture and on each postinjection blood sample. Prepare a standard from the stock-labeled red cells by diluting 2 mL of the labeled cells into a 100-mL volumetric flask. Again, the exact volume must be known. Therefore, the syringe should be weighed pre- and postdilution on an analytical balance. Do not rinse the standard syringe into the water. Bring the volume in the flask up to the line using distilled water. Mix well by inverting and shaking. Pipette duplicate 1-mL aliquots of the standard into counting tubes labeled "standard whole blood." Pipette 1 mL whole blood from each postinjection sample into a counting tube labeled "sample whole blood."

If the ascorbic acid-labeling method was used, centrifuge the remaining stock-labeled red cell mixture and each postinjection sample at 1500 *g* for 10 min. Pipette 1 mL plasma supernatant from each sample into labeled counting tubes. The standard counting tube should be labeled "standard plasma" and the sample counting tubes should be labeled "sample plasma."

Counting

Set the scintillation spectrometer to count ^{51}Cr. Count each 1-mL sample for sufficient time to ensure no more than a 1% counting error. Adjust all samples to net counts per minute by subtracting the patient background from the patient samples and room background from the standard samples.

Calculations

If the wash method was used, the following equation is used for the calculations:

$$\text{TRCV} = \frac{\text{volume injected (net standard counts} \times \text{dilution factor)}}{\text{net whole blood sample counts}} \times \text{decimal hematocrit.}$$

TRCV is calculated separately for each postinjection blood sample.

If the ascorbic acid-labeling method was used, the equation in Figure 18.3 is used for the calculations. Again, TRCV is calculated separately for each postinjection blood sample.

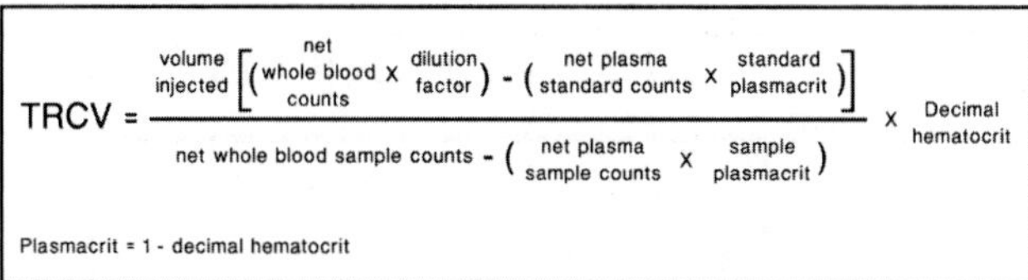

Figure 18.3 Total red cell volume calculation (ascorbic acid-labeling method).

Table 18.1 Normal Blood Volume Values (Milliliters per Kilogram)

Volume	Men	Women
Total blood volume	55–80	50–75
Total red cell volume[a]	22–35	20–30
Total plasma volume	30–45	30–45

[a]95% confidence limits. Valid only at sea level.

Sources of Error

Infiltration of the labeled red cells will cause erroneously high results. Likewise, damaged erythrocytes or excessive binding of the ^{51}Cr by leukocytes or platelets will yield spuriously high values. Falsely low results are caused by a failure to obtain a preinjection blood sample in a patient who has previously received radioactive tracers. All blood samples must be mixed well before hematocrit determinations and pipetting of samples. ^{51}Cr should not be added to the ACD solution before the patient's blood is added to the vial. Dextrose contained in the ACD solution acts as a reducing agent and inhibits red cell labeling.

Table 18.2 Adjustments for Fat Tissue

Ideal weights:	Male: 5 ft tall = 110 lb + 6 lb for every inch over 5 ft
	Female: 5 ft tall = 100 lb + 5 lb for every inch over 5 ft
Calculated weight:[a]	Example: 6 ft man weighing 275 lb
Ideal weight calculations:	5 ft = 110 lb + (6 lb/in × 12 in) = 182 lb
Difference between ideal and actual weight:	275 lb − 182 lb = 93 lb overweight
Twenty-percent vascularity of amount overweight:	93 lb × 0.2 = 18.6 lb
Calculated weight:	Ideal weight + 20% of amount overweight: 182 lb + 18.6 lb = 200.6 lb

[a]Includes 20% vascularity of fat.

Normal Ranges

The interpretation of TRCV and TPV depends upon a comparison between the measured volumes and normal values. The most common method is to estimate in terms of body weight (mL/kg). The normal values published by the International Panel on Standardization in Hematology are shown in Table 18.1.

Because fat is almost avascular, blood volume is closely related to lean tissue mass and not weight. Therefore, blood volumes vary considerably, even among healthy individuals with identical height and weight. In patients with conditions such as cachexia, heart or renal failure with edema, ascites, or obesity, an even greater variation in lean tissue mass must be taken into consideration.

Blood volume varies with body size, body type, sex, disease state, basal metabolic rate, nutritional state, and amount of physical work, because all of these factors affect the lean body mass. Also, blood volume varies with the season, arterial oxygen content, and changes in body position.

In healthy persons within the ideal weight range, lean body mass makes up a constant fraction of total weight. In these individuals, blood volume correlates well with weight. When fat is excessive (obesity) or deficient (emaciation, cachexia), corrections must be made to obtain an adjusted ideal weight. Because fat has a vascularity of approximately 20%, adjustments can be calculated to permit a comparison of an individual's blood volume with normal values (Table 18.2).

From a precise measurement of red cell or plasma volume and the venous hematocrit, the volume of the other compartments and, therefore, total blood volume can be calculated in normal individuals. Normally, there is a fixed relationship between the whole-body hematocrit and venous hematocrit, represented by a ratio of 0.89:0.92. The whole-body hematocrit is usually lower than the venous hematocrit because of variations in blood vessel size throughout the body.

Most patients referred to nuclear medicine for red cell and plasma volume measurements are ill, and the predicted normal relationship between whole-body and venous hematocrits will most likely not be present. In patients with splenomegaly, the ratio of whole-body hematocrit to venous hematocrit may be unpredictably increased to more than 1.0. In patients with polycythemia, plasma volume abnormalities as well as red cell volume abnormalities may be present. Therefore, in clinical situations, total blood volume can be reliably measured only by performing simultaneous independent measurements of red cell volume and plasma volume.

Red Cell Survival

The red cell survival study determines the mean survival time of ^{51}Cr-labeled autologous red cells in patients with hemolytic anemia.

Materials

^{51}Cr is labeled to red blood cells with the ascorbic acid-labeling technique. Chromium activity is adjusted to 55.5 kBq (1.5 μCi)/kg of body weight, with a minimum activity of 1.85 MBq (50 μCi). Equipment for collecting blood samples and injecting the radiopharmaceutical must be prepared in advance and includes gloves, 20-gauge needles, syringes, and labeled heparinized blood collection tubes.

Tracer Administration/Sample Collection

After labeling, the red cells are injected, and the first blood sample is drawn 24 hr later. This time period permits removal of cells that were damaged during the labeling procedure from the circulation, as well as clearance from the blood of any injected plasma activity. Heparinized blood samples are obtained from the patient every other day for the next 3 weeks.

Sample Handling

On the day of collection, 5 mL of well-mixed whole blood is pipetted into a labeled counting tube. A pinch of saponin powder is added to the tube and mixed to lyse the red cells. These samples are then stored at 4°C until the last day of the study. Hematocrit determinations also are made on each sample on the day of collection.

Sample Counting

On the last day of the study, all samples are counted on a scintillation spectrometer with settings of 280–360 keV for ^{51}Cr. Samples are counted long enough to give a counting error of 1% or less.

Calculations

To calculate the mean half-time of disappearance of the labeled red cells, the net counts per minute of each sample are plotted on semilogarithmic paper as a function of time (Fig.18.4). The best straight line is drawn through all the points. The half-time is obtained by extrapolating the line to time zero, which is the *y* intercept. Divide the *y* intercept value by 2. At this value on the *y* axis, draw a straight line parallel to the *x* axis until it intersects the best straight line drawn through the data points. Drop a perpendicular line to the *x* axis. This value is the mean survival time of the labeled red blood cells.

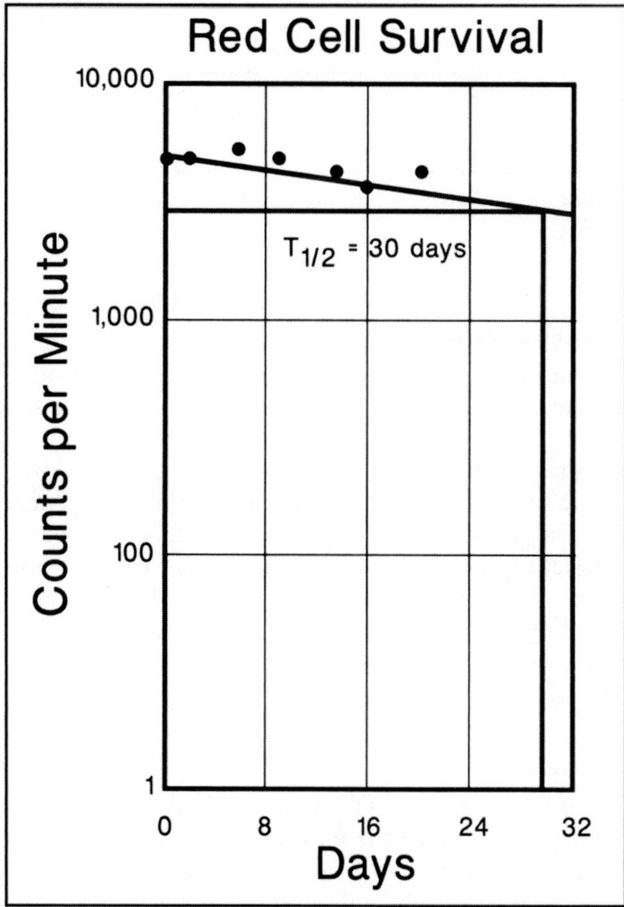

Figure 18.4 Red cell survival graph shows normal half-time of 30 days. (Reprinted, with permission, from McIntyre, 1972, p. 107.)

Sources of Error

Determining the mean red cell life span is useful only in a patient who is in steady state with regard to the rate of production and destruction of red cells. Performing a hematocrit on each sample during the study provides an assessment of this steady-state condition. ^{51}Cr-labeled red cell survival time will falsely appear to be shorter if the patient loses blood during the study. If the patient receives blood transfusions during the study, the mean survival time will appear shortened.

Normal Values

The mean half-time of normal ^{51}Cr-labeled red cells is 25–35 days. As normal red cells age, they are removed from the circulation at a rate of 1% per day. Therefore, the true mean survival time of a normal random red cell population is 50–60 days. If this normal 1% per day removal is coupled with the 1% per day elution of ^{51}Cr from the red cells, the combined mean half-time is 25–

35 days. Tables are available for correction of this elution, but they are derived from studies in normal individuals. The elution rate is known to vary in disease states. Therefore the use of these tables is questionable.

Splenic Sequestration

This test determines whether the spleen is the site of red cell destruction in a patient who has evidence of increased red cell destruction. A splenic sequestration study is routinely performed in conjunction with a red cell survival study.

Materials

Use ^{51}Cr-labeled red cells, 55.5 kBq (1.5 μCi)/kg of body weight. A scintillation probe equipped with a flat-field collimator is used as the counting device.

Patient Preparation

Counting begins 24 hr after injection of the ^{51}Cr-labeled red cells. The patient is placed on the examining table (in the positions described in the next paragraph), and the skin is marked with indelible ink. Transparent tape is placed over each anatomical location, and the patient is instructed not to remove or wash off the marks. Counting continues every other day for 3 weeks.

Counting

The following anatomical locations are marked for counting:

- Precordium: with the patient in the supine position, the detector is centered over the left, third intercostal space at the sternal border.
- Liver: with the patient in the supine position, the detector is placed over the ninth and tenth ribs on the right midclavicular line.
- Spleen: with the patient in the prone position, the detector is placed two-thirds of the distance from the spinal process to the lateral edge of the body, at the level of the ninth and tenth ribs.

The same counting geometry must be present each time the patient is counted. Sufficient counts should be collected to give a counting error of 5% or less.

Calculations

Results are expressed as the ratio of the net organ counts per minute to the net precordium counts per minute for each day. These ratios are then plotted on linear graph paper as a function of time (Fig. 18.5).

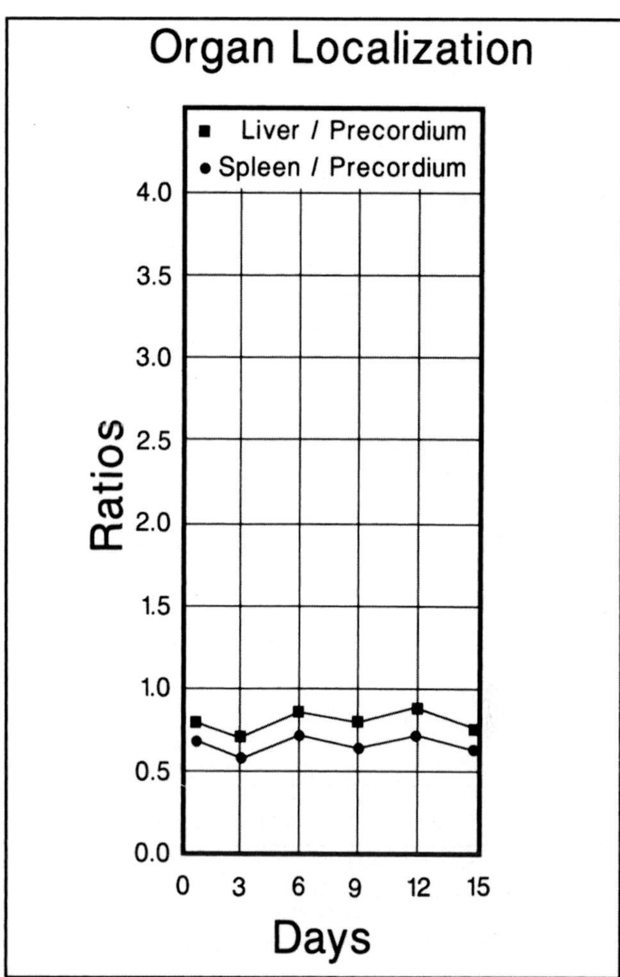

Figure 18.5 Organ localization of ^{51}Cr–red blood cells. Graph depicts normal liver-to-precordium and spleen-to-precordium ratios, which are about 1:1 or less. (Reprinted, with permission, from McIntyre, 1972, p. 107.)

Sources of Error

Inconsistent counting geometry from day to day will cause spurious results. Blood loss or transfusion during the counting interval also will affect results adversely.

Normal Values

The normal spleen-to-precordium ratio is between 0.5 and 1.0, and the normal liver-to-precordium ratio is 0.5. An initial spleen-to-precordium ratio greater than 2.0 indicates an increased splenic blood pool. A progressive, gradual increase over the course of the study indicates active splenic sequestration of the labeled red cells.

Table 18.3 Causes of Vitamin B_{12} Deficiency

I. Inadequate intake
II. Malabsorption
  A. Secondary to gastric abnormalities
    1. Absence of intrinsic factor
      a. Congenital
      b. Addisonian pernicious anemia
      c. Total gastrectomy
      d. Subtotal gastrectomy
    2. Excessive excretion of hydrochloric acid: Zollinger–Ellison syndrome
  B. Secondary to intestinal malabsorption
    1. Destruction, removal, or functional incompetence of ileal mucosal absorptive sites
    2. Competition with host for available dietary vitamin B_{12}
      a. *Diphylibothrium latum* (fish tapeworm)
      b. Small-bowel lesions associated with bacterial stagnation (jejunal diverticula, strictures, blind loops, etc.)
    3. Pancreatic insufficiency
    4. Drug therapy[a]
      a. Paraaminosalicylic acid (PAS)
      b. Neomycin
      c. Colchicine
      d. Calcium-chelating agents
  C. Genetic abnormality in transport protein transcobalamin II

[a]Although any of these agents may produce abnormalities in vitamin B_{12} absorption, only patients on long-term PAS therapy have been reported to develop clinical evidence of vitamin B_{12} deficiency.
(Reprinted, with permission, from McIntyre, 1975, p. 81.)

Table 18.4 Parameters Involved in Absorption of Dietary Vitamin B_{12} in Humans

1. Available for human nutrition only in animal food sources.
2. Binding of vitamin B_{12} by intrinsic factor produced by gastric mucosa.
3. Normal ileal mucosal absorptive sites in the presence of ionic Ca^{2+} and pH of ileal contents >6.0.
4. Normal "transport" protein (transcobalamin II) to convey vitamin B_{12} from ileal absorptive sites to areas of active utilization and storage.

The same parameters apply to absorption of tracer amounts of radioactive vitamin B_{12} used in absorption studies. (Reprinted, with permission, from McIntyre, 1975, p. 81.)

Vitamin B_{12} Absorption: Schilling Test

While Schilling's test kits are not currently available, historically these kits have been removed from the market only to return at a later point. The historical significance of this study is that it was one of the first nuclear medicine studies showing the importance of truly metabolic information that nuclear medicine could provide.

The consequences of untreated vitamin B_{12} deficiency are extremely serious and include certain hematological abnormalities, such as anemia and neurological defects, and, if the condition is untreated, can result in death. In the early stages, the symptoms of the deficiency are vague and insidious.

The most common causes of vitamin B_{12} deficiency are summarized in Table 18.3. Most cases of vitamin B_{12} deficiency are the result of some disorder causing malabsorption. A deficiency in intrinsic factor, a protein secreted by the parietal cells of the stomach, is the most common cause of malabsorption.

Table 18.4 summarizes factors necessary for human absorption of dietary vitamin B_{12}. The absorption of this vitamin through the terminal ileum depends on the stomach's secretion of intrinsic factor, which exists as a dimer and binds two molecules of vitamin B_{12}. The intrinsic factor itself is not absorbed at the sites in the terminal ileum but is required in an active transport mechanism. Ionic calcium and an ileal content pH greater than 6 are also required. Once absorption takes place, a normal transport protein, transcobalamin II, must be present in the blood to convey the B_{12} to areas of the body for utilization or storage.

Vitamin B_{12} Absorption Test: Stage I

Materials

The procedure requires 18.5–22.2 kBq (0.5–0.6 μCi) cobalt-57 (^{57}Co)-labeled vitamin B_{12}. It is important that this oral dosage be in the range of 0.25–2.0 μg of vitamin B_{12}, the amount that might be present in a typical meal. Quantities above this level may be absorbed by a mechanism not dependent on the presence of intrinsic factor. Labeled urine containers large enough to hold a 24-hr sample are also needed.

Patient Preparation

The patient should have nothing to eat after midnight before the test and should remain fasting for 2 hr after the oral dosage of ^{57}Co-labeled vitamin B_{12}. The patient should not receive enemas or laxatives or be scheduled for a barium enema or intravenous pyelogram for the duration of the study. Because of the effects of hepatobiliary recirculation, treatment doses of vitamin B_{12} should be discontinued 2–3 days before starting the Schilling test.

Dose Administration/Sample Collection

The ^{57}Co-labeled vitamin B_{12} capsule is administered orally with water. Two hours later, 1 mg of stable cyanocobalamin (vitamin B_{12}) is given intramuscularly. Nonradioactive vitamin B_{12}, sometimes referred to as the "flushing dose," causes temporary saturation of the normal binding sites in the plasma and results in renal excretion of a portion of the absorbed tracer dose. Excretion of radioactive vitamin B_{12} is maximal between 8 and 12 hr after administration of the flushing dose. Two 24-hr urine collections are obtained, one for each 24-hr period. The patient should be instructed to collect all urine during this period.

Sample Handling

After mixing each 24-hr collection well, the total volume and specific gravity of each sample are measured. Two 5-mL aliquots are pipetted from each 24-hr urine collection into labeled counting tubes. A standard is prepared from the reference standard solution supplied with the capsules.

Sample Counting

All samples are counted with a scintillation spectrometer set to count ^{57}Co. Each sample is counted for a sufficient time to ensure no more than a 1% counting error. All sample counts are adjusted to net counts per minute by subtracting the room background radiation.

Calculations

The percentage of the administered dose excreted is calculated for each 24-hr urine sample using the following equation:

$$\% \text{ excreted} = \frac{\text{net cpm urine sample (urine volume/sample volume)}}{\text{net cpm standard} \times \text{standard dilution factor}} \times 100.$$

Normal Values

Percentage of ^{57}Co excreted on day 1 is ≥9% and on day 2 is ≤1%.

Sources of Error

The major problem encountered with this test is its dependence on complete 24-hr urine collections. The loss of just one urine collection may cause falsely low results. The test depends on normal urinary function. In patients with abnormal urinary retention, such as in benign prostatic hypertrophy, the amount excreted in the first 24 hr will be reduced. Significant amounts of radioactivity will continue to be excreted for the next 24–48 hr, so that the total excretion will eventually be within normal limits. For this reason, it is recommended that two separate 24-hr urine specimens be collected after the "flushing" injection of cyanocobalamin. Excretion of other previously administered radionuclides can cause erroneously high results.

Vitamin B_{12} Absorption Test: Stage II

If the absorption of ^{57}Co vitamin B_{12} is low when compared with values in normal individuals, then a second absorption test is performed by giving hog intrinsic factor along with the oral dose of labeled vitamin B_{12}. This test determines whether the malabsorption is the result of the absence of intrinsic factor.

Materials

In addition to the materials described in stage I, a 10-mg dosage of intrinsic factor is needed; it is usually provided with the commercially available Schilling test kit.

Patient Preparation

See stage I.

Dose Administration

The ^{57}Co-labeled vitamin B_{12} and intrinsic factor are administered orally with water simultaneously. The remainder of the test is the same as described for stage I.

Normal Values

Percentage of ^{57}Co excreted on day 1 is ≥9% and on day 2 is ≤1%.

Sources of Error

When the radioactive vitamin B_{12} and the intrinsic factor are given in separate capsules, there may be incomplete binding of the two in the stomach, which gives a false-negative stage II Schilling test. It is recommended that the radioactive vitamin B_{12} and intrinsic factor be mixed together in water before administration.

If hog intrinsic factor is used, a negative result does not completely rule out intrinsic factor-dependent malabsorption, because some patients who have been exposed previously to hog intrinsic factor (present in many multivitamin preparations) may have antibodies against it.

Vitamin B_{12} deficiency can produce small bowel megaloblastosis with atrophy, which may cause ileal malabsorption. If a stage II study is performed before vitamin B_{12} therapy is started and the ileum is allowed to heal, a false-negative result will be obtained.

Vitamin B_{12} Absorption: Stage III

Having determined that the stage II Schilling test is truly abnormal, other causes of malabsorption must be investigated. If bacterial overgrowth is suspected, treatment with a broad spectrum antibiotic followed by a repeat stage I Schilling test is performed. If pancreatic insufficiency is suspected, a repeat stage I Schilling test can be performed after the administration of pancreatic extract.

References and Further Reading

Drew HH, Scheffel U, McIntyre PA, 2004. Hematopoietic system. In: Christian PE, Bernier DR, Langan JK, eds. *Nuclear Medicine and PET Technology and Techniques,* 5th ed. St. Louis, MO: Mosby; 520–535.

Fudenberg H, Baldini M, Mahoney JP, Dameshek W, 1961. The body hematocrit/venous hematocrit ratio and the splenic reservoir. *Blood.* 17:71–73.

Haurani FI, Sherwood N, Goldstein F, 1964. Intestinal malabsorption of vitamin B_{12} in pernicious anemia. *Metabolism.* 13:1342–1348.

Huff RL, Feller DD, 1956. Relation of circulating red cell volume to body density and obesity. *J Clin Invest.* 35:1–4.

International Committee for Standardization in Hematology, 1971. Recommended methods for radioisotope red cell survival studies. *Br J Haematol.* 21:241–250.

International Committee for Standardization in Hematology, 1973. Standard techniques for the measurement of red cell and plasma volume. *Br J Haematol.* 17:71–73.

International Committee for Standardization in Hematology, 1981. Recommended methods for the measurement of vitamin B_{12} absorption. *J Nucl Med.* 22:1091–1093.

McDonald JW, Barr RM, Barton WB, 1975. Spurious Schilling test results obtained with intrinsic factor enclosed in capsules. *Ann Intern Med.* 83:827–829.

McIntyre P, 1972. Radioactive tracers in hematologic disease: I. *Hosp Pract.* 7:94–108.

McIntyre P, 1975. Use of radioisotope techniques in the clinical evaluation of patients with megaloblastic anemia. *Semin Nucl Med.* 5:79–94.

Wright RR, T'no M, Pollycove M, 1975. Blood volume. *Semin Nucl Med.* 5:63–77.

CHAPTER 19 **Radionuclide Therapy**

Kathy Thomas, Ann Steves, and Norman Bolus

The most commonly used radionuclides for therapy include iodine-131 (^{131}I), phosphorous-32 (^{32}P), strontium-89 (^{89}Sr), samarium-153 (^{153}Sm), and yttrium-90 (^{90}Y) (Table 19.1). The technologist's responsibility in radionuclide therapy is dependent on state and/or federal regulations as defined by the user's radioactive materials license (RML). Regardless of Nuclear Regulatory Commission (NRC) or agreement state regulations pertaining to the use of radionuclides, the role of the technologist will include patient education and the preparation and safe handling of the required radiopharmaceutical. This chapter addresses those practices.

Table 19.1 Radioactive Therapeutic Agents

Agent	Principal use
^{131}I–sodium iodide	Hyperthyroidism
	Thyroid carcinoma
^{32}P–sodium phosphate	Polycythemia vera
	Certain leukemias
	Skeletal metastases
^{32}P–chromic phosphate	Peritoneal and pleural effusions
^{89}Sr–strontium chloride	Skeletal metastases
^{153}Sm–lexidronam	Skeletal metastases
^{90}Y–ibritumomab tiuxetan	Non-Hodgkin's lymphoma
^{131}I–tositumomab	Non-Hodgkin's lymphoma
^{90}Y–microspheres	Hepatic carcinoma

Patient Education/Preparation

Successful radionuclide therapy relies, in part, on the full cooperation of the patient. In most cases, the technologist's participation in patient education and preparation will reinforce information provided by the referring or treating physician. Patient education and preparation is procedure specific. In all cases, information should include the reason for the procedure, the length of the procedure, the physical requirements during the procedure, and pre- and post-treatment instructions, as well as contact information if the patient has questions or needs assistance after the procedure.

Radioiodine Therapy

Before 1997, patients receiving more than 1110 megabecquerels (MBq) (30 mCi) of ^{131}I were hospitalized. In 1997, the NRC revised Title 10 of the Code of Federal Regulations (10 CFR 35.75) to allow the release of patients immediately after radionuclide therapy providing the total effective dose equivalent from the patient to an individual does not exceed 5 millisieverts (mSv) (0.5 rem) in any 1 year. NRC release guidelines include the following statement:

> A licensee shall provide the released individual, or the individual's parent or guardian, with instructions, including written instructions, on actions recommended to maintain doses to other individuals as low as is reasonably achievable if the total effective dose equivalent to any other individual is likely to exceed 1 mSv (0.1 rem). If the total effective dose equivalent to a nursing infant or child could exceed 1 mSv (0.1 rem), assuming there were no interruption of breast-feeding, the instructions must also include:
>
> 1. Guidance on the interruption or discontinuation of breast-feeding; and
> 2. information on the potential consequences, if any, of failure to follow the guidance.
> 3. A licensee shall maintain a record of the basis for authorizing the release of an individual in accordance with § 35.2075(a).
> 4. The licensee shall maintain a record of instructions provided to a breast-feeding female in accordance with § 35.2075(b).

However, many agreement state facilities continue to use the older release criteria that state that the patient may be released either when the activity levels within the patient drop below 1110–1221 MBq (30–33 mCi) or dose rates at 1 meter (m) from the patient drop below 50 μSv/hr (5 mrem/hr). Therefore, on the basis of revised NRC guidelines, patient and hospital personnel education, room preparation, and patient monitoring for ^{131}I therapy are dependent on whether the procedure is scheduled as an inpatient or outpatient procedure.

Inpatient High-Dosage Radioiodine Therapy

Regardless of the patient's diagnosis, the use of high-dosage radioiodine therapy in an inpatient setting requires specific treatment room preparation and patient and personnel education.

Patient Education

It is important that the patient understand what to expect during hospitalization and how the experience will differ from other hospital stays; time taken to explain what the patient can expect will be time well spent:

- Minimal contact: Although necessary nursing care will be provided, nursing personnel will minimize the amount of time spent in contact with the patient. Visitors will be provided with specific rules regarding the time they may remain in the patient's room and the distance that must be maintained from the patient. Children and pregnant women will not be allowed to visit the patient.
- Confinement: Some patients may have difficulty being confined to a small area. They should be encouraged to bring materials to provide some diversion during their confinement. However, patients must understand that materials may become contaminated and it may be necessary to retain those items at the hospital for a period of time after the patient's discharge. Access to a television and telephone can lessen the feelings of isolation that the patient may experience. It is important to stress that the patient must remain in the isolation room until it has been determined that emitted radiation levels are within acceptable limits. The technologist should avoid predicting when the patient will be released from isolation.
- Excretion: Large amounts of the radioiodine will be excreted in the urine. Human excreta may be disposed of through the sewer system. The patient should be instructed to flush the toilet three or four times after each use to dilute the radioactivity.

Room Preparation

Sources of contamination include airborne ^{131}I and radioactivity in the patient's urine, perspiration, and saliva. To minimize contamination and facilitate decontamination of the treatment room after patient discharge, floors, countertops, and other porous surfaces should be covered with plastic-backed absorbent paper. Plastic covers should be placed over chairs. The use of a plastic mattress cover is recommended. Plastic wrap should cover any item the patient may come in contact with, including knobs, handles, telephone, nurse call light, bed controls, and TV remote control. Most of the radioactive contamination will be found on the bathroom fixtures and floor, so these should receive special attention.

The patient's linen should be kept in a container in the patient's room and monitored for contamination before it is sent to the hospital laundry. Trash, including eating utensils and uneaten food, should be collected for monitoring before disposal.

After radioiodine administration, the isolation room should be posted with a "Caution: Radioactive Material" sign. When the patient is discharged, the isolation room should be decontaminated and monitored before housekeeping personnel prepare the room for another patient (as defined by the institution's radiation safety guidelines).

Instructions to Hospital Personnel

All nursing personnel should be issued film badges and instructed on how to wear them. No pregnant personnel should be assigned to care for the therapy patient. Safe exposure times for visitors and assigned personnel should be determined and posted in the patient's chart or on the patient's door. Personnel should be instructed to wear shoe covers and gloves when entering the isolation room.

The names and telephone numbers of the nuclear medicine physician and radiation safety officer should be included with detailed instructions placed in the front of the patient's chart. Hospital personnel should be encouraged to call on these individuals should any question or unusual circumstance arise.

Patient Monitoring/Area Surveys

The patient is monitored with a portable ionization chamber to determine safe exposure times for personnel and visitors and when the patient can be released from isolation.

Daily area surveys of hallways, stairwells, and rooms adjacent to the patient's isolation room should be conducted and recorded to ensure that the dose to any individual in these unrestricted areas does not exceed 20 μSv (2 mrem) in 1 hr and 1 mSv/year (100 mrem/year). If the measured dose rate exceeds 2 mrem/hr, the length of time that visitors or nursing personnel can remain in the room must be calculated. For example, if the survey meter measurement at the bedside is 15 mrem/hr, how long can a visitor or nurse remain at the point where the reading was made? Because 2 mrem in any 1 hr is the exposure limit for nonoccupational individuals,

$$\frac{15 \text{ mrem}}{60 \text{ minutes}} = \frac{2 \text{ mrem}}{X}$$

$$X = \frac{2 \text{ mrem } (60 \text{ min})}{15 \text{ mrem}}$$

$$X = 8 \text{ min.}$$

The radiation dose rate will decrease with increasing distance. Therefore, the farther visitors stand from the bedside, the longer they will be able to remain in the room.

To ensure that patients in adjacent rooms do not receive more than 2mrem in an hour, measurements should be made to ascertain that exposure limits for nearby patients are not exceeded. This requires that a therapy patient be placed in a private room.

To determine when a patient can be released from isolation, daily radiation measurements are compared with the initial measurement recorded immediately after the patient received the radioiodine. The dose rate at the time of administration is measured at a distance of at least 3 m. Subsequent measurements are made at the same distance. The dose rate measurements are related to the number of millicuries retained in the patient:

$$\frac{\text{initial dose rate}}{\text{millicuries administered}} = \frac{\text{subsequent dose rate}}{\text{millicuries retained}}.$$

For example, a patient receives 3.7 gigabecquerels (GBq) (100 mCi) of ^{131}I. Immediately after the administration, the dose rate at 3 m measures 150 mrem/hr. Twenty-four hours later, the dose rate at 3 m measures 50 mrem/hr. How many millicuries remain in the patient?

$$\frac{150 \text{ mrem/hr}}{100 \text{ mCi}} = \frac{50 \text{ mrem/hr}}{X \text{ mCi}}$$

$$X = \frac{100 \text{ mCi } (50 \text{ mrem/hr})}{15 \text{ mrem}}$$

$$X = 1.23 \text{ GBq } (33.3 \text{ mCi})$$

Patient Discharge Instructions

Patients continue to excrete measurable amounts of radioiodine in their saliva, urine, and perspiration for about 7–10 days after administration of radioiodine. NRC regulations require that patients be instructed in techniques that will minimize the radiation dose to family members or other individuals with whom the patient may come in contact. The most likely routes of radioiodine transfer should be reviewed with the patient along with the following guidelines (refer to your institution's radiation safety guidelines for patient discharge instructions).

For 7–10 days:

1. Intimate personal contact should be avoided. Do not share a bed with anyone. Avoid close contact with children, such as holding or kissing.
2. Maintain a distance of 1–2 m from others.
3. Use separate bathroom facilities, if available. The toilet should be flushed two to three times after each use.
4. Spilled urine or other bodily fluids should be cleaned up immediately with tissue paper and flushed down the toilet.
5. Wash hands thoroughly after using the bathroom.
6. Use a single set of plates, cups, and silverware during the week and wash those items separately from the family's dishes. Do *not* use disposable eating utensils, including utensils, plates, or cups.
7. Clothes, towels, and linen should not be shared and should be washed separately.
8. Avoid eating foods that can become contaminated with saliva (e.g., chicken, ribs, fruit with a core, etc.).

Outpatient High-Dosage Radioiodine Therapy

Patient Assessment

Additional patient assessment is necessary in the selection of patients for high-dose radioiodine therapy. Candidates for high-dose outpatient radioiodine therapy must be:

- mentally alert and physically able to take care of themselves with little assistance from others,
- able to walk to the bathroom and use the toilet without spilling urine on the toilet or floor,
- able to travel from the hospital to the home residence using private transportation or a taxi,
- able to minimize public contact for the first 2–3 days after treatment, and
- able to understand and follow written guidelines to minimize radiation exposure to others following therapy.

Patient Preparation

1. Patients must discontinue use of iodide-containing preparations, iodine supplements, thyroid hormones, and other medications that potentially affect the ability of thyroid tissue to accumulate iodide for a sufficient period of time before therapy.
2. For thyroid cancer patients, experts recommend a low-iodide diet for 7–10 days before administration of therapy to improve iodine uptake.
3. The patient should be fasting to enhance the absorption of the iodine from the stomach.
4. Before treatment, the technologist can determine whether the patient has difficulty swallowing by asking the patient to drink a small amount of water.
5. The treating physician will explain the procedure, treatment, complications, side effects, therapeutic alternatives, and expected outcome and obtain a written informed consent to treat before administration of the therapy.

Radiation Safety Considerations for Handling Liquid ^{131}I

If liquid ^{131}I is selected for therapy, it is recommended that a sealed-vial delivery system be used to minimize exposure to volatile ^{131}I fumes and to eliminate the possibility of contamination from a spilled vial. Capsule containers should be initially opened in a properly vented fume hood, checked for removable contamination, and then stored in the fume hood until the time of use.

Phosphorus-32 Therapy

^{32}P is a pure β emitter and has a half-life of 14.3 days. It emits a β particle with a maximum energy of 1.72 megaelectron volts (MeV) and has a mean energy of 0.70 MeV and an average penetrating range of 3.0 mm in soft tissue. The nuclear medicine technologist should be aware of the technical considerations associated with administration of a pure β- or β-/γ-emitting radiopharmaceutical.

^{32}P–Sodium Phosphate

^{32}P–sodium phosphate is a clear, colorless solution intended for intravenous administration. Dosages range from 37 to 740 MBq (20 mCi), depending on the pathology being treated. ^{32}P–sodium phosphate is used for the treatment of polycythemia vera and the control of bone pain resulting from metastatic disease in the skeleton. Technical considerations similar to those for ^{89}Sr therapy should be adhered to during ^{32}P–sodium phosphate therapy. These considerations are discussed in the section on bone pain therapy.

^{32}P–Chromic Phosphate

(Note that this procedure is performed very rarely, if at all, anymore.) ^{32}P–chromic phosphate suspension is a blue-green colloidal solution intended for intracavitary use only. If this agent is mistakenly administered intravenously, the colloidal particles will be taken up by the Kupffer cells of the liver, thereby causing severe localized radiation damage. Dosages range from 222 to 740 MBq (6–20 mCi).

^{32}P-colloidal is introduced into the peritoneal or pleural cavities. Once administered, the agent remains in the cavity into which it was introduced. However, drainage from the instillation site or dressings covering the site should be considered radiation hazards and handled appropriately. All supplies used during the instillation (gloves, needles, tubing) should be disposed of as radioactive waste.

Pain Therapy

Radionuclide therapy is used to treat bone pain associated with metastatic bone disease. Radiopharmaceuticals approved by the U.S. Food and Drug Administration (FDA) to treat bone pain due to osteoblastic metastasis include ^{89}Sr–chloride, ^{153}Sm–lexidronam, and ^{32}P–sodium phosphate. The goal of this therapy is palliative and thus to improve the patient's quality of life by restoring his or her ability to resume the activities of daily living. The nuclear medicine technologist's responsibilities occur primarily at the time of radiopharmaceutical administration.

^{89}Sr–Chloride

^{89}Sr–chloride is an analog of calcium that is rapidly cleared from the blood and localizes in the bone. It preferentially localizes in the areas of active osteogenesis, remaining in the metastatic sites longer than in normal bone (about 50 days and 14 days, respectively). ^{89}Sr has a physical half-life of 50.5 days. It emits a β particle with a maximum energy of 1.46 MeV, a mean energy of 0.58 MeV, and an average penetrating range of 2.44 mm in soft tissue.

Therapeutic dosages range from 1.5 to 2.2 MBq/kg (40–60 μCi/kg) and are injected intravenously. Repeat therapy is at 12-week intervals (blood count dependent).

^{153}Sm–Lexidronam

^{153}Sm–lexidronam is a phosphate compound concentrating in bone mineral. ^{153}Sm has a physical half-life of 46.7 hr (1.9 days). It emits a β particle with a maximum energy of 0.81 MeV, mean energy of 0.23 MeV, an average penetrating range of 0.6 mm in soft tissue, and a β emission with a photopeak of 0.103 MeV. The therapeutic dosage is 37 MBq/kg (1 mCi/kg) injected intravenously. Repeat therapy is at 12-week intervals (blood count dependent).

^{32}P–Sodium Phosphate

^{32}P accumulates mainly in the hydroxyapatite crystal of the bone and the remainder in nonosseous tissue. The therapeutic dosage is 185–370 MBq (5–10 mCi) administered intravenously or 370–444 MBq (10–12 mCi) orally. Repeat therapy is at 12-week intervals (blood count dependent).

Patient Preparation for Bone Pain Therapy

- Recent bone scan (4–8 weeks) documenting increased osteoblastic activity should have been performed.
- To avoid severe leukopenia or thrombocytopenia, no long-acting myelosuppressive chemotherapy (e.g., nitrosoureas) or full dosages of other forms of myelosuppressive chemotherapy or systemic radiotherapy should be administered for 6–8 weeks or 4 weeks, respectively, before treatment or for 6–12 weeks thereafter.
- To reduce the probability of combined myelotoxicity from external and internal radiation sources, no external beam hemibody radiation should be administered in the 2–3 months before treatment.
- Complete blood counts should be performed 7 days before treatment (recommended values to reduce the chance of infection and bleeding: platelet counts $\geqslant$60,000–100,000/μL, leukocyte counts

≥2400–3000/μL, and absolute granulocyte counts ≥2000/μL).

- Negative pregnancy test in women of childbearing age should have been performed (no breast-feeding).
- Fasting is *not* required before administration. Hospitalization is *not* required after treatment.
- Venous access should have been established and verified (intravenous catheter or running intravenous line) before administration of radiopharmaceutical (slow intravenous push with continuous verification of intravenous patency to avoid infiltration). After administration of radiopharmaceutical, flush syringe and line with 0.9% normal saline.

Radiation Safety Considerations in Bone Pain Therapy

- Use plastic or plastic/tungsten or plastic/lead syringe shield.
- Catheterize incontinent patients for 3–5 days after therapy. Two-thirds of the administered dose is excreted in urine and the remainder in feces. Activity in urinary excretion is greatest in the first 2 days after administration. Gloves should be worn to handle soiled garments or patient excretion (urine, feces, saliva, or blood).
- Accurate calibration of ^{32}P, ^{89}Sr, or ^{153}Sm may be obtained from *Guidelines for the Calibration of Metastron (^{89}Sr–Chloride Injection)*, or use a dose calibrator specifically configured to quantitate β emissions. (^{153}Sm–lexidronam has a γ emission at 103 keV for calibration.) Because it is not possible to directly assay a β emitter in most dose calibrators, the NRC does not require that patient dosages containing pure β emitters be measured before administration if the dosages are supplied as a unit dosage from the manufacturer or licensed radiopharmacy. However, if the β-emitting radiopharmaceuticals are not received as a unit dosage, the licensee must assay them directly, using special instrumentation capable of the assay, or must assay them indirectly using a combination of measurements and calculations with available instrumentation. Refer to the references at the end of this chapter for additional information for the assay of β emitters.

Instructions to Patients

For 7 days:

- use condoms for sexual relations,
- wash hands thoroughly after using the toilet,
- avoid transfer of bodily fluids (saliva, blood, urine, stool), and
- clean up spilled urine and dispose of blood-contaminated material so that others will not inadvertently handle it.

Up to 12 months after treatment:

- use effective contraceptive methods.

Radioimmunotherapy for Non-Hodgkin's Lymphoma

Radioimmunotherapy combines a monoclonal antibody directed against a specific protein found on tumor cells with a β-emitting radionuclide to deliver a targeted dose of radiation directly to the tumor cell. When the radioactive tracer binds to the antigen expressed by the tumor, it delivers radiation to the cells it binds to as well as to nearby tumor cells and tumor cells that do not express the antigen or are poorly vascularized, bulky tumors. Because the path-length of β-emitting radionuclides is limited, ranging from 0.8 to 5.0 mm in tissue, the radiation absorbed dose to adjacent normal tissues is minimized.

^{90}Y–Ibritumomab Tiuxetan (Zevalin)

^{90}Y–ibritumomab tiuxetan (Zevalin) is a murine IgG_1 κ monoclonal antibody that targets the CD20 antigen. ^{90}Y has a physical half-life of 64.1 hr (2.67 days). It emits a β particle with a maximum energy of 2.281 MeV and an average penetrating range of 5 mm in soft tissue.

The therapeutic dosage is calculated on the basis of patient's weight and platelet count (0.3 mCi/kg for platelet counts between 100,000 and 149,000 μL; 0.4 mCi/kg for platelet counts ≥150,000 μL); the maximum dosage is not to exceed 32 mCi.

Patient Preparation

- Recent bone marrow biopsy to determine the extent of lymphoma in bone marrow (not to exceed 25%).
- Recent blood count to determine platelet count (must be ≥100,000 μL).
- Negative serum pregnancy test for women of childbearing age.
- Whole-body scan with indium-111 Zevalin at 2–24 hr and again at 48–72 hr to confirm biodistribution of monoclonal antibody during the week preceding treatment.
- Fasting not required before treatment.
- Infusion of rituximab, 250 mg/m^2 intravenously (completed no more than 4 hr before administration of the therapeutic dosage of ^{90}Y–ibritumomab tiuxetan.

- Venous access established and verified (intravenous catheter or running intravenous line) before administration of radiopharmaceutical.
- ^{90}Y–ibritumomab tiuxetan administered intravenously over 10 min with continuous verification of intravenous line patency to avoid infiltration—after administration of radiopharmaceutical, flush syringe and line with a minimum of 10 mL 0.9% normal saline.

Radiation Safety Considerations/ Instructions to Patient

Refer to those associated with bone pain therapy.

^{131}I–Tositumomab (Bexxar)

Tositumomab is a murine IgG_{2a} λ monoclonal antibody directed against the CD20 antigen, which is found on the surface of normal and malignant β lymphocytes. ^{131}I has a physical half-life of 8.04 days. It emits a range of β particles with a maximum energy of 606.3 keV.

The therapeutic dosage is calculated on the basis of patient platelet count. If the patient has greater than or equal to 150,000 platelets/mL, then an activity to deliver 75 centigrays (cGy) of ^{131}I to the whole body is given and 35 mg tositumomab is administered intravenously over 20 min. If the patient has a platelet count between 100,000 and 150,000/mL, then an activity to deliver 65 cGy of ^{131}I to the whole body is given and 35 mg tositumomab is administered intravenously over 20 min.

Usage and Patient Preparation

Patient preparation includes the following considerations:

- The Bexxar therapy is indicated for treatment of patients with CD20 antigen-expressing non-Hodgkin's lymphoma that has relapsed or is refractory. The therapy is also indicated for patients with low-grade, follicular, or transformed non-Hodgkin's lymphoma, including patients with Rituximab-refractory non-Hodgkin's lymphoma (this helps to determine the effectiveness of the Bexxar therapeutic alone or indicates the need for chemotherapy and Rituximab).
- This therapy is not indicated for the initial treatment of patients with CD20 positive non-Hodgkin's lymphoma.
- Recent blood count to determine platelet count must be ≥100,000 μL.
- Serum pregnancy test for women of childbearing age must be negative.

Proceed as described:

- Day −1: Patient begins thyroprotective regimen, which continues through 14 days post-therapeutic dose
- Day 0: Premedication with acetaminophen and diphenhydramine. *Dosimetric step*: IV infusion of 450 mg tositumomab over 60 min followed by IV infusion of 5.0 mCi Iodine ^{131}I–tositumomab (35 mg) over 20 min.
- Day 2, 3, or 4: Whole-body dosimetry and biodistribution
- Day 6 or 7: Whole-body dosimetry and biodistribution
- If biodistribution is acceptable then you proceed to the *therapeutic step*:
- Calculate patient-specific dose on the basis of platelet level.
- Day 7 up to day 14: Premedication with acetaminophen and diphenhydramine; IV infusion of 450 mg tositumomab over 60 min followed by therapeutic dose of Iodine ^{131}I–tTositumomab (35 mg) over 20 min.

Radiation Safety Considerations/ Instructions to Patient

Refer to safety considerations associated with ^{131}I therapy and continue thyroprotective regimen for 14 days post therapeutic dose.

Unresectable Hepatocellular Carcinoma

^{90}Y Microspheres (TheraSphere) Glass Microspheres

TheraSphere consists of insoluble glass microspheres where ^{90}Y is an integral constituent of the glass. The mean sphere diameter ranges from 20 to 30 μm. Each milligram contains 22,000–73,000 microspheres. ^{90}Y is a pure β emitter with a half-life of 64.2 hr (2.67 days) and the average β emissions are 936.7 keV.

Usage and Patient Preparation

- Prior to administration patient should undergo hepatic arterial catheterization using balloon catheterization or other appropriate angiographic techniques to prevent extrahepatic shunting.
- ^{99m}Tc MAA (75–150 MBq [2–4 mCi]) is administered into the hepatic artery to determine the extent of A-V shunting to the lungs and to confirm the absence of gastric and duodenal flow.
- Activity required for a particular dose to liver should be between 80 and 150 Gy (8,000 rad to 15,000 rad) and is calculated by:

$$\text{Activity required (GBq)} = [\text{desired dose (Gy)}][\text{liver mass (kg)}]/50.$$

- Liver volume is determined using CT or ultrasound.
- Actual dose to liver is calculated by:

$$\text{Dose (Gy)} = 50[\text{injected activity (GBq)}][1 - F]/\text{liver mass (kg)},$$

where F is the fraction of injected activity shunted to the lungs, as measured by ^{99m}Tc–MAA with a maximum amount being $F \times A = 0.61$ GBq (18.4 mCi).
- ^{90}Y microspheres are injected into arterial catheter and remain fixed as close as possible to tumor site.

Radiation Safety Considerations

Use standard precautions to ensure that the microspheres do not contaminate the work area. Survey with an appropriate survey meter and wipe check to ensure that contamination did not occur.

References and Further Reading

Bender JM, Dworkin HJ, 1993. Iodine-131 as an oncology agent. *J Nucl Med Technol.* 21:140–150.

Bexxar (Tositumomab), 2010. Prescribing information. Brentford, Middlesex, United Kingdom: GlaxoSmithKline.

Clarke MT, Galie E, 1993. Radionuclide therapy of osseous metastatic disease. *J Nucl Med Technol.* 21:3–6.

Dickinson CZ, Hendrix NS, 1993. Strontium-89 therapy in painful bony metastases. *J Nucl Med Technol.* 21:133–137.

Early PJ, Sodee DB, 1995. *Principles and Practice of Nuclear Medicine.* 2nd ed. St. Louis, MO: Mosby; 331–333, 752–756.

Miller KL, Bott SM, Velkley DE, Cunniungham DE, 1979. Review of contamination and exposure hazards associated with therapeutic uses of iodine. *J Nucl Med Technol.* 7:163–168.

Parthasarathy KL, Crawford ES, 2002. Treatment of thyroid carcinoma: emphasis on high-dose ^{131}I outpatient therapy. *J Nucl Med Technol.* 30:165–171.

Silberstein EB, Taylor AT Jr., 2001. Society of Nuclear Medicine procedure guidelines for bone pain treatment 2.0. In: *Society of Nuclear Medicine Procedure Guidelines Manual.* Reston, VA: Society of Nuclear Medicine; 111–116.

Silberstein EB, Alavi A, Balon HR, Becker DV, Brill DR, Clarke SE, Divgi C, Coldsmith SJ, Lull RJ, Meier DA, Royal HD, Siegal JA, Waxman AD, 2002. Procedure guideline for therapy of thyroid disease with I-131 (sodium iodide). In: *Society of Nuclear Medicine Procedure Guideline* Reston, VA: Society of Nuclear Medicine.

Steves AM, 1999. Radiation protection in nuclear medicine. In: Dowd SB, Tilson ER, eds. *Practical Radiation Protection and Applied Radiobiology.* 2nd ed. Philadelphia, PA: WB Saunders; 276–281.

TheraSphere, 2010. Yttrium-90 Glass Microspheres package insert. Ottawa, ON, Canada: MDS Nordion.

Thompson MA, 2001. Radiation safety precautions in the management of the hospitalized ^{131}I therapy patient. *J Nucl Med Technol.* 29:61–66.

Zevalin (ibritumomab tiuxetan), 2002. Prescribing information. San Diego, CA: IDEC Pharmaceuticals.

PART II

Advanced Information and Post Primary Certification Primers

CHAPTER 20 Advanced Nuclear Cardiology Review

Amy Byrd Brady

Nuclear cardiology has become a major component of nuclear medicine. Many technologists are solely focused on performing cardiac studies. Board-certified nuclear medicine technologists who have had at least 2 years of fulltime experience in nuclear medicine along with a few additional requirements may be eligible to sit for the nuclear cardiology specialty board exam. Information regarding this specialty exam, such as the exam application and an exam content outline, can be found on the Nuclear Medicine Technology Certification Board website (http://www.nmtcb.org) under the specialty exams tab. Prior to taking the exam, it is essential to review topics such as instrumentation, quality control, patient care, the cardiovascular system, pathology, electrocardiogram (ECG), emergency care, radiopharmaceuticals, and interventional drugs. The Society of Nuclear Medicine's website (http://www.snm.org) and the American Society of Nuclear Cardiology's website (http://www.asnc.org) provide a great resource for approved cardiac imaging and stress procedures. Another excellent resource for preparing for this exam is the Nuclear Cardiology Technology Study Guide, which is available at the Society of Nuclear Medicine website. This chapter focuses on introducing topics such as cardiac shunts, metaiodobenzylguanidine (MIBG) imaging, β-methyl-*p*-(I-123)-iodophenyl-pentadecanoic ([^{123}I]BMIPP) imaging, ECG interpretation, and building an enhanced knowledge from where previous chapters of this review book have left off.

Equipment

Equipment is a necessary component in nuclear cardiology and should be properly chosen for the specific purpose of its use. Once the equipment has been chosen, it is essential to have and maintain a first-class quality assurance (QA) plan for the equipment to produce high-quality imaging.

Planar Imaging

While planar imaging is no longer the standard approach used for myocardial perfusion imaging, it can be a great alternative for patients who are unable to have single-photon emission computed tomography (SPECT) imaging due to body habitus or an inability to remain in the position needed for SPECT imaging (see Fig. 20.1). For cardiac imaging, a small-field-of-view scintillation camera is practical. When using the 10-in. field of view (FOV) with a matrix of 128 × 128, the result is about 2 mm of pixel spacing. A 15-in. FOV camera should be zoomed using a magnification of 1.2–1.5 so that the pixel size is close to 2 mm.

Energy windows around the photopeak should always be symmetric. The energy peak and window settings are camera specific and should be established for each individual camera. In general, a 20% window is standard when using ^{99m}Tc. For ^{201}Tl, a 30% window around the 70-keV peak and a 15% window around the 167-keV peak are sufficient.

As far as collimation, it is recommended that a parallel-hole collimator be used for planar imaging. When using ^{99m}Tc, the low-energy, high-resolution collimator is usually best. When using ^{201}Tl, a low-energy, medium-resolution (all-purpose) collimator is best as the counting statistics become limited with a high-resolution collimator.

SPECT Imaging

SPECT imaging cameras incorporate many variables that dictate their performance. Single-head cameras are widely used; however, the benefit of adding additional detectors is evident. Each detector added to a system doubles the acquired counts, which in turn reduce the acquisition time (see Fig. 20.2).

Another variable in SPECT imaging is the orbit of the detector. A more traditional orbit used has been circular with step-and-shoot motion using a rotational range of 180° or 360°. When a 180° orbit is recommended for

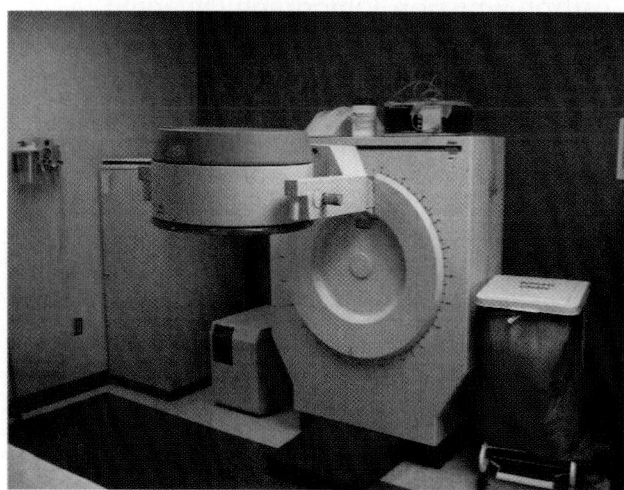

Figure 20.1 Typical gamma camera used for planar imaging. (Courtesy of Cheryl Counce from Brookwood Medical Center, Birmingham, AL.)

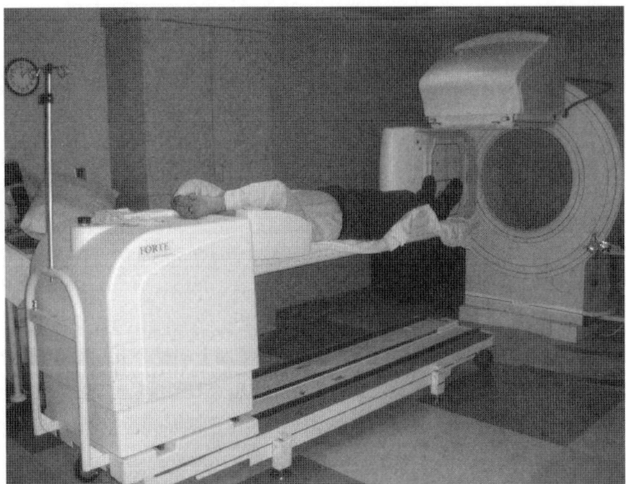

Figure 20.2 Typical SPECT gamma camera. (Courtesy UAB Medical West, Bessemer, AL.)

SPECT imaging, having two detectors separated by 90° as they rotate around the heart is the ideal method. When a 360° orbit is used, having three detectors separated by 120° from each other is also preferred. A more modern orbit used in most SPECT imaging systems today is the elliptical or noncircular orbit. The elliptical reduces the distance from the camera to the body by following the body contour, which in turn improves spatial resolution.

The combination of both SPECT and computed tomography (CT) add a range of potential and integration. The SPECT apparatus usually contains a large FOV and dual detectors. The CT apparatus include nondiagnostic units that are used for anatomical location and attenuation correction only. The CT apparatus may even include multislice units, which can perform stand-alone diagnostic scans.

Positron Emission Tomography Imaging

Most dedicated positron emission tomography (PET) cameras consist of rings of small detectors. Four commonly used crystal types include bismuth germinate (BGO), gadolinium oxyorthosilicate (GSO), lutetium oxyorthosilicate (LSO), and lutetium yttrium orthosilicate (LYSO). PET scanners mainly rely on CT scans for attenuation correction but can also use rotating-rod sources of germanium-68/gallium-68. The rotating-rod sources produce a transmission scan prior to or following the emission scan. The rotating-rod sources add approximately 3–8 min of scan time.

Quality Control

Quality control is the portion of quality assurance in which tests are performed to identify equipment problems and it should be completed prior to acquiring patient studies. Agencies such as the American College of Radiology (ACR) and the Intersocietal Commission for the Accreditation of Nuclear Medicine Laboratories (ICANL) require proof of a nuclear cardiology facility's performance of quality control.

The first step in creating a quality control plan for a nuclear cardiology facility is acceptance testing. Acceptance testing is completed once upon equipment installment and upon any major upgrades. It is recommended that the equipment perform as specified by the manufacturer according to National Electrical Manufacturers Association (NEMA) guidelines.

The next step in creating a well-designed quality control plan is to establish routine checks that can be closely monitored to note changes in performance parameters. A quality control plan must be established for planar imaging, SPECT imaging, sealed-source SPECT/transmission computed tomography (TCT) systems, X-ray-based SPECT/CT systems, dedicated PET imaging, and PET/CT imaging.

Planar Imaging Quality Control

Planar imaging includes four quality control tests: energy peaking, uniformity test, resolution and linearity test, and a sensitivity test (see Fig. 20.3). Energy peaking is used to confirm that the camera is counting photons having the correct energy. Uniformity is used to confirm that the camera's sensitivity response is uniform across the detector's face. Manufacturers may suggest whether uniformity be completed intrinsically or extrinsically. If uniformity is performed intrinsically, the radioactive point source should be positioned at a distance at least five times the crystal's useful field of view (UFOV). Resolution and linearity tests are performed to check the camera's spatial resolution and its change over time, along with the detector's ability to image straight lines.

SPECT Imaging Quality Control

SPECT imaging includes all of the general quality control tests required for planar images plus a center of rotation (COR), a high-count extrinsic flood-field uniformity correction, and a Jaszczak SPECT phantom test

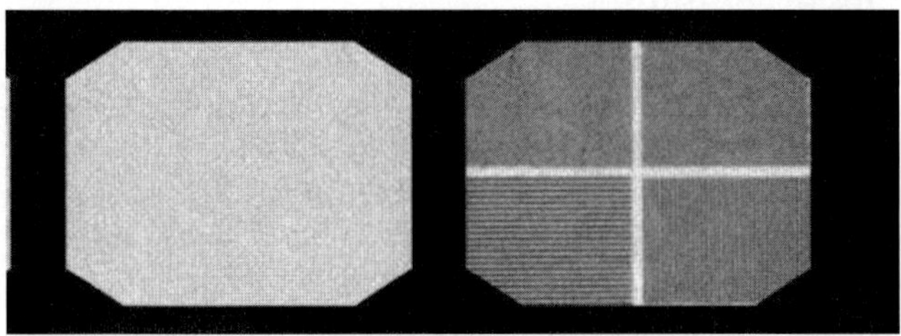

Figure 20.3 Typical uniformity and linearity test. (Courtesy of Saint Vincent's East Medical Center, Birmingham, AL.)

(see Figs. 20.4 and 20.5). The COR is a measure performed to ensure that the center field of view of the camera detector matches with the software of the computer. A ^{99m}Tc source can be used to perform the COR test on each detector head. COR testing should be performed in all detector formats if images are acquired in detector formations other than 180°. The accuracy of the COR alignment should be performed weekly and new COR calibrations should be performed after the camera is serviced, following power surges or outages, and for the computer after upgrades in the software. An error in the COR can reduce spatial resolution and image contrast through blurring of the image. An error can also cause significant artifacts in the image concerning the apex of the heart. A high-count extrinsic flood-field uniformity correction should be performed as directed by the manufacturer. The high-count flood is used to ensure that the efficiency of photon detection is constant across the surface of the collimated detector. It is recommended that 30–100 million count images be acquired for each detector and a deficiency in the flood can lead to characteristic "ring" artifacts in SPECT imaging. A Jaszczak SPECT phantom test is used to determine the 3D contrast, resolution, and uniformity of the camera. It is recommended by NEMA that the 30 million count acquisition and section reconstruction using a Jaszczak SPECT phantom should be completed quarterly.

Sealed-Source SPECT/TCT Systems Quality Control

Sealed-Source SPECT/TCT Systems includes all of the SPECT imaging quality control tests plus energy peaking, transmission source mechanics, and source strength. Energy peaking is completed to confirm that the camera is counting photons in the proper energy windows. A check of transmission source mechanics is performed to confirm the operation of the source shutter and translating mechanics, and a reference "blank" transmission scan should be acquired. It is recommended that the transmission source mechanics scan is performed weekly and possibly daily. The source strength is performed on systems using a 153-gadolinium (^{153}Gd) transmission source to evaluate the transmission-to-cross-talk ratio (TCR) value. Source strength should be performed at least monthly along with a baseline scan when the transmission source is installed or replaced.

X-Ray-Based SPECT/CT Systems Quality Control

X-ray-based SPECT/CT systems include all of the SPECT imaging quality control tests plus additional quality control specific to CT imaging. The CT imaging quality controls include calibration and field uniformity. Calibration is performed with a special phantom, which includes inserts of known CT numbers. A CT imaging system is considered not calibrated when the error is greater than 5 Hounsfield units. Field uniformity is performed to ensure a uniform response throughout the FOV.

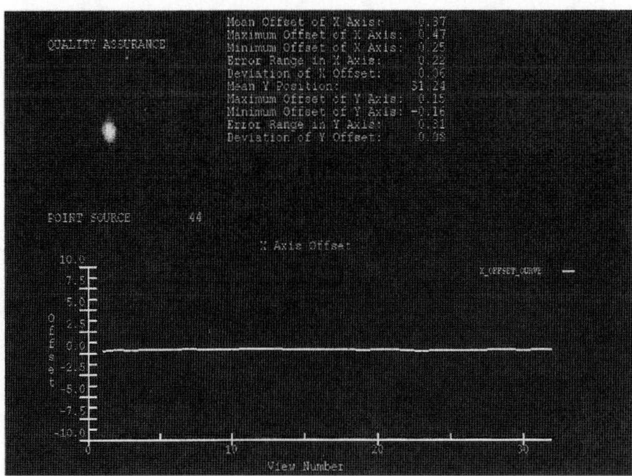

Figure 20.4 Results of a COR analysis. (Reprinted, with permission, from Alessi *et al.*, 2010.)

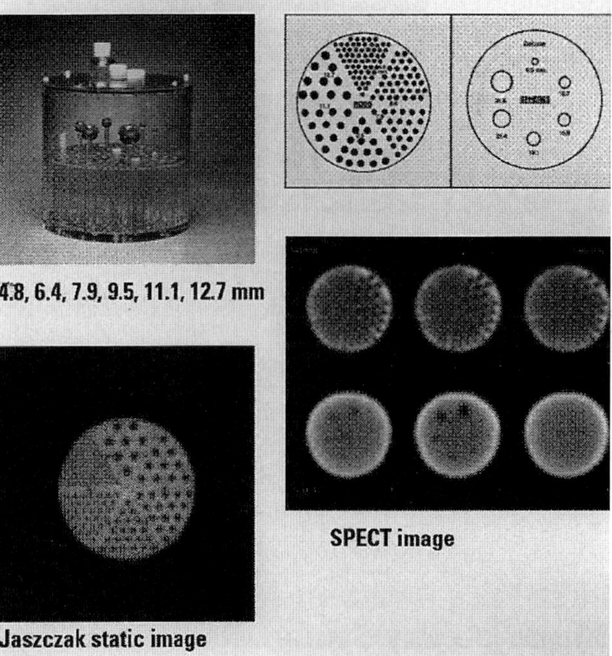

Figure 20.5 Photograph and diagrams of Jaszczak phantom showing the variable size of rods and spheres as well as the image result of static and SPECT phantom for camera QC. (Reprinted, with permission, from Alessi *et al.*, 2010.)

Combined SPECT/CT Quality Control

Combined SPECT/CT systems include all of the SPECT imaging and CT imaging quality control tests. However, when the SPECT/CT system is combined, the CT portion must additionally perform registration, attenuation correction accuracy, and misregistration consequences.

Dedicated PET Imaging Quality Control

Suggested quality controls for PET imaging includes acceptance testing, sensitivity, transverse resolution, scatter fraction, accuracy of attenuation correction, and any other test recommended by the manufacturer. Sensitivity is performed to monitor sensitivity changes and proper operation of the scanner. It is recommended that sensitivity be performed daily or at least weekly. Transverse resolution is performed using a point source or rod source. It is recommended that transverse resolution be performed annually. It is also recommended that scatter fraction and accuracy of attenuation correction be performed annually.

PET/CT Imaging Quality Control

The quality control of the PET portion of PET/CT includes all of the suggested quality controls for PET imaging. The quality control of the CT portion of PET/CT also includes calibration and field uniformity.

Combined PET/CT Quality Control

Quality control for combined PET/CT systems includes the individual PET and CT portions as mentioned and also registration and attenuation correction accuracy.

Dynamic Cardiac Imaging

Dynamic cardiac imaging is beneficial when evaluating the heart's ability to function (especially in patients with a known cardiac disease). Indications for dynamic cardiac imaging are included in Table 20.1. Dynamic cardiac imaging can be performed by the first-pass radionuclide angiography study and/or by the equilibrium radionuclide angiogram (ERNA) study. See Figure 20.6 for examples of kinesis, hypokinesis, akinesis, and dyskinesis.

Table 20.1 Indications for Dynamic Cardiac Imaging

1. Assess either left or right ventricular ejection fraction (EF) at rest and/or during exercise.
2. Evaluate regional wall-motion abnormalities, such as hypokinesia, akinesia, and dyskinesia (aneurysm), during rest or during exercise (Fig. 20.6).
3. Evaluate ventricular function (EF and wall motion):
   - before cardiac catherization
   - after a myocardial infarction
   - in patients with valvular disease
   - to monitor patients on doxorubicin and related chemotherapy agents
   - to evaluate responses to therapies, including exercise, angioplasty, open heart or cardiac bypass surgery, and others.
4. Estimate cardiac output, ventricular volumes, and other cardiac functional parameters.
5. Assess diastolic function of the left ventricle, such as peak-filling rate and time to peak-filling rate.
6. Evaluate and quantify left-to-right or right-to-left cardiac shunts.

Reprinted, with permission, from Crawford and Husain (2003).

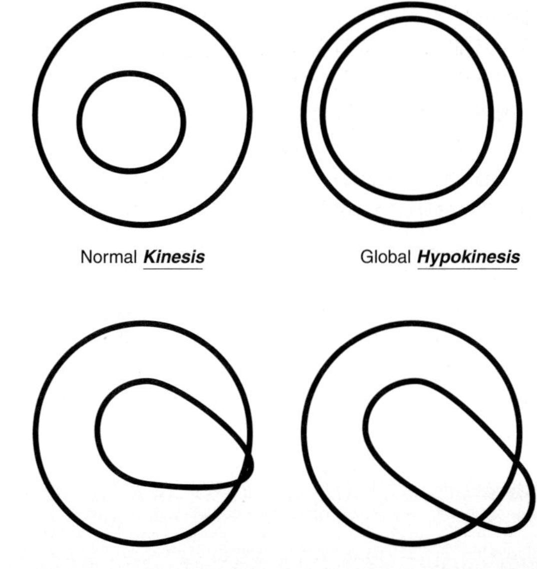

Figure 20.6 Wall-motion terms where kinesis is movement, hypokinesis is low wall motion, akinesis is motionless, and dyskinesis is an outward motion during systole (Crawford and Husain, 2003).

First-Pass Radionuclide Angiography Study

A first-pass study looks at both left and right ventricular function either at rest or stress. The first-pass study also evaluates cardiac shunts, which refer to the movement of blood across the septum. Shunts are usually a congenital defect that typically close as the patient matures. If surgery is needed, a first-pass study can verify resolution of the shunting after repair or calculate the amount of residual shunting if the repair is not complete. A cardiac shunt can be either right-to-left or left-to-right.

Acquisition Protocols When Assessing Left and Right Ventricular Function

Radionuclides commonly used when determining either left or right ventricular function in first-pass studies include [^{99m}Tc]diethylaminetriamine pentaacetic acid (DTPA), [^{99m}Tc]pertechnetate, [^{99m}Tc]sestamibi, and [^{99m}Tc]tetrofosmin. A standard dose of 925 MBq (25 mCi) is commonly used for both rest and exercise studies; however, lower doses may be adequate. A bolus injection of the radionuclide should be pushed through a three-way stopcock connected to an intravenous catheter that has been placed in the antecubital or external jugular veins. Note that the radionuclide bolus should be pushed rapidly over 2–3 sec when assessing left ventrical (LV) function such that the full width at half maximum (FWHM) of the bolus is less than 1 sec. A time–activity curve of the frames can be used to show the bolus flowing through the superior vena cava and determine the integrity of the bolus. If a bolus is fragmented and/or the FWHM is greater than 1 sec, then the study should be repeated. For right ventrical (RV) function, the radionuclide bolus should be pushed slightly slower over 3–4 sec to achieve a FWHM of 2–3 sec for the superior vena cava curve. For both LV and RV function, the radionuclide injection is followed by a 10- to 20-mL saline flush.

When imaging a patient for a first-pass study, the patient can be lying supine or sitting upright. A common imaging position used for LV function is the upright, straight anterior view. With this view, overlap of anatomic structures may occur. To eliminate this overlap a right anterior oblique (RAO) can be used. When evaluating EF of the right ventricle, a shallow RAO is recommended to eliminate overlapping anatomic structures such as the left ventricle. The camera should be positioned as close to the patient's chest as possible to optimize resolution and maximize count-rate detection. The heart must be centered in the field of view. See Figure 20.7 for proper positioning.

A first-pass study's imaging time per frame is very short; therefore, a high-sensitivity collimator is standard. In general, most systems support a matrix size of 64 × 64 for the acquisition but other matrices have been used. A 15% energy window around the 140-keV photopeak of ^{99m}Tc is standard. Images are commonly acquired at 25 msec/frame with a total of 1500–2000 frames. While gating is not essential for a first-pass study, it is preferred for assistance in the determination of the end-diastolic frames that may be hard to reliably identify.

Processing and Results When Assessing Left and Right Ventricular Function

Processing in nuclear cardiology has become more and more automated and faster over the past years. With new technology and software, the technologist should still be observant when processing to ensure accurate results. Processing a first-pass study involves the creation of the initial time–activity curve (TAC), beat selection, creation of the initial representative cycle, background correction, creation of final representative cycle, and possibly motion correction.

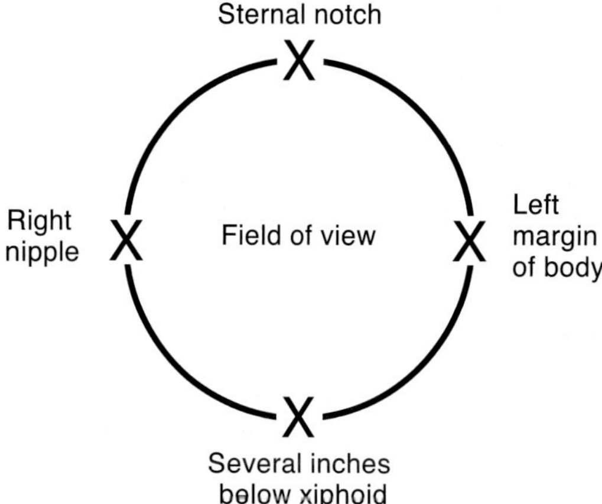

Figure 20.7 Anatomical landmarks used to position a first-pass study. (Reprinted, with permission, from Crawford and Husain, 2003.)

To create the initial TAC, the technologist should draw an initial ventricular region of interest (ROI). For beat selection, the technologist must identify the first and last beats to include in the representative cycle. When correcting background, the lung frame method is preferred; however, the periventricular method is a standard in many single-head gamma cameras. Once complete, the background correction should be applied to the initial representative cycle. The frames displaying the end diastolic and end systolic should be viewed and modified as needed. A final ROI should be drawn. The EF of the left ventricle is calculated from the final background-corrected representative cycle [(end-diastolic counts − end-systolic counts)/end-diastolic counts]:

$$\%\,\mathrm{EF} = \frac{\mathrm{net\ EDC} - \mathrm{net\ ESC}}{\mathrm{net\ EDC}} \times 100.$$

The left ventricular ejection fraction (LVEF) has a normal accepted range of 50–80% for a resting study. The LVEF under stress conditions for most normal individuals is 56% or greater. When using separate end-diastolic and end-systolic ROIs, the normal range for right ventricular ejection ranges from 40 to 65% in a rest study. RVEF usually increases during exercise but may actually decrease in patients with proximal right coronary artery lesions and/or pulmonary hypertension.

Cardiac Shunts

Cardiac shunts are most often found as a congenital defect, which usually closes on its own as a patient matures.

However, if the shunt does not close, surgery may be needed. Cardiac shunt evaluations are most often performed on pediatric patients and, therefore, the radioactive dose should be adjusted accordingly. While a nuclear medicine shunt evaluation is useful, ultrasound, Doppler imaging, and a cardiac catheterization are most currently used for shunt evaluation and quantification.

A right-to-left shunt occurs when a malformation allowing communication between the two sides of the heart is complicated by a lesion or condition that increases the right-sided pressure to greater than that of the left side. Blood that is shunted from the right side to the left bypasses the pulmonary arterial circulation and is prematurely returned to the systemic circulation without being oxygenated. Left untreated, a right-to-left shunt will cause cyanotic heart disease. A standard dose of 74–185 MBq (2–5 mCi) of [^{99m}Tc]macroaggregated albumin (MAA) can be used to evaluate a right-to-left shunt in the first-pass study. If a shunt is detected, there will be a premature visualization of the aorta before the lungs. The right heart may seem enlarged when compared to the left heart. The percentage of right-to-left shunting can be approximated by comparing the total body counts and total lung count (Fig. 20.8).

A left-to-right shunt occurs when the ductus arterious, which is a connection allowing blood to bypass the lungs in a developing fetus, does not close following birth. This shunt allows oxygenated blood from the left heart to flow back to the lungs. When imaging a first-pass study to evaluate a left-to-right shunt, a 370- to 555-MBq (10- to 15-mCi) dose of any of the ^{99m}Tc radiopharmaceuticals listed above is standard. Note that the FWHM of a good radionuclide bolus should be 3 sec or less. The total amount of frames acquired should bc 2000 and a matrix size of 64 × 64 or 32 × 32 is appropriate to use. If the shunt is detected, blood will return prematurely to the pulmonary circulation. Evaluation of the pulmonary TAC from the first-pass study may also detect the shunt. A normal pulmonary TAC will have a single large peak that is then followed by a small peak. An abnormal pulmonary TAC will show the initial peak of the TAC to have a bump on the downslope (Fig. 20.9).

To quantitate the left-to-right shunt, several methods such as the C_2/C_1 method, the area ratio method, and the gamma variate method can be used. An example of the C_2/C_1 method is given in Figure 20.10.

$$\%\ \text{Right to Left Shunt} = \frac{\text{Whole Body Counts} - \text{Lung Counts}}{\text{Whole Body Counts}} \times 100$$

Figure 20.8 Right-to-left shunt quantitation. (Reprinted, with permission, from Alessi *et al.*, 2010.)

Pulmonary Time Activity Curves

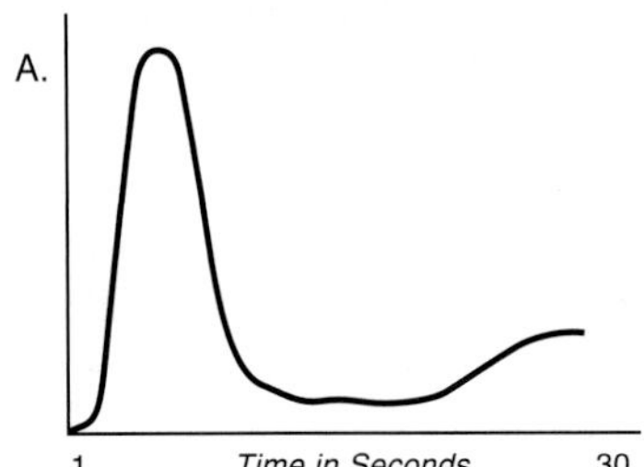

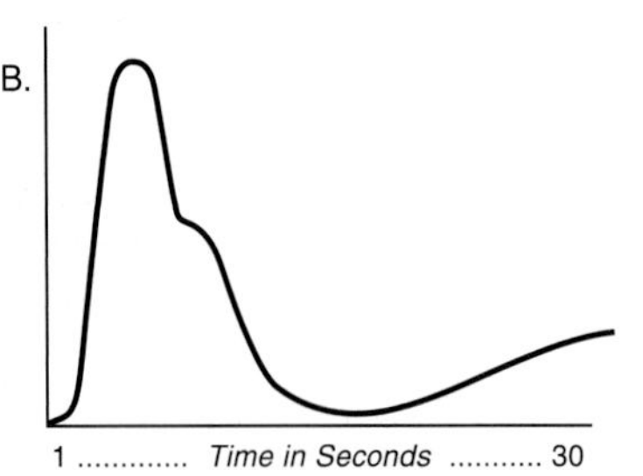

Figure 20.9 Pulmonary time–activity curves. (A) Normal curve. (B) Curve demonstrating a left-to-right shunt. (Reprinted, with permission, from Crawford and Husain, 2003.)

Equilibrium Radionuclide Angiogram (ERNA) Study

As previously mentioned in the cardiovascular system chapter of this review book, many names have been given to gated blood-pool imaging and it is important to recognize and become familiar with all of the names. A planar ERNA is used to primarily determine LV function at rest and/or during exercise stress or pharmacologic intervention. Ventricular function includes evaluating wall motion, EF, and other parameters of systolic and diastolic function. SPECT ERNA can also be used to determine both global and regional ventricular function at rest and/or during pharmacologic intervention.

Acquisition Protocols

The radionuclide used in ERNA studies is ^{99m}Tc-labeled red blood cells. For resting studies, the standard dosage is approximately 740–925 MBq/70 kg (20–25 mCi/70 kg) body weight. For exercise studies, the standard dosage is approximately 925–1295 MBq/70 kg (25–35 mCi/70 kg). The three techniques for labeling red blood cells include in vivo, in vitro, and modified in vivo/in vitro (Table 20.2). Poor labeling of the red blood cells results in an accumulation of ^{99m}Tc-free pertechnetate in the mucosa of the stomach and in the thyroid gland. Causes of poor labeling include certain medications such as heparin and when "old" [^{99m}Tc]pertechnetate of low specific activity is used.

When available for resting studies, it is best to use a parallel-hole collimator with high resolution and spatial resolution of approximately 8- to 10-mm FWHM. When performing a time-limited stress study such as the bicycle exercise, the low-energy all-purpose (LEAP) collimator should be used. However, if

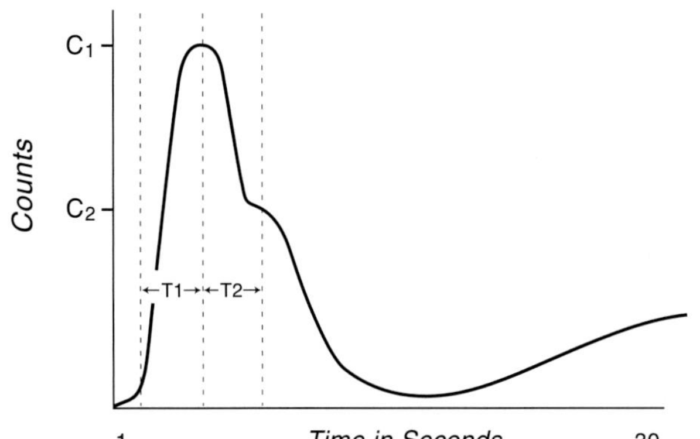

Figure 20.10 C_2/C_1 method for quantification of left-to-right shunts. T1, time interval from the beginning of the rise of the pulmonary curve to the maximum count; T2, time interval equal to T1 following T1; C_1, count level at the end of T1; and C_2, count level at the end of T2. (Reprinted, with permission, from Crawford and Husain, 2003.)

performing both a rest and stress study the same collimator should be used for both. In this case, the LEAP is recommended. A slant-hole collimator is best when performing a caudal tilt of 10° to 15°. Most ERNA studies are performed using a matrix zoomed 64 × 64. The standard energy window is ±10% of the 140 keV. While frame mode is standard, list-mode acquisition is a good option as it offers increased beat-length windowing flexibility.

In general, the ERNA study gathers data from many consecutive cardiac cycles that are all overlapped. The cardiac cycle is divided into a predetermined number of frames or images that generally ranges from 16 to 32. When a patient is connected to a three-lead ECG to the camera, the computer will start to acquire data when it sees the R wave and the time of the acquisition will be redirected to frame 1. This process is called "gating" and will continue until the information count density has been acquired. The data from all the cardiac cycles are basically overlapped to form a composite or summary image of the heart. The normal R–R interval is first computed and a tolerance limit of ±10% is usually chosen. If the R–R interval is shorter than normal, the data will not be acquired into one of the latter frames. If the R–R interval is longer than normal, the data acquisition will pause and wait for the next R wave.

Positioning

The three main views needed when assessing the wall motion of the left ventricle are the LAO, anterior, and left lateral or posterior oblique. The patient should be in the supine position or in the right lateral decubitus position (Figs. 20.11 and 20.12).

The 45° LAO view is used to visualize the septum. Depending on the patient, the 45° angle may vary slightly. The orientation should be that the long axis of the ventricle is vertical with the apex pointing down and the left ventricle on the right side of the image. A caudal tilt of approximately 10° to 15° can be used to help separate the atria from the ventricle (Fig. 20.13).

Image Display and Processing

The multiple-view ERNA is usually displayed as an endless-loop simultaneously in zones of the computer screen. Use of a linear gray scale is recommended when the views are displayed. A smoothing process (or Gaussian nine-point smoothing) is used to remove statistical fluctuations from the image. To determine the EF, an LV volume curve must be generated from manually drawing the ROI over the end diastole and end systole (Figs. 20.14, 20.15, and 20.16). Background must also be

Table 20.2 Techniques for Labeling Red Blood Cells

Labeling method	Technique	Problems	
In vivo	1. A "cold" pyrophosphate (PYP) kit reconstituted with saline is administered IV to the patient 2. 10–30 min later, Inject [^{99m}Tc]pertechnetate IV 3. Pertechnetate tags to the RBCs within 15 min	Not all of the [^{99m}Tc]pertechnetate tags to the RBCs	Not Recommended
In vitro	1. A blood sample is collected from the patient 2. RBCs are labeled in a vial outside of the patient 3. Permits washing of RBCs to remove unbound pertechnetate before readministration to patient (takes about 25 min)	Manipulation of the RBCs; sterility	Preferred
Modified in vivo/in vitro	1. Administer reconstituted cold PYP to the patient's IV 2. After 15–20 min, withdraw a blood sample into a heparinized syringe containing [^{99m}Tc]pertechnetate 3. Incubate the blood in the syringe for about 10 min, mixing frequently 4. Reinject the labeled blood cells		Standard

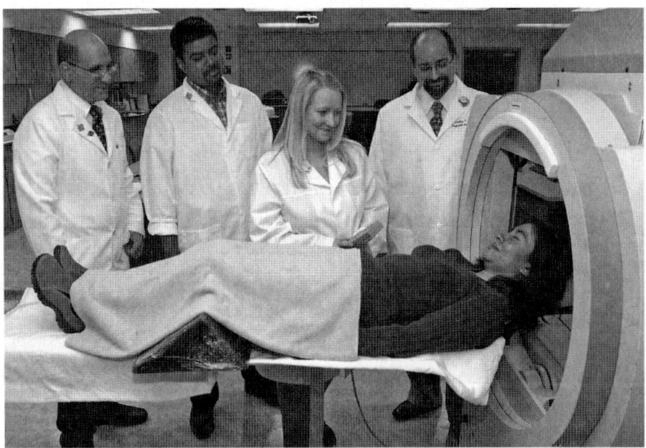

Figure 20.11 Setting a patient up for ERNA scan and assessing patient comfort prior to imaging. (Courtesy of UAB NMT Program Library, Birmingham, AL.)

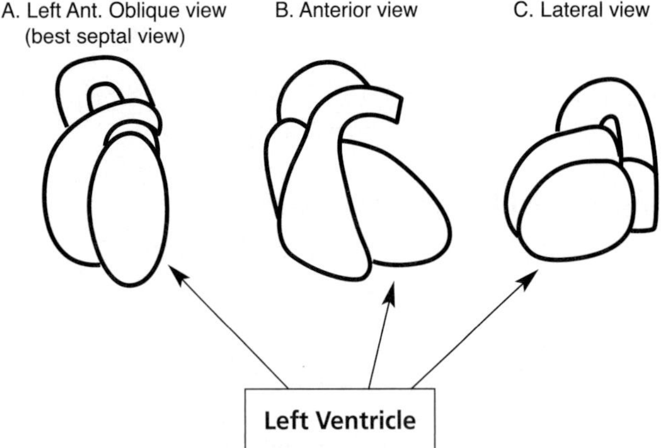

Figure 20.12 Proper positioning of commonly used views for an ERNA study (Crawford and Husain, 2003).

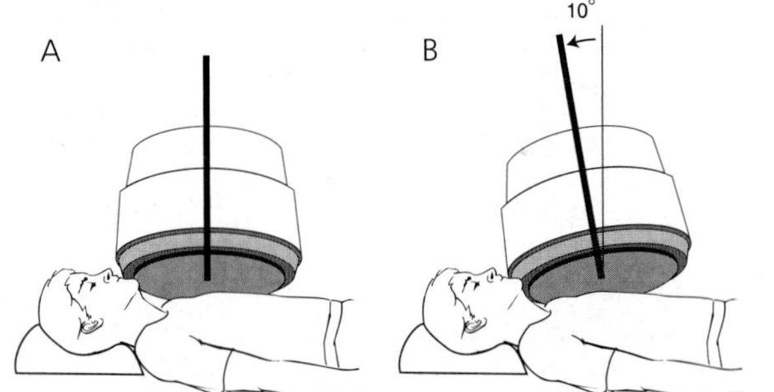

Figure 20.13 Caudal tilt of the camera. In both pictures the camera is angled 45°. (A) No caudal tilt. (B) The camera is angled with a 10° caudal tilt. It is tilted back toward the head of the imaging table at approximately 10°. (Reprinted, with permission, from Crawford and Husain, 2003.)

taken into consideration. An ROI ~5–10 mm away from the end-diastolic border and in the 2 o'clock to 5 o'clock area should be drawn to determine background. Once background is established, a background correction should be applied by simply subtracting background counts from LV ROI counts. The LVEF can then be determined by using the following equation:

$$\text{LVEF} = \frac{\text{EDV} - \text{ESV}}{\text{EDV}} \times 100.$$

Both a global and regional ejection fraction can be determined. The global EF is the entire ventricular volume. To evaluate regional EF, the ventricle must be divided into segments. The regional EF is helpful when evaluating regional wall motion.

When assessing ventricular function with stress, the baseline ERNA images should be displayed side-by-side with the stress images, which help in determining changes.

Myocardial Infarct-Avid Imaging, MIBG Imaging, and [^{123}I]BMIPP Imaging

While myocardial perfusion imaging is the most routinely performed nuclear cardiac study, other infrequent cardiac studies provide beneficial information for patients with not only cardiovascular disease but other diseases that affect the heart and vascular system as well. This section briefly reviews myocardial infarct-avid imaging, MIBG, and [^{123}I]BMIPP studies.

Myocardial Infarct-Avid Imaging

Chest pain is one of the top reasons most people go to the emergency department. While most patients can be diagnosed with an acute myocardial infarction, few patients will have results that are indeterminate. For those patients, a myocardial infarct-avid test would be beneficial. Radiopharmaceuticals used are [^{99m}Tc]PYP and [^{111}In]antimyosin (Table 20.7). Please note that [^{111}In]antimyosin is not currently available. When using [^{99m}Tc]PYP, the window of maximum diagnostic yield is 48–72 hr after the infarct. However, positive results can be seen as early as 12 hr post-infarct. When using [^{111}In]antimyosin, the window of maximum diagnostic yield is 18–24 hr after the infarct.

MIBG Imaging

[^{123}I]MIBG is a sympathetic nerve imaging drug typically used to diagnose neuroendocrine tumors. However, developments in cardiac imaging have led to the ability to detect abnormalities in patients with heart failure using [^{123}I]MIBG. Patients with heart failure have a decreased ability for norepinephrine synthesis, storage, and

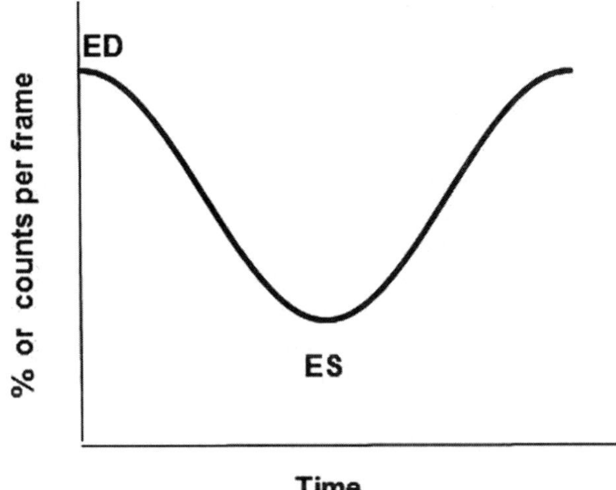

Figure 20.14 ERNA volume curve where ED is end diastolic and ES is end systolic.

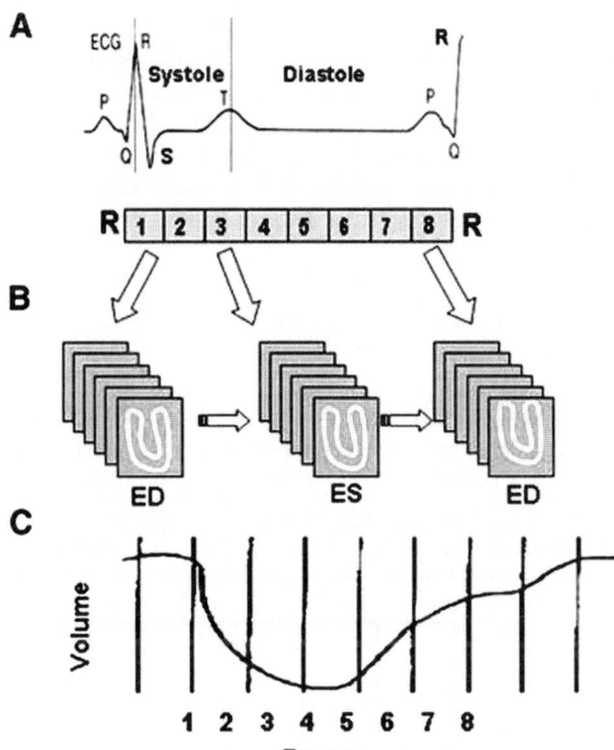

Figure 20.15 Principle of ECG-gated acquisition. R–R interval on ECG, representing one cardiac cycle, is typically divided into eight frames of equal duration (A). Image data from each frame are acquired over multiple cardiac cycles and stored separately in specific locations ("bin") of computer memory (B). When all data in a bin are added together, image represents a specific phase of cardiac cycle. Typically, a volume curve is obtained, which represents endocardial volume for each of eight frames (C). ED, end diastole; ES, end systole. (Reprinted, with permission, from Asit and Hani, 2004.)

release. This decreased ability results in an increase and higher concentration of circulating norepinephrine that is stored in granules in the presynaptic nerve terminals, which causes chronic stimulation. MIBG is thought to localize to myocardial sympathetic nerves due to its structural similarity to norepinephrine and uptake in the catecholamine storage granules, which reflect the extent of sympathetic innervation in the myocardium. Therefore, uptake of [^{123}I]MIBG is usually associated with diseases that result in heart failure or possibly fatal ventricular arrhythmias.

A typical dose of 370 MBq (10.0 mCi) [^{123}I]MIBG is given intravenously and planar images of the anterior chest are obtained at both 10-min and 4-hr postinjection. SPECT images may also be useful. A radius of 180°, RAO to LAO, should be used with a minimum of 60 stops at 30 sec per stop. A 64 × 64 matrix should be utilized. Uptake of [^{123}I]MIBG is measured by defining the heart-to-mediastinum uptake ratio and assessing the washout rate over time. Heart failure patients have a low heart-to-mediastinum ratio and high or increased washout (Fig. 20.17).

[^{123}I]BMIPP Imaging

[^{123}I]BMIPP is used as an "ischemic memory tracer" to identify significant ischemia in patients with coronary artery disease (CAD) by assessing fatty acid metabolism. An intravenous injection of 111–148 MBq (3–4 mCi) [^{123}I]BMIPP is a typical protocol. A LEAP or LEHR collimator is recommended along with a ±20% energy

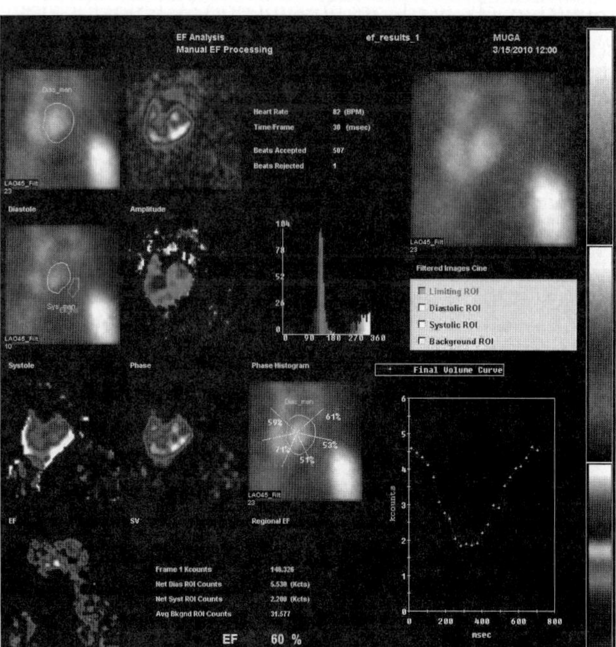

Figure 20.16 ERNA study with an EF of 60%. (Courtesy of Jim Nance from Citizen's Baptist Medical Center,Talladega, AL.)

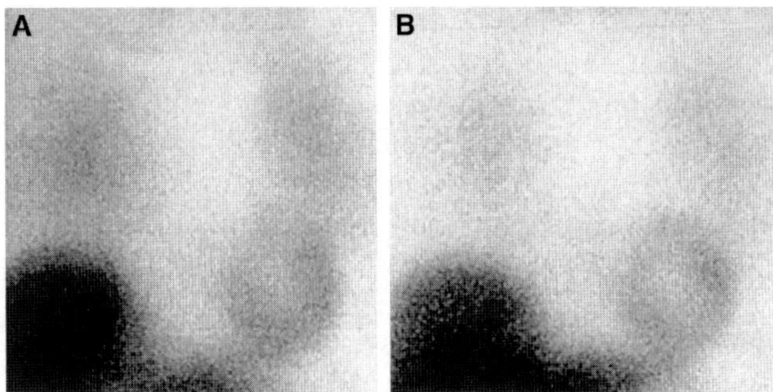

Figure 20.17 [^{123}I]MIBG uptake on (15-min) planar images (A) and delayed (4-hr) planar images (B). (Reprinted, with permission, from Scott and Kench, 2004.)

window around the 159 keV of ^{123}I. Planar images of the anterior chest are obtained 15–30 min postinjection along with a 4-hr-delayed image. SPECT images may also be useful and a radius of 180°, RAO to LAO, should be used with a minimum of 60 stops at 30 sec per stop. A 64 × 64 matrix should be utilized. A positive [^{123}I]BMIPP study will be evident within 20–30 min of the ischemic event and will stay positive for up to 2 weeks.

Emergency Care and ECG Interpretation

All employees in a nuclear cardiology facility should have basic life support (BLS) cardiopulmonary resuscitation (CPR) training. When conducting exercise and pharmacologic stress testing, at least one technologist should be trained in advanced care life support (ACLS) CPR along with an available physician. ACLS is an extension of BLS designed for healthcare providers who participate directly or indirectly in the resuscitation of a patient. ACLS guidelines are published by the American Heart Association and were last updated in 2010. The current ACLS guidelines use algorithms that are a set of instructions presented in the form of a flowchart to standardize treatment and increase effectiveness. Knowledge of pharmacology along with ECG interpretation is essential in ACLS training.

ECG interpretation is an invaluable skill used in nuclear cardiology. This section builds upon the cardiac electrical conduction system in the cardiovascular system chapter and reviews basic ECG interpretations.

In 1903, Willem Einthoven invented the first electrocardiogram machine. Today, there are many ECG monitors on the market but they all record electrical conduction through the heart. Electrodes are used to detect the electrical activity generated by the myocardial cells. The ECG monitor has one positive electrode, one negative electrode, and one ground electrode. ECG paper is used to print out heart rhythms and measure particular events such as the heart rate (Fig. 20.18). The paper is marked off in a grid on which each small square is 1 mm in length and represents 0.04 sec. The larger square is 5 mm in length and represents 0.20 sec.

When interpreting an ECG, one should become very familiar with what is normal (Fig. 20.19). It is also important to evaluate five important items from an ECG. First, evaluate the P wave for size, shape, and location in the waveform. If the P wave precedes the QRS complex, the electrical impulse is being initiated by the sinoatrial (SA) node. Absence of P waves or abnormality in their position relative to the QRS complex indicates that the pulse is starting outside the SA node and that an ectopic pacemaker is present. Second, evaluate the atrial rhythm and determine the atrial rate. This can be accomplished by measuring the P–P intervals and comparing. P waves should occur at regular intervals. Also, count the number of P waves in 30 large squares (or 6 sec) and multiply by 10 to obtain the atrial beats per minute. Third, the duration of the PR interval should be calculated. Simply count the number of small squares between the beginning of the P wave and the beginning of the QRS complex then multiply by 0.04 sec. A normal PR interval is between 0.12 and 0.20 sec or approximately 3–5 small squares. The forth step is to evaluate the ventricular rhythm and determine the ventricular rate. Measure the R–R intervals and compare. The R waves should occur at regular intervals. To find the ventricular rate, count

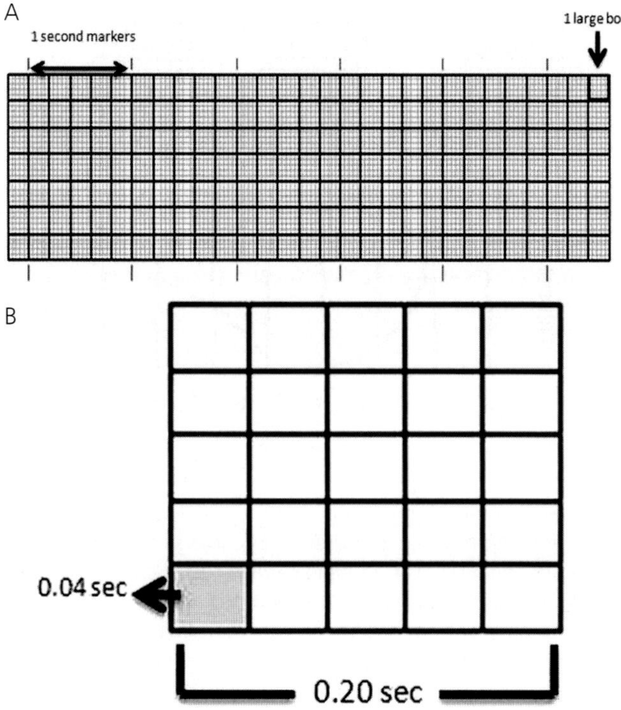

Figure 20.18 (A) ECG paper. (B) One large box on ECG paper that represents 0.20 sec. The small boxes represent 0.04 sec.

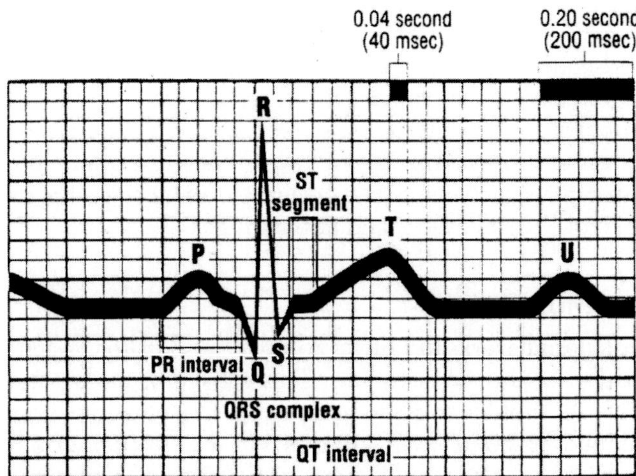

Figure 20.19 Basic ECG interpretation demonstrating the P wave, QRS complex, T wave, U wave, PR interval, ST segment, and QT interval. (Courtesy of the UAB NMT Teaching Files, Birmingham, AL.)

the small squares between two R waves. Each small square equals 0.04 sec; 1500 squares equal 1 min. Divide 1500 by the number of squares counted. Also check that the QRS complex is an appropriate shape for the particular lead used. The fifth step is to calculate the duration of the QRS complex. Count the small squares between the beginning and end of the QRS complex and multiply by 0.04 sec. A normal QRS complex is less than 0.12 sec or three fine lines on the ECG paper.

Appendix F includes an ECG interpretation guide. The guide is a quick review of normal sinus rhythm, rhythms originating in the SA node, rhythms originating in the atria, rhythms originating in the junction, heart blocks, rhythms originating in the ventricles, bundle branch blocks, and pacemakers.

Stress Protocols and Radiopharmaceuticals

Both exercise stress and pharmacologic stress tests are great protocols in the diagnosis of CAD.

Exercise Stress Test

Exercise is the preferred method for patients who are able to exercise and can reach at least 85% of the age-adjusted maximal predicted heart rate and five metabolic equivalents (METS). Exercise modalities include the treadmill or the upright bicycle. Although the treadmill is the most widely used, the bicycle is preferred when completing a dynamic first-pass study. Clinical indications and contraindications for the exercise stress test given by the ASNC are listed in Tables 20.3 and 20.4.

Table 20.3 Clinical Indications for an Exercise Stress Test

1. Detection of obstructive coronary artery disease in the following patients:
   a. patients with an intermediate pretest probability of CAD based on age, gender, and symptoms
   b. patients with high-risk factors for CAD
2. Risk stratification of post-myocardial infarction patients before and after discharge
3. Risk stratification of patients with chronic stable CAD into a low-risk category that can be managed medically or into a high-risk category that should be considered for coronary revascularization
4. Risk stratification of low-risk acute coronary syndrome patients and of intermediate-risk acute coronary syndrome patients 1–3 days after presentation
5. Risk stratification before noncardiac surgery in patients with known CAD or those with high-risk factors for CAD
6. To evaluate the efficacy of therapeutic interventions and in tracking subsequent risk on the basis of serial changes in myocardial perfusion in patients with known CAD.

Modified from Henzlova *et al*. (2009).

Table 20.4 Contraindications for an Exercise Stress Test

Absolute contraindications
1. High-risk unstable angina
2. Decompensated or inadequately controlled congestive heart failure
3. Uncontrolled hypertension (blood pressure >200/110 mm Hg)
4. Uncontrolled cardiac arrhythmias
5. Severe symptomatic aortic stenosis
6. Acute pulmonary embolism
7. Acute myocarditis or pericarditis
8. Acute aortic dissection
9. Severe pulmonary hypertension
10. Acute myocardial infarction (<4 days)
11. Acutely ill for any reason
Relative contraindications
1. Known left main coronary artery stenosis
2. Moderate aortic stenosis
3. Hypertrophic obstructive cardiomyopathy or other forms of outflow tract obstruction
4. Significant tachyarrhythmias or bradyarrhythmias
5. High-degree atrioventricular (AV) block
6. Electrolyte abnormalities
7. Mental or physical impairment leading to inability to exercise adequately
8. If combined with imaging, patients with complete left bundle branch block (LBBB), permanent pacemakers, and ventricular preexcitation (Wolff–Parkinson–White syndrome) should preferentially undergo pharmacologic vasodilator stress test (not dobutamine stress test)

Modified from Henzlova *et al*. (2009).

In addition to providing information about exercise capability, an exercise stress test can be used to assess risk in patients with known or suspected CAD. The Duke Treadmill Score is a prediction of CAD in a patient with chest pain undergoing an exercise stress test. The calculation for the Duke Treadmill Score is given in Table 20.5.

Procedure

Patient preparations for an exercise stress test include nothing to eat for 2 hr before the test. Certain blood pressure medications may need to be discontinued prior to a stress test but this is dependent upon the referring physician. A patient who is scheduled later in the day should eat a light breakfast. An 18- to 20-gauge intravenous catheter should be inserted and secured before starting radiopharmaceutical injection during the exercise stress. The patient's electrocardiogram should be monitored continuously during the exercise test and into the recovery phase for at least 5 min or until the resting heart rate is <100 beats/min and/or any exercise-induced ST-segment changes have resolved. Both the blood pressure and heart rate should be recorded at least every 3 min during exercise and into the recovery phase. Note that obtaining a maximum of 85% of the target heart rate is not an indication for termination of the stress test. The radiopharmaceutical should be injected at peak exercise and the patient should continue for at least 1 min postinjection. Indications for early termination of the exercise stress can be found in Table 20.6.

Pharmacologic Stress Agents

While the exercise stress test is the preferred method of choice, not all patients are able to exercise due to physical problems or medications. A sufficient alternate to the stress test is a pharmacologic stress. The most commonly used pharmacologic stress agents are adenosine, dipyridamole, regadenoson, and dobutamine.

Adenosine

Adenosine works as a direct coronary vasodilator by activation of the A2A receptor. This activation results in a 3.5- to 4-fold increase in blood flow. The adenosine dose should be given at an infusion rate of 140 μg/kg/min over 6 min. The radiopharmaceutical should be administered 3 min after the start of the adenosine infusion. With an adenosine concentration of 3 mg/mL, the total volume needed for a specific patient is calculated by

$$\text{total volume (mL)} = 0.28 \times \text{total body weight (kg)}.$$

The infusion rate is calculated as

$$\frac{0.140\ (\text{mg/kg/min}) \times \text{total body weight (kg)}}{\text{adenosine concentration (3 mg/mL)}}.$$

Dipyridamole

Dipyridamole increases adenosine levels in the tissue, which indirectly causes coronary artery vasodilation that induces hyperemia. The plasma half-life of dipyridamole

Table 20.5 Duke Treadmill Score: A Prediction of Coronary Heart Disease in a Patient with Chest Pain Undergoing a Treadmill Stress Test

Duke Treadmill Score = Exercise Time − (5 × ST-Segment Deviation) − (4 × Angina Index)
Exercise time is based on standard Bruce protocol using minutes. ST segment deviation is measured 60–80 msec after the J point. If the amount of exercise-induced ST-segment deviation is less than 1 mm, the value entered into the score for ST deviation is 0. Angina index is 0 if no exercise angina occurs, 1 if exercise angina occurs, and 2 if angina is the reason the patient stopped exercising.
Interpretation
Score >5: Low risk Score −10 to 4: Intermediate risk Score <−10: High risk

Table 20.6 Indications for Early Termination of Exercise

1. Moderate-to-severe angina pectoris
2. Marked dyspnea or fatigue
3. Ataxia, dizziness, or near syncope
4. Signs of poor perfusion (cyanosis and pallor)
5. Patient's request to terminate the test
6. Excessive ST-segment depression (>2 mm)
7. ST elevation (>1 mm) in leads without diagnostic Q waves (except for leads V_1 or augmented voltage right arm, aVR)
8. Sustained supraventricular or ventricular tachycardia
9. Development of left bundle branch block (LBBB) or intraventricular conduction delay that cannot be distinguished from ventricular tachycardia
10. Drop in systolic blood pressure of >10 mm Hg from baseline, despite an increase in workload, when accompanied by other evidence of ischemia
11. Hypertensive response (systolic blood pressure >250 mm Hg and/or diastolic pressure >115 mm Hg)
12. Technical difficulties in monitoring the electrocardiogram or systolic blood pressure

Modified from Henzlova *et al.* (2009).

is 15–30 min. A dipyridamole dose of 0.56 mg/kg should be given intravenously over a 4-min period (142 μg/kg/min).

Regadenoson

Regadenoson works as a coronary vasodilator by activating the A2A adenosine receptor. The recommended dose is 5 mL (0.4 mg).

Dobutamine

Dobutamine increases the heart rate, blood pressure, and myocardial contractility by direct β_1 stimulation. The dobutamine dose is incrementally infused starting at a dose of 5–10 μg/kg/min, which is increased at 3-min intervals to 20, 30, and 40 μg/kg/min. The dobutamine half-life is about 2 min.

Radiopharmaceuticals and Interventional Drugs

Radiopharmaceuticals used for planar and SPECT myocardial perfusion imaging include ^{201}Tl and ^{99m}Tc agents ([^{99m}Tc]sestamibi and [^{99m}Tc]tetrofosmin). Radiopharmaceuticals used for myocardial PET perfusion imaging include [^{18}F]FDG, [^{82}Rb]chloride, [^{13}N]ammonia, and [^{15}O]water (Table 20.7). Also, many interventional drugs, such as the pharmacologic stress agents, are used in nuclear cardiology. Some of the commonly used drugs are listed in Table 20.8.

Planar and SPECT Imaging Protocols and Image Review

Both planar and/or SPECT imaging can be acquired using ^{201}Tl, [^{99m}Tc]sestamibi, or [^{99m}Tc]tetrofosmin.

^{201}Tl Imaging Protocols

When only using ^{201}Tl for myocardial perfusion imaging, the stress test is conducted first. Whether the stress test was performed as physical exercise or using a pharmacologic agent, imaging should start 5 to 7 min post-injection of the radiopharmaceutical. A typical dose of 74–148 MBq (2–4 mCi) of ^{201}Tl should be administered when performing the stress test. If a second injection of ^{201}Tl is used for the rest, then a dose of 92.5–111 MBq (2.5–3 mCi) should be given at stress while 37–55.5 MBq (1.0–1.5 mCi) should be given with the second injection at rest. After stress, the delayed rest and redistribution images can be acquired 3–4 hr after the injection (Table 20.9). Both the rest and stress images are then compared. Due to the redistribution of ^{201}Tl, areas of the myocardium that were hypoperfused at stress may show significant improvement in the delayed study. If there is uniform uptake throughout the myocardium with no areas of hypoperfusion, then the study is negative. If the stress images along with the 3- to 4-hr-delayed rest images both show an area of hypoperfusion, then a fixed perfusion defect has occurred. The fixed perfusion defect may be due to chronic ischemia, hibernating

Table 20.7 Common Radiopharmaceuticals Used in Nuclear Cardiology

Radiopharmaceutical	Half-Life	Dose	Typical Usage
^{201}Tl	73.1 hr	92.5–148 MBq/2.5–4 mCi (depending on procedure)	Myocardial perfusion imaging; can detect hibernating myocardium
[^{99m}Tc]Sestamibi and [^{99m}Tc]tetrofosmin	6 hr	370–1110 MBq/10–30 mCi	Myocardial perfusion imaging
^{99m}Tc-labeled red blood cells	6 hr	925–1295 MBq/25–35 mCi (depending on procedure)	ERNA imaging
[^{18}F]FDG	110 min	370 MBq/10 mCi	PET myocardial perfusion imaging; can detect hibernating myocardium
[^{82}Rb]Chloride	75 sec	1850–2220 MBq/50–60 mCi	PET myocardial perfusion imaging
[^{13}N]Ammonia	10 min	666–740 MBq/18–20 mCi	PET myocardial perfusion imaging
[^{15}O]Water	122 sec	370 MBq/10 mCi	PET myocardial perfusion imaging
[^{123}I]MIBG	13.2 hr	370 MBq/10 mCi	Used to evaluate heart failure and cardiac dyssynchrony
[^{111}In]Antimyosin (not commercially available)	67.92 hr	74 MBq/2 mCi	Myocardial infarct-avid imaging
[^{99m}Tc]PYP	6 hr	555–925 MBq/15–25 mCi	Myocardial infarct-avid imaging
[^{123}I]BMIPP	13.2 hr	111–148 MBq/3–4 mCi	Used to identify significant ischemia in patients with CAD

Table 20.8 Common Interventional Drugs Used in Nuclear Cardiology

Drug	Usage
Adenosine	Direct coronary artery vasodilator used in myocardial perfusion stress testing
Regadenoson	An A2A adenosine receptor agonist that is a coronary vasodilator; used in myocardial perfusion pharmacologic stress testing
Dipyridamole	Indirect vasodilator used in myocardial perfusion pharmacologic stress testing
Dobutamine	A catecholamine that increases heart rate and myocardial contractility, used in myocardial perfusion pharmacologic stress testing
Aminophylline	Used to reverse the side effects of vasodilator stress testing and bronchial asthma (e.g., bronkodyl, theolair, Theo-Dur, elixophyllin)
Atropine	Used to increase the heart rate by blocking the parasympathetic system; patients are administered 0.5–1.0 mg atropine to increase heart rate by 15 beats/min; administration of 0.6–1.2 mg of atropine will increase heart rate by 25 beats/min
Esmolol	Used for the alleviation of the severe side effects of dobutamine administration; esmolol decreases the force of cardiac contraction and decreases the heart rate
Acetylsalicylic acid (aspirin)	Used for mild to moderate pain relief, fever reduction, and inflammation reduction; also used to prevent blood clot formation, heart attacks, and strokes
Anticoagulants	Stop blood from clotting and prevents coagulation; used to stop thrombosis in deep vein thrombosis, pulmonary embolism, myocardial infarction, stroke, atrial fibrillation, and in patients with mechanical prosthetic valves
Antiarrythmics	Used to treat ventricular tachycardias and other ventricular arrhythmias, atrial fibrillation, atrial flutter, and supraventricular tachycardias (e.g., amiodarone, lidocaine, esmolol, verapamil, procainamide)
β-Blockers	Used for the treatment of myocardial infarction, angina, hypertension, hypertrophic cardiomyopathy, congestive heart failure, glaucoma, cardiac arrhythmias, thyrotoxicosis, and prevention of migraines (e.g., atenolol, propranolol, esmolol, carvedilol)
Calcium channel blockers	A class of drugs that disrupts the calcium conduction of calcium channels and effects excitable cells in the body such as cardiac muscle; calcium channel blockers are used to decrease blood pressure, control heart rate, and reduce chest pain in patients with angina pectoris (e.g., verapamil, nifedipine, and diltiazem)
ACE inhibitors	Used in the treatment of hypertension and congestive heart failure (e.g., captopril, zofenopril, enalapril, ramipril)
Nitrates	Used to dilate the arteries, increase blood flow, and reduce chest pain (e.g., nitroglycerin)
Cholesterol-lowering drugs	The four types of cholesterol-lowering drugs include statins, fibrates, niacin, and bile acid sequestrants, used to lower "bad cholesterol" and increase "good cholesterol"
Diuretics	Used to elevate the rate of urination and for the treatment of hypertension, fluid retention states, kidney diseases, heart failure, and pulmonary edema
Digoxin	Used to suppress supraventricular arrhythmias such as atrial fibrillation and atrial flutter and/or to treat or prevent heart failure

myocardium, or scarred tissue. With ^{201}Tl, an 18- to 24-hr-delayed redistribution scan may be useful as it sometimes shows improvement in the areas of hypoperfusion, which is usually the case in hibernating but viable myocardium (Table 20.10).

[^{99m}Tc]Sestamibi and [^{99m}Tc]Tetrofosmin Imaging Protocols

Unlike ^{201}Tl, [^{99m}Tc]sestamibi and [^{99m}Tc]tetrofosmin do not redistribute but remain fixed in the myocardium. Either the rest or stress can be performed first and can be performed as a 1-day protocol or as a 2-day protocol. Although both of the ^{99m}Tc-labeled tracers have similar characteristics, tetrofosmin has a more rapid liver clearance than sestamibi. When using [^{99m}Tc]sestamibi, use of a minimum delay of 15–20 min for exercise, 45–60 min for rest, and 60 min for a pharmacologic stress is recommended. When using [^{99m}Tc]tetrofosmin, use of a minimum delay of 10–15 min for exercise, 30–45 min for rest, and 45 min for pharmacologic stress is recommended.

Two-Day Protocol

It is optimal to perform stress and rest imaging on separate days. However, for most patients, a 2-day study is not practical. The advantage of a 2-day protocol is almost complete effective decay of the tracer between studies (Fig. 20.20).

One-Day Protocol

Due to the possible impracticality of the 2-day protocol, most studies are performed using the 1-day protocol. The 1-day protocol requires the injection of a low-dose (296–444 MBq/8–12 mCi) and an injection of a high dose (888–1332 MBq/24–36 mCi) of the radiopharmaceutical. When using a 1-day protocol, it is important to avoid "cross talk" or "shine-through" from the first dose

Table 20.9 Thallium Imaging Procedure Options

Procedure 1	1. Administer 148 MBq (4 mCi) ^{201}Tl at peak stress. 2. Acquire a stress scan immediately after the ^{201}Tl injection (beginning within 5–7 min). 3. Acquire a 3- to 4-hr-delayed (redistribution) scan. 4. When a fixed defect is identified, acquire a 24-hr-delayed (redistribution) scan.
Procedure 2	1. Administer 92.5–111 MBq (2.5–3.0 mCi) ^{201}Tl at peak stress. 2. Acquire a stress scan immediately after the ^{201}Tl injection (beginning within 5–7 min). 3. Acquire a 3- to 4-hr-delayed (redistribution) scan. 4. When a fixed defect is identified, administer 37–55.5 MBq (1.0–1.5 mCi) ^{201}Tl the same day. 5. Perform a rest scan 10 min later.
Procedure 3	1. Administer 148 MBq (4 mCi) ^{201}Tl at peak stress. 2. Acquire a stress scan immediately after the ^{201}Tl injection (beginning within 5–7 min). 3. Acquire a 3- to 4-hr-delayed (redistribution) scan. 4. When a fixed defect is identified, administer 111–148 MBq (3–4 mCi) ^{201}Tl on a subsequent day. 5. Perform a rest scan 10 min later.
Procedure 4	1. Administer 92.5–111 MBq (2.5–3.0 mCi) ^{201}Tl at peak stress. 2. Acquire a stress scan immediately after the ^{201}Tl injection (beginning within 5–7 min). 3. Immediately after completion of the stress scan, administer 37–55.5 MBq (1.0–1.5 mCi) ^{201}Tl. 4. Acquire a rest scan 3–4 hr later.

Modified from Crawford and Husain (2003).

into the second dose. To accomplish this, use a 3:1 stress/rest dose ratio with a 2-hr delay and a 3.5 to 4:1 ratio with no delay. When using a 1-day stress–rest protocol, a 3- to 4-hr delay is needed. The reason for this delay is the high dose given at first, which takes longer to achieve the 4:1 ratio. See Figure 20.21 for both rest–stress and stress–rest 1-day protocols.

Dual-Isotope Imaging Protocol

Dual-isotope imaging is the use of ^{201}Tl for the initial rest imaging and a ^{99m}Tc-labeled tracer for stress imaging. Although the total time of the rest–stress dual-isotope protocol is less than the 1-day ^{99m}Tc protocol, the patient receives a higher radiation dose with the dual-isotope method. Figure 20.22 displays a standard dual-isotope protocol. Another protocol allows for the ^{201}Tl

Table 20.10 Clinical Significance of ^{201}Tl Images

Stress study	3- to 4-hr-delayed study	24-hr-delayed study	Clinical interpretation
Normal	Normal		Coronary artery disease unlikely
Abnormal	Normal		Stress-induced ischemia
Abnormal	Abnormal	Normal	Chronic ischemia
Abnormal	Abnormal	Abnormal	Fixed defect, nonviable, or scar tissue

Reprinted, with permission, from Crawford and Husain (2003).

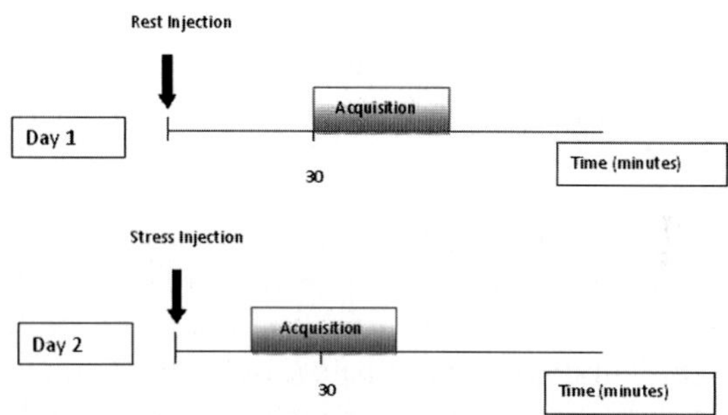

Figure 20.20 ^{99m}Tc two-day stress imaging protocol. Either stress or rest can be performed first.

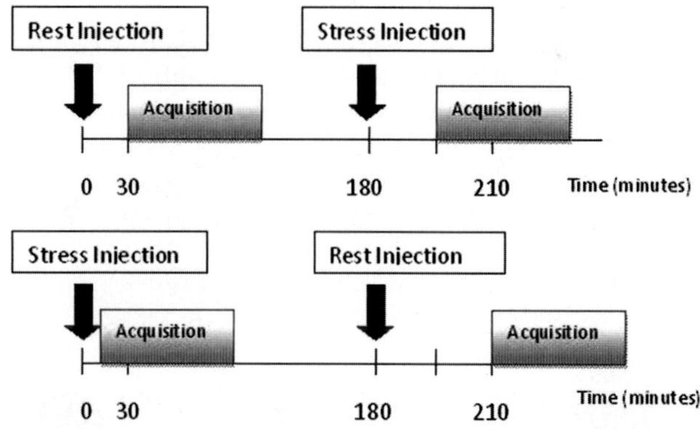

Figure 20.21 ^{99m}Tc one-day stress imaging protocol.

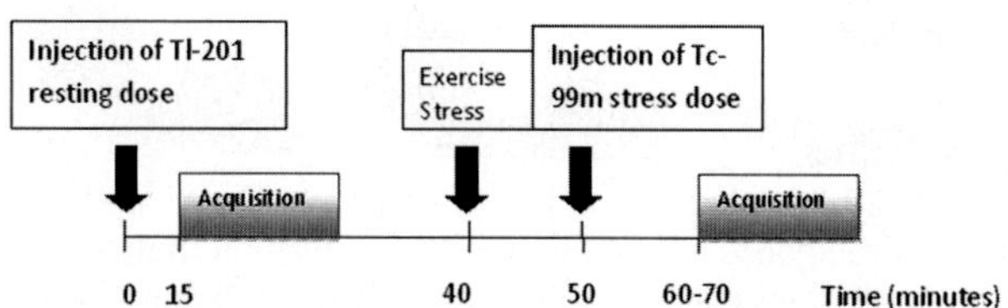

Figure 20.22 ^{201}Tl/^{99m}Tc one-day stress imaging protocol.

stress imaging to be performed first and a ^{99m}Tc-labeled tracer for the rest imaging.

Image Review

When it comes to myocardial perfusion imaging, SPECT imaging is preferred; however, SPECT may not always be an option. Some patients must be imaged at bedside due to medical issues and some patients may be too obese for the SPECT imaging table. Therefore, a sufficient alternative is planar imaging. Standard planar imaging views include LAO, anterior, and a right-side decubitus 90° left lateral. A normal planar myocardial perfusion scan is shown in Figure 20.23. When available, SPECT imaging is preferred and is used to evaluate regional myocardial perfusion. Planar and SPECT images are usually performed with the patient in a supine position. This positioning can sometimes result in diaphragmatic (abdominal or breast) attenuation of photons from the inferior wall of the left ventricle. When this occurs, imaging in the prone or left lateral position may produce a better result.

When the myocardial perfusion study is complete, it should be initially reviewed for possible artifacts due to attenuation, patient motion, imaging processing problems, and overall image quality before the visual or quantitative analysis is completed. Patient motion can be detected by reviewing the cine display. All data should then be reconstructed using either a filtered backprojection or iterative reconstruction algorithm. When reviewing the SPECT images, one should become familiar with the different planes. The transverse plane usually cuts the image of the heart horizontally and divides an organ from inferior to superior. The sagittal plane is usually a longitudinal section that divides an organ from right to left, and the coronal plane is usually longitudinal and divides from front to back (Fig. 20.24). Sectional views of the heart are then made, creating the short axis, horizontal long axis, and the vertical axis (Fig. 20.25). A normal SPECT perfusion study is shown in Figure 20.26 and an abnormal SPECT perfusion scan is shown in Figure 20.27.

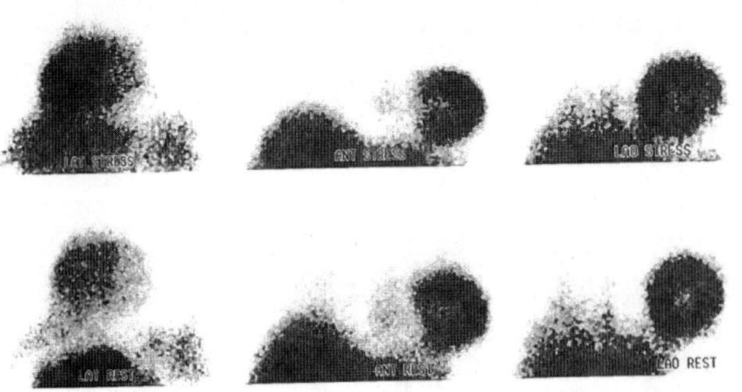

Figure 20.23 A normal [^{99m}Tc]sestamibi planar perfusion study. Top: Images made after the stress injection. Bottom: Images made after injection of sestamibi at rest. (Reprinted, with permission, from Crawford and Husain, 2003.)

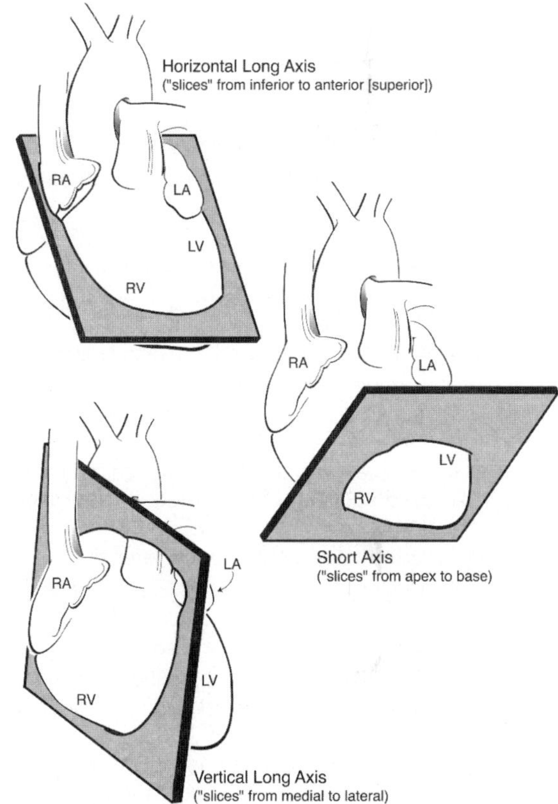

Figure 20.24 Tomographic planes of the heart. (Reprinted, with permission, from Crawford and Husain, 2003.)

When reviewing myocardial perfusion images, a simple interpretation of "normal" or "abnormal" should be more detailed, including the degree of decreased radiotracer uptake. While a visual assessment of the images allows one to detect defects in the anterior, septum, inferior, and lateral walls, a segmental scoring system allows for a more quantitative analysis. Perfusion defects are then scored using a five-point system in which 0 represents normal; 1, 2, and 3 represent mild, moderate, and severe reduction, respectively; and 4 represents the absence of detectable radiotracer uptake. These segmental scores are automatically determined by computer software and are reproducible.

The lung:heart ratio compares with lower resting LVEF, a higher pulmonary capillary wedge pressure, and a lower cardiac index. When looking at the lung:heart ratio, an increased lung uptake after thallium perfusion imaging can be an indicator of poor prognosis. When using a ^{99m}Tc-labeled tracer following an exercise stress, increased lung uptake can indicate severe and extensive CAD and reduced ventricular function. Normal values of the lung:heart ratio for ^{201}Tl is <0.51 and for [^{99m}Tc]sestamibi is <0.44.

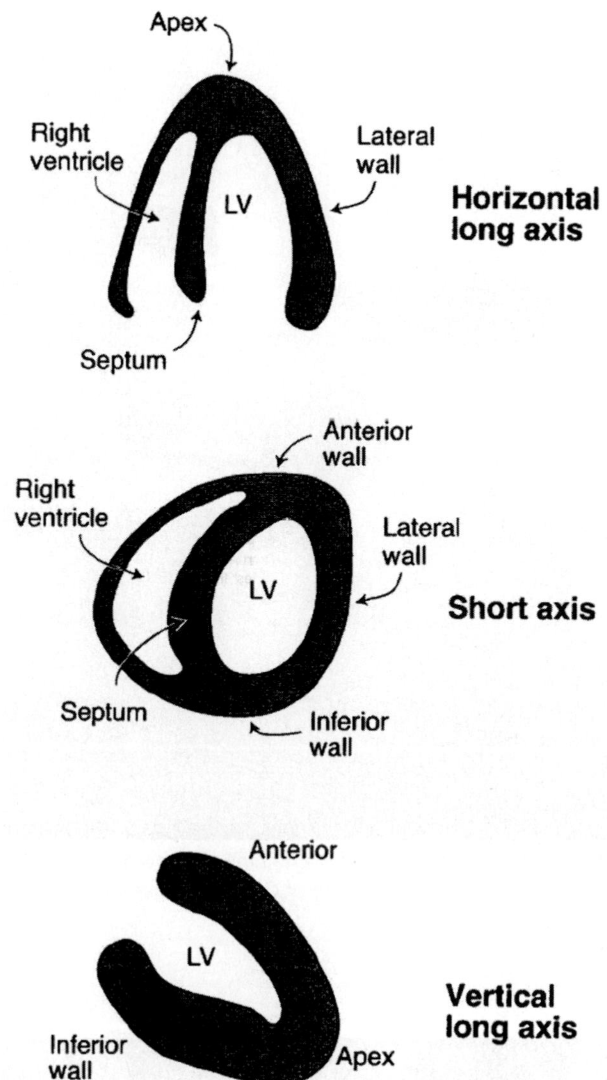

Figure 20.25 Walls of the heart seen in each sectional view. (Reprinted, with permission, from Crawford and Husain, 2003.)

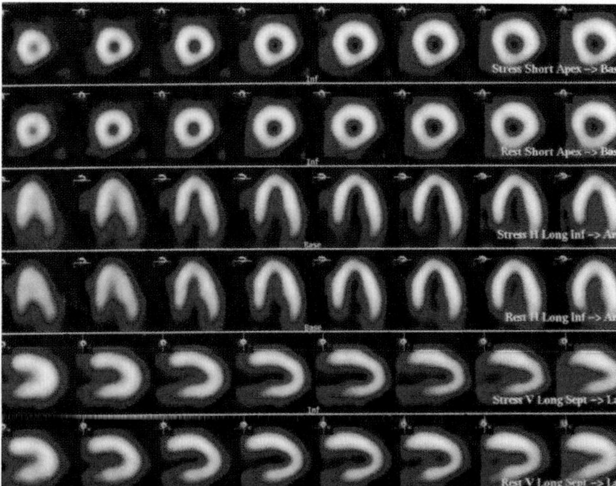

Figure 20.26 Normal stress–rest SPECT perfusion study. (Reprinted, with permission, from Crawford and Husain, 2003.)

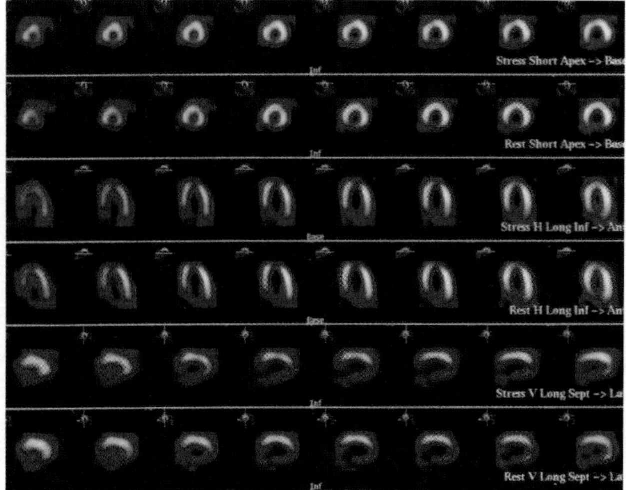

Figure 20.27 Stress–rest perfusion study with a fixed defect. A fixed inferior wall defect is seen in the short axis and vertical long axis slices. (Reprinted, with permission, from Crawford and Husain, 2003.)

Polar maps of ventricular perfusion provide a 2D representation of the 3D myocardium for comparisons of rest and stress studies, follow-up of a patient over time, or comparison between patients. When viewing a polar map, one should imagine looking at the myocardium from the apex with the anterior LV wall at the top and the septal wall to the left. The apex is always the center of every polar map and the base is always mapped to the peripheral circumference (Fig. 20.28).

Cardiac PET Imaging

Cardiac PET imaging is a reimbursable study that assesses myocardial perfusion, left ventricular function, and viability. PET offers better resolution than SPECT imaging, which in turn produces better-quality images. PET imaging can be performed only by pharmacologic stress. PET imaging protocols may vary from place to place but examples of standard protocols are given in Table 20.11. When using FDG in assessing myocardial viability, blood glucose levels should be between 120 and 160 mg/dL. If the levels are lower than 120 mg/dL, then an oral glucose loading of 100 g glucose should be administered.

References and Further Reading

Alessi AM, Farrell MB, Grabher BJ, Hyun MC, Johnson SG, Squires P, 2010. *Nuclear Cardiology Technology Study Guide.* Reston, VA: Society of Nuclear Medicine.

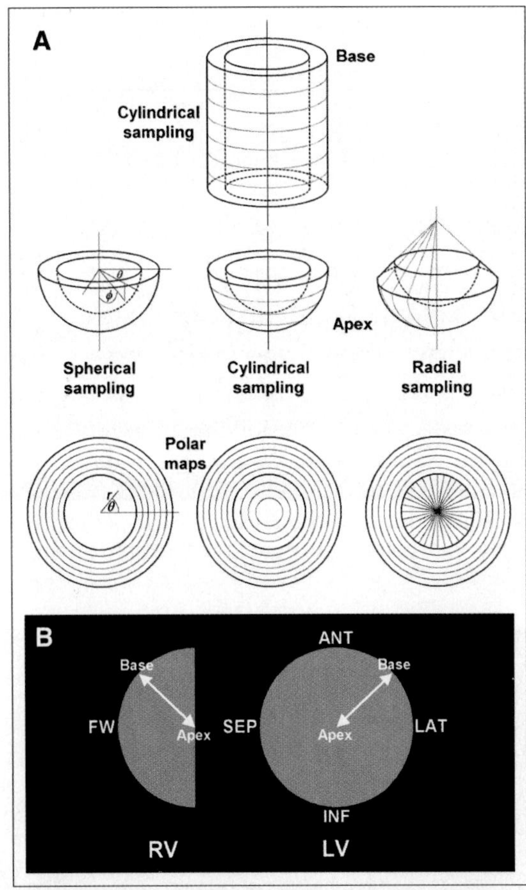

Figure 20.28 Polar-mapping conventions. (A) Three methods for mapping 3D myocardium in 2D polar maps: Cedars-Sinai Medical Center, Emory University, University of Michigan, and Baylor College of Medicine. Basal and midventricular walls are mapped by cylindric sampling in all methods. Apex is mapped by spheric, cylindric, and radial sampling, respectively. (B) Orientations of polar maps for RV and LV. In LV polar map, anterior (ANT) wall is at top, septal (SEP) wall is at left, inferior (INF) wall is at bottom, lateral (LAT) wall is at right, apex is at center, and base is at circumference. In blood pool SPECT, RV also is mapped to hemipolar map for RV free wall (FW). (Reprinted, with permission, from Lin *et al.*, 2006.)

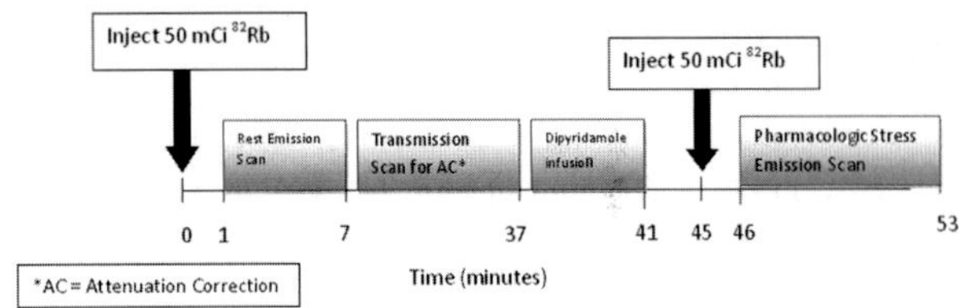

Figure 20.29 ^{82}Rb rest/stress imaging protocol.

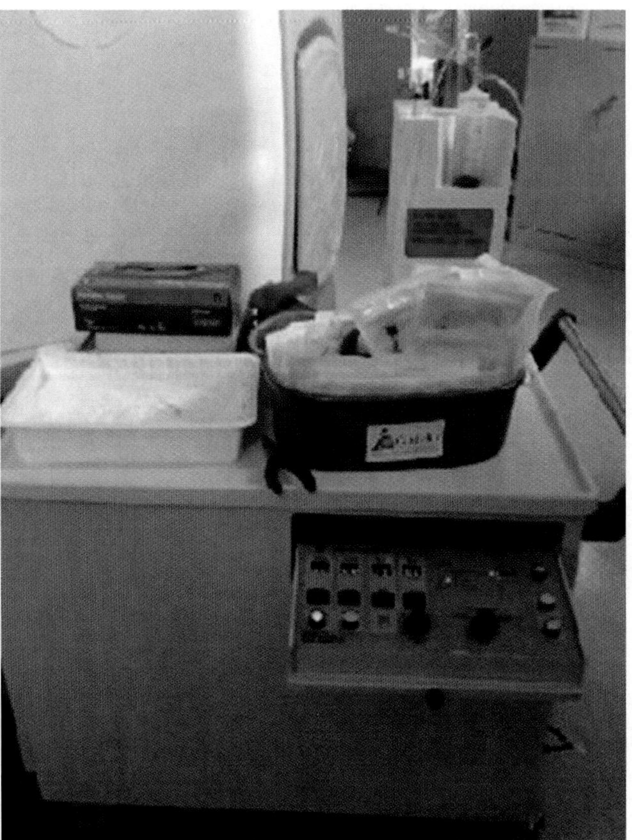

Figure 20.30 Infusion cart containing a generator used for ^{82}Rb cardiac imaging. (Courtesy of Cardiovascular Associates—Trinity, Birmingham, AL.)

A

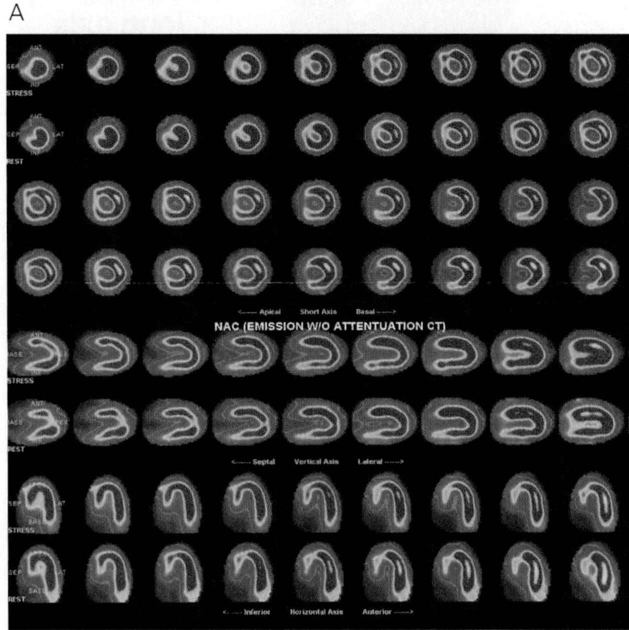

Figure 20.31 ^{82}Rb rest–stress images. (A) Emission images without attenuation correction. (B) Emission images with attenuation correction. (C) Gated image. (Courtesy of Cardiovascular Associates—Trinity, Birmingham, AL.)

Table 20.11 Cardiac PET Imaging Protocols

^{82}Rb-rest and pharmacologic stress perfusion imaging (Fig. 20.30)	1. Perform position scan. 2. Administer ^{82}Rb dose using the generator infusion system (Fig. 20.29). 3. Wait 70 sec before starting acquisition after ^{82}Rb infusion is complete. 4. Obtain rest emission scan. 5. Obtain transmission scan for attenuation correction after the completion of the rest emission scan. 6. Perform pharmacologic stress study. 7. Administer dose of ^{82}Rb via the infusion pump system. 8. Obtain stress emission scan 70 sec after the ^{82}Rb infusion is completed.
[^{13}N]Ammonia rest and pharmacologic stress perfusion imaging (Fig. 20.31)	1. Perform position scan. 2. Obtain transmission scan for attenuation correction. 3. Administer dose of [^{13}N]ammonia. 4. Acquisition of emission (rest scan) begins immediately after the administration of the radiopharmaceutical. 5. Patient remains in position for approximately 1 hr after injection to allow adequate decay before pharmacologic stress. 6. Upon completion of the decay time, the pharmacologic stress is performed. 7. Administer the second dose of [^{13}N]ammonia. 8. Acquire a second emission scan (stress scan) immediately after administration of radiopharmaceutical.
[^{18}F]FDG imaging (Fig. 20.32)	1. Complete a resting scan using [^{13}N]ammonia, ^{82}Rb, ^{201}Tl, or a ^{99m}Tc-labeled myocardial perfusion agent. 2. Perform position scan. 3. Obtain transmission scan for attenuation correction. 4. Administer [^{18}F]FDG. 5. Acquire emission data; multiple frame dynamic acquisition. 6. Obtain additional static images as needed.

Modified from Crawford and Husain (2003).

B

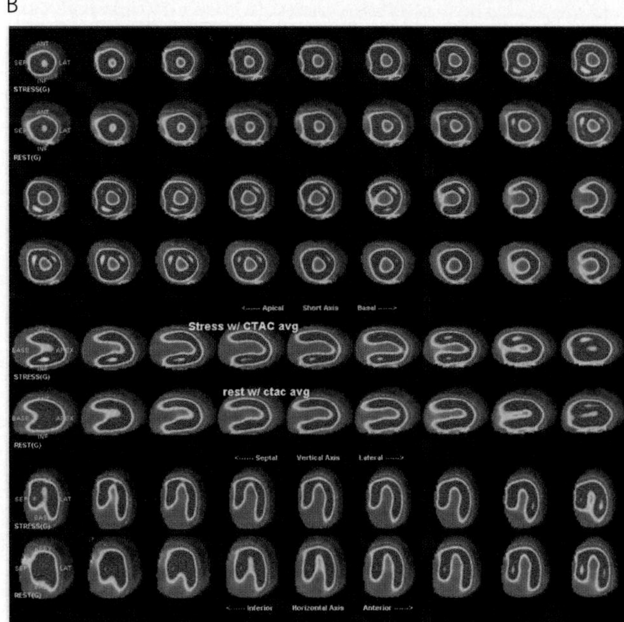

Figure 20.31 *(Continued.)*

C

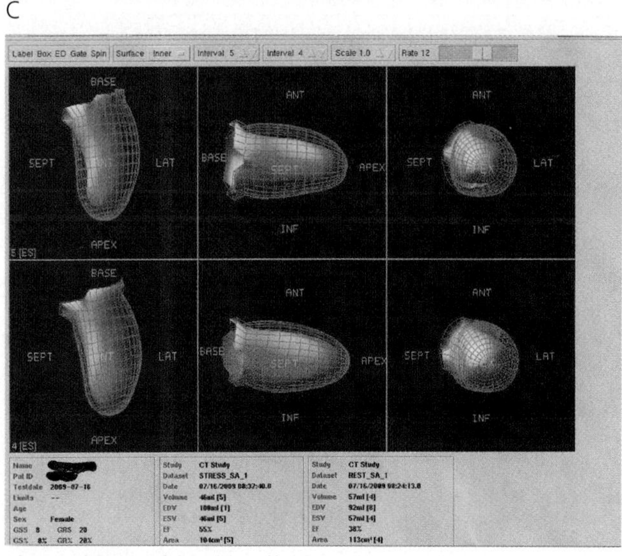

Figure 20.31 *(Continued.)*

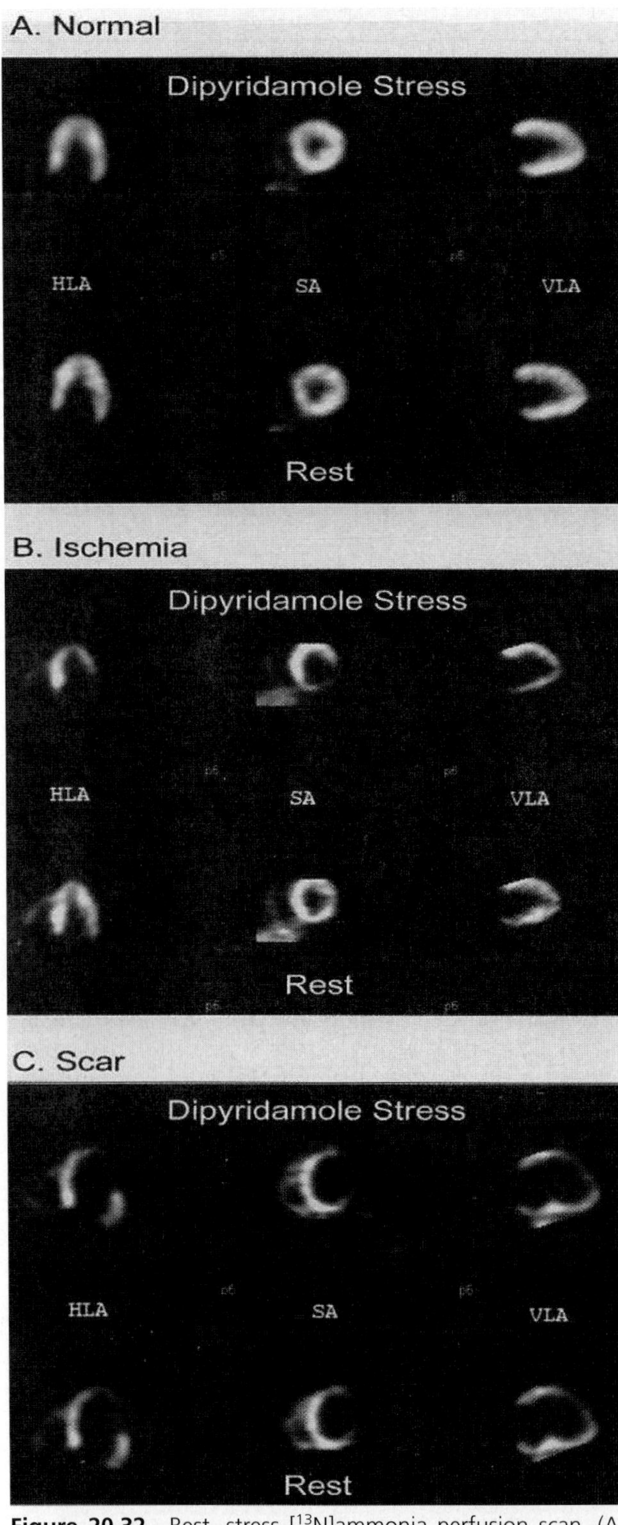

Figure 20.32 Rest–stress [^{13}N]ammonia perfusion scan. (A) Normal study. (B) Inferolateral/lateral wall ischemia. (C) Fixed defect. These images show lateral wall scar. (Reprinted, with permission, from Crawford and Husain, 2003.)

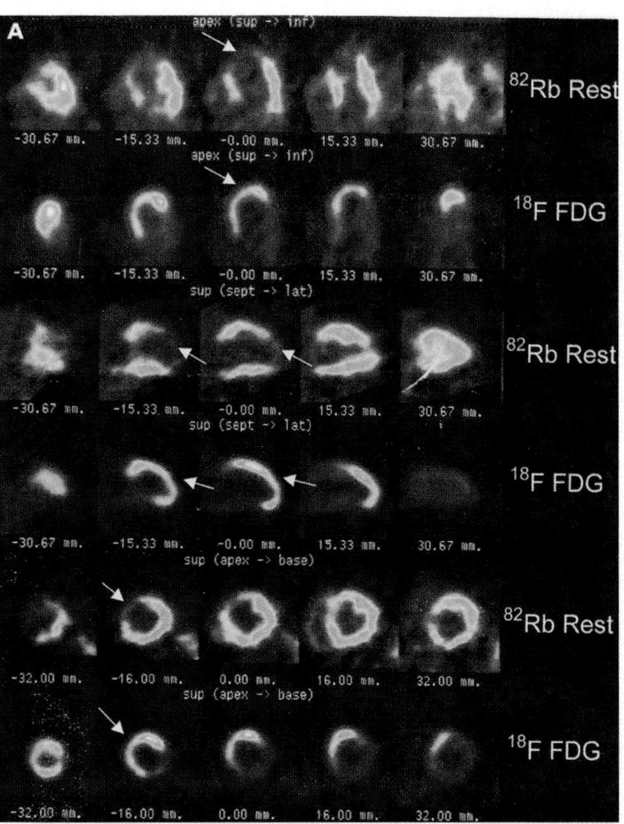

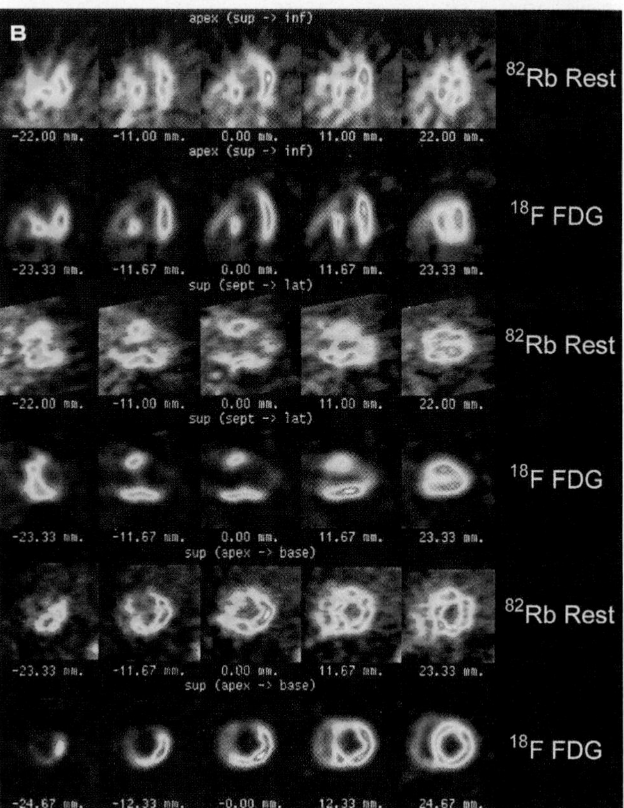

Figure 20.33 ^{82}Rb rest/[^{18}F]FDG stress/viability study. (A) Hibernating myocardium. (B) Matching defect. No viability. (Reprinted, with permission, from Crawford and Husain, 2003.)

Asit K, Hani A, 2004. Gated myocardial perfusion SPECT: Basic principles, technical aspects, and clinical applications. *J Nucl Med TS.* 32:179–187.

Crawford E, Husain S, 2003. *Nuclear Cardiac Imaging: Terminology and Technical Aspects.* Reston, VA: Society of Nuclear Medicine.

Henzlova MJ, Cerqueira MD, Hansen CL, Taillefer R, Yao SS, 2009. ASNC imaging guidelines for nuclear cardiology procedures. Stress protocols and tracers. Available at: http://www.asnc.org/imageuploads/ImagingGuidelinesStressProtocols021109.pdf.

Iskandrian AE, Verani MS, 2003. *Nuclear Cardiac Imaging Principles and Applications.* 3rd ed. Oxford, UK: Oxford University Press.

Lin GS, Hines HH, Grant G, Taylor K, Ryals C, 2006. Automated quantification of myocardial ischemia and wall motion defects by use of cardiac SPECT polar mapping and 4-dimensional surface rendering. *J Nucl Med Technol.* 34:3–17.

Scott LA, Kench P, 2004. Cardiac autonomic neuropathy in diabetic patients: Does ^{123}I–MIBG imaging have a role to play in early diagnosis? *J Nucl Med Technol.* 32:66–71.

Advanced Nuclear Cardiology Questions

1. Which of the following is not an indication for early termination of an exercise stress test based on the American Society of Nuclear Cardiology (ASNC) guidelines?

   a. The patient reaches target heart rate early
   b. Severe angina pectoris
   c. Excessive ST depression (>2 mm)
   d. Drop in systolic blood pressure

2. Vasodilator agents such as adenosine, dipyridimole, and regadenoson produce stimulation of which receptors?

   a. A1
   b. A2A
   c. A2B
   d. B1

3. Adenosine induces direct coronary arteriolar vasodilation through specific activation of the receptor. This results in an increase in myocardial blood flow by how many fold?

   a. 0.5–2
   b. 2–3
   c. 3.5–4
   d. 5–10

4. The ASNC guidelines indicate that adenosine should be given as a continuous infusion at a rate of ________ μg/kg/min over a 6-min period.

   a. 140
   b. 220
   c. 100
   d. 60

5. The combination of low-level exercise during an adenosine infusion results in which of the following?

   a. Increase in patient side effects
   b. Reduction in patient side effects
   c. Decrease in accuracy of results
   d. Significant increase in heart rate

6. Dobutamine infusion results in a direct β1 and β2 stimulation with a dose-related increase in heart rate, blood pressure, and myocardial contractility.

   a. True
   b. False

7. When performing a planar equilibrium radionuclide angiocardiography (ERNA), an LAO view with a caudal tilt of what degree is helpful in separating the atria from the ventricle?

   a. 5–8
   b. 1–4
   c. 20–25
   d. 10–15

8. Which of the following is the preferred method for planar ERNA?

   a. In vivo
   b. In vitro
   c. Modified in vivo
   d. Modified in vitro

9. What type of uptake in the myocardium has been well validated as an indicator of myocardial viability?

   a. Sestamibi
   b. MDP
   c. MAA
   d. FDG

10. At what distance should a radioactive point source be from an uncollimated camera when performing an intrinsic flood?

   a. One FOV
   b. Two FOVs
   c. Three FOVs
   d. Four FOVs
   e. Five FOVs

Answers

(1) a, (2) b, (3) c, (4) a, (5) b, (6) a, (7) d, (8) b, (9) d, (10) e

CHAPTER 21 Advanced PET Imaging Review

Dusty M. York

Physics of Positron Emission and Annihilation

Positron emission tomography (PET) is an advanced imaging modality used to image physiologic processes within the body. The emergence of PET, as the functional modality of choice for diagnosis, staging, therapy monitoring, and assessment of cancer recurrence, has led to considerable growth in this field. PET imaging is not intended to take the place of anatomic imaging, but to add to the biological evaluation of the processes taking place in the body.

PET consists of imaging positron-emitting radiopharmaceuticals. Positron emitters are neutron-deficient isotopes that achieve stability through the nuclear transformation of a proton into a neutron. These positron-rich nuclei then expel a positron, which is essentially a positively charged electron and a neutrino, from the nucleus of the atom. The positrons travel a very short distance before pairing up with an electron. The average positron range in matter depends on the positron's energy and material characteristics. Upon reaching the end of its path, the positron will annihilate with an atomic electron. In the annihilation, electrons and positrons convert their masses into energy and produce a pair of 511-keV photons traveling in opposite directions 180° apart, as seen in Figure 21.1.

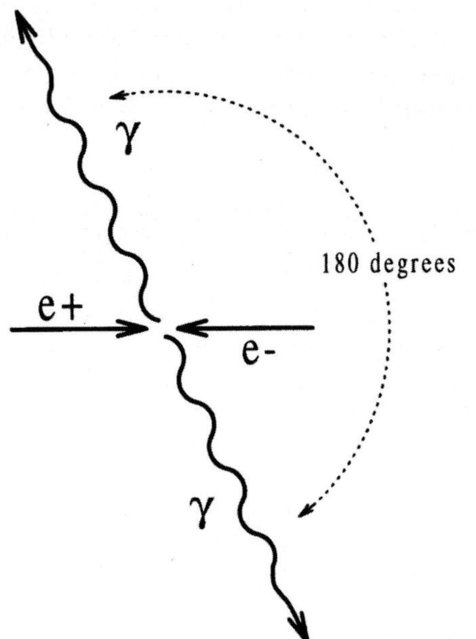

Figure 21.1 Electron–positron annihilation, producing two 511-keV photons departing in opposite directions. (Reprinted, with permission, from Turkington, 2001.)

PET Radionuclides

Radiopharmaceuticals utilized in PET imaging are proton rich, which requires a device that can add protons to the nucleus. Medical cyclotrons are the most common devices used to produce PET radiopharmaceuticals. In a cyclotron, charged particles, such as protons, are accelerated in circular paths in "dees" under a vacuum by means of an electromagnetic field. Radiopharmaceuticals produced by this method include ^{11}C, ^{13}N, ^{15}O, and ^{18}F. The majority of PET radiopharmaceuticals are cyclotron produced; two exceptions are gallium-68 and rubidium-82, which are both generator produced. Gallium-68 is produced by the $^{68}Ge-^{68}Ga$ generator and is routinely used as a standard sealed source for calibration of PET systems, but its clinical use is very limited. Table 21.1 provides a list of common radionuclides used in PET.

PET Radionuclides at a Glance

[^{18}F]Sodium Fluoride

Fluorine-18 is produced by irradiation of [^{18}O]water with protons in a cyclotron and recovered as [^{18}F]sodium fluoride by passing the irradiated water target mixture through a carbonate-type anion-exchange resin column. The water passes through, the ^{18}F is retained on the column, and is then removed by elution with a potassium carbonate solution. [^{18}F]sodium fluoride is most commonly used for the synthesis of [^{18}F]fluorodeoxyglucose; it is also approved by the FDA for bone scintigraphy.

[^{18}F]Fluorodeoxyglucose (FDG)

[^{18}F]FDG is the most utilized PET radiopharmaceutical and can be given credit for the growth of PET over the last 20 years. [^{18}F]FDG is a glucose analog in which the

Table 21.1 PET Radionuclides

Nuclide	$T_{1/2}$	B+ range, max (mm)	Production method
^{15}O	2 min	8.0	Cyclotron
^{13}N	10 min	5.0	Cyclotron
^{11}C	20 min	3.8	Cyclotron
^{18}F	110 min	2.2	Cyclotron
^{82}Rb	75 sec	15.5	Generator ($^{82}Sr-^{82}Rb$)

hydroxyl group on the 2-carbon of a glucose molecule is replaced by a fluoride atom. [^{18}F]FDG is an excellent indicator of glucose uptake and cell viability. Like glucose, [^{18}F]FDG is taken up into living cells by facilitated transport and then phosphorylated by hexokinase. Unlike glucose, [^{18}F]FDG cannot undergo further metabolism and remains trapped in the cells.

The most commonly used method for the production of [^{18}F]FDG involves the method developed by Hamacher *et al.* (1986). This method utilizes a nucleophilic substitution reaction (Fig. 21.2). Nucleophilic substitution is a chemical reaction involving the addition of a highly negatively charged molecule into an electron drawing group attached to the parent molecule through an unstable chemical bond. Synthesis of [^{18}F]FDG can be carried out in many different controlled synthesizers; the process consists of roughly the same stages to include the following: removal of ^{18}F from the [^{18}O]water dispensed from the cyclotron by ammonium anion exchange. The retained ^{18}F is eluted with an acetonitrile solution of Kryptofix and potassium carbonate. Kryptofix is used to increase the reactivity of the ^{18}F-labeled anion. The next step involves evaporation of residual [^{18}O]water from the ^{18}F with acetonitrile. This is followed by addition of mannose triflate into the ^{18}F with acetonitrile, where the nucleophilic substitution takes place. The ^{18}F-labeled ion approaches the mannose triflate, while the triflate group leaves the protected mannose molecule to form [^{18}F]FDG. After the nucleophilic replacement of the triflate group by ^{18}F, the acetyl groups can easily be removed by hydrolysis to produce [^{18}F]FDG. The final step involves hydrolysis, which consists of removing the protective acetyl groups to form [^{18}F]FDG and purification of the final product (Fig. 21.2). Most automatic synthesizers can produce [^{18}F]FDG of over 95% routinely. [^{18}F]FDG has a half-life of 110 min allowing availability in most areas. [^{18}F]FDG is primarily used for oncology applications.

[^{18}F]Fluorodopa

6-[^{18}F]Fluoro-3,4-dihydroxy-phenylalanine ([^{18}F]fluorodopa) is cyclotron produced. There are several methods of synthesizing 6-[^{18}F]fluorodopa. [^{18}F]Flurodopa is commonly produced by fluorodemetallation using electrophilic fluorinating agents. [^{18}F]Flurodopa is used for the assessment of the presynaptic dopaminergic function in the brain.

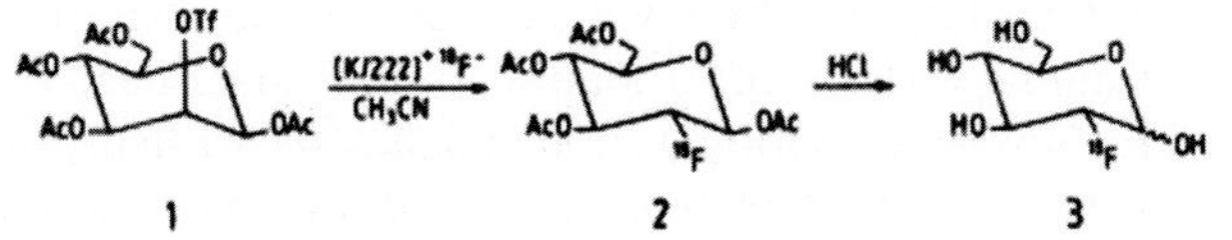

Figure 21.2 Reaction scheme depicting synthesis of FDG. (Reprinted, with permission, from Hamacher *et al.*, 1986, p. 236.)

[^{18}F]Fluorothymidine (FLT)

[^{18}F]Fluorothymidine (FLT) is prepared by nucleophilic reaction between [^{18}F]fluoride and a precursor that is prepared by standard organic synthesis. Thymidine is incorporated into DNA and provides a measure of cell proliferation; [^{18}F]FLT is used for in vivo diagnosis and characterization of tumors in humans.

[^{15}O]Water

[^{15}O]Oxygen is produced in the cyclotron by the ^{15}N (*p*, *n*) ^{15}O reaction, and the irradiated gas is transferred to a [^{15}O]water generator, which is then mixed with hydrogen and passed over a palladium/charcoal catalyst at 170°. The $H_2{}^{15}O$ vapor is then trapped in saline for injection to the patient. The short half-life of approximately 2 min limits the use and availability of [^{15}O]water. This tracer is most commonly used for myocardial and cerebral blood flow studies.

[^{13}N]Ammonia

Nitrogen-13-labeled ammonia is cyclotron produced by the ^{16}O (*p*, α) ^{13}N nuclear reaction. This reaction is performed using a solution of ethanol in water to yield ^{13}N in the form of ammonia. ^{13}N has a half-life of approximately 10 min and is primarily used as a myocardial perfusion imaging agent.

[^{11}C]Carbon

Carbon-11 is generally produced by the ^{10}B (d, *n*) ^{11}C or ^{14}N (*p*, *n*) ^{11}C or ^{14}N (*p*, α) ^{11}C nuclear reactions. A number of ^{11}C-labeled compounds have been synthesized as PET radiopharmaceuticals. The most common are discussed briefly below. [^{11}C]Acetate, a tracer used in the study of myocardial metabolism, is currently being evaluated for use as a prospective agent in the evaluation of prostate cancer. [^{11}C]Glucose is also used to study metabolism. Carbon-11-labeled C-L-methionine has been used for the detection of different types of malignancies. [^{11}C]Raclopride is primarily used to detect various neurologic and psychiatric disorders. Carbon-11 has a half-life of 20 min.

[^{82}Rb]Rubidium Chloride

[^{82}Rb]Rubidium chloride is available from the ^{82}Sr–^{82}Rb generator, which is supplied monthly. ^{82}Rb is eluted with saline and must by checked for ^{82}Sr and ^{85}Sr breakthrough daily before the start of its use for patient studies. The allowable limit for ^{82}Sr is 0.74 kBq/37 MBq (0.02 μCi/mCi ^{82}Rb) and for ^{85}Sr is 7.4 kBq/37 MBq

(0.2 μCi/mCi ^{82}Rb). ^{82}Rb has a very short half-life of 75 sec and is administered to the patient by way of an infusion pump connected directly to the generator. ^{82}Rb is used for myocardial perfusion imaging.

Quality Control for [^{18}F]FDG

Since [^{18}F]FDG is the most widely used and distributed PET radiopharmaceutical, it is important to discuss the quality control requirements specific to this agent. Due to the short half-life of [^{18}F]FDG, all the required tests cannot be completed prior to release of the [^{18}F]FDG product. Prerelease U.S. Pharmacopeia (USP) quality control testing for PET radiopharmaceuticals includes a visual inspection, identity testing, pH, radiochemical and chemical purity, and residual solvent analysis. Sterility testing and bacterial endotoxin test (BET) are required postrelease for every production of [^{18}F]FDG radiopharmaceutical prepared for human use.

Visual Inspection

[^{18}F]FDG should appear as a clear and colorless solution without particulate matter.

Identity Testing

The radionuclidic identity can be confirmed measuring the half-life of the product. This test is performed using a dose calibrator and involves decay analysis over a defined period of time. The acceptable half-life of [^{18}F]FDG is 109.7 min with an allowable range of 105–115 min. Radionuclidic purity should be determined with γ spectroscopy. A multichannel analyzer (MCA) is used to determine the presence of any γ photon energy other than that characteristic of ^{18}F, which includes 511 keV, 1.02 MeV, or Compton scatter. The radionuclidic purity must be 99.9%.

pH

The pH value of an injectable should be as close to the physiological pH as possible. The pH of [^{18}F]FDG must be between 4.5 and 7.5. This test is performed using pH papers.

Radiochemical Purity

The radiochemical purity of a radiopharmaceutical is the fraction of the total radioactivity in the desired chemical form in the radiopharmaceutical. The radiochemical purity of [^{18}F]FDG can be determined by using silica gel thin layer chromatography (TLC) plates developed in acetonitrile:water (95:5). The R_f values should be confirmed per the validation process. [^{18}F]FDG (R_f = 0.4), [^{18}F]fluoride (R_f = 0.6). Acceptable radiochemical purity is ≥90%.

Chemical Purity

The chemical purity of a radiopharmaceutical is the fraction of the material in the desired chemical form. A series of chemical purity tests may be required, if any of the following agents are used in the synthesis of [^{18}F]FDG: Kryptofix, acetonitrile, ethanol, or ether. If the synthesis involves Kryptofix, the USP requires determination of the concentration prior to releasing the final product. The current USP-approved method utilizes silica gel TLC developed in a mixture of ethanol and water. The developed plate is dried and an iodine vapor chamber is used for visualization. A yellow spot indicates the presence of Kryptofix. The Kryptofix concentration must be less than 50 μg/mL. The maximum concentration of other solvents is as follows: acetonitrile must be 0.04 mg/mL, ethanol 5 mg/mL, and ether 5 mg/mL.

Sterility

Sterility indicates the absence of any viable bacteria or microorganisms in a radiopharmaceutical preparation. Postrelease sterility testing must be performed for each batch of [^{18}F]FDG. The product must be inoculated on both soybean casein digest medium and fluid thioglycollate within 24 hr. The sterility test takes 14 days to complete, which does not allow for prerelease results. Since [^{18}F]FDG is released and injected into patients before sterility results are available, the final product is passed through a 0.22-μm filter to ensure sterility.

Bacterial Endotoxins Limulus Amoebocyte Lysate (LAL Test)

The Bacterial Endotoxin Test (BET) is a test for pyrogens. The bacterial endotoxins level is tested using the LAL test. The sensitivity of the test is given in endotoxin units (EU). BET should be <175 EU/mL. Most testing kits require an incubation period of 20–60 min. Therefore, it is unlikely that the test will be completed before release of the product.

Radiation Protection in PET

PET requires special consideration regarding radiation safety. A basic understanding of radiation safety techniques should be incorporated to keep clinical and occupational exposures as low as reasonably achievable (ALARA). Considerations should be incorporated in the design and setup of all PET facilities. PET/CT facilities can be even more challenging with the incorporation of shielding due to the CT component. Within a PET imaging department, the majority of exposure to personnel results from the injected patient; therefore, planning adequate shielding can be a challenge. When planning a PET department, it is important to consider exposure of all personnel surrounding the

PET department and plan for the appropriate amount of shielding to be incorporated. The scanner room, preparation room, and possibly a postinjection waiting area, such as a quiet room, may need to be considered for shielding.

To keep exposure to the technologist as low as reasonably achievable the technologist should consider time, distance, and shielding. The time the technologist is exposed to the source, which includes the injected patient, should be limited. The technologist should explain the procedure and request a thorough patient history prior to injecting the patient. This will limit the time spent after injection with the patient. Technologists should maximize the distance between themselves and the patients and should use tongs or remote manipulators, if possible, when handling doses. The dose rate is inversely related to the square of the distance from the source. Finally, the technologist should ensure proper shielding techniques when measuring doses and performing injections. Shielding devices require thicker shielding material. Doses should be prepared and measured behind a lead shield. Syringe shields should be utilized when injecting patients. Tungsten is preferable over lead for syringe shields used in PET. The 511-keV photons have a half-value layer of 4 mm in lead compared to 3 mm in tungsten.

PET Instrumentation

PET Detectors

PET imaging systems utilize scintillation crystals, but several additional considerations are necessary beyond those pertaining to general nuclear medicine. An ideal PET scintillation detector would have the following characteristics: has high density to stop the high-energy photons, has very efficient scintillation, which produces a large amount of light, and is an exceptionally fast scintillator. Most scintillation crystals are lacking at least one of these ideal characteristics. Table 21.2 lists several scintillation crystals that have been used as PET detectors, along with some properties of each.

The sodium iodide detector remains the detector of choice in single-photon emission tomography because of its excellent energy resolution and higher light output. The density of the NaI(Tl) detector is its limiting factor for PET application; it is not very effective at stopping the high-energy photons used in PET.

Several other detector materials have resulted in greater success. In the early PET scanners, bismuth germinate ($Bi_4Ge_3O_{12}$) or BGO were utilized. BGO detectors have a high density, which means they are more efficient at stopping the high-energy photons utilized in PET. However, the decay time and light yield of BGO are both limiting factors. BGO also has poor energy resolution, which requires energy windows to be wider than preferred. The latest detectors include lutetium orthosilicate (Lu_2SiO_5[Ce] or LSO), yttrium orthosilicate ($Lu_{1.9}Y_{0.5}SiO_5$[Ce] or YLSO), and gadolinium orthosilicate (Gd_2SiO_5[Ce] or GSO). These new detectors are all doped with cerium (Ce) to improve their scintillation efficiency; all have a greater light output and shorter decay times, when compared to BGO.

A couple of new scintillators are being evaluated for time of flight (TOF) PET. These detectors include barium fluoride (BaF_2) and lanthanum bromide ($LaBr_3$). Both of these detectors are faster scintillators and have shorter decay times. TOF systems can accurately estimate an annihilation event location along the coincidence line of response (LOR), by measuring the difference in the arrival times of the annihilation photons at the opposing detectors. TOF imaging can be performed with some of the other faster scintillators, but is more accurate with one of the more advanced scintillators. The main benefit to TOF-PET is a significant improvement in the signal-to-noise ratio in the reconstructed 3D image.

Table 21.2 PET Scintillation Detectors

Property	NaI(Tl)	BGO	GSO	LSO	YLSO
Density (g/cm^3)	3.7	7.1	6.7	7.4	7.1
Emission intensity (relative to NaI[Tl])	100	15	25	75	80
Decay time (ns)	230	300	50	40	40
Hygroscopic	Yes	No	No	No	No

Scanner Design

The basic primary component of a PET system is two opposed crystals connected to a coincidence circuit. The annihilation photons detected in PET are simultaneously released in 180° opposite directions. To be considered a valid event, the two annihilation photons must both be detected within a very short coincidence timing window of 5–12 ns. The detectors used for coincidence detection identify an annihilation photon pair and determine an LOR path representing the path of the photon pair (Fig. 21.3).

The detectors used in PET are composed of small cube-shaped crystals about 4 mm in size and 20–30 mm in length. PET scanners typically have 18–40 rings of detectors for a total of approximately 10,000–25,000 small detectors. Electronically the scintillation crystals are organized into detector blocks with multiple detectors coupled to a single photo multiplier tube.

Types of Events in PET

True coincidences or true events occur when two annihilation photons from a single annihilation interaction are

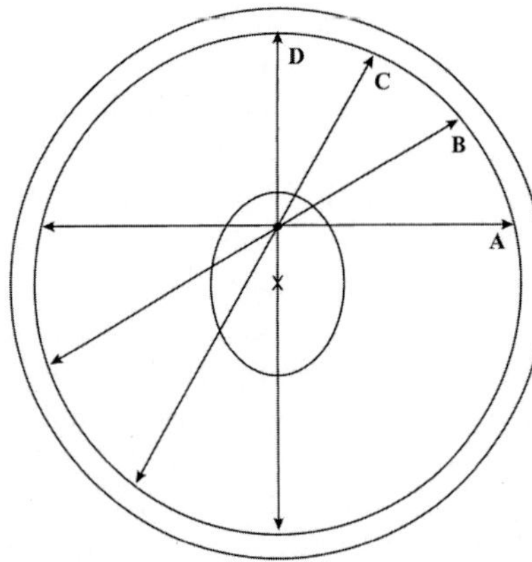

Figure 21.3 An illustration of four LORs that pass through a single point. (Reprinted, with permission, from Fahey, 2002, p. 40.)

detected within the timing window. Several other possibilities exist, such as random coincidences and scatter coincidences (Fig. 21.4). Random coincidences or random events occur when two single events from two separate annihilations are detected within the timing window. When this happens, a false event is recorded. The randoms rate increases relative to the square of the dosage. Processing software attempts to estimate these false events and applies corrections during reconstruction; another method to reduce the randoms rate is reducing the coincidence timing window. Utilizing a fast scintillator, such as LSO, also decreases random coincidences. Another type of event is known as a scatter event. Scatter events arise from the scatter of annihilation photons between their origin and the detectors. Scatter is affected by the distribution of radioactivity, size, and density of the object as well as their location relative to the detector. Randoms and scatter events are inevitable in imaging and corrections are essential, if quantitative results are to be obtained.

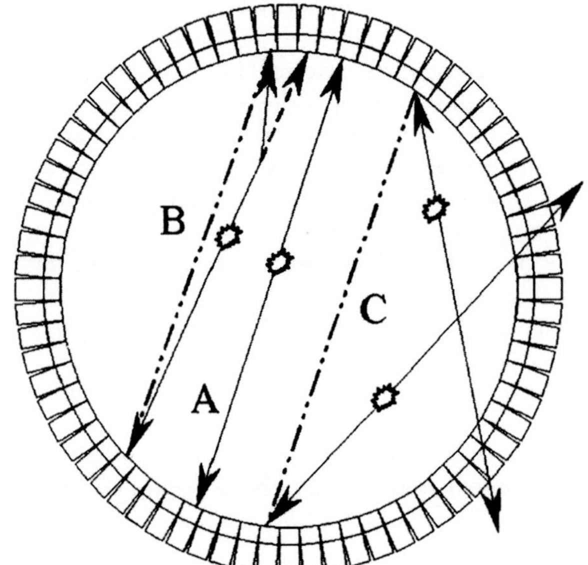

Figure 21.4 Graphic representation of true (A), scatter (B), and random events (C). (Reprinted, with permission, from Tarantola, 2003.)

Attenuation Correction

Attenuation correction is critical for both visual and quantitative accuracy of PET images. Attenuation will vary from patient to patient since the makeup and size of the patient's body varies. The only way to accurately evaluate the attenuation coefficient is to pass a beam of radiation through the body and measure the attenuation. If the system is an independent PET system without the CT component, this is performed by rotating a radioactive rod source around the patient. This attenuation image is known as a transmission image. The radioactive sources are usually ^{68}Ge or ^{137}Cs, which are housed within the gantry and extended through the use of a robotic system only for the transmission portion of the exam. A transmission image will need to be performed for each bed position along with an emission image. These images are usually interlaced by performing emission–transmission–transmission–emission (ETTE) to reduce total scan time. With the advent of CT into our PET scanner design, the CT scan replaces the need for the transmission scan. The transmission scan data are reconstructed into an attenuation correction map for each slice.

2D and 3D Imaging

Some PET scanners have thin rings of lead or tungsten, known as septa, positioned between the rings of the detectors. The scanner has the capability to operate with the septa extended and in use, which is known as 2D mode. Retracting the septa places the scanner in 3D mode. While operating in 2D mode, the septa serve to limit the FOV of events to those within the same detector ring and to reduce the number of scatter and random coincidence events. When the septa are retracted in 3D mode, more annihilation events can be detected across the detector rings resulting in a drastic increase in sensitivity (Fig. 21.5). Unfortunately, at the cost of increasing the detection of true events we also increase the detection of scatter and random events. Correction techniques are crucial in the processing of 3D data. Many of today's scanners no longer have the capability to operate in 2D mode; with the introduction of faster detectors, timing windows can be reduced to help decrease the errors produced in 3D imaging. Along with the image quality being enhanced in 3D imaging, the gantry opening also

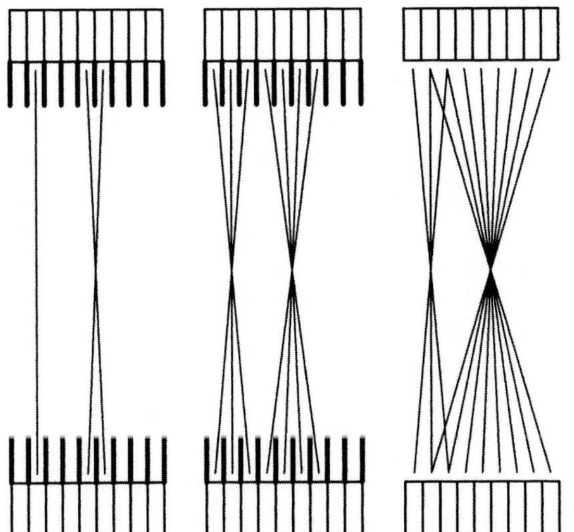

Figure 21.5 Multiring PET acquisition modes. Left: Examples of simple 2D direct and cross planes. Middle: Extended 2D direct and cross planes for increased efficiency. Right: Full 3D acceptance. The acceptance is greater for radiation in the middle of the axial FOV than for radiation near the end. (Reprinted, with permission, from Turkington, 2001.)

increases due to the removal of the septa, allowing larger patients to benefit from PET imaging. With the initiation of these faster scintillators along with improvements in correction techniques, 3D imaging has evolved into routine clinical use.

Data Collection and Analysis

Reconstruction Algorithms

During image reconstruction, data must first be reformatted into sinograms. A sinogram is simply a plot of counts registered in each LOR. PET data sets may be reconstructed with either analytic or iterative techniques. The analytic method of performing filtered backprojection is probably the simplest way to perform reconstruction and definitely the fastest. However, filtered backprojection tends to create artifacts and results in increased image noise. Another method of reconstruction is known as iterative reconstruction. Iterative reconstruction algorithms estimate image values and perform repeated calculations. This ongoing repetition of estimations takes considerably more time, but can be accommodated by today's faster computers. 3D image reconstruction demands more reconstruction considerations and is essentially converted into a 2D approximation before further reconstruction. This 3D to 2D conversion is referred to as rebinning. Iterative techniques are usually preferred for 3D image applications. The completed image from iterative reconstruction techniques results in less noise and artifacts than filtered backprojection.

Two iterative algorithms important to PET are maximum-likelihood expectation maximization (MLEM) and ordered subset expectation maximization (OSEM). It is important to note that both of these algorithms require a substantial amount of computations to complete and are both time consuming when compared to filtered backprojection. MLEM was one of the first iterative algorithms introduced. MLEM requires many iterations utilizing the entire data set, which is very time consuming. OSEM is a faster and more efficient iterative algorithm. OSEM uses selected subsets of the data, which results in fewer iterations and reduces the amount of time required.

Performance Evaluations

The National Electrical Manufacturers Association (NEMA) has developed guidelines on how some performance parameters, such as spatial resolution and sensitivity, should be evaluated and presented. These guidelines are used to make a better assessment of system performance.

Scatter Fraction

Scatter fraction is a measure that indicates a PET tomograph's sensitivity to scatter coincidences. It is defined as the ratio of scatter coincidences to total counts:

$$\text{Scatter fraction (SF)} = \frac{S(0) = 8 \times S(4.5) + 10.75 \times S(9)}{T_{\text{tot}}(0) = 8 \times T_{\text{tot}}(4.5) + 10.75 \times T_{\text{tot}}(9)}$$

where S is the number of the scattered counts per unit activity and T_{tot} is the total number of counts (true + scattered) per unit activity.

Several factors affect the scatter fraction, such as acquisition mode, energy mode, and the geometry of the scanner. The desire is to achieve a low scatter fraction. This value allows the user to verify that the scatter correction techniques utilized are accurate.

Noise Equivalent Count Rate

The noise equivalent count rate (NEC) is a measure of signal-to-noise ratio. The NEC is defined as

$$\text{NEC} = \frac{T^2}{T + S + 2fR}$$

where T, S, and R are the true, scatter, and random coincidence counting rates, f is the fraction of the sinogram width produced by the phantom, and the factor 2 comes from online randoms subtraction.

Quantitative Image Analysis

Quantitative uptake value of a radiopharmaceutical can be measured in an attempt to more thoroughly analyze radiotracer distribution. The degree of radiotracer uptake is a determining factor used to evaluate malignant from benign processes. Standardized uptake values (SUVs) give the user a better quantitative uptake ratio. Malignant processes will typically demonstrate higher SUVs when compared to normal tissue. SUVs require close attention to detail from the technologists to ensure accurate information regarding time of dose, activity administered, injection time, patient height and weight, and the time when images were actually obtained. The SUV is most often calculated utilizing the weight-based calculation:

$$\text{SUV} = \frac{\text{ROI activity in mCi/mL}}{\text{injected activity in mCi/mL/patient weight in g}}$$

Another factor in the accuracy of SUV values is cross calibration between the tomograph obtained and the dose calibrators used to measure dose activity. Imaging parameter selection can also affect SUV values. Dual-point imaging may be performed followed by SUV determination. SUV values of malignant processes tend to increase or remain constant while SUV values of infectious processes tend to decrease on the delay images. There is still much controversy regarding the accuracy of SUVs, but it is still widely recognized.

PET Scanner Calibration and Quality Control

Quality control on a PET camera is required and consists of a series of tests performed to ensure that the equipment is operating efficiently. A description of the various quality control procedures follows and is summarized in Table 21.3.

Energy Window Calibration

Energy window calibration is typically performed only after repairs or during quarterly preventive maintenance. This application is performed to ensure that the energy window is correctly positioned around the 511-keV energy of PET radionuclides.

Coincidence Timing Calibration

The coincidence timing window should be evaluated during quarterly preventive maintenance to ensure uniform timing windows for all detectors. Typical PET timing windows are set around 5–12 ns. As timing windows are extended, significantly more random and scatter events are accepted.

Normalization

The normalization calibration is an evaluation of the correction factors that are applied to every study. This calibration procedure is performed by using the radioactive rod sources housed in the gantry, or if the scanner does not have these sources, a ^{68}Ge canister source is used. This calibration requires a long acquisition to provide good statistical data and ultimately decrease the noise as much as possible. Therefore, the calibration is usually performed overnight and usually takes a minimum of 6 hr to complete. A normalization calibration for 3D mode may need to be acquired separately. This calibration can be compared to performing a high-count uniformity correction on gamma cameras. Normalization calibrations are performed quarterly and after repairs.

Blank Scan

The blank scan is performed daily to make certain the scanner is operating properly. The blank scan is essentially a transmission scan without a patient in the gantry, hence the name blank scan. This scan is used to identify equipment failures prior to imaging patients. The blank scan is performed by acquiring a short, approximately 30 min, acquisition of the transmission rod sources housed in the gantry or a ^{68}Ge canister source. The sinogram is then evaluated for obvious malfunctions. Since the detector blocks are visualized along a diagonal in the sino-

Table 21.3 PET/CT Scanner Quality Control

Test[a]	Recommended testing frequency[b]
Energy window calibration	Quarterly
Coincidence timing calibration	Quarterly
Normalization	Quarterly
Blank scan	Daily
Absolute activity calibration	Quarterly
CT uniformity	Daily

[a]These tests should also be performed after repair or preventive maintenance.
[b]Camera manufacturers may recommend other testing frequencies.

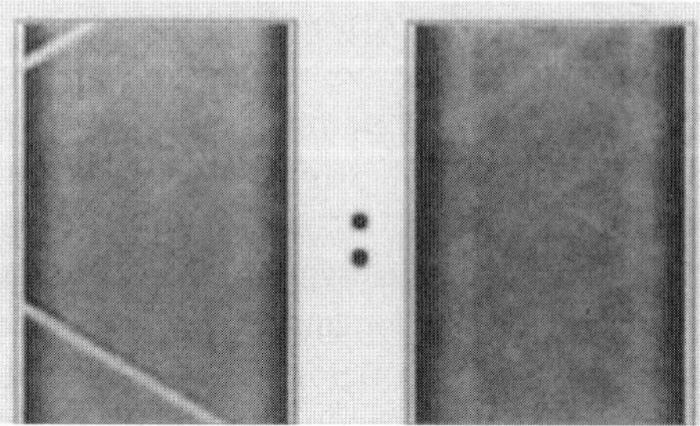

Figure 21.6 Left: An example of an abnormal blank scan indicating detector failure. Right: A normal blank scan. (Reprinted, with permission, from Buchert *et al.*, 1999, p. 1658.)

gram, any malfunctions will be visualized as a diagonal line. Figure 21.6 is an image of abnormal and normal blank scans.

Absolute Activity Calibration

Absolute activity calibration, also known as well-counter calibration or cross calibration, is performed to obtain quantitative information about radioactivity. Essentially this is a method to convert counts per second per voxel into microcuries per milliliter. This calibration is vital to quantitative analysis in PET. To calculate standard uptake values this calibration must be performed. Ideally, cross calibration with the dose calibrator used in the PET department would also be performed. This calibration is performed by taking a known amount of activity and adding this to a known volume in a water-filled phantom. The phantom is imaged and reconstructed, the count rate per voxel is determined, and a calibration factor is calculated. Absolute activity calibration should be performed quarterly or after major service, but only after all other calibrations have been performed.

CT Quality Control Requirements

When utilizing a PET/CT scanner, quality control requirements are necessary for the CT component of the system as well. These include CT calibration and field uniformity. Calibration is performed to assure that accurate CT numbers are expressed in Hounsfield units. Calibration of the CT system is critical for the use of CT images for PET attenuation correction. CT system calibration is performed with a special calibration phantom that includes inserts of known CT numbers. This calibration is typically performed by the service engineer and checked daily by the technologist with a water-filled phantom. Field uniformity is evaluated to confirm a uniform response throughout the field of view.

There are also other particular quality control considerations when utilizing a PET/CT system. These should include an evaluation of the registration accuracy when fusing the two modalities, as well as evaluation of attenuation correction accuracy when performing a CT for attenuation correction.

Imaging Applications

Oncology Applications

[^{18}F]FDG Metabolism

[^{18}F]FDG is very similar to naturally occurring glucose. [^{18}F]FDG essentially serves as an external marker of cellular glucose metabolism. This is important, especially in oncology applications, due to the fact than many types of cancer cells utilize glucose at higher rates than normal cells. The body is ultimately able to distinguish [^{18}F]FDG from normal glucose and therefore allows a "trapping" of [^{18}F]FDG for imaging purposes.

Naturally occurring glucose goes through a series of steps in order to be metabolized in the body. Glucose is transported to cells by glucose transporters (GLUT), and there are several types of glucose transporters. The most important transporters for FDG appear to be GLUT1 and GLUT4. GLUT1 is expressed in almost all cell types. GLUT4 is an insulin-sensitive transporter and is present in the myocardium and skeletal muscle. Overexpression of GLUT1 transporters is usually demonstrated in many cancerous processes and supports the increased uptake of FDG in cancerous cells. Once [^{18}F]FDG is transported into the cell along with naturally occurring glucose, the cell begins the breakdown process. Once inside the cell, hexokinase initiates the conversion of FDG to FDG-6 phosphate. The first step of conversion is performed by adding a phosphate group. FDG experiences the same process and is thus transformed into FDG-6 phosphate. The next step is to transform the glucose component into fructose; FDG-6 phosphate cannot be transformed into fructose and thus remains trapped in the cell.

[^{18}F]FDG Normal Biodistribution

The normal whole-body distribution of FDG is summarized here. At initial review of a whole-body PET scan, the most significant areas of uptake are the brain, kidneys, and bladder. Within the central nervous system uptake increases throughout the brain, demonstrating high uptake in the cortex, basal ganglia, thalamus, cerebellum, and brainstem. The white matter and spinal fluid typically demonstrate low uptake. The elevated uptake in the area of the brain limits the ability of FDG for oncology brain applications. The cardiovascular system demonstrates variable uptake in the left ventricular myocardium, but usually no uptake in the right ventricle and atria. The gastrointestinal system demonstrates variable uptake in the stomach, small intestine, colon, and rectum. The reticuloendothelial system and lymphatic system demonstrate low- to mid-grade uptake in the liver and spleen along with an absence of uptake in normal lymph nodes. Variable activity can be present in the tonsils, as well as in thymic and adenoid tissue. The genitourinary system demonstrates moderate uptake due to excretion of [^{18}F]FDG in the urine. Skeletal muscle uptake should be low, but can be affected by activity prior to and immediately after injection. Uptake in the bone marrow and lungs is typically very low in a normal patient. An example of an [^{18}F]FDG PET scan can be seen in Figure 21.7.

There are a variety of normal variations as well. Skeletal muscle uptake can be affected by exercise or tension

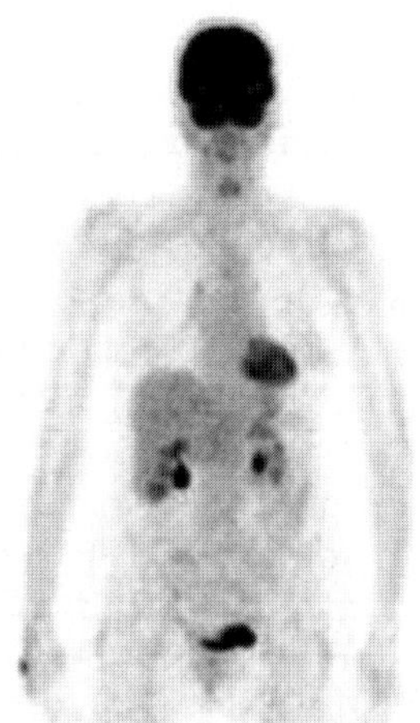

Figure 21.7 [^{18}F]FDG PET scan. (Reprinted, with permission, from Schwarz *et al.*, 2009.)

causing increased uptake. Symmetrical uptake in the neck and supraclavicular region has been identified to result from brown fat uptake. Uptake in brown fat results from the process of thermogenesis; this uptake can be reduced with the administration of benzodiazepines or simply by providing a warm blanket to the patient prior to injection of FDG and during the uptake phase. Myocardial activity commonly varies, but can be regulated by diet. The majority of fasting patients will demonstrate very little to no ventricular activity. Addition of a low-carbohydrate diet prior to the study can aid in the elimination of ventricular activity. The area of the mouth can also demonstrate variable uptake due to the accumulation of FDG in the salivary glands. The muscles in the facial area are also a possible site of uptake if the patient talks or grinds his or her teeth during the uptake phase. Variable uptake in the colon is also a very common problem, which is assumed to be caused by peristalsis. [^{18}F]FDG uptake is typically enhanced by inflammatory induced changes, which could include surgical incisions, arthritis, and a variety of other inflammatory conditions. Patients undergoing a PET scan after recent therapy can also demonstrate unusual findings. Patients having undergone radiation therapy can demonstrate inflammatory changes; thus imaging should be delayed for at least 4–6 months after completion of radiation if possible. Uniform diffuse increased bone marrow activity can be seen with bone marrow recovery after chemotherapy; this usually resolves by 1 month after therapy. An additional reason for increased bone marrow uptake results from patients taking hematopoietic growth factors or other bone-stimulating medications.

Many malignant processes avidly utilize [^{18}F]FDG, although there are several applications in which [^{18}F]FDG PET is of little or no benefit, such as prostate cancer. Other areas of limitation include hypometabolic malignancies, urologic cancers, and very small lesions. Therefore, obtaining a thorough patient history and understanding normal biodistribution is imperative in interpreting PET studies.

Indications

Numerous oncology applications have been proven to benefit from PET imaging. The most frequent applications are in staging of disease, assessment, and monitoring of treatment response, and evaluation of tumor recurrence. Single pulmonary nodules were the first oncology-approved indication by the Centers for Medicare and Medicaid Services (CMS). CMS currently recognizes the following indications for oncologic PET imaging:

- Breast (staging, restaging, and monitoring)
- Cervix (staging, restaging)
- Colorectal (diagnosis, staging, restaging)
- Esophagus (diagnosis, staging, restaging)
- Head and neck (excluding thyroid and CNS) (diagnosis, staging, restaging)
- Lymphoma (diagnosis, staging, restaging)
- Melanoma (diagnosis, initial staging excluding regional lymph nodes, restaging)
- Non–small cell lung (diagnosis, staging, restaging)
- Thyroid (only covered for restaging of follicular cell types)

CMS is currently evaluating new indications and has proposed many new changes. The CMS approvals should be reviewed frequently for updated information regarding approved indications. CMS is also willing to accept several additional indications if they can be supported by evidence development.

Procedures

Patient preparation. Patient preparation for PET scans utilizing [^{18}F]FDG for oncology applications is a very important process. The utilization of correct patient preparation steps will enhance image quality. An example of a commonly used protocol follows.

Prior to arrival in the department, patients should be instructed to fast, except for water, for at least 4–6 hr before the administration of [^{18}F]FDG to decrease the physiologic glucose levels and to reduce serum insulin levels to near basal levels. Hydration with water is encouraged prior to imaging to reduce bladder radiation dose and to improve image quality by reducing urinary artifacts. There are a variety of additional factors that may enhance image quality. Some examples include encouraging a low-carbohydrate/high-protein diet prior to the exam, which can decrease myocardial uptake. Patients' avoidance of strenuous exercise the day of the study may reduce muscle uptake, thus decreasing the possibility for image artifact. If intravenous contrast is administered, the patient should be screened for a history of iodinated contrast material allergy, use of metformin for the treatment of diabetes mellitus, and a history of renal disease.

Prior to injection of [^{18}F]FDG, several steps should be followed. A thorough patient history is performed prior to injection, allowing time for the patient to ask questions and relax. Prior to injection the patient should be placed in a quiet room. These are dedicated uptake rooms, which provide a quiet, warm, low-lit environment. The room is usually equipped with a recliner or a stretcher to promote a resting position. The patient should remain in a latent state during injection and the subsequent uptake period. Quiet room characteristics promote resting and help prevent muscular uptake. Patients can be provided with a warm blanket to help reduce the uptake of brown fat. Brown fat is usually represented as bilateral uptake in the areas of the supraclavicular region as seen in Figure 21.8. Brown fat uptake has also been shown to be reduced by pharmacological intervention with diazepam. To reduce brown fat uptake, 5–10 mg of diazepam can be administered orally 1 hr prior to injection of [^{18}F]FDG. An intravenous catheter should be placed for the [^{18}F]FDG administration. The size of the IV should be considered if IV contrast is to be administered. The blood glucose level should be checked prior to [^{18}F]FDG administration. The IV line can be used to gain a small amount of blood for glucose testing with the glucose meter. High glucose levels compete with [^{18}F]FDG uptake. This can substantially degrade image quality and the accuracy of the results obtained. It is preferred that glucose levels be $\leqslant$150 mg/dL but scans are usually performed as long as levels are $\leqslant$200 mg/dL. Special consideration needs to be given to diabetic patients. Recommended protocols for diabetic patients include imaging Type I diabetes patients early in the morning, after an overnight fast. Type II diabetics may require the administration of insulin the morning of the exam. If insulin is administered, the injection of [^{18}F]FDG must be

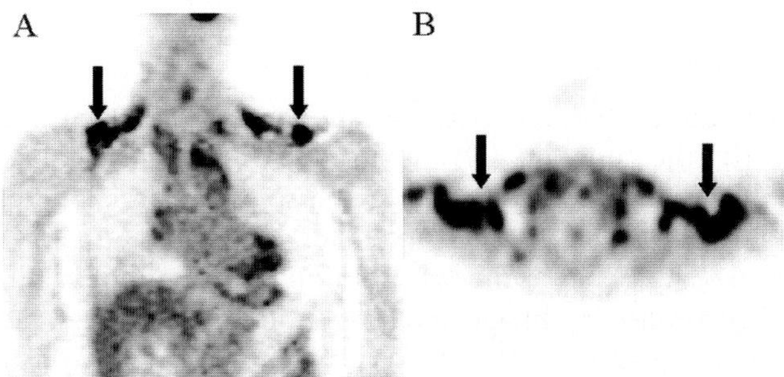

Figure 21.8 Uptake in the supraclavicular region representing brown fat uptake. (Reprinted, with permission, from Cohade *et al.*, 2003.)

delayed for at least 1 hr and is ultimately dependent upon the type and route of administration of insulin. Patients who present with elevated blood glucose levels may demonstrate inhomogeneous activity resulting in poor image quality; thus it is important to document the blood glucose level.

If a PET/CT scan is to be performed, an intraluminal gastrointestinal contrast agent may be administered to provide adequate visualization of the gastrointestinal tract.

Image acquisition. The majority of oncology PET exams are positioned and acquired from the skull base to the mid-thigh. This scan typically requires five to eight bed positions depending on the dimensions of the scanner field of view and the patient's height. This particular body survey is recommended for most tumor types. For imaging tumors with a high likelihood of scalp, skull, or brain involvement or lower extremity involvement, whole-body imaging is performed. Whole-body imaging includes the entire body to include the skull and all extremities. Whole-body imaging should always be performed on patients who present with an indication of melanoma.

For optimal imaging of the body, on a standard PET scanner, the patients may be scanned with their arms by their sides for comfort. When performing PET/CT the arms should be elevated over the head, if possible; if placed along the patient's sides, beam-hardening artifacts over the torso may be produced. For optimal imaging of the head and neck, the arms should be positioned along the sides. The patient should urinate prior to image acquisition to limit the radiation dose to the renal collecting system and bladder. The acquisition usually begins at the level of the mid-thigh in order to image the pelvis before the bladder has time to refill. If evaluating the pelvis, some facilities recommend bladder catheterization.

The CT component of a PET/CT exam can be performed for either attenuation correction purposes or as a diagnostic scan. If the CT scan is performed for attenuation correction, a low milliampere-second setting is recommended to reduce the radiation dose to the patient. If performing a diagnostic CT, standard settings are recommended. The CT scan may be performed with intravenous and/or oral contrast for many indications. When performing a CT scan as part of a PET/CT exam, the position of the diaphragm on the PET emission images should match closely that of the CT transmission images. A diagnostic CT scan of the chest is generally acquired during end-inspiration breath holding; this technique is contraindicated for PET/CT because it may result in considerable respiratory motion misregistration on the images. Many protocols recommend a mid-inspiration breath hold, while others recommend that the patient continue shallow breathing during the CT acquisition.

The PET scan or actual emission image should be performed at least 45 min postinjection of [^{18}F]FDG. Most protocols recommend imaging 60–90 min postacquisition. The emission scan typically takes 3–5 min per bed position, resulting in a total acquisition time of approximately 14–40 min on an average patient. Increased bed acquisition times may be beneficial for large patients.

Image interpretation. Images are usually displayed in the axial, coronal, and sagital planes, as well as the maximum-intensity projection images for review in a 3D cine mode. When performing PET/CT, CT images, PET images, and fusion images are available in all three planes, as well. PET images should always be reviewed with and without attenuation correction. Nonattenuation-corrected images are especially useful when reviewing scans with an indication of melanoma. Some subcutaneous lesions could be missed on attenuation-corrected images and thus be visualized on nonattenuation-corrected images. Nonattenuation-corrected images may also be useful in evaluating artifacts created from the use of CT.

Many normal structures in the body avidly take up [^{18}F]FDG so the ability to recognize normal biodistribution is critical in image interpretation. A variety of normal variants of [^{18}F]FDG have been seen, and PET is often utilized along with other conventional methods to make a diagnosis.

[^{18}F]Sodium Fluoride Bone Imaging

[^{18}F]Sodium fluoride is a PET radionuclide used primarily for the evaluation of metastatic bone disease. Studies suggest that [^{18}F]sodium fluoride is more accurate than planar imaging or SPECT with [^{99m}Tc]MDP for localizing and characterizing both malignant and benign bone lesions. [^{18}F]Sodium fluoride is well localized in the skeleton and results in superb image quality. [^{18}F]Sodium fluoride demonstrates a rapid uptake in bone and fast clearance from soft tissue allowing imaging to commence 15–30 min postinjection of the radiopharmaceutical. A potential limitation of [^{18}F]sodium fluoride is the inability to yield a study equivalent to a three-phase bone scan. [^{18}F]Sodium fluoride does not accumulate in acute inflammatory processes in soft tissue and is therefore not useful for three-phase evaluation. An image of an [^{18}F]sodium fluoride bone scan can be found in Figure 21.9.

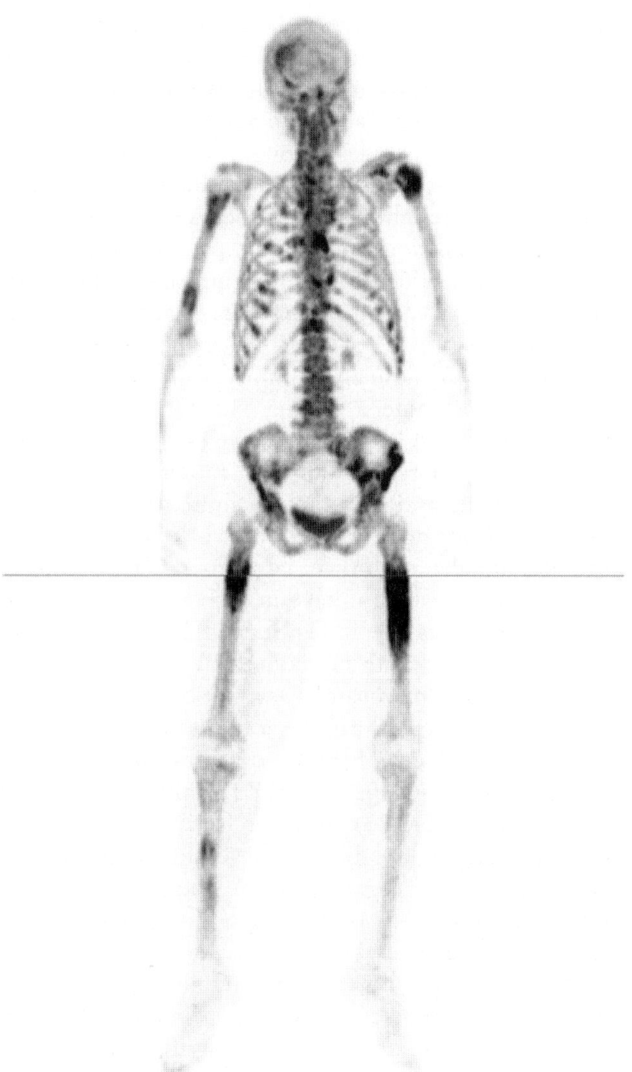

Figure 21.9 [^{18}F]Sodium fluoride bone scan demonstrating diffuse metastatic disease. (Courtesy of The Medical Center at Bowling Green, Bowling Green, KY.)

Cardiac Applications

Positron emission tomography was first established for clinical research in neurology and cardiology applications. PET has the capability to assess myocardial perfusion and viability.

Cardiac Perfusion Assessment

Myocardial perfusion studies are commonly performed with the use of [^{82}Rb]chloride or [^{13}N]ammonia. [^{15}O]Water has also been used to assess myocardial blood flow, but currently the Centers for Medicare and Medicaid Services has limited approval to [^{82}Rb]ammonia and [^{13}N]ammonia. Image interpretation follows the same criteria as in general SPECT imaging. Normal myocardial perfusion demonstrated on stress images implies absence of significant coronary artery disease. Abnormal myocardial perfusion on stress images suggests the presence of coronary artery disease. If the stress-induced imaging defect persists on the corresponding rest images, it suggests the presence of an irreversible myocardial injury. If the defect on the stress images resolves on the rest images, it suggests the presence of stress-induced myocardial ischemia. Patient preparation for PET myocardial perfusion imaging should follow the same criteria as in SPECT imaging. The stress protocols should also follow the same protocols as those utilized in SPECT imaging. Pharmacologic stress is the preferred method for PET myocardial perfusion studies due to the short half-lives of the PET radionuclides utilized, although some facilities have incorporated supine bicycle and treadmill exercise with success. The American Society of Nuclear Cardiology has published guidelines for PET myocardial perfusion and metabolism clinical imaging and these are summarized in the following reading.

^{82}Rb Perfusion Imaging

^{82}Rb perfusion imaging requires the purchase of a ^{82}Sr–^{82}Rb generator, which must be replaced every 4 weeks. ^{82}Rb is eluted from the generator with 10–50 mL of normal saline and the generator can be eluted every 5 min, if necessary. A dose of 20–40 mCi of ^{82}Rb is adequate for rest–stress myocardial perfusion imaging. ^{82}Rb does have poorer resolution when compared to ^{18}F and ^{13}N, due to the long positron range it expresses, but is still an acceptable imaging agent. When performing an ^{82}Rb study, scout scanning is recommended prior to the actual study for positioning purposes. The scout scan can be performed with a transmission scan or a low-dose CT. Rest imaging should be performed prior to stress imaging to reduce the effects the stress testing may have. ^{82}Rb is typically infused over a period of 30 sec followed by the initiation of imaging at 70–90 sec postinfusion. If the patient suffers from reduced ventricular function, imaging may be delayed to begin at 90–110 sec postinfusion.

13N Ammonia Perfusion Imaging

^{13}N has a very short half-life of 10 min and requires an on-site cyclotron and radiochemistry synthesis capability to be utilized as a myocardial perfusion agent. As with ^{82}Rb, a scout scan is recommended prior to imaging. The typical dose of [^{13}N]ammonia for rest/stress imaging is 10–20 mCi per dose with the initiation of imaging at 1.5–3 min postinfusion.

Cardiac Metabolic Imaging

The myocardium can utilize many substrates for metabolism, primarily free fatty acids and glucose. Under the fasting state and aerobic conditions, fatty acids are the preferred fuel in the heart. In the case of reduced oxygen supply or anaerobic conditions experienced during an ischemia or infarction, the myocardium favors glucose. [^{18}F]FDG is the pharmaceutical of choice when performing a PET myocardial viability study. Another tracer that has been used is ^{11}C, but at this time only [^{18}F]FDG is FDA approved.

The goal of viability imaging with [^{18}F]FDG is to encourage the heart's preferential use of glucose. There are a variety of protocols for performing an [^{18}F]FDG viability study; the most common utilize glucose loading, by either an oral or intravenous method. The purpose of glucose loading is to switch the nutrient substrate utilized in the heart from free fatty acids to glucose. The myocardium typically utilizes free fatty acids in the fasting state. The patient should arrive at the department after fasting for at least 6 hr prior to the exam. Standardization of the metabolic environment is necessary for clinical myocardial metabolic imaging. Oral glucose loading with 25–100 g is the most common method, but IV loading has also been used with great success. Diabetic patients pose a challenge to the traditional glucose loading protocol due to limited ability to produce endogenous insulin or because they are less likely to respond to insulin stimulation. Therefore, this method is often not effective in diabetic patients. An alternate technique is the hyperinsulinemic–euglycemic clamp method. The clamp method is performed by infusing insulin for the duration of the study while simultaneously infusing glucose. This dual infusion is performed to maintain blood glucose at baseline levels. The clamp method is more effective at stabilizing the metabolic environment in diabetic patients, but is time and labor intensive. Another option for encouraging the use of glucose is to administer a nicotinic acid derivative. Unfortunately, no FDA-approved agents are available at this time.

Upon completion of patient preparation to stimulate glucose metabolism, [^{18}F]FDG can be administered. Typically, 5–15 mCi is injected and imaging is delayed until at least 45 min postinjection. Images are displayed in the same views as customarily viewed in myocardial perfusion imaging to include short axis, vertical long axis, and horizontal long axis. For interpretation, metabolism images are typically compared to resting perfusion images. These images are reviewed for match or mismatched patterns. Matched reduction in perfusion and [^{18}F]FDG accumulation is indicative of nonviability. A mismatch representing decreased perfusion with relatively normal [^{18}F]FDG uptake suggests viability in the mismatched area. Myocardial metabolism images obtained from [^{18}F]FDG can be compared to SPECT images with technetium or thallium agents (Fig. 21.10). However, it is recommended, when possible, to compare these images to either an [^{82}Rb]chloride or a [^{13}N]ammonia perfusion study. This is because the attenuation correction will influence consistency in the images.

Neurologic Applications

PET studies conducted on the brain evaluate glucose metabolism, neuroreceptor binding, and cerebral blood flow. These neurologic applications include the evaluation of specific disease states, such as epilepsy, dementia, movement disorders, and tumors, as well as assisting in treatment planning. Research evaluating the use of PET in brain trauma, drug effects, and neuropsychiatric disease is ongoing.

One of the major concerns when performing brain imaging is patient preparation due to the way stimuli affect brain images. The patient should undergo all of the previous [^{18}F]FDG imaging preparations and precautions mentioned, as well as avoiding caffeine, alcohol, or drugs that may affect cerebral glucose metabolism. Thirty minutes pre- and postinjection, the patient should be placed in a quiet, dimly lit room in a comfortable position. In addition, the intravenous access site must be placed in the patient at least 10 min prior to radiopharmaceutical injection. Any external stimulation can result in increased metabolic activity in various regions of the brain. A delay in sedation, preferably at least 30 min post-radiopharmaceutical injection, is also recommended. Imaging typically begins 30–60 min postinjection.

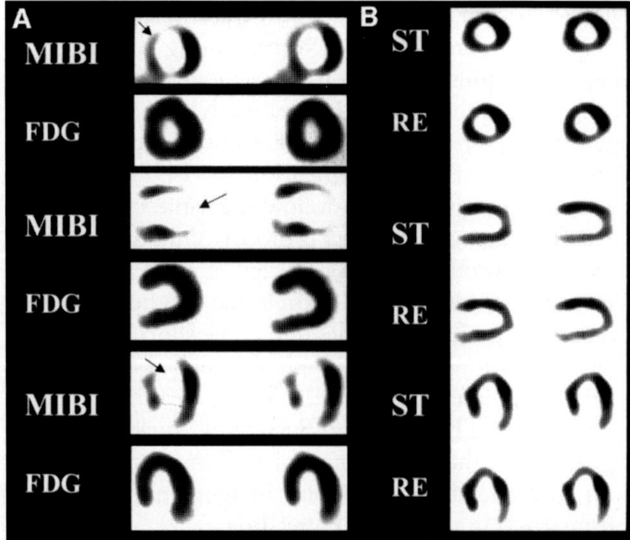

Figure 21.10 [^{99m}Tc]MIBI SPECT and FDG PET images of patient with MI. (A) Perfusion–metabolism mismatch at apex, anterior, septal, and inferoposterior walls (arrows) before revascularization indicating viable tissue. (B) After CABG, perfusion defects of segments improved significantly and size of left ventricle decreased. EF increased from 30 to 42%. ST, stress; RE, rest. (Reprinted, with permission, from Xiaoli *et al.*, 2001.)

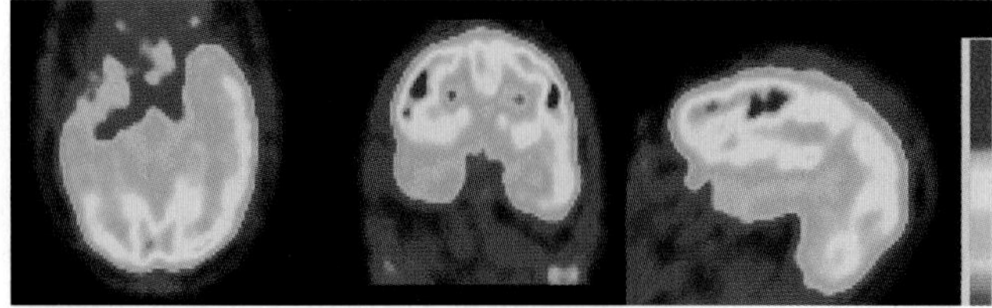

Figure 21.11 [^{18}F]FDG image of patient with partial epilepsy in the right temporal lobe. (Reprinted, with permission, from O'Brien *et al.*, 2001.)

[^{18}F]FDG for Glucose Metabolism

The brain undergoes dramatic changes between birth and adulthood; however, as early as at 8 months, glucose utilization resembles that of an adult. The brain then continues a normal aging pattern. During adulthood, the brain relies almost entirely on glucose oxidation for energy metabolism and this energy metabolism is tightly connected to neuronal activity. As a rule, regional cerebral blood flow (rCBF) and local cerebral glucose metabolism are proportional to each other. The metabolic activity in gray matter, as compared to white matter, is approximately at a ratio of 4:1. When evaluating metabolism in the brain, the cerebellum is 10–30% less metabolically active than the cerebral cortex, the basal ganglia activity is normally 10–30% greater than that of the cortex, and cerebral cortical activity is typically midway in intensity between normal basal ganglia and the cerebellum.

[^{18}F]FDG brain imaging can be useful in epileptic seizure imaging and the evaluation of the interictal phase because of areas of hypometabolic activity in seizure foci (Fig. 21.11). To ensure that the patient is not administered the radiopharmaceutical in a post-ictal state, continuous electroencephalogram (EEG) monitoring is recommended beginning 2 hr before injection and at least 20 min postinjection. The preferable time elapsed between last known seizure and injection of the approximately 5–20 mCi of [^{18}F]FDG is at least 6 hr. The region of interictal hypometabolism almost always correlates with the EEG. If the patient is injected during the ictal state, an area of hypermetabolic activity will be in the seizure foci.

[^{18}F]FDG uptake depends on the specific disorder or disease state and can vary widely. Most tumors will have an increased uptake of [^{18}F]FDG, while dementia or necrotic areas will demonstrate decreased activity. As a rule, the location of the decreased activity depends on the cause of dementia. For example, in Alzheimer's disease (Fig. 21.12) decreased areas of uptake are found primarily in the parietal, temporal, and frontal lobes, whereas in Pick's disease the frontal and temporal lobes are most widely affected. Huntington's disease, as well as Parkinson's disease, affects the striatum of the forebrain (Fig. 21.13). Patients with Lewy bodies dementia demonstrate decreased uptake in the occipital, parietal, and temporal lobes. These variances are what allow neurological PET imaging to differentiate the various disease states.

It is important to realize that normal uptake of [^{18}F]FDG varies considerably. A reason for this variance 2is that the normal brain itself is not completely symmetrical. In addition, distribution of [^{18}F]FDG is also affected by patient activity during the uptake phase. An example of this phenomenon is the appearance of increased auditory cortical activity observed in patient studies obtained in a noisy room. Medications and substances that alter cerebral metabolism include sedatives, antiepileptics, amphetamines, chemotherapy for brain tumors, anticholinesterase drugs for memory impairment, psychotropics, narcotics, corticosteroids, and cocaine. Most medications affect the brain globally, rather than regionally. However, some medications do affect the brain regionally, and therefore, the patient should refrain from using them, if at all possible.

It is also important to understand that normal brain metabolism patterns in children differ considerably from those in adults. In the normal newborn, the sensorimotor cortex is metabolically more active when compared with the rest of the cerebral cortex, producing a pattern that resembles progressive Alzheimer's disease. Therefore, it is important to understand the normal appearance of cerebral metabolism of [^{18}F]FDG in PET to accurately interpret images.

[^{18}F]DOPA for Movement Disorders

Although [^{18}F]FDG may be useful in the differential diagnosis of the various movement disorders, another ^{18}F agent has proven very useful in this patient population. [^{18}F]6-Fluoro-L-DOPA ([^{18}F]DOPA) is widely used to investigate dopaminergic function. Decreased [^{18}F]DOPA uptake has been reported in the striatum in movement disorders, such as Parkinson's disease.

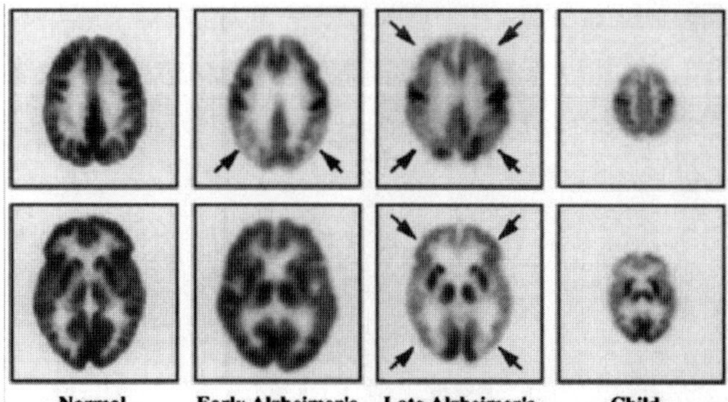

Figure 21.12 PET [^{18}F]FDG study of glucose metabolism in Alzheimer's disease in various stages compared to the normal glucose metabolism of a child. (Reprinted, with permission, from Phelps, 2000.)

Advances in Neurological PET Imaging

Research to find further uses for the more readily available PET radiopharmaceuticals is ongoing; however, other agents are being researched and utilized when feasible for the facility and when appropriate for the patient population. These agents include [^{15}O]H_2O for determining regional cerebral blood flow, [^{15}O]O_2 for monitoring oxygen metabolism, and various ^{11}C agents that have been utilized as dopamine transporters, receptors, or other neuroreceptor binders.

Artifacts

A variety of image artifacts can manifest in PET images; when utilizing a PET/CT system there is the chance for a greater number of artifacts. The most common artifacts will be discussed here.

Preprocedure artifact concerns relate to medications, prosthetics, therapeutic effects, and exercise, as discussed previously in patient preparation factors that affect normal biodistribution.

Partial Volume Effect

Another concern in PET imaging is the ability to accurately determine the activity concentration in regions or volumes that are small compared with the resolution of the PET scanner. PET systems have limited spatial resolution, which ultimately results in small object activity concentration being underestimated in comparison to larger objects of equal activity concentration. When this occurs it is recognized as the partial volume effect. The size of an object needs to be approximately three times

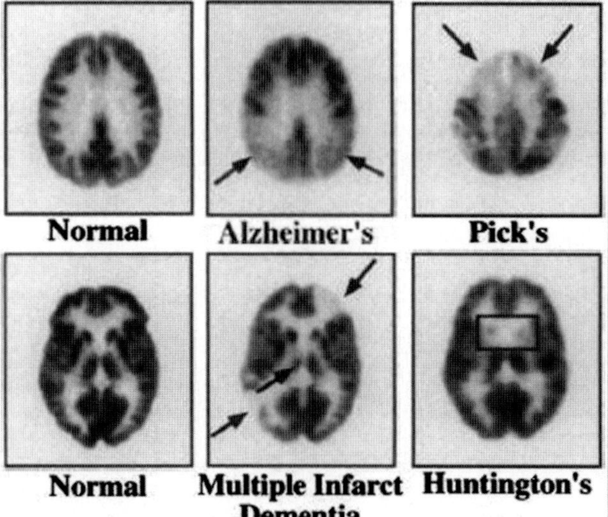

Figure 21.13 PET studies of glucose metabolism for differential diagnosis of dementias. (Reprinted, with permission, from Phelps, 2000.)

greater than the image resolution for the activity to be accurately represented.

Metallic Artifacts

Metallic artifacts (Fig. 21.14) result in high CT numbers or Hounsfield units, which in turn results in high PET attenuation coefficients and leads to an overestimation of activity in the actual PET scan.

Respiratory Motion or Mismatch

Respiratory motion or mismatch is due to the difference in breathing cycles that occur between the PET and CT scans. CT scans are usually acquired in a certain phase of the breathing cycle, whereas PET is an average of many breathing cycles. This difference creates a respiratory motion artifact. This artifact is often expressed as curvilinear cold areas at the base of the lungs, where the lungs and diaphragm meet, as seen in Figure 21.15.

Contrast Media

Contrast media also produce high CT numbers similar to metallic implants. This overestimation can create an overcorrection and can falsely increase areas of activity on the PET scan, as demonstrated in Figure 21.16.

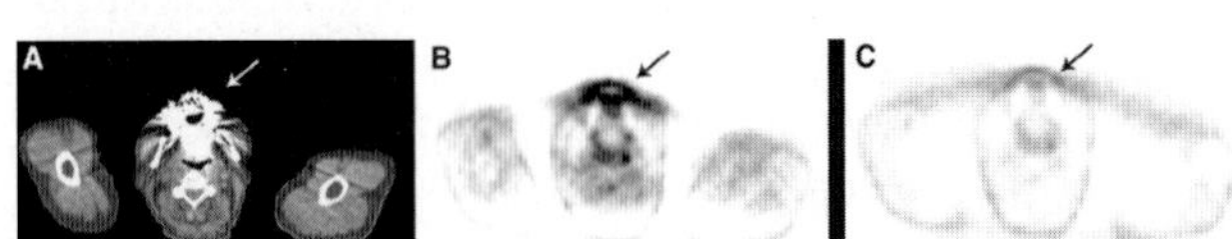

Figure 21.14 (A) High-density metallic implants generate streaking artifacts and high-CT numbers (arrow) on CT image. (B) High-CT numbers will then be mapped to high-PET attenuation coefficients, leading to overestimation of activity concentration. (C) PET images without attenuation correction help to rule out metal-induced artifacts. (Reprinted, with permission, from Sureshbabu and Mawlawi, 2005.)

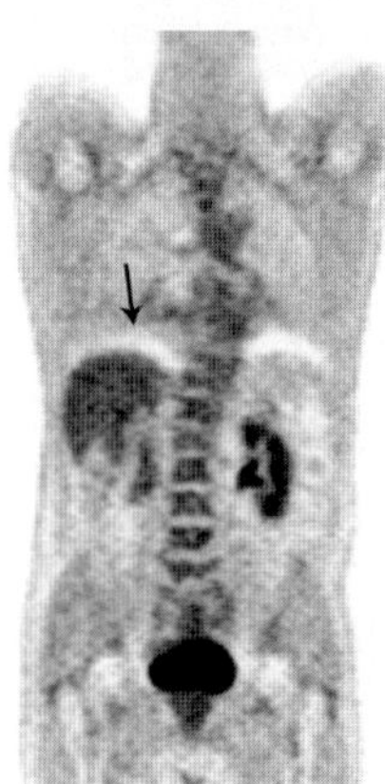

Figure 21.15 A curvilinear cold artifact is a result of respiratory mismatch on a PET image due to the use of CT attenuation correction. (Reprinted, with permission, from Sureshbabu and Mawlawi, 2005.)

Truncation Artifact

A truncation artifact (Fig. 21.17) results from the difference in the size of the field of view of the CT compared to the PET. The CT field of view is significantly smaller, averaging 50 cm, compared to 70 cm in PET. These artifacts typically manifest in larger patients or patients imaged with their arms down by the sides. The truncation artifact is produced because the patient extends beyond the field of view of the CT scan; this extended anatomy is truncated and not represented in the reconstructed image. This results in no attenuation correction for these corresponding areas. Truncation can also create a streaking artifact at the edge of the image and results in a rim of high activity at the truncation edge. The best way to prevent this artifact is by making sure that the patient is positioned at the center of the field of view with the arms above the head.

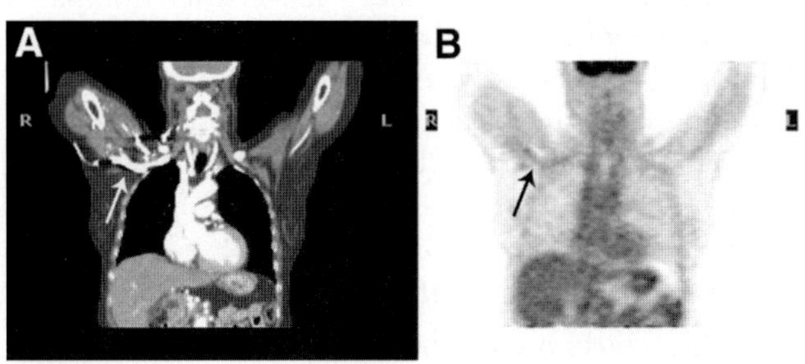

Figure 21.16 CT scan shows IV contrast medium in right subclavian vein (A). Radiotracer uptake is increased in corresponding region of PET image (B). (Reprinted, with permission, from Sureshbabu and Mawlawi, 2005.)

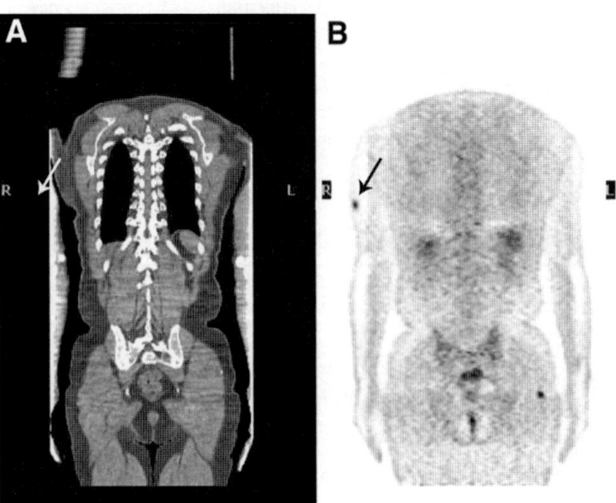

Figure 21.17 CT image is truncated at sides (A) and biases PET attenuation–corrected image (B). (Reprinted, with permission, from Sureshbabu and Mawlawi, 2005.)

Image Misalignment

Image misalignment can result between a mismatch between the PET and CT scans and even between the emission and transmission image of a dedicated PET system. This can cause a visual misregistration, and attenuation correction map may cause PET artifacts and distort standard uptake values.

References and Further Reading

Abouzied MM, Crawford ES, Nabi HA, 2005. ^{18}F-FDG imaging: pitfalls and artifacts. *J Nucl Med Technol.* 33:145–155.

Buchert R, Bohuslavizki KH, Mester J, Clausen M, 1999. Quality assurance in PET: evaluation of the clinical relevance of detector defects. *J Nucl Med.* 40:1657–1665.

Cohade C, Osman M, Pannu HK, Wahl RL, 2003. Uptake in supraclavicular area fat ("USA-Fat"): description of ^{18}F-FDG PET/CT. *J Nucl Med.* 44:170–176.

Daniel HS, Silverman MD, 2004. Brain ^{18}F-FDG PET in the diagnosis of neurodegenerative dementias: comparison with perfusion SPECT and with clinical evaluations lacking nuclear imaging. *J Nucl Med.* 45:594–607.

Delbeke D, Coleman RE, Guiberteau MJ, Brown ML, Royal HD, Siegals BA, Townsend DW, Berland LL, Parker JA, Hubner K, Stabin MG, Zubal G, Kachelriess M, Cronin V, Holbrook S, 2006. Procedure guideline for tumor imaging with ^{18}F-FDG PET/CT 1.0. In: *Society of Nuclear Medicine Procedure Guidelines.* Reston, VA: Society of Nuclear Medicine.

Dilsizian V, Bacharach SL, Beanlands RS, Bergmann SR, Delbeke D, Gropler RJ, Knuuti J, Schelbert HR, Travin MI, 2009. PET myocardial perfusion and metabolism clinical imaging. In: *ASNC Imaging Guidelines for Nuclear Cardiology Procedures.* Bethesda, MD: American Society of Nuclear Cardiology.

Fahey FH, 2002. Data acquisition in PET imaging. *J Nucl Med Technol.* 30:39–49.

Grant FD, Fahey FH, Packard AB, Davis RT, Alavi A, Treves ST, 2007. Skeletal PET with ^{18}F-fluoride: applying new technology to an old tracer. *J Nucl Med.* 49:68–78.

Habbian MR, Delbeke D, Martin WH, Sandler MP, Vitola JV, 2008. *Nuclear Medicine Imaging: A Teaching File.* Philadelphia, PA: Lippincott Williams & Wilkins; 164, 168, 170, 182, 184, 198.

Hamacher K, Coenen HH, Stocklin G, 1986. Efficient stereospecific synthesis of NCA 2-[^{18}F]fluoro-2-deoxy-D-glucose using aminopolyether supported nucleophilic substitution. *J Nucl Med.* 27:235–238.

Kamo H, McGeer PL, Harrop R, McGeer EG, Calne DB, Martin WRW, Pate BD, 1987. Positron emission tomography and histopathology in Pick's disease. *Neurology.* 37:439–445.

Kipper MS, Tartar M, 2004. *Clinical Atlas of PET: With Imaging Correlation.* Philadelphia, PA: Saunders; 1–5, 369–372, 411–415.

Knesaurek K, Machac J, Krynyckyi BR, Almeida OD, 2003. Comparison of 2-dimensional and 3-dimensional ^{82}Rb myocardial perfusion PET imaging. *J Nucl Med.* 44:1350–1356.

Lin EC, Alavi A, 2005. *PET and PET/CT: A Clinical Guide.* New York, NY. Thieme; 21–73, 159–167.

Neary D, Snowden JS, Shields RA, Burian AW, Northen B, MacDermott N, Prescott MC, Testa HJ, 1987. Single photon emission tomography using ^{99m}Tc–HM-PAO in the investigation of dementia. *J Neurol Neurosurg Psychiatry.* 50:1101–1109.

O'Brien TJ, Hicks RJ, Ware R, Binns DS, Murphy M, Cook MJ, 2001. The utility of a 3-dimensional, large-field-of-view, sodium iodide crystal-based PET scanner in the presurgical evaluation of partial epilepsy. *J Nucl Med.* 42:1158–1165.

Oehr P, Biersack HJ, Coleman E, 2004. *PET and PET-CT in Oncology.* New York, NY: Springer; 30–46, 59–64.

Phelps ME, 2000. PET: the merging of biology and imaging into molecular imaging. *J Nucl Med.* 41:664.

Phelps ME, 2006. *PET: Physics, Instrumentation, and Scanners.* New York, NY: Springer; 32–67, 101–106.

Prekeges J, 2011. *Nuclear Medicine Instrumentation.* Boston, MA: Jones & Bartlett; 187–238.

Saha GB, 2004. *Fundamentals of Nuclear Pharmacy.* 5th ed. New York, NY: Springer; 144–148.

Schwarz JK, Grigsby PW, Dehdashti F, Delbeke D, 2009. The role of ^{18}F-FDG PET in assessing therapy response in cancer of the cervix and ovaries. *J Nucl Med.* 50:64S–73S.

Sureshbabu W, Mawlawi O, 2005. PET/CT imaging artifacts. *J Nucl Med Technol.* 33:156–161.

Tarantola G, Zito F, Gerundini P, 2003. PET instrumentation and reconstruction algorithms in whole-body applications. *J Nucl Med.* 44:756–769.

Turkington TG, 2001. Introduction to PET instrumentation. *J Nucl Med Technol.* 29:4–11.

Valk PE, Delbeke D, Bailey DL, Townsend DW, Maisey MN, 2006. *Positron Emission Tomography Clinical Practice.* London: Springer; 1–78.

Xiaoli Z, Ziu-Jie L, Qingyu W, Shi R, Gao R, Liu Y, Hu S, Tian Y, Guo S, Fang W, 2001. Clinical outcome of patients with previous myocardial infarction and left ventricular dysfunction assessed with myocardial ^{99m}Tc-MIBI SPECT and ^{18}F-FDG. *J Nucl Med.* 42:1166–1173.

Yu, S, 2006. Review of ^{18}F-FDG synthesis and quality control. *Biomed Imaging Intervention J.* 2(4):e57.

Advanced PET Imaging Questions

1. Positron emitters are:

   a. Proton-deficient isotopes
   b. Neutron-rich isotopes
   c. Neutron-deficient isotopes
   d. Electron-rich isotopes

2. The pH of [^{18}F]FDG is:

   a. Between 2.0 and 4.5
   b. Between 4.5 and 7.5
   c. Between 7.5 and 9.0
   d. Between 9.0 and 11.5

3. Which of the following shields is better to use for PET agents than lead?

a. Air
b. Aluminum
c. Depleted uranium
d. Tungsten

4. Which of the following PET crystals has the highest density?

a. LSO
b. GSO
c. NaI(Tl)
d. BGO

5. To reduce the possibility of brown fat artifacts in [^{18}F]FDG PET imaging one can use what to reduce the effect of the possible artifact?

a. Water (ask the patient to drink a cold cup of water prior to imaging)
b. A warm blanket (for the patient's shoulders prior to imaging)
c. Blood transfusion (give the patient a transfusion of blood prior to imaging)
d. Exercise (ask the patient to exercise his or her arms prior to imaging)

6. Which of the following PET agents is best for imaging Parkinson's disease?

a. ^{15}O
b. [^{18}F]FDG
c. L-[^{18}F]DOPA
d. [^{13}N]Ammonia

Answers

(1) c, (2) b, (3) d, (4) a, (5) b, (6) c

CHAPTER 22 Magnetic Resonance Imaging Primer

Chalonda Jones-Thomas

There are various types of imaging: images made with reflected electromagnetic radiation, such as photography; images made with transmitted electromagnetic radiation, such as radiographs; and images made with emitted electromagnetic radiation, such as magnetic resonance imaging (MRIs). MRI, originally known as nuclear magnetic resonance (NMR), originates from signals given off from the nuclei of hydrogen (primarily water molecules) in the patient's body. The MRI phenomenon is based on the quantum physics of nuclear spin. Nuclei with odd number of neutrons, protons, or both will have a net magnetic moment and therefore become NMR active. Unlike most imaging modalities, magnetic resonance image is a non-ionizing clinical imaging modality. Magnetic resonance (MR) is a phenomenon involving magnetic fields and radiofrequency (RF) electromagnetic waves. This section outlines the basic principle of MRI to give the reader the background for more specialized topics.

Brief MRI History

In 1946, Felix Bloch proposed a Nobel Prize–winning paper about the properties of atomic nucleus. Bloch's theory stated that the nucleus behaves like a magnet. He explained that as a proton spins around its own axis a magnetic field is formed. If a hydrogen atom or water molecule is placed in a high field of magnetic radiation, the molecule and hydrogen atoms would line up within the field line. If the magnetic field were cut off, the hydrogen would spin down to a resting state and give off radiofrequencies in the process. These radiofrequencies could be captured and each will be unique depending on the amount of hydrogen in a molecule. The radiofrequencies are then combined to form the MR image. This is how an MR image is actually formed. The knocking one hears associated with an MRI unit is actually the radiofrequencies associated with the magnetic field being turned off and on very rapidly. But it was not until the 1950s that Bloch's theories were verified experimentally. Bloch's theories about nucleus behavior were widely used in academia and research. It was not until the late 1960s, when Raymond Damadian discovered that malignant tissues have NMR parameters different than those of normal tissue, that MR was considered for the clinical setting. In 1977, Damadian and his colleagues conducted the first MR scan on a human, which took nearly 5 hr to complete. The name *nuclear magnetic resonance* was changed to *magnetic resonance imaging* because it was believed the word nuclear would frighten the public and emphasize an untruth that ionizing radiation was a part of the MR imaging technique. Eventually, MRI became a recognized imaging modality in and of itself.

In the 1980s MRI scanners were in almost every major facility. Since that time scanners have steadily evolved and become more sophisticated. Advancement of applications for MRI includes: open MRI, MR angiography (MRIa), perfusion/diffusion, spectroscopy, functional imaging (MRIf), breast MRI, and most recently positron emission tomography (PET)/MRI.

Requirement for MRI

A strong magnetic field is required to generate the MR signal used to create the MR image. The magnetic field strength used in MRI is many thousands of times greater than the earth's magnetic field. The magnetic field is represented by the *M* in MRI. An external energy source must occur to stimulate the patient's tissue and generate an MR signal. This external energy source is a radiotransmitter that is similar to commercial AM radio broadcast. This external energy is radiofrequency energy. For MR imaging to be produced, material in the human body must be able to respond appropriately to the external magnetic field and the external RF energy source. Hydrogen is the most suitable material in the human body for MR imaging for two main reasons: (1) it is abundant within the human body, and (2) hydrogen contains an odd number of protons (atomic and mass number 1). Both of these characteristics allow the maximum amount of magnetization to occur in the body.

The Hydrogen Proton

Protons are positively charged particles. Hydrogen contains one positively charged proton that spins about its own axis. The moving hydrogen nucleus generates a magnetic field and acts as a bar magnet. The magnet of each hydrogen nucleus has a north and south pole of equal strength. Therefore, all hydrogen protons in the human body have magnetic properties. The north and south axis of each nucleus is represented by a magnetic moment. The magnetic moment of each nucleus has vector properties (i.e., size and direction). The direction of the nucleus is denoted by an arrow. Normally, the human body usually does not experience magnetic forces. This is because the proton dipoles are randomly oriented in space and the net magnetic effects are canceled (Fig. 22.1).

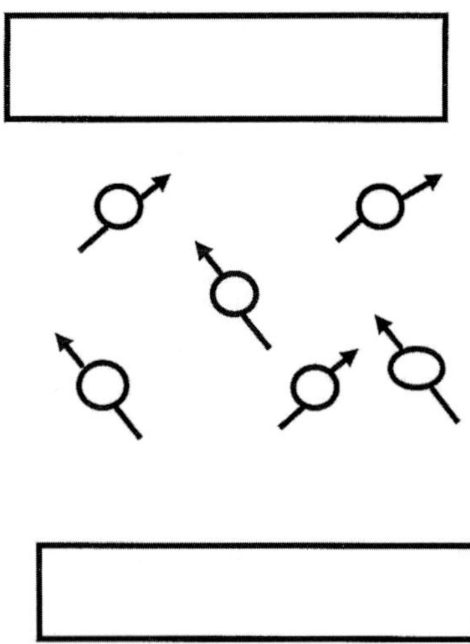

Figure 22.1 Random dipoles naturally in space.

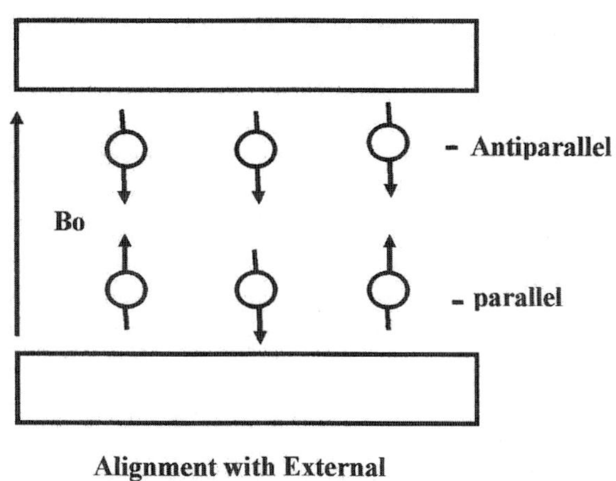

Figure 22.2 Protons aligning either in parallel or antiparallel in the presence of a strong magnetic field.

When a patient is placed in a strong external magnetic field, the protons experience a strong magnetic field from the MRI. The protons of the hydrogen align parallel, which is in the same direction as the magnetic field, or antiparallel, which is in the opposite direction of the magnetic field. The hydrogen protons that are parallel to the magnetic field are referred to as low-energy state or spin-up nuclei. The hydrogen protons that are antiparallel are referred to as high-energy state or spin-down nuclei (Fig. 22.2). The result of the protons aligning either parallel or antiparallel is referred to as the net magnetic moment. Simply stated, the net magnetic moment is the sum of magnetic effects of all the protons exposed to the main magnetic field. Because there are more protons in the low-energy state than in the high-energy state, the overall net magnetization occurs in the parallel direction. This overall net magnetization is also called equilibrium magnetization.

Two factors determine which hydrogen proton aligns parallel and which proton aligns antiparallel: (1) the strength of the external magnetic field, and (2) the thermal energy level of the nuclei. Low-thermal-energy nuclei do not have enough energy to oppose the magnetic field. High-energy nuclei have enough energy to oppose the magnetic field. As the magnetic field increases (i.e., going from a 1 Tesla, T, magnet to a 3-T magnet) fewer nuclei will have the energy to oppose the magnetic field that results in more low-energy nuclei. You can compare the protons' action to a person swimming upstream because this requires much more energy to overcome the water's effect. So, to oppose the stream you have to use more or higher energy. If you don't have enough energy, you are forced to go with the flow. There are more protons aligned parallel or in the low-energy state than antiparallel or high-energy state. In a 1.0-T system there are approximately six per million more protons in the low-energy state and in a 1.5-T system there are nine per million more protons in the lower-energy state. This is one reason a 1.5-T MRI system produces better images than a lower-field MRI system does.

Precession

As stated previously, MRI was called NMR due to the fact that nuclei of certain elements have a magnetic moment when placed in a magnetic field. The nuclei tend to line up with the magnetic field. To be more precise, the nuclei do not line up perfectly. The law of quantum physics mechanics states that nuclei align at an angle to the direction of the field. The magnetic moment wobbles around the main magnetic field at an angle and behaves similarly to a spinning top. Unlike a spinning top the magnetic moment wobbles very quickly. This wobbling motion is known as precession. The precessional frequency is also referred to as the resonant frequency. As the magnetic field increases so does the precessional or resonant frequency (the rate of spin) (Fig. 22.3).

The precessional frequency is important because at the precessional frequency the RF energy transmits the patient's body, which tilts the net magnetization of nuclei. The patient's nuclei also generate a signal at the precessional frequency. To differentiate tissues in MRI (i.e., normal from pathology) the RF must knock the nuclei out of alignment. Once the RF energy is removed from the nuclei, the nuclei relaxes back into position or equilibrium.

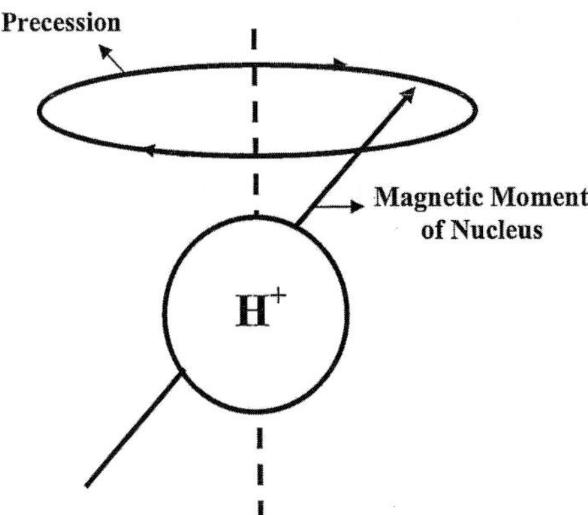

Figure 22.3 Precessional spin of proton.

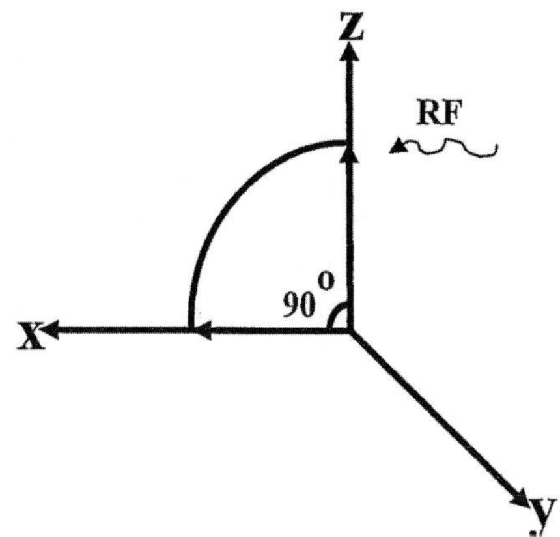

Figure 22.4 A 90° flip angle allows the nuclei to have adequate energy for the longitudinal NMV to completely transfer into the transverse plane.

Resonance

Once a brief pulse of radiofrequency, or RF pulse, energy disturbs the protons by moving the protons net magnetization out of alignment, resonance may occur. This is representated by the *R* in MRI. Resonance, a phenomenon that permits the efficient transfer of energy from one object or system to another, causes the receiving object or system to oscillate at the same frequency as the sender. The RF pulse transmitted from the RF coil into the patient's body must be at the same resonant frequency of the precessing hydrogen nuclei for the energy to be absorbed. The nucleus gains energy and resonates if the energy is the same as the precessional frequency. If the energy is different from the precessional frequency, a resonance does not occur. So only MR active nuclei with the same presessional frequency of water will resonate. At resonance, this absorption of energy will result in the net magnetization vector (NMV) to move out of alignment from the main magnetic field (B_0). A signal from the patient's body cannot be detected unless the NMV is moved from B_0.

B_0 is located in the longitudinal direction. The plane that is perpendicular to B_0 or the longitudinal plane is called the transverse plane. Once the imaging professional applies RF energy to the patient, the NMV of the nuclei is tilted out of alignment as it continues to precess in the transverse plane. The angle that the NMV moves from B_0 is called the flip angle. The stronger the RF pulse, the longer the pulse is applied, the farther the NMV will move from the longitudinal plane into the transverse plane. A 90° flip angle allows the nuclei to have adequate energy for the longitudinal NMV to completely transfer into the transverse plane (Fig. 22.4). On the other hand, if the flip angle is less than 90°, only part of the NMV is transferred in the transverse plan. A signal is generated despite the amount of NMV placed in the transverse plane.

Relaxation Processes

When the RF pulse is turned off, the NMV nuclei return back to B_0, also known as equilibrium. Protons prefer to align with the main magnetic field. For hydrogen nuclei to return back to B_0, hydrogen nuclei must lose energy given to them by the RF pulse. The process of energy loss is called relaxation. There are two types of main relaxations in MR: T_1 relaxation, also referred to as spin lattice or longitudinal relaxation, and T_2 relaxation, also referred to as spin–spin or transverse relaxation. Although both T_1 and T_2 relaxation occur concurrently, they also occur independently of one another.

T_1 relaxation dissipates energy from the nuclei to the surrounding molecular environment (lattice). The rate the energy dissipates from the nuclei is unique to the tissue type, thus tissues can be distinguished from one another on an image. T_1 is the time it takes 63% of the longitudinal magnetization to recover in the tissue (Fig. 22.5). For example, during evaluation of an image of the brain, the white matter has very short T_1 relaxation and cerebrospinal fluid has very long T_1 relaxation. Therefore, on a T_1-weighted image the white matter will appear bright and the cerebrospinal fluid will appear dark.

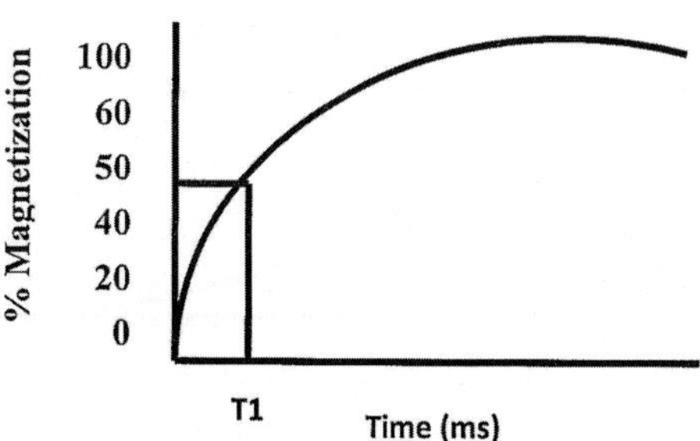

Figure 22.5 T_1 is the time it takes 63% of the longitudinal magnetization to recover in the tissue.

The differences between T_1 of tissues are sampled each time the NMV is moved into the transverse plane.

On the other hand, T_2 relaxation is defined as the amount of time it takes for the transverse magnetization to decay to 37% of the entire spin–spin interaction (Fig. 22.6). T_2 relaxation or T_2 decay is caused by the nuclei exchanging energy with other neighboring nuclei. Tissues with longer T_2 relaxation times appear bright on a T_2-weighted image. In this case, during evaluation of the brain in an image, the cerebrospinal fluid, which has a long T_2 relaxation time, will appear bright on a brain image, and the white matter, which has a short relaxation time, will appear dark on a T_2-weighted image.

Remember:

- T_1 and T_2 occur independently, but occur simultaneously.
- T_1 occurs along the *z*axis and T_2 occurs along the *X–Y*-plane.
- T_2 occurs much more quickly than T_1.

Image Weighting

Unlike other imaging modalities, contrast in MRI is described in terms: T_1, T_2, and proton density. There are areas of the body that have a high signal (which appear white on an image), areas of the body that have a low signal (which appear dark on the image), and areas of the body that have an intermediate signal (which appear as shades of gray on an image).

T_1 weighting mainly depends on the differences between fat and water (along with all other tissues with intermediate signals). The number of times the signal is repeated is called repetition time (T_R). T_R controls how far the NMV recovers before it is excited by the next RF pulse. For a T_1-weighted image to be received, the T_R must be short enough so neither fat nor water has enough time to fully return to B_0. Therefore, T_R controls the amount of T_1 weighting.

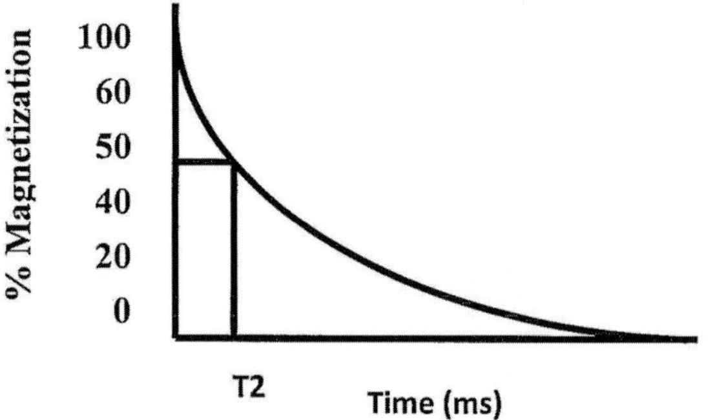

Figure 22.6 T_2 relaxation is defined as the amount of time it takes for the transverse magnetization to decay to 37% of the entire spin–spin interaction.

T_2 weighting depends mainly on the differences between fat and water (along with all other tissues with intermediate signals). The number of times that the signal is echoed is called echo time (T_E). T_E controls the amount of T_2 decay that is allowed to occur before a signal is received. For a T_2 image to be acquired the T_E must be long enough for both fat and water to decay. T_E controls the amount of T_2 weighting. For T_2 the T_E must be long.

Proton density (PD) depends mainly on the difference in the number of protons per unit volume in the patient. Proton density is always present in an image to some extent. To accomplish a PD-weighted image, T_1 and T_2 must be diminished. To decrease T_1 and T_2 contrast and increase PD contrast, the T_R has to be long enough for both water and fat to fully recover. The T_E has to be short; therefore, neither fat nor water has time to decay and T_2 weighting is diminished.

Acquisition

While a more in-depth look of the physics of MRI is necessary for MRI technologists, this brief overview covers the basics of MRI physics. The next aspect is the acquisition and how image formation occurs. This is represented by the *I* in MRI. During the relaxation process the spins release the excess energy, which was gained from the RF pulse, in the shape of RF waves. To produce an image, the released energy needs to pick up these waves before disappearing into space. The released RF energy must be picked up by the coil for a signal to be produced. This is accomplished by the RF receiver coil. The receiver coil can be the same unit as the transmitting RF coil. If the receiving RF coil does not pick up adequate RF energy, a diagnostic image will not occur. This is why the RF coils are at right angles to B_0. Next, the received signal is acquired into the computer and a quarter of a second later an image appears on the screen of the console. Much more computing is involved in the development of the image, but that is beyond the scope of this section.

Advantages of MRI

Traditional nuclear medicine technology and X rays do not show anatomical information very well. The overall contrast resolution is poor. To enhance the image, either contrast media (X ray) must be introduced in the patient or advanced instrumentation techniques (NMT) must be used to increase resolution. MRIs have proven clinically useful because the magnetic resonance signal offers a greater information density than those available through other imaging modalities (i.e., ultrasound, X-ray CT, nuclear medicine, etc.). Also, the overall contrast resolution (the ability to distinguish the differences between tissues)

Table 22.1 Comparison of Spatial Resolution and Contrast Resolution for Nuclear Medicine, Ultrasound, CT, and MRI Imaging

	Nuclear medicine	Ultrasound	Radiography	Computed tomography	Magnetic resonance imaging
Spatial resolution (mm)	5	2	0.1	0.5	0.5
Contrast resolution (mm at 0.5% tissue difference)	20	10	10	4	1

is an advantage of MRI (Table 22.1). The system's multiplanar imaging capabilities are also an advantage. The MR system is able to directly acquire images in the following planes: (1) axial or transverse, (2) sagittal, (3) coronal, and (4) oblique. When acquiring MR images, no special angulations of the patient or reformatting of images is required from the axial plane, unlike in other modalities. Technically, an MRI acquisition can be imaged in any plane preferred for the scan. Another advantage of MRI, as stated before, is that it does not use ionizing radiation.

MR Safety

MRI is generally a safe procedure, but if education about the strong magnetic fields and RF pulses are ignored, the results can lead to patient injury and even death. The invisible magnetic field, which comes from the center of the unit and runs in circles or ellipses out from the bore of the magnetic, has a strong pulling force, and when any ferromagnetic object is within the magnetic field the object will become attracted to the bore of the magnet, which concentrates the constant magnetic field strength. The magnetic field is never turned off and is produced via a superconducting magnetic coil. The higher the magnetic field strength, the stronger the attraction or pull on the ferromagnetic object toward the bore of the magnet, and the more massive the object, the greater the force upon impact within the bore of the magnet. Therefore the object could affect the patient while he/she is having a scan. A 1.5-T magnet can result in an object "flying" at a speed of up to 40 miles per hour. Unfortunately in the past, while rare, injury and even one recorded death have occurred due to staff bringing ferromagnetic material into the MR suite. The death occurred when an oxygen tank was being rushed into the MR suite during a sudden cardiopulmonary arrest and a "code" was called for a patient. The "code team" who responded was unaware of the potential problem with the ferromagnetic oxygen tank.

All individuals who enter the MR suite must be screened to ensure their safety. This includes patients, family members, staff members, and anyone else who will be entering the MR suite. Education about the risks associated with various types of implants, devices, and ferromagnetic objects that can be harmful once an individual enters the suite is needed. The technologist's responsibility is to be aware continuously of and attentive to everyone who enters the suite, by not only visually checking each individual but also by obtaining information and documentation about these objects to provide the safest MR setting.

Safety of the patient should be everyone's concern. Therefore, ideally the patient should be checked more than once. The referring physician department should check the patient before the patient arrives at the MRI department, if possible, and once the patient arrives at the MRI suite the technologist should check the patient immediately before the patient enters the department. The technologist should never assume that the patient has been checked. A screening form should be provided in every MR department to address concerns of cardiac pacemakers or other electrical, magnetic, or mechanical devices.

The energy from the radiofrequency pulses that emits from the RF coils causes heating of tissues from the electric field component of the RF wave. The testes and eyes are the most vulnerable tissues because of the lack of heat dissipation of these tissues. It is important to remember that the pulse sequence used has a great impact on the heat dissipated. A 180° pulse needs four times more power than a 90° pulse. Therefore, spin-echo sequences with multiple 180° pulses pose *significant* heating risks. The FDA limit for RF exposure is measured as either an increase in body temperature or as a specific absorption rate (SAR). FDA limitation is an increase of 1°C in the core body temperature. Knowledge of proper technical factors can decrease a patient's SAR.

There are five types of hazards in MRI:

1. *Projectile*: objects with ferrous magnetic material are pulled toward the magnet (object examples include oxygen tanks, IV poles, scissors, stethoscopes, pens, traction weights, hair pins).
2. *Twisting* (any ferromagnetic objects aligning with the magnetic field-torque):
   a. Cerebral aneurysm clips and cochlear implants twists inside the patient can cause damage.
   b. Magnetic devices and implants that are loose can rip from their foundation causing the device to fail or injury to the patient.
3. *Burns*:
   a. Burns to the patient are usually caused by

electrically conductive material inside the magnet bore.

b. Looped MR accessories, such as RF coil leads, pulse oximeter cable, and ECG leads can become heated and may cause serious burning of the skin of a patient who is under sedation.
c. Although rare, tattoos, and permanent eye liner can become heated and result in burns.

4. *Metal-induced image artifact and possible "tugging" or "pulling"*:
   a. Metal can twist or be tugged or pulled in the body. Depending on where this is, it could adversely affect the patient and could be a contraindication for performing an MRI. Also, metal causes artifacts (signal void) in the areas where there is metal (even small metal fragments such as shrapnel can cause rather large signal loss).
   b. Signal voids can also hide pathology or be misrepresented as pathology.
5. *Device malfunction*:
   a. There have been reports of patient-controlled analgesic (PCA) and infusion pumps reversing flow despite the flow appearing normal to the user.
   b. Electrocardiogram waveform distorted due to the static magnetic field.
   c. Pacemakers and ventilators can pace or ventilate at the wrong point in the cycle resulting in a wrong pacing or in the ventilator delivering inadequate inspiratory pressure.

Conclusion

MRI is complex subject matter. This primer only begins to scratch the surface. The purpose of this chapter is to give the reader a basic understanding of MRI. With the advancements in the field of imaging, fusion of imaging modalities has become a reality. With future PET/MRI imaging possibly becoming more popular, it is important for nuclear medicine personnel to have a basic understanding of MRI advantages and disadvantages, challenges, and hazards.

References and Further Reading

Rink PA, 2001. *Magnetic Resonance in Medicine.* 4th ed. Malden, MA: Blackwell Science.

Westbrook C, Roth CK, Talbot J, 2005. *MRI in Practice.* 3rd ed. Malden, MA: Blackwell Publishing.

We give special thanks to the illustrator, Trameze Jones, for this section on MRI.

Magnetic Resonance Imaging Questions

1. Why are hydrogen atoms so useful in making MRI images?

   a. Hydrogen atoms have a low gyromagnetic ratio
   b. Hydrogen atoms have a high natural abundance in the body
   c. Hydrogen atoms have an integer spin quantum number that makes them "MR visible"
   d. Hydrogen atoms have two protons that resonant symmetrically better than other atoms

2. In a T_1-weighted image sequence, fat or white matter will look:

   a. Dark
   b. White
   c. Gray
   d. Light gray

3. In a T_2-weighted image sequence, fluid will look:

   a. Dark
   b. White
   c. Gray
   d. Light gray

4. In a T_1-weighted image sequence, fluid will look:

   a. Dark
   b. White
   c. Gray
   d. Light gray

5. Clinical magnetic resonance imaging utilizes electromagnetic waves from what part of the electromagnetic spectrum?

   a. Radiowave region
   b. Microwave region
   c. X-ray region
   d. Infrared region

6. Which type of magnetism describes a type of material that is very easily magnetized and/or interacts very strongly with a magnetic field?

   a. Ferromagnetic
   b. Paramagnetic
   c. Diamagnetic
   d. Anamagnetic

Answers

(1) b, (2) b, (3) b, (4) a, (5) a, (6) a

PART III

Preparation for Primary Certification Examination

Computer-Adaptive Testing

In July 1996, the Nuclear Medicine Technology Certification Board (NMTCB) began offering a computer-adaptive test (CAT) for classification in association with ACT, Inc., the college entrance exam. The CAT for classification is designed to render a pass/fail decision. In a CAT of this type, examinees are *not* rank ordered along a score scale to make a precise and accurate classification decision. To administer a CAT for classification, the items themselves are ranked at the decision point on the score scale according to their ability to classify accurately and quickly. Each item in the item pool is associated with the information on its difficulty (the proportion of examinees answering an item correctly) and discrimination (the ability of an item to distinguish between passing and failing individuals) levels. An item that has a difficulty level at or near the passing score and has good discrimination will be a better item for decisionmaking than another item that is too difficult or too easy or has little ability to discriminate between those examinees who should pass and those who should fail. ACT, Inc., psychometric staff obtained item response theory (IRT) statistics for all items in the item pool.

A "classification" CAT is still adaptive in that those examinees whose abilities are far from the passing score (in either direction) will require fewer test items for classification than those whose ability is at or near the passing score. The test will adapt by test length rather than by item difficulty. For the classification CAT, the type of items that are administered to each and every candidate are the same: there are no "difficult items for better candidates" or "easier items for poorer candidates." All examinees receive the same type of test items. Each examinee answers a total of 90 items, and the items are different for each examinee.

Items for the classification CAT are selected in the following approximate proportions for each of four content domains of nuclear medicine technology:

1. radiation safety (15%),
2. instrumentation (20%),
3. clinical procedures (45%), and
4. radiopharmacy (20%).

Decisions for pass/fail were based on the passing score from the benchmark examination administered in September 1993. The September 1993 examination was the first test developed under the current test blueprint. The algorithm used in the classification CAT adjusts for differences in test form difficulty. For example, candidates that receive a CAT that is easier relative to the benchmark exam must answer more items correctly to receive a passing score. Conversely, if a candidate receives a set of items that is more difficult, they would be required to answer fewer questions correctly to pass the exam. In essence, each CAT administered is equalized so the passing level is appropriate for the set of items selected for administration to each candidate.

The CAT for classification, while providing a high degree of confidence in the pass/fail decision, does not allow the same analysis of individual performance and subgroup performance obtained with the paper and pencil exam. In the past, because all examinees who sat at the same administration of a test took the same test, comparative information was obtained. Because the primary purpose of the CAT exam is to classify candidates as pass or fail, CAT for classification selects items that are optimal for minimizing errors in classification, a critical consideration in an occupation-certification program. Candidates whose ability estimates are close to the passing score require more items to make a pass/fail decision, whereas those who are clearly significantly above the pass/fail mark need fewer items. Candidates are required to answer every item as it is presented.

Editors' note: Some questions are not counted toward the final score but are merely "test" questions that may or may not appear on future exams. The examinee has no way of knowing which questions are counted toward the final pass/fail decision.

Note: From the Nuclear Medicine Technology Certification Board website at http://www.nmtcb.org

How to Use the Practice Examinations

This section contains seven 100-question practice examinations with annotated answers. Each examination includes multiple-choice questions that cover the areas of radiopharmacy, instrumentation, clinical procedures, and radiation protection. The best way to prepare for a certification examination is to review the latest task analysis published by the certification agency. The task analysis is a list of all tasks that practitioners should be able to perform, and questions on these tasks will be included on the exam. Candidates should compare their knowledge with those tasks on the list and review material from areas in which they feel the least comfortable.

Because certification examinations in nuclear medicine technology (NMT) are given nationally, knowledge of federal regulations only (including the U.S. Nuclear Regulatory Commission, the U.S. Department of Transportation, and the U.S. Food and Drug Administration [FDA]) is tested and only FDA-approved radiopharmaceuticals and diagnostic procedures are included. Certain topics may not be included on the exam, even though they are taught in NMT programs (for example, historical information about the development of the nuclear medicine specialty).

After candidates have reviewed the material to be presented on the examination, the questions in this section may serve as a "mock" certification exam. After reading each question carefully, choose the best option from the choices given. Note that not all possible options may be given or the best option overall may not appear in the list of choices. As the directions on certification exams state, choose the *best* answer from the options provided. If you are unsure of an answer, first eliminate any choices that are obviously incorrect. Then, review the remaining choices to determine whether any contain clues that might indicate the correct answer or that rule out other choices as incorrect. If the question deals with a topic with which you are totally unfamiliar, an "educated guess" may be impossible. In such a case, make a note to review material on this topic. An explanation of each answer and a reference are provided for each question.

Many of the questions involve calculations. A calculator and decay factor tables for the radionuclides commonly used in nuclear medicine will be necessary to answer some of these questions. The incorrect answers offered for calculations are often chosen to mimic frequently made mistakes. Be certain that you have done the complete calculation and are not choosing the answer to an intermediate step in the solution.

Also be careful of questions or answers containing negatives (those containing the words "not" or "except"). Read carefully. Certification examination questions are not designed to be "tricky" but, instead, to separate individuals who are well prepared and know the information from those who do not.

Acronyms commonly used in nuclear medicine practice have not been spelled out in the questions and answers. The terms for which they stand have been covered in the body of the text for this volume, and these acronyms should be familiar to every nuclear medicine technologist.

The questions and answers in this book have been reviewed for clarity and accuracy. The references are, for the most part, the most readily available and current at the time this text was prepared. Nuclear medicine has always been a dynamic and sometimes rapidly changing field. At times, the task analyses of the certification agencies lag behind current practice, in large part as a result of the complications of the test development process. The authors have attempted to balance task analysis content with state-of-the-art clinical practice. Nevertheless, the reader should be mindful that certain content in this publication may become outdated quickly.

Examination 1

1. Before tracer administration, all of the following preparations are required for a 27-year-old woman referred for total-body bone imaging *except*:

a. explaining the procedure to the patient
b. answering the patient's questions
c. ruling out pregnancy
d. removing attenuating materials from the patient

2. Which of the following structures normally appear as areas of increased activity on the bone images of children?

a. diaphyses of the long bones
b. breast tissue
c. costochondral junctions and epiphyseal plates
d. lumbar spine and cranium

3. If tracer concentration is visualized in the skeleton, stomach, thyroid, and salivary glands on a bone image, the most likely explanation for these findings is that the:

a. patient was imaged too soon after tracer administration
b. radiopharmaceutical contained excess free [^{99m}Tc]pertechnetate
c. patient's renal function is compromised
d. incorrect radiopharmaceutical was administered

4. For interpretation of nuclear medicine lung images, a chest X ray is required to:

a. determine cardiac size
b. rule out a pulmonary embolus
c. rule out previous lung surgery
d. rule out possible causes of the patient's symptoms

5. The image shown here was obtained after the administration of [^{99m}Tc]MAA. Which of the following is the most likely explanation for the quality of this lung perfusion image?

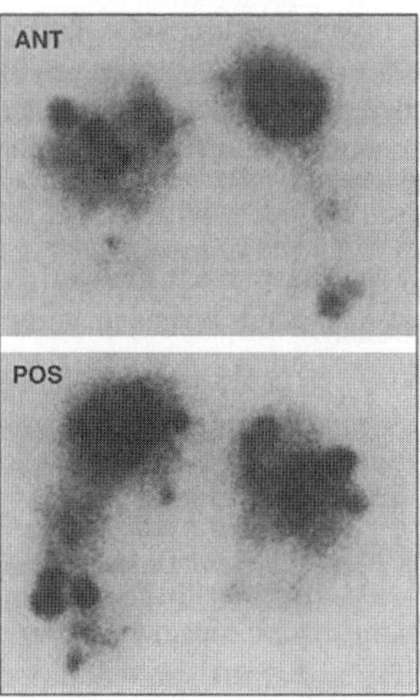

a. The image shows lung pathology.
b. Blood clotted to MAA particles was injected intravenously.
c. There is radioactive contamination on the patient's skin or camera detector.
d. Too many MAA particles were administered to the patient.

6. The purpose of a charcoal filter in a xenon delivery unit is to absorb:

a. bacteria
b. carbon dioxide
c. moisture
d. xenon gas

7. Radionuclide venography may be performed with which of the following radiopharmaceuticals?

a. [^{99m}Tc]pentetate
b. [^{99m}Tc]pertechnetate
c. [^{99m}Tc]exametazime
d. [^{99m}Tc]MAA

8. If ectopic thyroid tissue is suspected, the technologist can expect to find it most commonly in which of the following areas?

a. in the brain
b. at the base of the tongue
c. in the mediastinum
d. at the base of the tongue or in the mediastinum

9. During parathyroid imaging, images of the chest as well as the neck are obtained to:

a. correct the image series for patient motion
b. visualize ectopic parathyroid tissue
c. visualize substernal thyroid tissue
d. diagnose hyperparathyroidism

10. When performing a gated equilibrium cardiac study, which of the following anatomical views best separates the right and left ventricles?

a. left lateral
b. left posterior oblique
c. left anterior oblique
d. anterior

11. In preparation for a ^{201}Tl stress test, patients are instructed to fast to:

a. prevent gastrointestinal upsets during exercise
b. minimize tracer uptake in the gastrointestinal tract
c. enhance myocardial tracer uptake
d. standardize test conditions among patients

12. Which of the following agents used for pharmacologic stress testing remains in the plasma for the greatest length of time?

a. dobutamine
b. adenosine
c. dipyridamole
d. nitroglycerin

13. SPECT liver imaging with [^{99m}Tc]sulfur colloid is performed how soon after tracer administration?

a. immediately
b. 10–15 min
c. 30–45 min
d. 1–2 hr

14. Significantly increased serum bilirubin levels will most likely cause which of the following to be visualized on hepatobiliary images?

a. colon
b. kidneys
c. lungs
d. spleen

15. Localization of a Meckel's diverticulum can be accomplished with which of the following radiopharmaceuticals?

a. [^{67}Ga]citrate
b. [^{99m}Tc]pentetate
c. [^{99m}Tc]pertechnetate
d. [^{99m}Tc]sulfur colloid

16. In infants, 24-hr images are sometimes performed over what area to demonstrate gastroesophageal reflux?

a. lung fields
b. lower esophagus
c. stomach
d. upper small intestine

17. Effective renal plasma flow (ERPF) is measured with which of the following radiopharmaceuticals?

a. [^{99m}Tc]pentetate
b. [^{99m}Tc]disofenin
c. [^{99m}Tc]medronate
d. [^{99m}Tc]mertiatide

18. Evaluating the quality of a bolus injection is best accomplished by which of the following techniques?

a. visually inspecting the bolus
b. calculating the cardiac transit time
c. generating a time–activity curve for the superior vena cava
d. imaging the injection site for residual activity

19. Which of the following is/are *not* normally visualized on a ^{67}Ga image acquired 72 hr after tracer administration?

a. kidneys
b. lacrimal glands
c. sternum
d. liver

20. Which of the following statements about "transmission-based precautions" is *false*?

a. These precautions are applied when a patient is known to be infected with a communicable disease.
b. These precautions must be implemented in the case of diseases such as varicella, tuberculosis, and mumps.
c. These precautions replace "standard precautions."
d. These precautions include guidelines for airborne, droplet, and contact transmitted diseases.

21. Which of the following statements about pentetreotide is *true*?

a. It is labeled with ^{99m}Tc.
b. It is a labeled antibody.
c. It exhibits no human antimurine antibody (HAMA) effect.
d. It is excreted exclusively through the kidneys.

22. The purpose of using acetazolamide in conjunction with a brain agent is to:

a. tranquilize the patient
b. evaluate cerebrovascular ischemia
c. localize the area of the brain from which seizures arise
d. localize brain tumors

23. The technologist's responsibilities during tracer administration for a cisternogram include:

a. performing the lumbar puncture
b. obtaining consent to perform the procedure
c. monitoring the patient for any adverse reactions to the procedure
d. ensuring that personnel and the surroundings are not contaminated with radioactivity

24. Sodium phosphate ^{32}P may be used to treat which of the following conditions?

a. liver metastases
b. polycythemia vera
c. rheumatoid arthritis
d. malignant effusions

25. Supersaturated potassium iodide solution may be administered to the patient for therapy with which of the following radiopharmaceuticals?

a. [^{153}Sm]lexidronam
b. [^{89}Sr]chloride
c. [^{131}I]sodium iodide
d. [^{131}I]tositumomab

26. The first step that a technologist should initiate when an adult patient experiences cardiac arrest is to:

a. perform chest compressions
b. establish an airway
c. call for help
d. perform rescue breathing

27. [^{111}In]Pentetreotide should *not* be administered through an intravenous line containing:

a. a total parenteral nutrition mixture
b. 0.9% sodium chloride
c. dextrose and water
d. glucose

28. Dual-isotope gastric emptying studies use which of the following radiopharmaceuticals for each phase of gastric emptying?

	Liquid phase	Solid phase
a.	[^{99m}Tc]Sulfur colloid	[^{111}In]Pentetate
b.	[^{111}In]Pentetate	[^{99m}Tc]Sulfur colloid
c.	[^{201}Tl]Thallous chloride	[^{99m}Tc]Sestamibi
d.	[^{99m}Tc]Pentetate	[^{99m}Tc]Sulfur colloid

29. Proper placement of a urine collection bag includes:

a. placing it across the patient's lower legs to keep it near the level of the bladder
b. placing it on the stretcher near the patient's feet so that it is out of the field of view of the camera
c. hanging it from an IV pole and raising it above the level of the bladder
d. hanging it from the imaging table so that it is lower than the level of the bladder

30. Which of the following radiopharmaceuticals can be used to assess vesicoureteral reflux by the indirect method?

a. [^{99m}Tc]pertechnetate
b. [^{99m}Tc]sulfur colloid
c. [^{99m}Tc]albumin
d. [^{99m}Tc]pentetate

31. If 0.02μg/kg of cholecystokinin is needed for a hepatibiliary study, what volume needs to be drawn for a 175-lb patient with a solution of 10 μg/mL available to draw from?

a. 0.115 mL
b. 0.159 mL
c. 0.175 mL
d. 0.192 mL

32. Parenteral administration of a drug or radiopharmaceutical would include all of the following routes *except:*

a. intravenous
b. intramuscular
c. subcutaneous
d. oral

33. The red cell survival test is most often performed on a patient with suspected:

a. pernicious anemia
b. intestinal malabsorption
c. iron deficiency anemia
d. hemolytic anemia

34. A technologist confirms a referring physician's request for a nuclear medicine procedure for a hospitalized patient by

a. locating the order for the test in the patient's medical record
b. telephoning the patient's physician for confirmation
c. asking the patient why he/she came to the nuclear medicine department
d. conferring with the nuclear medicine physician

35. Which type of collimator should be used for organ counting during a red cell sequestration study?

a. low-energy, high-sensitivity parallel hole
b. high-energy, low-resolution parallel hole
c. pinhole
d. flat field

36. If a plasma volume has been determined to be 15 L, which of the following events has most likely occurred?

a. completion of a satisfactory study
b. overhydration of the patient
c. leakage of tracer from the circulation
d. infiltration of the tracer

37. A biohazard warning label would be found on all of the following *except* a:

a. contaminated sharps container
b. refrigerator containing potentially infectious material
c. receptacle for contaminated laundry
d. unit of blood released for clinical use

38. The total blood volume may be calculated by dividing the plasma volume measured with labeled albumin by the:

a. hematocrit
b. plasmacrit
c. corrected hematocrit
d. corrected plasmacrit

39. If radioactivity in the circulation from a previous nuclear medicine test is unaccounted for, results of a plasma volume determination will be:

a. unaffected
b. falsely elevated
c. falsely decreased
d. impossible to predict

40. The recommended amount of captopril to be given orally an hour before renal imaging in a hypertension study is:

a. 10–15 mg
b. 15–20 mg
c. 25–50 mg
d. 55–100 mg

41. Imaging with [^{111}In]pentetreotide routinely includes what areas of the body?

a. head and chest
b. chest
c. abdomen
d. head to upper femurs

42. A patient scheduled for scintimammography has symptoms involving her left breast. Which of the following sites is the best choice for injection of the radiopharmaceutical?

a. right antecubital area
b. right carotid artery
c. left carotid artery
d. left hand

43. Based on the net counts data shown here:

Right lung: 175,362
Left lung: 325,672

what is the percentage perfusion to the right lung?

a. 30%
b. 35%
c. 54%
d. 65%

44. If 375 mCi ^{99m}Tc are present on the column of a ^{99}Mo/^{99m}Tc generator and after elution 342 mCi ^{99m}Tc are assayed in the elution vial, the approximate elution efficiency of the generator is:

a. 110%
b. 91%
c. 33%
d. 11%

45. Two-hundred fifty kilobecquerels are equivalent to how many microcuries?

a. 0.25 μCi
b. 6.76 μCi
c. 9.25 μCi
d. 9.250 μCi

46. If a ^{99}Mo/^{99m}Tc generator is eluted on Monday at 0600, the maximum ^{99m}Tc activity could next be eluted at what time?

a. 1200, Monday
b. 1800, Monday
c. 0600, Tuesday
d. 0600, Wednesday

47. According to the NRC, ^{99}Mo contamination in ^{99m}Tc eluate must be measured how often?

a. weekly
b. daily
c. after each elution
d. only after the first elution

48. The results shown here were obtained when ^{99m}Tc eluate was assayed for ^{99}Mo breakthrough at 0600, immediately after elution:

^{99}Mo: 10 μCi
^{99m}Tc: 416 mCi

Which of the following statements about this elution at 1700 is *true*?

a. The eluate should not be used to label compounds with ^{99m}Tc.
b. The eluate does not contain sufficient ^{99m}Tc activity.
c. The eluate may be administered to patients.
d. The eluate must not be administered to patients.

49. A technologist performs an aluminum ion breakthrough test on ^{99m}Tc eluate and obtains the following results: When the indicator paper is spotted with aluminum ion solution, a faint red color is observed, but when the paper is spotted with eluate, no color change is observed. These results indicate:

a. the absence of radionuclidic impurities in the eluate
b. that the aluminum ion concentration in the eluate is below the U.S. Pharmacopeia (USP) limit
c. that the eluate should be discarded
d. that the aluminum ion solution contains less aluminum than the eluate

50. All of the following procedures may be performed with [^{99m}Tc]sulfur colloid *except*:

a. gastric-emptying study
b. gastroesophageal reflux study
c. gastrointestinal-bleeding localization
d. Meckel's diverticulum localization

51. Based on the day's clinic schedule shown here:

Patient	Procedure
Patient A	Thyroid uptake and image
Patient B	Therapy for hyperthyroidism
Patient C	Cisternogram

the technologist should prepare or order which of the following radiopharmaceuticals?

a. [^{131}I]human serum albumin, [^{131}I]sodium iodide, and [^{99m}Tc]pertechnetate
b. [^{111}In]oxine and [^{123}I]sodium iodide
c. [^{123}I]sodium iodide, [^{131}I]sodium iodide, and [^{111}In]pentetate
d. [^{131}I]sodium iodide and [^{111}In]chloride

52. If an MAA kit must be reconstituted with 3.5 mL of [^{99m}Tc]pertechnetate, what are the consequences if only 2.0 mL are added to the kit?

a. Patients will receive fewer MAA particles per milliliter of [^{99m}Tc]MAA.
b. Patients will receive more MAA particles per milliliter of [^{99m}Tc]MAA.
c. Patients will receive the recommended number of particles if the correct activity is administered.
d. The resulting perfusion lung images will have the appearance of decreased tracer uptake.

53. Reconstituted "cold" pyrophosphate is administered to the patient in which red blood cell labeling method(s)?

a. in vitro method
b. in vivo method
c. modified in vivo method
d. both the in vivo method and the modified in vivo method

54. Which of the following radiopharmaceutical kit formulations is light sensitive?

a. sestamibi
b. oxidronate
c. mertiatide
d. exametazime

55. When performing radiochromatography on a radiopharmaceutical sample, the solvent front is located 8.5 cm from the origin and the radiochemical impurity is at the origin. What is the R_f value of the radiochemical impurity?

a. 0
b. 0.85
c. 1.0
d. 8.5

56. According to the USP, to be administered to patients, most ^{99m}Tc-labeled radiopharmaceuticals should have a radiochemical purity of at least what percentage?

a. 98%
b. 95%
c. 90%
d. 88%

57. A technologist must administer 8 mCi [^{99m}Tc]mebrofenin to a patient at 1100. On the basis of the vial label information shown here:

Calibration:	0700, August 4
Total activity:	100 mCi
Total volume:	8.5 mL
Concentration:	11.8 mCi/mL
Expiration:	1500, August 4

what volume of [^{99m}Tc]mebrofenin should be administered to the patient?

a. 0.13 mL
b. 0.68 mL
c. 0.92 mL
d. 1.1 mL

58. A technologist must administer 37 MBq [^{201}Tl]thallous chloride at 1000 on February 16. On the basis of the vial label information shown here:

Calibration:	1200, February 14
Total activity:	222 MBq
Total volume:	4.0 mL
Concentration:	55.5 MBq/mL
Expiration:	1200, February 17

what volume should be administered to the patient?

a. 0.44 mL
b. 0.84 mL
c. 1.0 mL
d. 2.3 mL

59. A technologist needs 4 mCi [^{201}Tl]thallous chloride at 0800 on June 29. The label on the radiopharmaceutical vial contains the following information:

Total activity:	10.0 mCi
Total volume:	5.5 mL
Assay:	1200, July 1

What volume is required to obtain the necessary activity on June 29?

a. 3.6 mL
b. 1.35 mL
c. 0.74 mL
d. 0.28 mL

60. Which radiopharmaceutical is used to label red blood cells with ^{99m}Tc?

a. [^{99m}Tc]albumin
b. [^{99m}Tc]exametazime
c. [^{99m}Tc]pertechnetate
d. [^{99m}Tc]pyrophosphate

61. Which of the following radiopharmaceuticals is used to label white blood cells with ^{99m}Tc?

a. [^{99m}Tc]bicisate
b. [^{99m}Tc]exametazime
c. [^{99m}Tc]pertechnetate
d. [^{99m}Tc]sestamibi

62. When [^{99m}Tc]exametazime is used to label white blood cells, which of the following reagents is omitted from its preparation?

a. [^{99m}Tc]pertechnetate
b. 0.9% sodium chloride
c. methylene blue stabilizer
d. ACD solution

63. Four millicuries of [^{201}Tl]thallous chloride is the prescribed unit dosage. According to the NRC, which of the following dose calibrator measurements verifies that a dosage within acceptable limits has been dispensed into the syringe?

I. 3.5 mCi
II. 4.0 mCi
III. 4.3 mCi
IV. 4.5 mCi

a. II only
b. II or III only
c. I, II, or III only
d. I, II, III, or IV

64. In labeling red blood cells with radiochromium, the order of components to be added to the vial containing ACD solution is:

a. patient blood, radiochromium, ascorbic acid
b. radiochromium, patient blood, ascorbic acid
c. radiochromium, ascorbic acid, patient blood
d. ascorbic acid, radiochromium, patient blood

65. If a unit dosage of [^{99m}Tc]MAA contains 148 MBq and 325,000 particles in 0.75 mL at 1000, approximately how many particles will be contained in 148 MBq at 1600?

a. 162,500
b. 325,000
c. 650,000
d. 866,666

66. If a unit dosage of radioactivity contains 4.5 mCi in 1.2 mL, how many milliliters must be removed so that 3.5 mCi remain in the syringe?

a. 0.93 mL
b. 0.78 mL
c. 0.42 mL
d. 0.27 mL

67. If a radiopharmaceutical kit must be reconstituted with 30 mCi contained in 5 mL and the eluate has an activity of 350 mCi in 7 mL, how many milliliters of preservative-free saline must be added?

a. 0.1 mL
b. 0.6 mL
c. 4.4 mL
d. 4.9 mL

68. What is the minimal centrifugation time needed if a protocol specifies 5000 *g* for 5 min, but the maximum relative centrifugal force that can be obtained is 2500 *g*?

a. 2 min
b. 2.5 min
c. 10 min
d. 12.5 min

69. According to the NRC, imaging rooms should be posted with which of the following signs?

a. No posting is required.
b. "Caution: Radioactive Materials"
c. "Caution: Radiation Area"
d. "Caution: High Radiation Area"

70. Which of the following exposure rates indicate that a package containing radioactive material must be labeled with a category III DOT label?

	At package surface	At 1 m
a.	56 mR/hr	3.5 mR/hr
b.	22 mR/hr	0.9 mR/hr
c.	1.5 mR/hr	1.0 mR/hr
d.	0.5 mR/hr	No detectable radiation

71. If a point source produces an exposure rate of 30 mR/hr at a distance of 15 cm, what is the exposure rate at 40 cm from the source?

a. 0.2 mR/hr
b. 4.2 mR/hr
c. 11.2 mR/hr
d. 22 mR/hr

72. If the half-value layer (HVL) for ^{131}I in lead is 0.3 cm, what is the minimum thickness of lead that is required to reduce the exposure rate of a ^{131}I source from 12 mR/hr to less than 2 mR/hr?

a. 0.3 cm
b. 0.6 cm
c. 0.9 cm
d. 1.2 cm

73. A patient receives a unit dosage of [^{89}Sr]chloride intended for another patient. Which of the following statements about this situation is *true*?

a. Because the patient received only a unit dosage of ^{89}Sr, no report to the NRC is required.
b. According to the NRC, this does not constitute a medical event, but a departmental record should be maintained.
c. The situation describes a medical event that needs to be reported only to the nuclear medicine supervisor and the authorized user.
d. The situation describes a medical event requiring notification of the NRC.

74. According to NRC regulations, the annual occupational dose limit to the eye is:

a. 500 mSv
b. 150 mSv
c. 50 mSv
d. 5 mSv

75. A vial of ^{133}Xe has been decayed in storage for 2 months. When the vial is monitored with a survey meter, the reading is twice the background radiation level. What should the technologist do next?

a. Remove any radiation symbols from the vial, then dispose of it.
b. Return the vial to storage.
c. Dispose of the vial as biohazardous waste.
d. Vent the radioactivity left in the vial into a fume hood.

76. According to the NRC, wipe tests of areas where radiopharmaceuticals are prepared or administered must be performed:

a. on a reasonable schedule
b. every day on which radiopharmaceuticals are used
c. weekly
d. only if contamination occurs

77. What is the measured exposure rate shown on the diagram of the G–M meter depicted here?

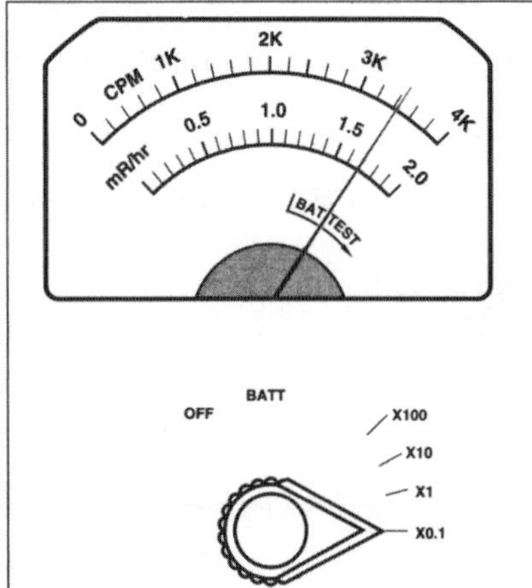

a. 0.17 mR/hr
b. 1.7 mR/hr
c. 17 mR/hr
d. 170 mR/hr

78. When opening packages containing radioactive material, which of the following steps should be performed *first*?

a. Visually inspect the package for damage or leakage.
b. Put on disposable gloves.
c. Verify the package contents against the packing slip.
d. Wipe test the package for contamination.

79. During cleanup of a radioactive spill, decontamination of the area must continue until:

a. no more contamination can be removed from the area
b. the exposure rate cannot be distinguished from background activity
c. the contamination is reduced to a small area
d. no one would receive the maximum allowable total effective dose equivalent (TEDE) if he/she remained in the area

80. Personnel must wear a radiation monitoring device during work hours if they are:

a. exposed to radiation at any time during work hours
b. exposed to radiation above background levels
c. likely to exceed 10% of the annual maximum allowable occupational exposure
d. likely to exceed the annual maximum allowable occupational exposure

81. A patient can be released after receiving a therapeutic radiopharmaceutical if no other individual is likely to receive an exposure dose, from being exposed to the patient, exceeding how many rems?

a. 0.1 rem
b. 0.2 rem
c. 0.5 rem
d. 5.0 rem

82. If a source of radioactive contamination produces an exposure rate of 3 mR/hr, how long will it take for the exposure rate to drop to a background exposure rate of 0.05 mR/hr?

a. 4 half-lives
b. 5 half-lives
c. 6 half-lives
d. 7 half-lives

83. According to the NRC, records of surveys must be retained for how many years?

a. 1 year
b. 3 years
c. 5 years
d. as long as the facility's license is in effect

84. Which of the following materials is recommended for shielding syringes containing positron-emitting radionuclides?

a. lead
b. plastic-lined lead
c. tungsten
d. steel

85. If a nuclear medicine technologist needs a diagnostic X ray, how should this exposure be included in his/her occupational exposure record?

a. The technologist should wear his/her radiation dosimeter during the X-ray examination.
b. The RSO will estimate the probable exposure and add it to the technologist's permanent record.
c. The RSO will supply a separate dosimeter for the technologist to wear during the X-ray examination.
d. The exposure from the X-ray examination must not be included in the occupational exposure record.

86. According to the standard of practice, if the results of a dose calibrator linearity test demonstrate that the measured values exceed the values by 12–15%, the technologist should:

a. replace the instrument
b. have the instrument repaired
c. use a correction factor to determine true activities
d. use the actual dose calibrator activity readings

87. A technologist measures a ^{57}Co standard in a dose calibrator on the following settings: ^{57}Co, ^{99m}Tc, ^{123}I, ^{131}I, ^{133}Xe, and ^{201}Tl, and then calculates the percentage difference between the calculated and measured activities. The technologist is assessing:

a. accuracy
b. constancy
c. linearity
d. geometric variation

88. A ^{137}Cs reference standard is counted daily with a scintillation spectrometer, using the same gain, window, and high voltage setting. On the basis of the data shown here:

Date	Net counts per minute
July 15	12,555
July 16	12,534
July 17	12,613
July 20	10,678

on July 20, the technologist should:

a. use the spectrometer for clinical studies
b. arrange for repair of the instrument
c. change the gain setting
d. recalibrate the operating voltage

89. According to the standard of practice, how often should dose calibrator linearity testing be performed?

a. annually
b. quarterly
c. monthly
d. daily

90. To repair the nonuniformity demonstrated on the intrinsic uniformity image shown here:

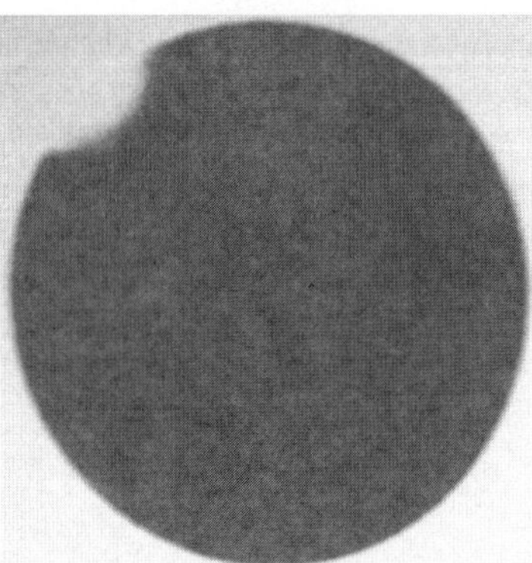

the service engineer will need to:

a. replace the crystal
b. replace a photomultiplier tube
c. repair the collimator
d. replace the x,y localization board

91. Which of the following sources is the most appropriate for assessing dose calibrator constancy?

a. ^{99m}Tc
b. ^{137}Cs
c. ^{125}I
d. ^{131}I

92. Which of the following statements about the effect of the filter-cutoff frequency is *true*?

a. The lower the cutoff frequency, the smoother the image.
b. The lower the cutoff frequency, the noisier the image.
c. Adjusting the cutoff frequency will not affect image appearance.
d. The cutoff frequency cannot be adjusted after the image has been acquired.

93. Temporal resolution is related to which of the following acquisition parameters?

a. percentage energy window
b. matrix size
c. framing rate
d. collimator

94. Temporal smoothing could be appropriately applied in which of the following studies?

a. whole-body bone image
b. gated-equilibrium cardiac function study
c. SPECT study of the liver
d. thyroid image

95. If an image is acquired into a 128 × 128 matrix on a scintillation camera with a 350-mm-diameter field of view, what are the dimensions of each pixel?

a. 0.37 × 0.37 mm
b. 2.73 × 2.73 mm
c. 3.14 × 3.14 mm
d. 5.9 × 5.9 mm

96. Which of the following instruments should be used to determine whether all removable contamination has been eliminated?

a. Geiger–Mueller counter
b. cutie pie (ionization chamber)
c. well counter
d. uptake probe

97. Which of the following matrix sizes and acquisition modes would be most appropriate for a blood flow study of the feet?

a. 64×64 byte
b. 64×64 word
c. 256×256 byte
d. 256×256 word

98. A daily uniformity flood for a scintillation camera should contain a minimum of how many counts?

a. 1–2 million
b. 3–5 million
c. 6–10 million
d. 20–30 million

99. As a pinhole collimator is moved farther away from the thyroid, how will it affect the image?

a. The gland will appear larger.
b. The gland will appear smaller.
c. Right and left are reversed.
d. There is no change in size or orientation.

100. During geometric variation testing of a dose calibrator, activity in a 1-mL syringe measures 253 μCi when the expected reading is 212 μCi. Which of the following correction factors should be applied to the measured reading?

a. 0.84
b. 1.19
c. 4.1
d. 23.3

Examination 2

1. Static bone imaging is routinely performed how long after tracer administration to an adult?

a. 30 min
b. 1 hr
c. 2–3 hr
d. 24 hr

2. Which of the following structures normally appear as areas of increased activity on the bone images of adults?

a. anterior iliac crests
b. glenoid fossa
c. sternoclavicular joints
d. all of the above

3. Which of the following conditions is visualized on a bone image as a photopenic area?

a. attenuation
b. tracer infiltration
c. acute myocardial infarction
d. osteomyelitis

4. It is safe to block a portion of the pulmonary circulation with MAA particles in patients with suspected pulmonary emboli because the:

a. number of injected particles blocks only a small number of precapillary arterioles
b. particles are made from albumin isolated from human serum
c. particles are rapidly phagocytized by lung macrophages
d. albumin is denatured before it is made into particles

5. A nebulizer is used to administer which of the following lung ventilation radiopharmaceuticals?

a. ^{81m}Kr gas
b. ^{133}Xe gas
c. [^{99m}Tc]pentetate
d. [^{99m}Tc]macroaggregated albumin

6. Which of the following radiopharmaceuticals may be used to image acute deep vein thrombosis in the lower extremities?

a. [^{99m}Tc]macroaggregated albumin (MAA)
b. [^{99m}Tc]arcitumomab
c. [^{131}I]iobenguane
d. [^{111}In]oxyquinoline

7. In performing radionuclide venography with [^{99m}Tc]MAA, the radiopharmaceutical is administered at what site?

a. antecubital area of either arm
b. either femoral vein
c. dorsal veins on top of each foot
d. either basilic vein

8. After total thyroidectomy, total-body imaging with radioiodine normally will demonstrate tracer concentration in which of the following areas?

a. liver, lungs, and bones
b. salivary glands, stomach, and bladder
c. liver, salivary glands, stomach, and lungs
d. bladder, liver, and brain

9. A parathyroid adenoma will concentrate which of the following radiopharmaceuticals?

a. [^{123}I]sodium iodide
b. [^{99m}Tc]pertechnetate
c. [^{99m}Tc]sestamibi
d. [^{99m}Tc]pertechnetate or [^{99m}Tc]sestamibi

10. When positioning a patient for an LAO view of a gated equilibrium ventricular function study, tilting the camera detector toward the patient's feet separates what two structures?

a. left ventricle and aorta
b. left ventricle and left atrium
c. left and right atria
d. left and right ventricles

11. Which tracer is excreted primarily via the hepatobiliary system?

a. [^{99m}Tc]sestamibi
b. [^{99m}Tc]exametazime
c. [^{99m}Tc]medronate
d. [^{201}Tl]thallous chloride

12. A cardiac stress test requires the placement of how many electrodes on the patient's body?

a. 3
b. 6
c. 10
d. 12

13. Visualization of bone marrow uptake on a [^{99m}Tc]sulfur colloid liver/spleen image is most likely the result of which of the following?

a. improper colloid particle size
b. insufficient tracer circulation time
c. liver dysfunction
d. overactive bone marrow

14. During hepatobiliary imaging, which structure will NOT be visualized if cystic duct obstruction is present?

a. common hepatic duct
b. common bile duct
c. gallbladder
d. small intestine

15. How long after the administration of [^{99m}Tc]pertechnetate does imaging begin for the localization of a Meckel's diverticulum?

a. immediately
b. 15–20 min
c. 1 hr
d. 2–3 hr

16. All of the following ^{99m}Tc-labeled radiopharmaceuticals may be appropriate for performing a left-to-right cardiac shunt examination using the first-pass method *except:*

a. sulfur colloid
b. pentetate
c. sestamibi
d. tetrofosmin

17. The glomerular filtration rate (GFR) is measured with which of the following radiopharmaceuticals?

a. [^{99m}Tc]pentetate
b. [^{99m}Tc]succimer
c. [^{99m}Tc]gluceptate
d. [^{99m}Tc]mertiatide

18. Radionuclide cystography is performed by the direct method using which of the following radiopharmaceuticals?

a. [^{99m}Tc]pentetate or [^{99m}Tc]medronate
b. [^{99m}Tc]pertechnetate or [^{99m}Tc]sulfur colloid
c. [^{99m}Tc]pertechnetate or [^{99m}Tc]mertiatide
d. [^{99m}Tc]gluceptate or [^{99m}Tc]sulfur colloid

19. Filtered [^{99m}Tc]sulfur colloid is required for which of the following examinations?

a. gastroesophageal reflux
b. gastric emptying
c. LeVeen shunt patency
d. lymphoscintigraphy

20. A patient with a nasogastric tube in place is transferred to the nuclear medicine department for an imaging procedure. The technologist should:

a. confirm physician orders for transfer and reestablish suction if required
b. remove the nasogastric tube because it will interfere with the imaging procedure
c. use the nasogastric tube to administer the radiopharmaceutical
d. cancel the study because the presence of a nasogastric tube precludes any imaging procedure being performed

21. The appearance of what structure indicates the beginning of the venous phase of a cerebral blood flow study?

a. anterior cerebral arteries
b. carotid arteries
c. nasopharynx
d. superior sagittal sinus

22. In performing cisternography, the purpose of acquiring the first image over the lower thoracic/lumbar spine is to ascertain:

a. the site of tracer administration
b. the flow rate of the cerebral spinal fluid
c. that the tracer was not infiltrated
d. that the spinal cord was not damaged during tracer administration

23. On Wednesday a patient had a ^{123}I thyroid study performed; a ^{125}I plasma volume is ordered to be performed on Thursday. Which of the following statements about the situation is correct?

a. The ^{123}I will not interfere with the plasma volume determination.
b. The blood volume determination should be postponed until the ^{123}I is decayed.
c. A baseline plasma sample should be collected before performing the plasma volume.
d. ^{131}I instead of ^{125}I-human serum albumin should be used for the plasma volume determination.

24. [^{89}Sr]Chloride is used to treat which of the following conditions?

a. bone pain
b. polycythemia vera
c. rheumatoid arthritis
d. malignant effusions

25. Whole-body imaging with [^{131}I]sodium iodide is optimally performed how long after tracer administration?

a. 12 hr
b. 18–24 hr
c. 48–72 hr
d. 96 hr or longer

26. A patient undergoing an imaging procedure indicates to the technologist that a seizure is impending. The most appropriate action for the technologist is to:

a. instruct the patient to breathe deeply to help increase oxygen levels in the brain
b. ignore the patient's concerns because the timing of seizures cannot be predicted
c. increase the number of physical restraints on the patient to prevent patient movement and injury
d. stop the imaging procedure and have the patient lie on the floor with a pillow supporting the head

27. After administration of [^{111}In]pentetreotide, which areas of the body should be imaged?

a. anterior and posterior chest
b. anterior and posterior abdomen
c. anterior and posterior whole body
d. anterior, posterior, and laterals of head and neck

28. Which of the following is the initial positioning for visualizing gastrointestinal bleeding with labeled red blood cells?

a. xiphoid in middle of field of view
b. symphysis pubis in middle of field of view
c. lower border of liver and spleen at top of field of view
d. lower esophagus at top of field of view

29. Which of the following tracers is preferred if a first-pass stress and rest cardiac function examination is to be performed on a patient?

a. [^{99m}Tc]pertechnetate
b. [^{99m}Tc]medronate
c. [^{99m}Tc]pentetate
d. [^{99m}Tc]sestamibi

30. Patient preparation for breast imaging with [^{99m}Tc]sestamibi includes which of the following?

a. explanation of the procedure
b. fasting for 8 hr before tracer administration
c. discontinuation of any medications
d. consumption of a fatty meal

31. Historically, a Schilling test may be ordered for a patient with suspected:

a. hemolytic anemia
b. pernicious anemia
c. iron deficiency anemia
d. lymphocytic anemia

32. Data derived from a first-pass cardiac examination and a region of interest drawn over the lung are used to generate the pulmonary time–activity curve shown here.

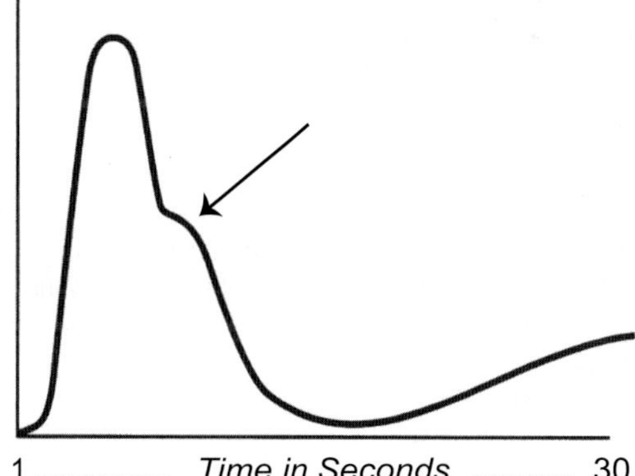

The arrow indicates:

a. first pass of activity through the lungs
b. second pass of activity through the lungs
c. activity prematurely returning to the lungs
d. activity returning from the systemic circulation

33. The proper route of administration for a lymphoscintigraphy exam is:

a. an intravenous injection
b. orally
c. an intrathecal injection
d. a subcutaneous injection

34. A patient's plasmacrit may be determined by:

a. multiplying the patient's hematocrit by 0.9
b. subtracting the decimal hematocrit from 1
c. finding the ratio of plasma volume to red blood cell volume
d. dividing 1 by the decimal hematocrit

35. During a red cell sequestration study, counts are obtained from all of the following organs *except* the:

a. liver
b. spleen
c. heart
d. kidneys

36. In performing a plasma volume with ^{125}I-albumin, three blood samples are collected at varying times after tracer administration and counted. These counts vs. time are plotted on semilog graph paper. The purpose of this graph is to:

a. give a visual representation of the data
b. obtain the half-time clearance value used in the calculations
c. correct for leakage of the radiopharmaceutical
d. show the decay of the radionuclide

37. Patient preparation for a thyroid uptake test may include discontinuation of antithyroid medications. Which of the following is one of these antithyroid drugs?

a. synthroid
b. potassium perchlorate
c. propylthiouracil
d. thyroxine

38. During a radiochromium red cell mass determination, an infusion set may be used to place a needle in the patient's antecubital vein. To maintain the patency of the infusion set tubing, what substance should be injected into the infusion set tubing?

a. heparin
b. normal saline
c. ACD solution
d. bacteriostatic water

39. A gastric-emptying study uses which of the following radiopharmaceuticals ?

a. [^{99m}Tc]medronate
b. [^{99m}Tc]disida
c. [^{99m}Tc]sulfur colloid
d. [^{99m}Tc]MAA

40. In the case of insulinoma, which of the following radiopharmaceuticals may cause hypoglycemia?

a. [^{111}In]pentetreotide
b. [^{99m}Tc]sestamibi
c. [^{67}Ga]citrate
d. [^{18}F]fluorodeoxyglucose

41. Which of the following structures is normally visualized on an image performed with [^{18}F]fluorodeoxyglucose?

a. thyroid
b. brain
c. pituitary gland
d. pancreas

42. The [^{14}C]urea breath test is used to:

a. detect the presence of peptic ulcers
b. detect the presence of *Helicobacter pylori* bacteria
c. identify gastric cancers
d. rule out Zollinger–Ellison syndrome

43. On the basis of the data shown here:

	Time	Counts/min
Capsule	0900	216,789
Background	0900	92
Thyroid	1500	94,954
Thigh	1500	521

what is the patient's thyroid uptake at 1500 if a [^{123}I]sodium iodide capsule administered to the patient is used as the standard?

a. 32%
b. 44%
c. 60%
d. 87%

44. If the elution efficiency of a ^{99}Mo/^{99m}Tc generator is 96% and 11.7 MBq ^{99m}Tc is present on the column, approximately how much activity will be removed during elution?

a. 0.46 MBq
b. 11.2 MBq
c. 11.7 MBq
d. 12.2 MBq

45. A dry-column generator is eluted with 5 mL of saline, and the eluate containing 863 mCi is collected into a 10-mL evacuated vial. What is the concentration of the eluate?

a. 172.6 mCi/mL
b. 86.3 mCi/mL
c. 57.5 mCi/mL
d. 5.79 mCi/mL

46. If no eluate is obtained during generator elution, the technologist should next:

a. attempt elution with another evacuated elution vial
b. contact the generator manufacturer
c. check the generator tubing for kinks or leaks
d. add more saline to the generator column

47. According to the NRC, records of ^{99}Mo concentration in ^{99m}Tc eluate must be maintained for how long?

a. 1 year
b. 3 years
c. 5 years
d. 10 years

48. According to the NRC, the concentration of what radionuclidic impurity must be determined after the first elution of a ^{99}Mo/^{99m}Tc generator?

a. Al^{3+}
b. free pertechnetate
c. ^{99}Mo
d. a and c

49. Based on the day's clinic schedule shown here:

Patient	Procedure
Patient A	Renal function study
Patient B	Total-body bone image
Patient C	Meckel's diverticulum localization
Patient D	Hepatobiliary study

the technologist should prepare or order all of the following radiopharmaceuticals *except:*

a. [^{99m}Tc]macroaggregated albumin
b. [^{99m}Tc]mebrofenin
c. [^{99m}Tc]medronate
d. [^{99m}Tc]mertiatide

50. According to NRC regulations, records of written directives must be maintained for how long?

a. 3 years
b. 5 years
c. 10 years
d. indefinitely

51. Which of the following radiopharmaceuticals should be prepared if a renal function study is being performed to determine the glomerular filtration rate?

a. [^{99m}Tc]gluceptate
b. [^{99m}Tc]mertiatide
c. [^{99m}Tc]pentetate
d. [^{99m}Tc]succimer

52. What is the final concentration of the [^{99m}Tc]sulfur colloid if the maximum activity is prepared with the following reagents?

Reaction vial	Lyophilized thiosulfate mixture
Sulfur colloid kit	
Syringe I	1.6 mL acid
Syringe II	1.6 mL buffer
Maximum activity to be added	400 mCi
^{99m}Tc volume to be added	1.0–3.0 mL
[^{99m}Tc]Pertechnetate	
Concentration	75.5 mCi/mL
Total volume	15 mL

a. 75.5 mCi/mL
b. 47.0 mCi/mL
c. 42.7 mCi/mL
d. 36.5 mCi/mL

53. Heating is required during the preparation of all of the following ^{99m}Tc-labeled radiopharmaceuticals *except*:

a. bicisate
b. mertiatide
c. sestamibi
d. sulfur colloid

54. To calculate the yield of a ^{99}Mo/^{99m}Tc generator, in what sequence should the following steps be performed?

I. Measure the amount of ^{99m}Tc activity eluted from the generator.
II. Determine the amount of ^{99}Mo activity present on the generator at a given time *t*.
III. Calculate the fraction of ^{99m}Tc activity eluted compared with the ^{99m}Tc activity present on the generator column.
IV. Determine how much ^{99m}Tc activity has formed by ^{99}Mo decay at a given time *t*.
V. Determine the elapsed time from calibration to time *t*.

a. V, II, IV, I, III
b. II, V, I, IV, III
c. IV, II, V, III, I
d. I, V, II, IV, III

55. When performing radiochromatography on a radiopharmaceutical sample, the locations of the radiochemical components on the chromatography strip are as shown here. What is the R_f value of hydrolyzed-reduced ^{99m}Tc if the solvent front is 12.6 cm from the origin?

Radiochemical component	Distance from origin
Hydrolyzed-reduced ^{99m}Tc	2.5 cm
[^{99m}Tc]pertechnetate	12.6 cm
^{99m}Tc-labeled radiopharmaceutical	0 cm

a. 0
b. 0.20
c. 0.25
d. 4.8

56. All of the following units are expressions of radiopharmaceutical specific activity *except*:

a. μCi/mg
b. kBq/mL
c. Ci/g
d. MBq/mole

57. A technologist needs 1 mCi [^{111}In]chloride at 0900 on May 18. The label on the radiopharmaceutical vial contains the following information:

Total activity: 3.0 mCi
Total volume: 3.0 mL
Assay: 1200, May 21

What volume is required to obtain the necessary activity on May 18?

a. 2.1 mL
b. 1.4 mL
c. 0.69 mL
d. 0.48 mL

58. If 25 μCi of a radiopharmaceutical are to be administered for each kilogram of body weight, approximately how much activity should be administered to a child weighing 15.5 kg?

a. 852 μCi
b. 0.39 mCi
c. 0.85 mCi
d. 1.6 mCi

59. For labeling red blood cells, the prescribed adult dosage of [^{99m}Tc]pertechnetate is 925 MBq ±10%. Which of the following dose calibrator readings obtained from the syringe containing the patient dosage would verify that the prescribed activity was dispensed?

a. 21 mCi
b. 28 mCi
c. 20 mCi
d. 25.5 mCi

60. When red blood cells are labeled with ^{99m}Tc using the in vivo method, in what order are the reagents injected into the patient?

a. Stannous pyrophosphate and [^{99m}Tc]pertechnetate are administered at the same time.
b. Stannous pyrophosphate is administered 15–30 min before [^{99m}Tc]pertechnetate.
c. Stannous pyrophosphate is administered 2–3 hr before [^{99m}Tc]pertechnetate.
d. [^{99m}Tc]pertechnetate is administered 15–30 min before stannous pyrophosphate.

61. If the following reagents are available, what volume of each reagent must be added together to prepare 20 mCi of [^{99m}Tc]succimer?

Succimer kit
2.2 mL succimer reagent: Use 1 part by volume to 2 parts of [^{99m}Tc]pertechnetate

[^{99m}Tc]Pertechnetate
Concentration: 20 mCi/mL
Total volume: 10 mL

	Succimer volume	*^{99m}Tc volume*
a.	0.5 mL	1.0 mL
b.	0.75 mL	0.5 mL
c.	1.0 mL	2.5 mL
d.	2.0 mL	4.5 mL

62. Venipuncture materials labeled with which of the following expiration dates may be used safely on August 10, 2005?

I. July 31, 2005
II. August 31, 2005
III. September 30, 2005
IV. October 1, 2006

a. IV only
b. III or IV only
c. II, III, or IV only
d. I, II, III, or IV

63. According to NRC regulations, all of the following information must appear in the record of ^{99}Mo concentration measurements *except*

a. ratio of ^{99}Mo to ^{99m}Tc activities
b. time and date of measurement
c. name of the individual making the measurement
d. dose calibrator make and model

64. According to the NRC, a written directive must be prepared for administration of which of the following radiopharmaceuticals?

a. 1 mCi [^{111}In]oxine
b. 5 mCi [^{131}I]sodium iodide
c. 10 mCi [^{67}Ga]citrate
d. 30 mCi [^{99m}Tc]sestamibi

65. If ^{99m}Tc eluate needs to be diluted to prepare other ^{99m}Tc-labeled products, the correct diluent is which of the following?

a. sterile saline containing 0.2% thiosulfate
b. preservative-free isotonic saline
c. bacteriostatic saline
d. distilled water

66. A unit dosage of [^{67}Ga]citrate calibrated for 0800 on July 9 contains 5 mCi in 2.6 mL. If 3 mCi are needed on July 10 at 0800, what volume should be retained in the syringe?

a. 0.7 mL
b. 1.1 mL
c. 1.5 mL
d. 1.9 mL

67. If a 2.5–Ci ^{99}Mo/^{99m}Tc generator is estimated to contain 268 mCi of [^{99m}Tc]pertechnetate, but 198 mCi are eluted, what is the approximate elution efficiency of the generator?

a. 74%
b. 26%
c. 11%
d. 8%

68. What is the volume contained in the syringe shown here?

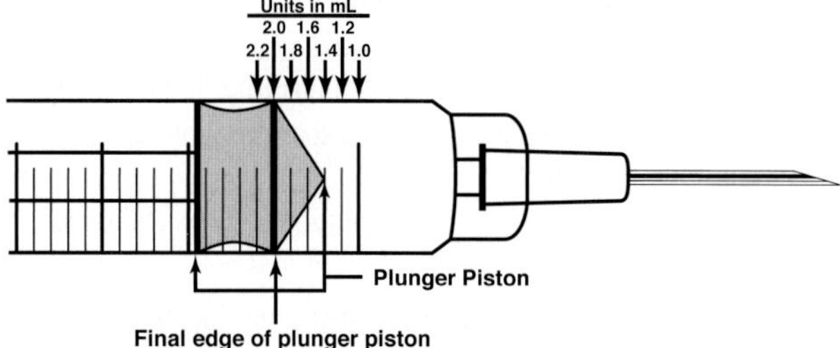

a. 1.4 mL
b. 1.6 mL
c. 1.8 mL
d. 2.0 mL

69. Which of the following federal (U.S.) agencies regulates the packaging and transport of radioactive materials?

a. Department of Transportation
b. Environmental Protection Agency
c. Food and Drug Administration
d. Nuclear Regulatory Commission

70. Which of the following exposure rates indicate that a package containing radioactive material must be labeled with a category II DOT label?

	At package surface	At 1 m
a.	65 mR/hr	5.5 mR/hr
b.	52 mR/hr	2.2 mR/hr
c.	35 mR/hr	1.0 mR/hr
d.	0.5 mR/hr	No detectable radiation

71. If the radiation intensity of a point source at 0.5 m measures 36 mR/hr, at what distance will the intensity be halved?

a. 0.5 m
b. 0.7 m
c. 2.2 m
d. 7.1 m

72. If the HVL of ^{60}Co in lead is 1.25 cm, what percentage of ^{60}Co photons is absorbed from a ^{60}Co source shielded with 2.5 cm of lead?

a. 25%
b. 50%
c. 75%
d. 87.5%

73. According to the NRC, a written directive is required for the administration of all of the following radiopharmaceuticals *except*:

a. 25 mCi [^{131}I]sodium iodide
b. 20 mCi [^{18}F]FDG
c. 15 mCi [^{32}P]sodium phosphate
d. 10 mCi [^{89}Sr]chloride

74. According to NRC regulations, the annual occupational dose limit to any organ or tissue other than the eye is:

a. 50 mSv
b. 5 mSv
c. 15 rem
d. 50 rem

75. According to NRC regulations, which of the following cannot be disposed of in the sewage system?

a. disposable diaper of a child who has received ^{67}Ga
b. feces from a patient who received ^{131}I therapy
c. unused [^{123}I]sodium iodide capsules
d. urine from a renal test

76. In performing a room survey with an end-window G–M counter, the technologist should *first*:

a. measure the room background
b. perform a battery check on the counter
c. measure each area designated on the survey diagram
d. perform a wipe test on each designated area

77. What is the maximum exposure rate that can be measured with the G–M meter shown below?

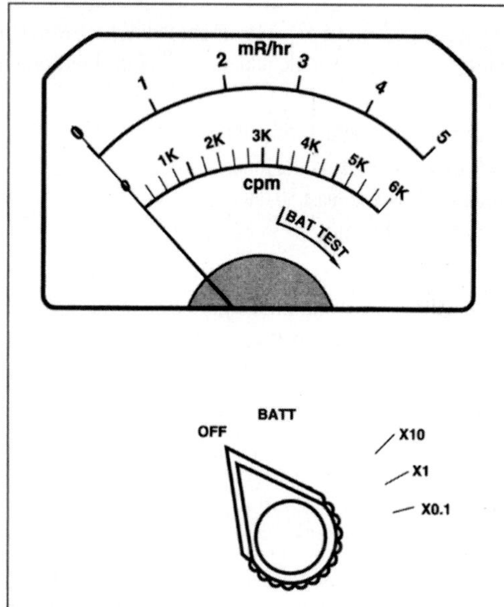

a. 5 mR/hr
b. 50 mR/hr
c. 500 mR/hr
d. 5000 mR/hr

78. A technologist monitors the empty carton from a shipment of [^{131}I]sodium iodide. The container measures 0.08 mR/hr, and room background measures 0.07 mR/hr. The technologist should next:

a. obliterate any radiation symbols and dispose of the container in regular trash
b. dispose of the container as radioactive waste
c. wipe test the container for contamination
d. notify the NRC

79. According to NRC regulations, in what areas can radioxenon be administered?

a. in any room that can be closed off with doors
b. only in rooms that have xenon alarm systems
c. only in imaging rooms that can be negatively pressurized
d. in any room where a G–M detector is available to use

80. When can a decay factor be used to calibrate a unit dosage in place of measuring the dosage in a dose calibrator?

a. A dose calibrator must be used to measure every dosage.
b. Only if a unit dosage was not manipulated after preparation and calibration.
c. Only if the dosage contains ^{99m}Tc.
d. Only if the dosage contains less than 1 mCi activity.

81. A patient received 5 mCi of [^{131}I]sodium iodide for treatment of hyperthyroidism. The patient should adhere to all of the following instructions *except*:

a. minimize close contact with others
b. wash hands after using the toilet
c. remain at home at least 30 days
d. drink plenty of liquids

82. After a ^{99m}Tc spill, decontamination procedures have not been able to remove all of the spilled material. If the current exposure rate is 32 mR/hr, how long will it take for the exposure rate to drop to 2 mR/hr?

a. 16 hr
b. 18 hr
c. 24 hr
d. 30 hr

83. If a patient must be hospitalized in isolation after receiving a high activity of ^{131}I, which of the following signs must be placed on the door of the isolation room?

a. "Authorized Personnel Only"
b. sign noting the length of time a visitor may stay in the room
c. "Reverse Isolation Procedures Required"
d. sign-in sheet to record name and age of each visitor

84. How soon after a medical event has occurred must the NRC be notified?

a. telephone notification no later than the following calendar day
b. telephone notification within 72 hr
c. written report within 5 regular workdays
d. written report within 30 calendar days

85. According to the NRC, written instructions must be provided to a patient who has received radionuclide therapy when:

a. the patient is a female of childbearing age
b. the patient resides with children younger than 18 years of age
c. another individual may receive an exposure greater than 0.1 rem from the patient
d. every patient must receive instructions, regardless of dosage

86. Which of the following statements about the shielding method of performing a dose calibrator linearity test is *true*?

a. When the shields are first used, the decay method must be used to confirm their accuracy.
b. Only a few microcuries of radioactivity are needed to perform the test.
c. Linearity must be tested more frequently if this method is used.
d. A different source activity is required for each shield combination.

87. The following dose calibrator constancy test results were obtained with a ^{57}Co reference source:

Radionuclide setting	Measured value	Calculated value
^{57}Co	56.6 μCi	57.8 μCi
^{99m}Tc	59.2 μCi	58.7 μCi
^{123}I	46.9 μCi	51.7 μCi
^{201}Tl	47.9 μCi	53.5 μCi

Which of the following measured values fall within the limits according to the standard of practice?

a. ^{57}Co, ^{99m}Tc, ^{123}I, ^{201}Tl
b. ^{57}Co, ^{99m}Tc, ^{123}I
c. ^{99m}Tc, ^{123}I, ^{201}Tl
d. ^{57}Co, ^{99m}Tc

88. Based on the graph shown here:

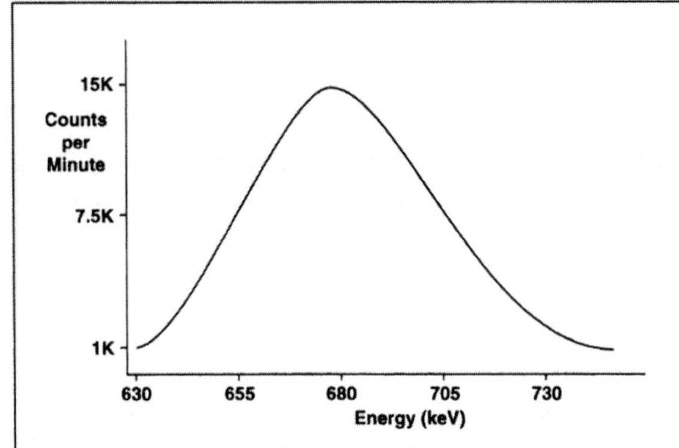

the full width at half maximum (FWHM) is:

a. 50 keV
b. 680 keV
c. 7500 cpm
d. 15,000 cpm

89. To perform a constancy test on a dose calibrator that is being used in a general nuclear medicine imaging department, the best choice of radionuclide settings on which to count the reference standard would include which of the following?

a. ^{123}I, ^{125}I, ^{131}I
b. ^{125}I, ^{57}Co, ^{137}Cs
c. ^{99m}Tc, ^{201}Tl, ^{123}I
d. ^{57}Co, ^{137}Cs, ^{131}I

90. The scintillation camera quality control image shown here:

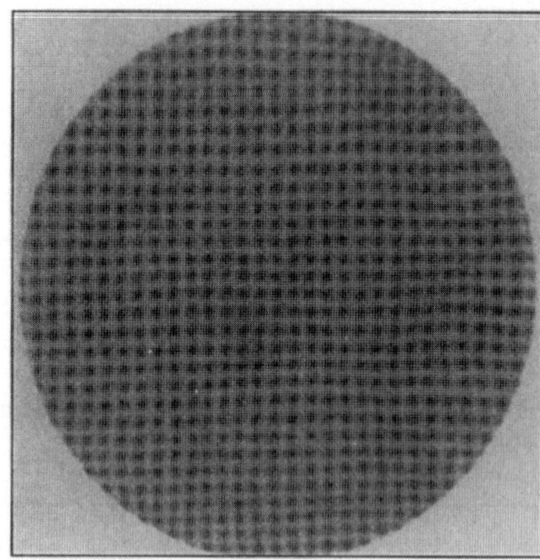

was obtained with which of the following transmission phantoms?

a. four-quadrant bar
b. Hine–Duley
c. orthogonal hole
d. parallel-line equal-space (PLES)

91. The following data were obtained during a dose calibrator accuracy test:

Radionuclide	Calculated value	Measured value
^{57}Co	80.6 μCi	71.0 μCi
^{137}Cs	62.3 μCi	55.9 μCi

On the basis of these results, which of the following statements is *true*?

a. The wrong radionuclides were used to perform this test.
b. Insufficient radioactivity was used to perform this test.
c. The instrument should be repaired or replaced.
d. The instrument accurately measures radionuclides of different energies.

92. Which of the following filters is a high-pass filter?

a. Butterworth
b. Hanning
c. Parzen
d. Ramp

93. In quantitating scintillation camera detector uniformity, the central field of view (CFOV) is defined as the diameter of the useful field of view (UFOV) times:

a. 0.75
b. 0.5
c. 0.33
d. 0.25

94. When the heart rate is 95 beats/min, what is the length of an average R–R interval?

a. 0.5 sec
b. 0.63 sec
c. 1 sec
d. 1.6 sec

95. To perform pixel calibration, two capillary sources are placed on the camera surface 15 cm apart. From an image acquired using a 128 × 128 matrix, an activity profile is generated on the computer. If the profile shows that there are 45 pixels between the two activity peaks, the pixel size is:

a. 0.02 cm
b. 0.33 cm
c. 3 cm
d. 42 cm

96. Coincidence loss is likely to occur when using a well counter if the:

a. energy of the radionuclide is below 50 keV
b. energy of the radionuclide is above 300 keV
c. activity of the source is below 1 μCi
d. activity of the source is above 2 mCi

97. To assure a maximum error of 2% at the 95% confidence level, all samples that are measured in a well counter should be counted for a time interval that produces at least:

a. 10,000 counts
b. 5000 counts
c. 1000 cpm
d. 500 cpm

98. If a ^{137}Cs source used to determine constancy of a dose calibrator was originally calibrated to contain 200 μCi on June 1, 1998, what would be the expected activity of the source on June 1, 2002 (1-year decay factor of 0.977; 2-year decay factor of 0.955)?

a. 195.4 μCi
b. 191.0 μCi
c. 186.6 μCi
d. 182.4 μCi

99. A ^{57}Co source used to determine dose calibrator constancy was originally calibrated to contain 325.8 μCi 35 days ago. If the source is measured today, the dose calibrator reading must fall within what range of activities to meet the accepted standard?

Days	^{57}Co decay factor
1	0.997
2	0.995
3	0.992
4	0.990
5	0.987
10	0.975
20	0.95
30	0.926
40	0.902

a. 238.2–357 μCi
b. 268.0–327.6 μCi
c. 271.5–331.9 μCi
d. 280.3–342.7 μCi

100. It has been determined that a correction factor of 1.15 must be used when a 5-mL syringe containing about 25 mCi is measured in a particular dose calibrator. If a unit dosage activity reads 26.2 mCi, what is the true activity?

a. 22.7 mCi
b. 25.1 mCi
c. 27.4 mCi
d. 30.1 mCi

Examination 3

1. Static bone imaging is performed several hours after tracer administration to permit:

a. maximum tracer uptake in the skeleton
b. blood clearance of excess tracer
c. tracer clearance from sites of infiltration
d. tracer clearance from normal bone tissue

2. For which of the following clinical indications would limited bone imaging ("spot" views) be most appropriate?

a. evaluate temporomandibular joint pain
b. evaluate Paget's disease
c. rule out skeletal metastases
d. history of child abuse; rule out occult fractures

3. Three- or four-phase bone imaging is particularly useful when which of the following conditions is suspected?

a. skeletal metastases
b. osteoporosis
c. osteomyelitis
d. stress fracture

4. The standard views performed in a lung perfusion study are:

a. anterior and posterior only
b. posterior and obliques only
c. anterior, posterior, and lateral of the affected lung
d. anterior, posterior, laterals, and obliques

5. Upon completion of an imaging procedure, the patient sits up quickly and complains of dizziness and feeling faint. The most appropriate action for the technologist would be to:

a. talk with the patient and have the patient breathe slowly and deeply
b. check vital signs
c. have the patient lie down again
d. have the patient stand and walk around the room

6. All of the following statements about performing a lung ventilation study with [^{99m}Tc]pentetate aerosol are *true, except*:

a. multiple projections may be obtained with one dose of tracer
b. the patient is disconnected from the nebulizer after inhalation of the aerosol
c. the patient is imaged while inhaling particles from the nebulizer
d. the face mask, tubing, and nebulizer must be disposed of as radioactive waste

7. The purpose of wrapping the legs with elastic bandages before performing a radionuclide venogram with [^{99m}Tc]MAA is to:

a. distend the veins in the feet
b. suppress superficial circulation
c. prevent blood clots from traveling to the lung
d. trap the tracer in the lower extremities

8. When the radiation level coming from a radioiodine therapy patient in isolation is measured, it should be measured:

a. every day
b. every day at the same time
c. at the same distance from the patient each time
d. every day and at the same distance from the patient each time

9. The function of a draw sheet is to provide:

a. warmth to the patient during the procedure
b. support for the patient during a stretcher to bed transfer
c. protection from infectious disease
d. patient privacy during an imaging procedure

10. A gated equilibrium ventricular function study can be performed with which of the following ^{99m}Tc-labeled tracers?

a. pentetate
b. medronate
c. pyrophosphate
d. human serum albumin

11. Which of the following diagrams is a correctly labeled representative slice of the horizontal long axis of the left ventricular myocardium?

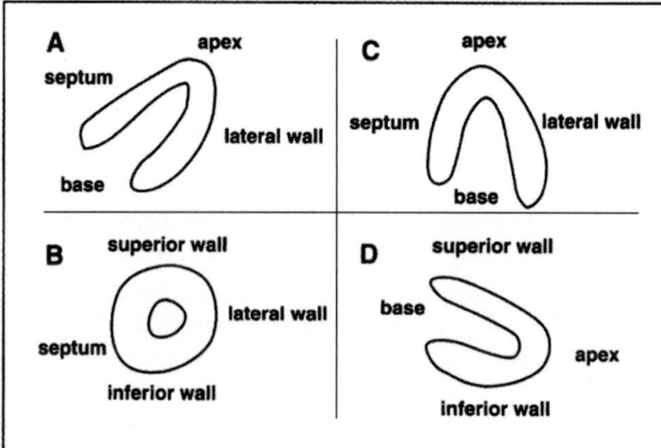

12. Stress–rest myocardial imaging performed with [^{99m}Tc]sestamibi requires two administrations of tracer, because the tracer:

a. does not redistribute once it has been taken up by the myocardium
b. rapidly washes out of the myocardium after administration
c. has too short a half-life to permit delayed imaging
d. must be administered immediately after its preparation

13. In a normal hepatobiliary study, which of the following structures will *not* be visualized?

a. liver
b. spleen
c. common bile duct
d. gallbladder

14. In preparation for hepatobiliary imaging, patients are required to fast to:

a. prevent renal uptake of the tracer
b. enhance liver uptake of the tracer
c. avoid stimulating the gallbladder
d. minimize the risk of radioactive emesis

15. To determine the patency of a LeVeen shunt, the radiopharmaceutical is administered into:

a. a vein
b. the peritoneal cavity
c. the intrathecal space
d. the shunt tubing

16. Which of the following is the correct patient/camera positioning for imaging a transplanted kidney?

	Patient position	Camera placement
a.	Upright	Anterior
b.	Upright	Posterior
c.	Supine	Anterior
d.	Supine	Posterior

17. In performing an effective renal plasma flow determination, the injection site should be imaged to:

a. quantitate the amount of tracer deposited at the injection site
b. rule out tracer infiltration
c. calculate the amount of injected activity
d. correct the kidney transit time of the tracer

18. Radionuclide cystography performed by the direct method requires which of the following?

a. intravenous injection of the tracer
b. use of a renal agent
c. catheterization of the patient
d. administration of furosemide

19. All of the following conditions may demonstrate uptake of ^{111}In-labeled leukocytes *except*:

a. osteomyelitis
b. dental abscess
c. pulmonary embolism
d. ostomy site

20. Signs/symptoms that a patient is going into anaphylactic shock include all of the following *except*:

a. hot, dry skin
b. pallor
c. restlessness
d. tachycardia

21. Which of the following radiopharmaceuticals crosses the intact blood–brain barrier?

a. [^{99m}Tc]bicisate
b. [^{99m}Tc]gluceptate
c. [^{99m}Tc]pentetate
d. [^{99m}Tc]pertechnetate

22. The patency of ventriculoperitoneal shunts may be assessed with which of the following tracers?

a. [^{111}In]chloride
b. [^{99m}Tc]pertechnetate
c. [^{99m}Tc]bicisate
d. [^{99m}Tc]MAA

23. According to the FDA, written informed consent must be obtained to administer which of the following radiopharmaceuticals?

a. [^{123}I]sodium iodide
b. [^{99m}Tc]sestamibi
c. [^{99m}Tc]bicisate
d. any IND

24. Patient preparation for [^{89}Sr]chloride therapy includes all of the following *except*:

a. nuclear medicine bone imaging
b. complete blood count
c. discontinuation of pain medication
d. renal function studies

25. Patient preparation for ^{131}I therapy for thyroid cancer includes all of the following *except*:

a. ruling out pregnancy
b. administering oral potassium iodide
c. reviewing isolation requirements
d. discontinuing breast-feeding

26. One verification method used to ensure that the correct radiopharmaceutical is being administered is to check the label found on the vial. The best times to check this label would include all of the following *except*:

a. before the vial is removed from the shelf
b. before the radiopharmaceutical is dispensed
c. after the vial is placed back on the shelf
d. after the radiopharmaceutical is administered to the patient

27. When dual-radionuclide myocardial perfusion imaging is performed, which of the following tracers is used for stress and which for rest?

	Stress	Rest
a.	[^{99m}Tc]Sestamibi	[^{201}Tl]Thallous chloride
b.	[^{201}Tl]Thallous chloride	[^{99m}Tc]Sestamibi
c.	[^{99m}Tc]Sestamibi	[^{99m}Tc]Teboroxime
d.	[^{99m}Tc]Sestamibi	^{99m}Tc-labeled red blood cells

28. If [^{99m}Tc]sulfur colloid is administered to demonstrate gastrointestinal bleeding, the bleeding can be best visualized how long after the radiopharmaceutical is administered?

a. 10–15 min
b. 20–30 min
c. 45 min–1 hr
d. Anytime up to 24 hr

29. Which of the following areas is the recommended injection site for a cardiac first-pass study?

a. median basilic vein
b. cephalic vein
c. axillary vein
d. dorsal vein

30. Patient preparation for a ^{131}I therapy includes:

a. having a low-iodine diet for 1 week prior to the therapy
b. having a high-iodine diet for 1 week prior to the therapy
c. consuming a low-carbohydrate diet for 3 days prior to the therapy
d. not consuming any salt for 1 week prior to the therapy

31. For a ^{67}Ga infection imaging, the proper route of administration of the radiopharmaceutical is what?

a. intravenously
b. intramuscularly
c. orally
d. by inhalation

32. Which of the following statements best describes the preferred injection and blood sampling site(s) when performing a plasma volume?

a. A butterfly placed in an antecubital vein should be used for injection of the radiopharmaceutical and subsequent blood sampling.
b. Intravenous injection should be performed in an antecubital vein, and subsequent blood samples should be obtained from the same vein.
c. Intravenous injection should be performed in an antecubital vein, and subsequent blood samples should be obtained from a different antecubital vein in the same arm.
d. Intravenous injection should be performed in an antecubital vein in one arm, and subsequent blood samples should be obtained from an antecubital vein in the opposite arm.

33. When administering an intravenous injection, the needle should be inserted into the vein at an angle of:

a. 90°
b. 45°
c. 15°
d. 5°

34. When counting ^{51}Cr red blood cell samples in a scintillation well counter, the window should be set around the photopeak at:

a. 81 keV
b. 159 keV
c. 320 keV
d. 511 keV

35. Which tomographic plane of the heart displays all walls of the left ventricle?

a. horizontal long axis
b. short axis
c. transaxial
d. vertical long axis

36. When performing a radioiodine thyroid uptake with an uptake probe, the most appropriate collimator to use is a:

a. low-energy, high-sensitivity parallel-hole collimator
b. converging collimator
c. straight-bore collimator
d. flat field collimator

37. Which of the following would *not* be in accordance with electrical safety guidelines?

a. use of three-pronged plugs and outlets
b. disconnecting an electrical plug from the wall by pulling on the cord
c. keeping walk areas free from electrical cords
d. not using frayed or kinked cords

38. Which of the following statements about the image of a left ventricle slice shown here is correct?

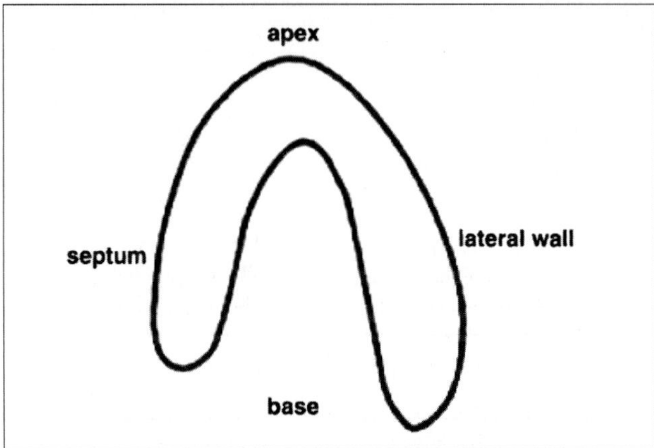

a. It is a correctly labeled image of a horizontal long-axis slice.
b. It is an incorrectly labeled image of a horizontal long-axis slice.
c. It is a correctly labeled image of a vertical long-axis slice.
d. It is an incorrectly labeled image of a vertical long-axis slice.

39. When using [^{18}F]FDG for PET imaging a consideration must be made for which of the following being a contraindication for performing the study?

a. blood glucose level of 200 mg/dL
b. blood glucose level of 120 mg/dL
c. high-iodine diet within past week
d. low-iodine diet within past week

40. A 1:25 dilution of a solution with a concentration of 10 μCi/mL is prepared. What is the tracer concentration in the dilution?

a. 0.04 μCi/mL
b. 0.25 μCi/mL
c. 0.4 μCi/mL
d. 2.5 μCi/mL

41. In preparation for [^{18}F]fluorodeoxyglucose (FDG) imaging, patients are required to fast to:

a. prevent hypoglycemic episodes
b. enhance cardiac uptake
c. maximize tumor uptake
d. eliminate the need for laxatives

42. Which of the following steps is performed before the administration of [^{90}Y]ibritumomab tiuxetan therapy?

a. determine PSA level
b. fasting for 8 hr
c. whole-body imaging with [^{111}In]ibritumomab tiuxetan
d. intravenous hydration for 4 hr

43. The size of a ^{99}Mo/^{99m}Tc generator is expressed as the total activity of:

a. ^{99}Mo on the column
b. ^{99m}Tc on the column
c. ^{99m}Tc eluted from the column
d. decay-corrected ^{99m}Tc available at time of elution

44. If 1.2 Ci of ^{99m}Tc are eluted from a generator in a 5.7-mL volume, what is the concentration of the eluate?

a. 210 mCi/mL
b. 475 mCi/mL
c. 32.4 MBq/mL
d. 5.7 GBq/mL

45. If 633 mCi are expected to be eluted from a wet-column generator, what volume evacuated vial should be used to obtain an eluate concentration of approximately 30 mCi/mL?

a. 5 mL
b. 10 mL
c. 15 mL
d. 20 mL

46. The maximum allowable limit of Al^{3+} in ^{99m}Tc eluate is set by the:

a. Nuclear Regulatory Commission
b. U.S. Pharmacopeia
c. Environmental Protection Agency
d. U.S. Department of Transportation

47. If the following measurements were obtained from an assay of ^{99m}Tc eluate:

^{99}Mo, 8 μCi
^{99m}Tc, 652 mCi

then the ^{99}Mo concentration in 1 mCi of ^{99m}Tc is:

a. 81.5 μCi/mCi
b. 8.0 μCi/mCi
c. 0.012 μCi/mCi
d. 0.000012 μCi/mCi

48. Increased levels of Al^{3+} in ^{99m}Tc eluate used to prepare [^{99m}Tc]sulfur colloid may cause the tracer to concentrate in the:

a. liver
b. lungs
c. red blood cells
d. thyroid

49. Which of the following radiopharmaceuticals may be ordered to treat bone pain caused by bony metastases?

a. [^{131}I]sodium iodide
b. [^{111}In]oxine
c. [^{32}P]chromic phosphate
d. [^{153}Sm]lexidronam

50. According to NRC regulations, reports of medical events sent to the NRC must include all of the following information *except*:

a. whether the patient or a relative was notified
b. a description of the incident
c. the referring physician's name
d. the patient's name

51. All of the following radiopharmaceuticals are prepared with reduced [^{99m}Tc]pertechnetate *except*:

a. [^{99m}Tc]sulfur colloid
b. ^{9}[^{99m}Tc]oxidronate
c. [^{99m}Tc]macroaggregated albumin
d. [^{99m}Tc]lidofenin

52. What is the approximate final concentration of the [^{99m}Tc]sulfur colloid if 125 mCi are prepared using the following reagents?

Sulfur colloid kit
Reaction vial: 0.5 mL acid
Syringe A: 1.1 mL thiosulfate mixture
Syringe B: 2.1 mL buffer
Maximum activity to be added: 400 mCi
^{99m}Tc volume to be added: 0.5–5.0 mL

[^{99m}Tc]pertechnetate
Concentration: 26.7 mCi/mL
Total volume: 8.0 mL

a. 14.9 mCi/mL
b. 15.8 mCi/mL
c. 21.3 mCi/mL
d. 33.8 mCi/mL

53. On the basis of the USP criteria, which of the following statements about the particle size of MAA preparations is *true*?

a. No particles should exceed 90 μm in diameter.
b. Some particles may be smaller than 10 μm.
c. All particles have the same diameter.
d. Up to 10% of the particles may exceed 150 μm in diameter.

54. An eluate of [^{99m}Tc]pertechnetate is assayed for ^{99}Mo contamination immediately after elution. If the ^{99}Mo breakthrough is determined to be 0.035 μCi ^{99}Mo/mCi ^{99m}Tc and the shelf life of the eluate is 12 hr, for how many hours after elution can the [^{99m}Tc]pertechnetate be administered to patients?

a. 6 hr
b. 8 hr
c. 12 hr
d. 18 hr

55. The radiochemical purity of a radiopharmaceutical is determined using a solvent/support media combination with the R_f values shown here:

Radiopharmaceutical: 0
Radiochemical impurity: 1.0

After the radiochromatography strip is developed and cut in half, the solvent front half of the strip counted 15,345 cpm and the origin half of the strip counted 55,632 cpm. What is the radiochemical purity of the sample?

a. 21.6%
b. 27.6%
c. 72.4%
d. 78.4%

56. On the basis of the radiopharmaceutical vial label information shown here, which of the preparations should the technologist administer on July 9 at 0800 to perform three-phase bone imaging?

	Vial	Radiopharmaceutical	Assay time/date	Expiration time/date
a.	A	[^{99m}Tc]Bicisate	0700/July 9	1900/July 9
b.	B	[^{99m}Tc]Medronate	0600/July 8	1400/July 8
c.	C	[^{99m}Tc]Oxidronate	0600/July 9	1400/July 9
d.	D	[^{99m}Tc]Pertechnetate	0600/July 9	1800/July 9

57. The standard adult dosage of [^{123}I]sodium iodide is 400 μCi ± 10%. On the basis of the vial label information shown here:

Total activity: 1 mCi
Number of capsules: 10
Activity/capsule: 100 μCi/capsule
Calibration: 1200, October 5

how many [^{123}I]sodium iodide capsules should be administered to the patient at 0800 on October 5?

a. four
b. three
c. two
d. The capsules may not be administered until 1200.

58. A technologist needs 185 MBq [^{131}I]sodium iodide solution on November 3. The label on the radiopharmaceutical vial contains the following information:

Total activity: 740 MBq
Total volume: 10 mL
Assay: 1200, October 28

What volume is required to obtain the necessary activity on November 3?

a. 0.42 mL
b. 1.5 mL
c. 4.2 mL
d. 4.6 mL

59. In labeling red blood cells with [^{51}Cr]sodium chromate, which of the following reagents is used to prevent the blood sample from coagulating?

a. ACD solution
b. EDTA
c. heparin
d. sodium fluoride

60. All of the following medications has been shown to interfere with in vivo ^{99m}Tc labeling of red blood cells *except*

a. doxorubicin
b. heparin
c. penicillin
d. lidocaine

61. [^{99m}Tc]pentetate was prepared using the following reagents:

Pentetate kit
Reconstituting volume: 1–8 mL [^{99m}Tc]pertechnetate
Activity range: 3–160 mCi

[^{99m}Tc]Pertechnetate
Concentration: 25.0 mCi/mL
Total volume: 5.0 mL

Which of the following dose calibrator readings would verify that the maximum activity of [^{99m}Tc]pentetate was prepared from the reagents available?

a. 100 mCi
b. 125 mCi
c. 160 mCi
d. 200 mCi

62. In the radiopharmacy laboratory, good radiation protection technique includes all of the following practices *except*

a. wearing disposable gloves when withdrawing unit doses
b. wiping the top of the vial with betadine solution before withdrawing a dose
c. manipulating needles, syringes, and vials containing radioactivity at arm's length
d. using syringe shields when preparing unit doses

63. If [^{99m}Tc]exametazime is prepared at 0900 to label white blood cells, it should be used no later than what time?

a. 0930
b. 1100
c. 1300
d. 1500

64. Upon visual inspection, a vial of [^{99m}Tc]medronate appears to be white and slightly turbid. Which of the following actions should the technologist perform next?

a. Prepare unit doses from the vial.
b. Adjust the pH of the preparation.
c. Prepare another vial of [^{99m}Tc]medronate.
d. Filter the preparation with a membrane filter.

65. On the basis of the chromatography results shown here:

	Origin	Solvent front
System 1	3 μCi HR-Tc	177 μCi [^{99m}Tc]pentetate + [^{99m}Tc]pertechnetate
System 2	275 μCi [^{99m}Tc]pentetate + HR-Tc	15 μCi [^{99m}Tc]pertechnetate

what is the percentage radiochemical impurity of the [^{99m}Tc]pentetate preparation?

a. 6.9%
b. 93.1%
c. 94.8%
d. 98.3%

66. If a 290 μCi/kg dose is needed, approximately how many millicuries should a 95-lb patient receive?

a. 5.8 mCi
b. 11.5 mCi
c. 12.5 mCi
d. 20 mCi

67. Of the following needles, which size is the most likely to cause coring of the rubber closure of a medication vial?

	Gauge	Length
a.	27	3/8 in.
b.	25	3/4 in.
c.	22	1 in.
d.	16	1.5 in.

68. According to NRC regulations, which of the following signs should be posted on the door of a radiopharmacy laboratory in which radiation levels have been measured to be 7.5 mR/hr?

a. No posting is required.
b. "Caution: Radioactive Materials"
c. "Caution: Radiation Area"
d. "Caution: High Radiation Area"

69. To determine the transportation index for a package containing radioactive material, the package must be monitored at:

a. the surface of the package
b. 6 in. from the surface
c. 1 m from the surface
d. 2 m from the surface

70. To comply with NRC regulations, personnel radiation exposure records must be maintained:

a. for 3 years
b. for 5 years
c. for 5 years
d. indefinitely

71. If a point source produces an exposure rate of 50 mR/hr at a distance of 1 foot, at what distance from the source will the exposure rate be reduced to 2 mR/hr?

a. 5 ft
b. 5.5 ft
c. 10 ft
d. 25 ft

72. An occupationally exposed worker who is required to wear a personal radiation monitor must wear it at work *except* when:

a. the worker leaves the nuclear medicine department
b. the worker is personally undergoing a radiographic or nuclear medicine procedure
c. badge readings are likely to exceed allowable limits
d. radiation exposure results from patients who had radioactive materials administered at another facility

73. According to the NRC, a written directive for the administration of 15 mCi of [^{131}I]sodium iodide must include the following information:

a. dosage
b. patient's thyroid uptake value
c. patient's birth date
d. lot number of the radiopharmaceutical

74. According to the NRC, the annual radiation exposure to members of the general public must be limited to no more than:

a. 500 mrem
b. 100 mrem
c. 50 mrem
d. 2 mrem

75. Which of the following materials is the best choice for shielding ^{32}P?

a. lead
b. plastic
c. tungsten
d. No shielding is required for ^{32}P.

76. A technologist is measuring room background with an end-window G–M survey meter. The meter shows the following reading:

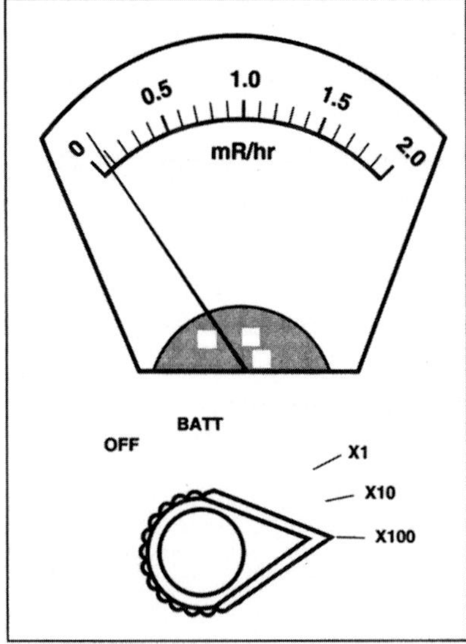

What should the technologist do next?

a. Choose another area of the room to measure background.
b. Record the meter reading as the room background.
c. Adjust the scale of the meter.
d. Recalibrate the survey meter.

77. During a routine room survey for radioactive contamination, a technologist identifies an area on the floor that exceeds the trigger level. Which of the following should the technologist do next?

a. Determine the identity of the radionuclide present in the contaminated area.
b. Ascertain the source of the contamination.
c. Perform a wipe test to determine if the contamination is removable.
d. Cover the area until it has decayed to background level.

78. In the case of a radioactive spill that involves contamination and life-threatening injuries to personnel, which of the following actions should be given priority?

a. decontamination of the victim
b. confinement of the radioactive spill
c. medical treatment of the seriously injured
d. notification of the radiation safety officer

79. Nurses caring for ^{131}I therapy patients who require isolation should be advised that the major sources of contamination include the patient's:

a. feces, urine, and blood
b. urine, saliva, and perspiration
c. blood and urine
d. sputum and blood

80. According to NRC regulations, a technologist cannot use a diagnostic dosage that exceeds 20% of the dosage prescribed by the authorized user unless:

a. there is no other radiopharmaceutical available
b. the patient weighs more than 20% over the standard reference weight
c. the authorized user approves the individual dosage
d. the patient's physician approves the individual dosage

81. If a woman who is breast-feeding needs ^{131}I therapy for treatment of thyroid cancer, how long must she suspend breast-feeding?

a. 48 hr
b. 1 week
c. She may not resume it with this child.
d. Suspension of breast-feeding is not necessary in this case.

82. According to the NRC, wipe test results must be reported as:

a. cpm
b. dpm
c. mR/hr
d. mrem/hr

83. Fifteen mrem is equivalent to how many mSv?

a. 0.0015
b. 0.015
c. 0.15
d. 1.5

84. A package containing radiopharmaceuticals is delivered before the nuclear medicine department opens. According to the NRC, the package must be checked in and monitored:

a. as soon as the department opens
b. within 3 hr after the department opens
c. within 6 hr after the department opens
d. within 24 hr of the time of delivery

85. On the basis of the following data:

Wipe test count: 375 cpm
Background count: 120 cpm

and a well-counter efficiency of 45%, the results of the wipe test in dpm are:

a. 49 dpm
b. 115 dpm
c. 255 dpm
d. 567 dpm

86. On the basis of the graph shown here:

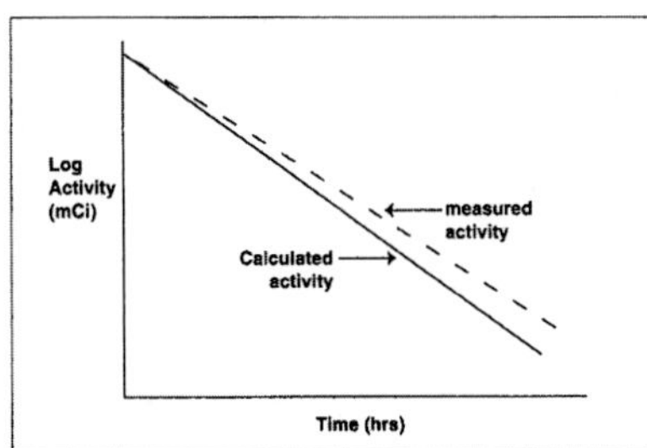

the dose calibrator linearity test results demonstrate that:

a. the instrument is operating linearly over the range of activities measured
b. lower activities are measured as accurately as higher activities
c. the instrument consistently gives higher readings than expected
d. the instrument should be used to measure only millicurie amounts of radioactivity

87. The calibration of a scintillation spectrometer yielded the following data:

Voltage	Net cpm
600	8,010
605	8,830
610	9,543
615	10,998
620	11,523
625	11,175
630	10,789
635	10,111
640	9,514
645	8,912
650	8,246

What is the operating voltage of this instrument?

a. 615
b. 620
c. 625
d. 630

88. An energy resolution test is performed on a scintillation spectrometer using ^{137}Cs. If the full width at half maximum (FWHM) is determined to be 53 keV and the photopeak energy is 662 keV, what is the percentage energy resolution of the instrument?

a. 0.08%
b. 8%
c. 1.3%
d. 12.5%

89. If a dose calibrator linearity test begins by assaying 50 mCi of [^{99m}Tc]pertechnetate, for how long should the test be carried out?

a. 24 hr
b. 48 hr
c. 66 hr
d. 72 hr

90. If a PLES transmission phantom is used, how many images must be acquired to assess linearity over the entire field of view of a scintillation camera?

a. one
b. two
c. three
d. four

91. According to the NRC, all dose calibrator quality control results must be retained for:

a. 1 year
b. 3 years
c. the life of the instrument
d. as long as the facility's license is in effect

92. What is the effect of changing the order of a Butterworth filter from 3 to 5?

a. The image will be smoother.
b. The image will be sharper.
c. The image will appear unchanged.
d. The star artifact will be eliminated.

93. A 256 × 256 matrix requires how much more computer memory than a 64 × 64 matrix?

a. 2 times more
b. 4 times more
c. 8 times more
d. 16 times more

94. Which of the following statements about an image acquired with zoom is *true*?

a. Background counts are increased.
b. Image resolution is increased.
c. More memory is required.
d. Contrast is decreased.

95. If a [^{99m}Tc]medronate bone image and a ^{111}In-tagged white blood cell image are acquired simultaneously with a 128 × 128-word mode matrix, how much computer memory is required to store the images?

a. 16 kB
b. 32 kB
c. 64 kB
d. 128 kB

96. An uptake probe would be used for which of the following studies?

a. plasma volume test
b. red cell mass
c. red cell survival
d. splenic sequestration

97. How much memory will be needed for a gated-equilibrium cardiac function examination that is acquired in 30 frames with a 128 × 128-byte mode matrix?

a. 491,520 bytes
b. 16,384 bytes
c. 3,840 bytes
d. 546 bytes

98. What energies will be accepted by a 15% window placed around a centerline of 159 keV?

a. 135–183 keV
b. 144–174 keV
c. 147–171 keV
d. 151–167 keV

99. A SPECT study is acquired using 60 projections over a 360° rotation. Each projection is acquired for 0.5 min. If the counting rate is 144,000 cpm, how many counts will be collected for the total acquisition?

a. 1,036,800
b. 4,320,000
c. 8,640,000
d. 25,920,000

100. Using a 125-μCi source, 30,500 cpm were collected during a camera sensitivity determination. If the background count is 1,200 cpm, what is the sensitivity of the instrument?

a. 234 cpm/μCi
b. 244 cpm/μCi
c. 29,300 cpm
d. 3,662,500 cpm

Examination 4

1. A [^{99m}Tc]medronate image of the region shown would best demonstrate which of the following structures?

I. iliac crests
II. distal femur
III. ischium
IV. thoracic vertebrae 10–12

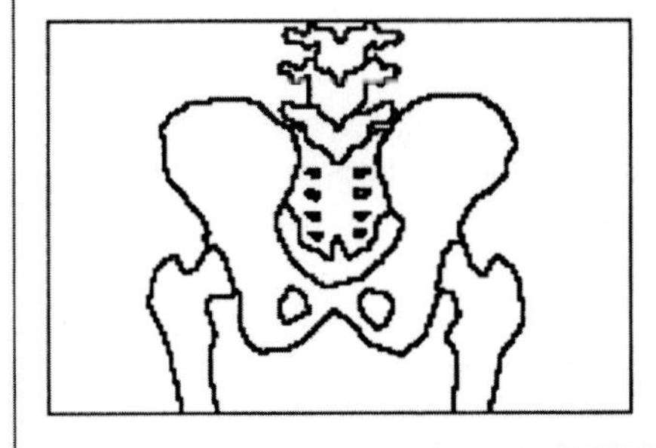

a. III only
b. I and III only
c. III and IV only
d. I, III, and IV only

2. In performing a bone image, which of the following views would best demonstrate an abnormality in the calcaneus?

a. lateral views of the patella
b. postvoid image of the pelvis
c. plantar view of the feet
d. anterior view of the distal humerus and radius

3. All of the following statements about four-phase bone imaging are *true, except*:

a. this study includes both dynamic and static imaging
b. the study may be performed with any blood pool agent
c. the patient is positioned under the camera before tracer administration
d. the third phase is performed 5–6 hr after tracer administration

4. Which of the following patients should receive fewer particles than typically administered for lung perfusion imaging?

a. 80-year-old woman with suspected pulmonary embolism
b. 65-year-old man with chronic obstructive pulmonary disease
c. 45-year-old man with right-to-left cardiac shunt
d. 25-year-old woman with asthma

5. Which of the following statements about the wash-in/washout method for performing xenon ventilation studies is *true*?

a. The patient rebreathes a mixture of xenon and oxygen during the wash-in phase.
b. The patient can be disconnected from the gas-trapping apparatus after the wash-in phase.
c. This method is not recommended for comatose patients.
d. It is not necessary to introduce oxygen or air into the xenon delivery system.

6. After the administration of [^{99m}Tc]pentetate aerosol with a face mask, radioactive contamination is likely to be found in all of the following areas *except*:

a. on the floor between the patient and nebulizer
b. around the patient's mouth
c. on the patient's chest
d. on the technologist's hands

7. Thyroid imaging may be performed with which of the following radiopharmaceuticals?

a. [^{99m}Tc]pertechnetate
b. [^{123}I]sodium iodide
c. [^{99m}Tc]sestamibi
d. [^{99m}Tc]pertechnetate or [^{123}I]sodium iodide

8. When performing a radioiodine thyroid uptake, nonthyroidal (body) background measurements may be taken over the:

a. lateral skull
b. mediastinum
c. abdomen
d. thigh

9. Pulse rates may be determined by all of the following methods *except*:

a. multiplying the respiration rate by 4
b. using a pulse oximeter
c. listening to the heart with a stethoscope
d. analyzing the electrocardiogram

10. Which of the following statements regarding the administration of oxygen is *false*?

a. Oxygen is classified as a drug.
b. Oxygen therapy may be ordered by a physician, nurse, athletic trainer, or respiratory therapist.
c. With the consent of a physician or nurse, an oxygen appliance may be removed from the patient if it interferes with the imaging procedure.
d. Orders for oxygen therapy must include the amount to be delivered, the type of oxygen appliance to be used, and whether administration is to be continuous or intermittent.

11. Treatment of the adverse effects induced by dipyridamole involves the administration of:

a. adenosine
b. aminophylline
c. acetazolamide
d. nitroglycerin

12. Which of the following must be discontinued for at least 24–36 hr before the administration of dipyridamole?

a. water
b. aspirin
c. insulin
d. theophylline

13. In a normal hepatobiliary study, excretion of the tracer into the intestine should occur a maximum of how long after tracer administration?

a. 5–10 min
b. 20–30 min
c. 45–60 min
d. 1–2 hr

14. Which of the following agents would be used to perform a gallbladder ejection fraction?

a. sincalide and [^{99m}Tc]disofenin
b. sincalide and [^{99m}Tc]sulfur colloid
c. morphine and [^{99m}Tc]lidofenin
d. morphine and [^{99m}Tc]mertiatide

15. For which of the following procedures is the radiopharmaceutical administered orally?

a. gastric emptying
b. gastrointestinal bleeding
c. salivary gland imaging
d. vesicoureteral reflux imaging

16. Patient preparation for functional renal imaging should include which of the following?

a. hydration of the patient
b. discontinuation of all medications
c. fasting for at least 2 hr before imaging
d. administration of furosemide 1 hr before imaging

17. Static renal imaging is performed about how long after the administration of [^{99m}Tc]succimer?

a. immediately
b. 30 min
c. 2 hr
d. 8 hr

18. Patient preparation for [^{67}Ga]citrate imaging may include administration of which of the following?

a. diuretics
b. potassium perchlorate
c. Lugol's solution
d. laxatives

19. A normal biodistribution of ^{111}In-labeled leukocytes will demonstrate the greatest tracer uptake at 24 hr after injection in which of the following sites?

a. bone marrow
b. liver
c. lung
d. spleen

20. A patient with diabetes who becomes hypoglycemic may exhibit all of the following signs and symptoms *except*:

a. weakness and shakiness
b. confusion
c. irritability
d. nausea and vomiting

21. Which of the following tracers may be used to confirm brain death?

a. [^{99m}Tc]exametazime
b. [^{99m}Tc]oxidronate
c. [^{99m}Tc]mertiatide
d. [^{201}Tl]thallous chloride

22. Counting cotton gauze that has been placed in a patient's nose after intrathecal tracer administration is most useful when which of the following conditions is suspected?

a. rhinorrhea
b. hydrocephalus
c. CSF shunt patency
d. blockage of CSF flow

23. Colloidal [^{32}P]chromic phosphate is administered by which of the following routes?

a. intraperitoneal
b. intravenous
c. subcutaneous
d. inhalation

24. Which of the following radiation safety measures should be used when performing ^{89}Sr therapy?

a. use of lead vial and syringe shields
b. urinary catheterization for incontinent patients
c. use of absorbent paper in isolation room
d. monitoring patient radiation levels weekly

25. On the basis of blood flow, which of the following is visualized as an area of high tracer concentration on a brain image performed with [^{99m}Tc]exametazime?

a. gray matter
b. white matter
c. pineal body
d. medulla oblongata

26. A technologist is performing a lung image on a patient known to have active tuberculosis. The most appropriate personal protective device the technologist should utilize is:

a. latex gloves
b. gown
c. lab coat
d. mask

27. The patency of a LeVeen shunt may be demonstrated with which of the following radiopharmaceuticals?

a. [^{99m}Tc]disofenin or [^{99m}Tc]sulfur colloid
b. [^{99m}Tc]MAA or [^{99m}Tc]sulfur colloid
c. [^{99m}Tc]pentetate or [^{99m}Tc]pertechnetate
d. [^{99m}Tc]albumin or ^{99m}Tc-labeled red blood cells

28. Which of the following is common to imaging gastroesophageal reflux in both adults and children?

a. [^{99m}Tc]Sulfur colloid is the tracer of choice.
b. The patient must fast starting at midnight before the test.
c. An abdominal binder is used to increase pressure over the abdomen.
d. The patient ingests dilute hydrochloric acid with the tracer.

29. The following studies are ordered for a patient:

I. ERPF determination
II. total-body bone imaging
III. [^{111}In]pentetreotide imaging

In which order should the studies be performed so that they do not interfere with one another and so that they can be accomplished in the shortest amount of time?

a. I, II, III
b. I, III, II
c. II, I, III
d. III, II, I

30. Historically, the function of intrinsic factor administered during a Schilling test was to:

a. increase urine output
b. facilitate the absorption of vitamin B_{12}
c. saturate the body's vitamin B_{12} storage sites
d. relieve patient anxiety

31. The region(s) of interest for detection of a left-to-right cardiac shunt is (are) drawn around which of the following structures?

a. superior vena cava
b. one or both lungs
c. left ventricle
d. right ventricle and great vessels

32. Which of the following sets of vital signs measurements represent normal values for an adult?

	Pulse (bpm)	Blood pressure (mm Hg)	Respirations (resp/min)	Temperature (oral, °F)
a.	45	85/45	10	97
b.	60	100/50	12	98.6
c.	75	120/80	17	98.6
d.	100	150/100	25	102

33. A common antecubital vein used for intravenous administration of a radiopharmaceutical is the:

a. cephalic
b. radial
c. brachial
d. ulnar

34. The ^{51}Cr red cell sequestration study is performed to identify abnormal destruction of red blood cells by the:

a. bone marrow
b. heart
c. liver
d. spleen

35. The difference in hematocrit values between the average whole-body hematocrit and the venous hematocrit is the result of:

a. the difference in vessel size
b. the variation in red blood cell diameter
c. the increased amount of blood in the extremities
d. plasma leakage

36. On the basis of the following counts per minute obtained from a thyroid uptake test:

Thyroid: 2876
Patient background: 563
Standard: 10,111
Room background: 124

the percentage radioiodine uptake is:

a. 3.5%
b. 4.3%
c. 23%
d. 28%

37. A technologist is asked to check the flow rate on a drip infusion on a patient in the department. An acceptable flow rate is how many drops per minute?

a. 1–5
b. 10–20
c. 40–60
d. 75–100

38. The total blood volume may be calculated by dividing the measured red cell volume by the:

a. hematocrit
b. plasmacrit
c. corrected hematocrit
d. corrected plasmacrit

39. The following data were collected for a plasma volume determination:

Net standard counts: 839,621 cpm
Standard dilution factor: 15
Net plasma counts: 2,528 cpm/mL

The calculated plasma volume in milliliters is:

a. 2214
b. 3321
c. 4516
d. 4982

40. If the concentration of a 1:2,000 dilution is 0.05 μCi/mL, what is the tracer concentration of the original solution?

a. 0.00025 μCi/mL
b. 10 μCi/mL
c. 25 μCi/mL
d. 100 μCi/mL

41. A patient scheduled for [^{18}F]FDG imaging has a measured blood glucose level of 100 mg/dL. Which of the following actions should the technologist perform next?

a. Reschedule the patient for a later time.
b. Administer insulin to lower the patient's blood glucose level.
c. Administer glucose to raise the patient's blood glucose level.
d. Proceed with the examination.

42. Based on the net counts shown here, what is the percentage gallbladder ejection fraction?

Maximum gallbladder counts: 185,632
Minimum gallbladder counts: 77, 203

a. 71%
b. 58%
c. 41%
d. 29%

43. After a ^{99}Mo/^{99m}Tc generator is eluted, it takes approximately how many hours for the ^{99m}Tc activity to build up to a maximum level?

a. 8 hr
b. 12 hr
c. 24 hr
d. the secular generator can be eluted only once

44. What is the total activity of 8 mL of ^{99m}Tc eluate that has a concentration of 2.0 MBq/mL?

a. 4 MBq
b. 6 MBq
c. 10 MBq
d. 16 MBq

45. A wet-column generator is equipped with all of the following parts *except* a(n):

a. alumina column
b. lead shield
c. charging port
d. collection port

46. According to the USP, the maximum allowable aluminum concentration in ^{99m}Tc eluate is not to exceed:

a. 0 μg/mL
b. 10 μg/mL
c. 20 μg/mL
d. 10 mg/mL

47. Which of the following statements about determining ^{99}Mo concentration in ^{99m}Tc eluate using the lead shield method is *true*?

a. The eluate is assayed only for ^{99}Mo.
b. The lead shield is used to absorb high-energy ^{99}Mo photons.
c. The unshielded eluate is assayed for ^{99}Mo and ^{99m}Tc by adjusting the dose calibrator settings.
d. The eluate in the lead shield is measured with the dose calibrator set to assay ^{99}Mo.

48. The test kit used to measure aluminum ion concentration in ^{99m}Tc eluate contains specially treated indicator paper and an aluminum solution with a concentration of approximately:

a. 2 μg/mL
b. 5 μg/mL
c. 10 μg/mL
d. 20 μg/mL

49. Which of the following pairs of radiopharmaceuticals may be used to perform lung perfusion and ventilation imaging?

a. [^{99m}Tc]sulfur colloid and [^{99m}Tc]pentetate aerosol
b. [^{99m}Tc]albumin and ^{133}Xe gas
c. [^{99m}Tc]macroaggregated albumin and ^{133}Xe gas
d. [^{99m}Tc]bicisate and [^{99m}Tc]pentetate aerosol

50. An eluate of [^{99m}Tc]pertechnetate is assayed for ^{99}Mo contamination at 0600 with the following results:

^{99}Mo: 15.5 μCi
^{99m}Tc: 250 mCi

At 1000, the eluate is used to prepare a ^{99m}Tc-labeled compound with a shelf life of 8 hr. What is the latest time that the ^{99m}Tc compound may be administered to patients?

a. 1400
b. 1500
c. 1700
d. 1800

51. If the following reagents are available:

Oxidronate kit
Maximum ^{99m}Tc activity to be added: 250 mCi
Reconstituting volume: 1.0–5.0 mL

[^{99m}Tc] Pertechnetate
Concentration: 35.0 mCi/mL
Total volume: 10 mL

what is the maximum amount of [^{99m}Tc]oxidronate (in mCi) that can be prepared from one kit?

a. 35 mCi
b. 175 mCi
c. 250 mCi
d. 350 mCi

52. Which of the following ingredients in a sulfur colloid kit are combined and heated?

a. [^{99m}Tc]pertechnetate and thiosulfate mixture
b. thiosulfate mixture and acid
c. [^{99m}Tc]pertechnetate, thiosulfate mixture, and acid
d. [^{99m}Tc]pertechnetate, thiosulfate mixture, acid, and buffer

53. When preparing to withdraw a unit dose of [^{32}P]chromic phosphate, the technologist visually inspects the radiopharmaceutical and notes that it is a blue-green color. The technologist should next:

a. contact the radiopharmaceutical manufacturer
b. reschedule the procedure
c. withdraw the unit dose
d. place the dose in radioactive waste for disposal

54. What is the concentration of [^{99m}Tc]succimer if 1.5 mL succimer reagent and 30 mCi [^{99m}Tc]pertechnetate (concentration is 18 mCi/mL) are mixed to prepare the radiopharmaceutical?

a. 20 mCi/mL
b. 17.6 mCi/mL
c. 14.3 mCi/mL
d. 9.4 mCi/mL

55. The tagging efficiency of a radiopharmaceutical is determined using the following solvent/support media systems:

	R_f values		
	Radiopharmaceutical	Free pertechnetate	Hydrolyzed-reduced ^{99m}Tc
System 1	0.0	0.9	0.0
System 2	1.0	1.0	0.0

After a chromatography strip containing a sample of the radiopharmaceutical was developed in each solvent, cut in half, and counted, the following results were obtained:

	Counts per minute	
	Solvent front half	Origin half
System 1	1,716 cpm	23,706 cpm
System 2	21,001 cpm	1,200 cpm

What is the tagging efficiency of the sample?

a. 92.8%
b. 87.9%
c. 12.1%
d. 6.7%

56. The label on an unopened vial states that the vial contains 10 mL of radiopharmaceutical with a concentration of 55.5 MBq/mL. When the technologist assays the vial in a dose calibrator, it measures 9 mCi. Which of the following actions should the technologist perform first?

a. Check the radionuclide setting on the dose calibrator.
b. Begin to prepare unit doses from the vial.
c. Perform an accuracy check on the dose calibrator.
d. Contact the radiopharmaceutical manufacturer.

57. A vial of [^{67}Ga]gallium citrate is calibrated to contain 5 mCi at 0600, Pacific Standard Time, on March 8. How much activity does the vial contain on March 9 at 1200, Eastern Standard Time?

a. 6.3 mCi
b. 4.9 mCi
c. 3.9 mCi
d. 3.7 mCi

58. A technologist needs 50 μCi [^{51}Cr]sodium chromate at 0800 on March 15. The label on the radiopharmaceutical vial contains the following information:

Total activity: 2.0 mCi
Total volume: 5.0 mL
Assay: 0600, March 18

What volume is required to obtain the necessary activity on March 15?

a. 0.07 mL
b. 0.12 mL
c. 0.86 mL
d. 1.2 mL

59. In labeling red blood cells with [^{51}Cr]sodium chromate, which of the following components is first added to the ACD solution?

a. [^{51}Cr]sodium chromate
b. blood sample
c. ascorbic acid
d. heparin

60. All of the following are advantages of the in vitro method of labeling red blood cells with [^{99m}Tc]pertechnetate *except*:

a. The red blood cells can be washed to remove substances from the plasma that may interfere with labeling.
b. A commercially manufactured kit that requires no cell separation by centrifugation is available.
c. Higher labeling efficiencies than with the in vivo method are possible.
d. In vitro labeling has the lowest risk of red cell hemolysis.

61. Which of the following equipment is needed to verify the size and number of MAA particles in a [^{99m}Tc]MAA preparation?

a. dose calibrator
b. limulus amebocyte lysate solution
c. chromatography strips, solvent, developing chamber
d. hemocytometer, light microscope

62. According to NRC regulations, records of patient dosage determinations must be retained for how long?

a. 3 years
b. 5 years
c. 10 years
d. indefinitely

63. During red blood cell labeling with ^{51}Cr, the purpose of adding ascorbic acid to the ACD (acid–citrate–dextrose)–whole blood solution is to:

a. prevent hemolysis of the red blood cells
b. maintain the pH of the mixture
c. prevent clot formation
d. reduce the chromate ion to a lower valence state

64. Upon visual inspection, a vial of [^{99m}Tc]MAA has a white, slightly cloudy appearance. Which of the following actions should the technologist perform next?

a. Prepare unit doses from the vial.
b. Prepare another vial of [^{99m}Tc]MAA.
c. Filter the preparation.
d. Adjust the pH of the preparation.

65. On the basis of the chromatography results shown here, what is the percentage radiochemical purity of the [^{99m}Tc]mertiatide preparation?

	Origin	Solvent front
System 1	107.5 μCi [^{99m}TC]mertiatide + HR-Tc	9.2 μCi [^{99m}Tc]pertechnetate
System 2	8.4 μCi HR-Tc	132.6 μCi [^{99m}Tc]mertiatide + HR-Tc

a. 13.9%
b. 86.1%
c. 92.1%
d. 94.0%

66. If an MAA kit contains approximately 6 million particles, what reconstituting volume is required to obtain 500,000 particles in 0.4 mL?

a. 0.03 mL
b. 0.21 mL
c. 4.8 mL
d. 12 mL

67. When assembling a needle and syringe for an intravenous administration, all of the following areas must remain sterile *except* the:

a. outer side of the syringe barrel
b. syringe tip
c. needle shaft
d. needle tip

68. The NRC defines an unrestricted area as one in which an individual will receive less than how many millirems in an hour?

a. 2 mrem
b. 5 mrem
c. 50 mrem
d. 100 mrem

69. A package containing radioactive material is monitored and found to produce 0.4 mR/hr at the surface and no detectable radiation exposure at 1 m from the surface. Which DOT label must be affixed to the outside of the package?

a. "Category I"
b. "Category II"
c. "Category III"
d. No DOT label is required.

70. The NRC requires that all of the following information be included in unit dosage measurement records *except* the:

a. date and time of measurement
b. dose calibrator make and model number
c. patient's name
d. radiopharmaceutical name

71. If the distance between a radiation point source and a survey meter is doubled, the measured radiation exposure rate is reduced:

a. to half of the original exposure rate
b. to one-quarter of the original exposure rate
c. to one-eighth of the original exposure rate
d. unpredictably

72. According to NRC regulations, which of the following radiopharmaceutical administration errors must be reported to the NRC?

a. A patient receives 18 mCi of [^{99m}Tc]pertechnetate when 20–25 mCi was prescribed.
b. A patient scheduled for bone imaging receives 20 mCi of [^{99m}Tc]pertechnetate instead of [^{99m}Tc]medronate.
c. Patient A receives a hepatobiliary scan dosage intended for patient B that results in a 20 rem exposure to the liver.
d. A patient receives a whole-body scan dosage of ^{131}I instead of ^{123}I for a thyroid uptake and scan that exceeds 50 rem exposure to the thyroid.

73. According to the NRC, a written directive for the administration of [^{89}Sr]chloride must include all of the following information *except*:

a. route of administration
b. radiopharmaceutical name
c. patient's Social Security number
d. signature of an authorized user

74. According to the NRC, the radiation dose to the fetus of a declared pregnant worker must not exceed how many rems during the pregnancy?

a. 500 rem
b. 50 rem
c. 5 rem
d. 0.5 rem

75. Which of the following monitoring techniques should be employed to rule out internal contamination after handling a radioiodine solution?

a. thyroid uptake 24 hr after handling the solution
b. urine counts 2–4 hr after handling the solution
c. plasma counts 24 hr after handling the solution
d. pocket dosimeter reading

76. When surveying for contamination, which of the following diagrams depicts the correct position of the probe of an end-window G–M meter in relation to the surface being monitored?

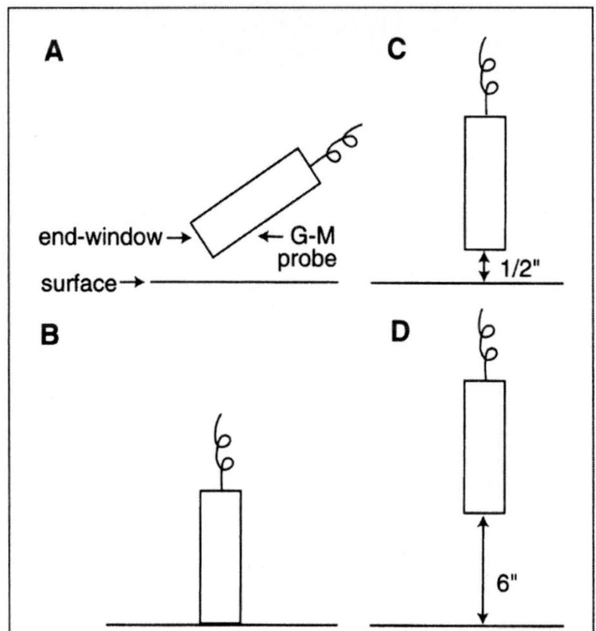

77. According to the NRC, packages with which of the following DOT labels must be checked for contamination using a wipe test?

a. yellow II only
b. white I and yellow II only
c. yellow II and yellow III only
d. white I, yellow II, and yellow III

78. The first step in the decontamination of personnel is to:

a. remove any articles of contaminated personal or protective clothing
b. wash contaminated areas of the skin with soap and water
c. remove the contaminated person from the site of the spill
d. immediately place the contaminated person in a shower

79. According to NRC regulations, a written directive must be retained:

a. for 1 year
b. for 3 years
c. for 5 years
d. indefinitely

80. According to the NRC, patient dosage records must be retained for how many years?

a. 1 year
b. 3 years
c. 5 years
d. as long as the facility's license is in effect

81. If a technologist stands next to a radioactive source that is producing an exposure rate of 0.5 mrem/hr for 20 min, what radiation dose does the technologist receive?

a. 0.17 mrem
b. 0.5 mrem
c. 10 mrem
d. 17 mrem

82. A wipe test gives a reading of 1,240 cpm with a background count of 410 cpm. If the efficiency of the instrument is 35%, what is the wipe test reading in dpm?

a. 35 dpm
b. 290 dpm
c. 2,371 dpm
d. 3,542 dpm

83. Ten millisieverts is equivalent to how many millirems?

a. 0.1
b. 1
c. 100
d. 1000

84. If a technologist received dosimeter readings that are nearly equal to the NRC limits, which of the following is the most appropriate action?

a. The technologist must cease working in a radiation area.
b. The technologist can work in a radiation area but must limit exposure.
c. The RSO must review the technologist's work habits.
d. The RSO must give the technologist a written warning.

85. How often must dose calibrator constancy be performed?

a. annually
b. monthly
c. weekly
d. daily

86. According to the NRC, records of survey meter calibration are retained for how long?

a. 3 years
b. 5 years
c. as long as the instrument is in use
d. as long as the facility license is in effect

87. The γ-ray spectrum shown here was obtained at a voltage of 800.

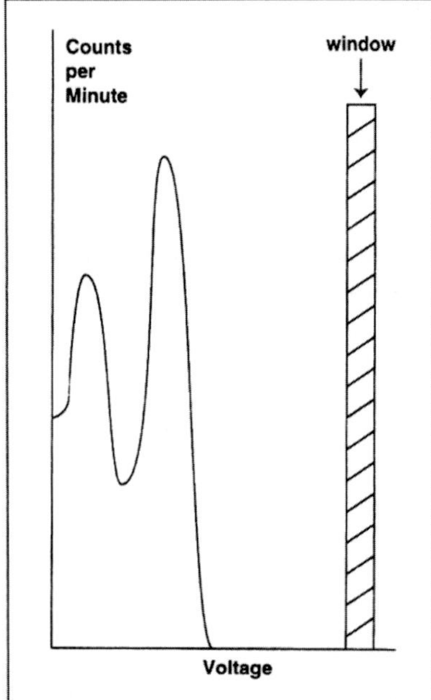

To move the photopeak into the window, which of the following actions should be taken?

a. The voltage should be increased.
b. The voltage should be decreased.
c. The window should be widened.
d. The window should be moved.

88. The following are the results of energy-resolution tests for the last four quarters:

Month	% energy resolution
January	9.5%
April	10.3%
July	10.9%
October	11.1%

According to these data, which of the following statements is *true*?

a. The energy resolution of the instrument is improving.
b. The energy resolution of the instrument is worsening.
c. The results indicate that the instrument should no longer be used.
d. The test should be performed with a different radionuclide.

89. According to the NRC, how often must survey meters be calibrated?

a. daily
b. before each use
c. monthly
d. annually

90. On the basis of the flood image shown here:

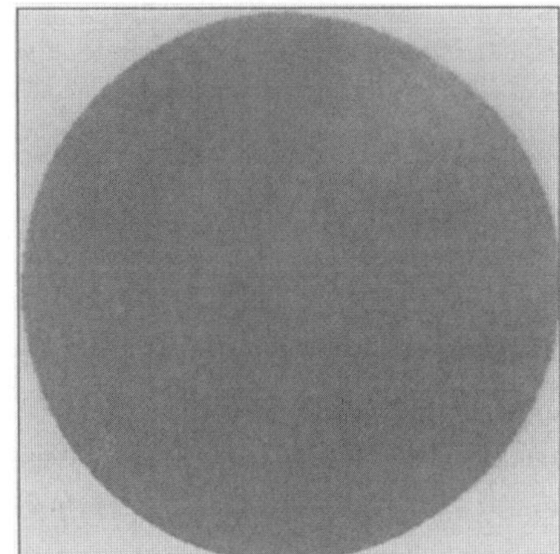

which of the following should the technologist do?

a. Check the radionuclide setting.
b. Reacquire the flood for more counts.
c. Arrange for service immediately.
d. Perform patient studies.

91. The standard of practice dictates that the center of rotation (COR) offset correction be performed how frequently on SPECT cameras?

a. daily
b. weekly
c. monthly
d. quarterly

92. How often should a uniformity flood be acquired on a scintillation camera?

a. daily
b. weekly
c. monthly
d. quarterly

93. Static frame mode acquisition is the most appropriate type of image acquisition for which of the following procedures?

a. first phase of a three-phase bone scan
b. left ventricular ejection fraction determination
c. thyroid imaging
d. renal function imaging

94. Which of the following radionuclide sources is used to acquire a uniformity correction flood?

a. ^{99m}Tc point source with collimator removed
b. ^{57}Co sheet source with collimator removed
c. ^{99m}Tc point source with collimator in place
d. ^{57}Co sheet source with collimator in place

95. It is recommended that high-count uniformity correction flood images be acquired how frequently?

a. daily
b. weekly
c. monthly
d. quarterly

96. Which of the following will increase the resolution of a "spot view" bone image obtained with a parallel-hole collimator?

a. increasing the pulse-height analyzer window width
b. moving the camera closer to the patient's body
c. using a high-sensitivity collimator instead of LEAP collimator
d. using fewer shades of gray to display the image

97. If a Butterworth filter is applied to an image and the order of the filter remains constant, which of the following cutoff frequencies (the frequency at which the filter magnitude drops below 0.5) will result in the smoothest image?

a. 0.50 cycles/pixel
b. 0.42 cycles/pixel
c. 0.33 cycles/pixel
d. 0.15 cycles/pixel

98. When a high activity of a radionuclide is used for a PET scan, image quality is degraded because:

a. deadtime decreases
b. random events increase
c. attenuation increases
d. noise increases

99. If a 20% window is set around a centerline of 364 keV, what energies will be accepted by the pulse-height analyzer?

a. 291–437 keV
b. 328–400 keV
c. 344–384 keV
d. 354–374 keV

100. A technologist changes the collimator on a gamma camera from a low-energy all-purpose collimator to a high-resolution collimator. If the same number of counts is acquired, how will the acquisition time change when the high-resolution collimator is used?

a. The acquisition time will be the same with both collimators.
b. The acquisition time will decrease.
c. The acquisition time will increase.
d. The effect on acquisition time is unpredictable.

Examination 5

1. A [^{99m}Tc]oxidronate image of the region shown would demonstrate all of the following structures *except* the:

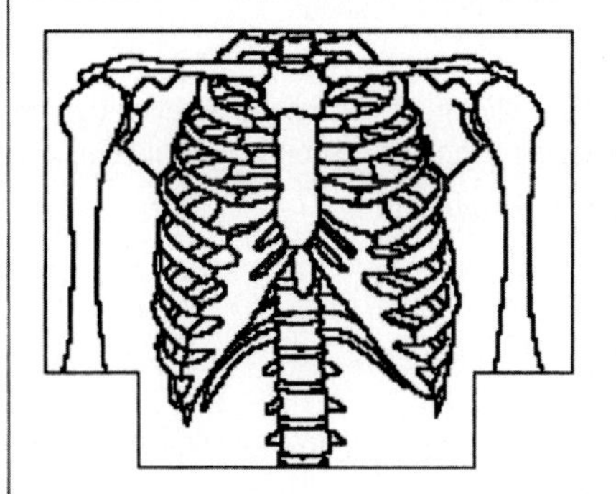

a. costochondral junctions
b. sternum
c. clavicles
d. acromion processes

2. For a patient undergoing bone imaging, all of the following information from the medical history is relevant to the interpretation of the bone image *except*

a. gallbladder sergery a year ago
b. abdominal surgery 10 days ago
c. radiation therapy to the breast 6 months ago
d. results of previous bone imaging procedures

3. If a patient is injected with [^{99m}Tc]MAA while in an upright position, which of the following is most likely to be seen on the perfusion lung images?

a. increased tracer activity in the lung apices
b. decreased tracer activity in the lung apices
c. decreased tracer activity in the lung bases
d. decreased tracer activity throughout both lungs

4. If the usual adult dosage of [^{99m}Tc]MAA is 4 mCi, a patient who has had a right pneumonectomy should receive what dosage?

a. 1 mCi
b. 2 mCi
c. 3 mCi
d. 4 mCi

5. Which one of the following steps would be appropriate during a standby-assist wheelchair transfer?

a. The wheelchair should be perpendicular to the imaging table.
b. The wheelchair footrests should be out of the way.
c. The wheelchair should be placed parallel to the imaging table.
d. The wheelchair should be unlocked.

6. Patient preparation for infection imaging using tagged white blood cells include:

a. fasting for at least 4 hr with a blood glucose level below 120 mg/dL
b. smoking cessation for at least 24 hr
c. discontinuation of certain medications
d. lab work and information concerning recent blood transfusions

7. Thyroid imaging may be performed with which of the following collimators?

a. flat field
b. pinhole
c. parallel hole
d. pinhole or parallel hole

8. In performing a thyroid uptake, a technologist collects the thyroid counts 5 cm from the surface of the patient's neck and the standard counts 20 cm from the surface of the neck phantom. What is the effect on the thyroid uptake value calculated from this data?

a. The uptake value will be accurate.
b. The uptake value will be falsely decreased.
c. The uptake value will be falsely increased.
d. The results are unpredictable.

9. The percentage left ventricular ejection fraction calculated from the net counts per minute shown here:

End diastole: 2,875
End systole: 2,162

is approximately:

a. 13%
b. 25%
c. 33%
d. 75%

10. When a technologist cares for a patient who is not known to have a communicable disease, all of the following infection control measures should be implemented *except*:

a. decontaminating imaging equipment with an antiseptic
b. wearing gloves when collecting a blood sample
c. handwashing before and after the nuclear medicine examination
d. using a needle recapping device

11. Normal sinus rhythm is characterized by which of the following?

I. 60–100 beats/min
II. R wave occurs at constant intervals
III. PR interval 0.12–0.20 sec long

a. I and II only
b. I and III only
c. II and III only
d. I, II, and III

12. After stress myocardial imaging with [^{201}Tl]thallous chloride, 1–1.5 mCi of [^{201}Tl]thallous chloride may be administered before rest myocardial imaging to:

a. improve patient throughput
b. demonstrate reversible ischemia more readily
c. demonstrate infarct size more precisely
d. minimize visualization of attenuation artifacts

13. If the gallbladder is not visualized within 60 min during hepatobiliary imaging, which of the following may be administered?

a. cimetidine
b. morphine
c. dobutamine
d. furosemide

14. Preparation of the patient for Meckel's diverticulum localization includes:

a. the administration of laxatives
b. fasting for at least 2 hr before imaging
c. an enema immediately before imaging
d. oral or intravenous hydration

15. Which of the following ^{99m}Tc-labeled agents is the preferred tracer for demonstrating intermittent gastrointestinal bleeding?

a. human serum albumin
b. lidofenin
c. red blood cells
d. sulfur colloid

16. Furosemide is sometimes administered during renal imaging to:

a. rule out transplant rejection
b. rule out ureteropelvic obstruction
c. enhance tracer uptake in an abnormal kidney
d. increase blood flow to the kidneys

17. Which of the following events is a normal response when furosemide is administered near the end of a renal function study?

a. Radioactivity is cleared from the renal pelvis into the bladder.
b. Radioactivity is taken up into the renal cortex.
c. Mechanical blockages in the renal collecting system are cleared.
d. The peak transit time of the radiopharmaceutical is shortened.

18. Early (6 hr after injection) ^{67}Ga imaging should be performed if which of the following conditions is suspected?

a. sarcoma
b. osteomyelitis
c. lymphoma
d. bronchogenic carcinoma

19. The most effective way of controlling the spread of infectious disease in a hospital setting is for the technologist to:

a. stay home when ill
b. wear gloves, mask, and hospital gown at all times
c. wash hands both before and after patient contact
d. maintain distance from each patient

20. [^{111}In]pentetreotide normally localizes in all of the following sites *except*:

a. pituitary gland
b. salivary glands
c. spleen
d. thyroid gland

21. SPECT brain imaging may begin how soon after the administration of [^{99m}Tc]exametazime?

a. immediately
b. 15–20 min
c. 1–2 hr
d. 24 hr

22. Radioactivity is visualized in all of the following areas during a normal cisternographic study *except* the:

a. cerebral convexities
b. basal cisterns
c. lateral ventricles
d. central canal

23. Patient preparation for instilling colloidal [^{32}P]chromic phosphate into the peritoneal cavity includes which of the following?

a. surgical placement of a LeVeen shunt to remove excess peritoneal fluid
b. introducing [^{99m}Tc]sulfur colloid into the cavity to confirm that the ^{32}P will disperse evenly
c. instructing the patient about isolation requirements
d. fasting for 8–12 hr before radiopharmaceutical administration

24. Patient preparation for post-thyroidectomy ^{131}I whole-body imaging for metastases may include all of the following *except*:

a. discontinuation of replacement thyroid hormone
b. administration of exogenous TSH
c. administration of 600–1000 mg of potassium perchlorate 2 hr before imaging
d. following a low-iodine diet for 1–2 weeks before imaging

25. The administration technique for [^{99m}Tc]bicisate includes which of the following?

a. direct venous stick
b. infusion at peak cardiac stress
c. bolus injection technique
d. minimize environmental stimuli

26. Which of the following instructions should be given to patients after administration of [^{18}F]FDG for PET imaging?

a. The patient may leave the imaging area and return in approximately 90 min.
b. The patient should rest quietly in a designated waiting area until imaging begins.
c. The patient may read or watch television until imaging begins.
d. The patient should consume a fatty meal to clear excess tracer from the hepatobiliary system.

27. In performing a gastric-emptying study, imaging should begin:

a. 15 min after meal consumption, then every 15 min for 1 hr
b. 1 hr after meal consumption, then every 15 min for the next hour
c. immediately after meal consumption, then every 5 min for at least 1 hr
d. immediately after meal consumption, then every 15 min for at least 2 hr

28. A patient with a chest tube arrives in the nuclear medicine department for an imaging study. The technologist should:

a. cancel the procedure because chest tube apparatus will interfere with the study
b. place the chest tube's external apparatus on a level lower than the patient's chest
c. place the chest tube's external apparatus on the imaging table next to the patient
d. hang the chest tube's external apparatus from an IV pole and raise it above the patient's chest

29. The following studies are ordered for a patient:

I. GFR determination [^{99m}Tc]pentetate
II. Schilling test [^{57}Co] 0.5 μCi
III. Thyroid uptake ([^{123}I]sodium iodide)

In which order should the studies be performed so that they do not interfere with one another and so that they can be accomplished in the shortest amount of time?

a. I, II, III
b. II, III, I
c. II, I, II
d. III, II, I

30. To help clear the thyroid, liver, and bowel when performing a cardiac perfusion study with sestimibi, a technologist should give what prior to imaging?

a. a fatty meal
b. a glass of cold water
c. dextrose intravenously
d. adenosine

31. A contraindication for performing a myocardial perfusion resting study is:

a. fasting for 4–12 hr prior to the study
b. drinking cold water prior to the study
c. having a nitroglycerin drip
d. being NPO for 4–12 hr prior to study

32. A postsurgery patient is in the nuclear medicine department for a study. The technologist notices that the patient's surgical dressing shows signs of drainage. The most appropriate action for the technologist is to:

a. remove the old dressing and replace it with a fresh one
b. reinforce the dressing with additional gauze and notify the appropriate medical personnel
c. terminate the study and transport the patient back to his/her room
d. complete the nuclear medicine procedure and ignore the dressing

33. If the hematocrit is 40% and a plasma-volume determination, performed with [^{125}I]-human serum albumin, is 3900 mL, what are the derived red cell and whole blood volumes, in milliliters?

	Red cell volume (mL)	Whole blood volume (mL)
a.	1,560	2,340
b.	2,340	6,240
c.	2,600	6,500
d.	5,850	9,750

34. During a red blood cell survival study, the first blood sample is taken 24 hr after the injection of the labeled cells. This 24-hr time period is needed to allow:

a. the radiochromium to decay to a level compatible with the scintillation detector
b. removal of any cells damaged during the labeling process
c. patient recovery from the radiopharmaceutical injection
d. uniform mixing of the labeled cells throughout the vascular system

35. If an anticoagulant is added to a blood sample, the fluid portion of the blood sample is known as:

a. plasma
b. serum
c. antiserum
d. blood complement

36. In a hospital setting, CPR *cannot* legally be administered to a patient in cardiac arrest when the:

a. patient has an infectious disease
b. patient's chart indicates DNR
c. patient is hallucinating
d. patient's chart indicates a terminal illness

37. Pentagastrin is commonly used in which of the following scans:

a. gastric emptying
b. deep vein thrombosis
c. LeVeen shunt patency
d. Meckel's diverticulum

38. Data collected from a red cell survival procedure are plotted on what type of graph paper?

a. linear
b. semilog
c. log–log
d. logit–log

39. Which of the following is *not* recommended *during* HMPAO/ECD administration?

a. dim the lights
b. inject using an IV line
c. talk calmingly to the patient while injecting
d. ask the patient to keep eyes and ears open

40. If a 1:50 dilution of a solution with a tracer concentration of 50 μCi/mL is prepared, followed by a 1:200 dilution of the 1:50 dilution, what is the final dilution?

a. 1:20
b. 1:50
c. 1:1,000
d. 1:10,000

41. Which of the following medical history is relevant to [^{111}In]capromab pendetide imaging?

a. breast-feeding schedule
b. mammogram results
c. PSA level
d. pregnancy status

42. On the basis of the data shown here:

	Total counts	No. pixels
Cardiac ROI	28,503	417
Background ROI	1,859	88

what are the net counts in the cardiac region of interest?

a. 28,065
b. 26,644
c. 19,694
d. 15,463

43. If a ^{99}Mo/^{99m}Tc generator is eluted at 0700 and again at 1300, the next day's ^{99m}Tc yield at 0700:

a. will be decreased
b. will be unaffected
c. will be increased
d. cannot be predicted

44. One hundred twenty-seven millicuries is equivalent to how many gigabecquerels?

a. 0.003 GBq
b. 4.70 GBq
c. 3,430 GBq
d. 4,699 GBq

45. All of the following factors affect the amount of ^{99m}Tc eluted from a ^{99}Mo/^{99m}Tc generator *except*:

a. the amount of ^{99}Mo activity present on the column
b. the time elapsed since the last elution
c. the elution efficiency of the generator
d. the saline volume used for elution

46. According to the NRC, the maximum allowable ^{99}Mo concentration in ^{99m}Tc eluate at the time of administration to the patient must not exceed:

a. 0.15 μCi ^{99}Mo/mCi ^{99m}Tc
b. 1 μCi ^{99}Mo/mCi ^{99m}Tc
c. 5 μCi ^{99}Mo/mCi ^{99m}Tc
d. 5 μCi in a unit dose

47. An eluate of [^{99m}Tc]pertechnetate is assayed for ^{99}Mo contamination with the following results:

^{99}Mo: 45 μCi
^{99m}Tc: 275 mCi

On the basis of this assay, the technologist should:

a. wait for the ^{99}Mo to decay to an acceptable level
b. use the eluate only for studies requiring other ^{99m}Tc-labeled agents
c. use the eluate for only the next 12 hr
d. discard the eluate

48. If a new generator is eluted several times and each time the amount of aluminum in the eluate exceeds the USP limit, the technologist should:

a. increase the elution volume
b. use the eluate for patients
c. contact the generator manufacturer
d. prepare kits with an additional oxidation agent

49. Which of the following ^{99m}Tc-labeled agents is approved for perfusion brain imaging?

a. apcitide
b. exametazime
c. succimer
d. tetrofosmin

50. The shelf life of most ^{99m}Tc-labeled radiopharmaceuticals is:

a. 4–6 hr
b. 6–8 hr
c. 10–12 hr
d. 16–18 hr

51. If the following reagents are available:

Disofenin kit
Maximum ^{99m}Tc activity to be added: 100 mCi
Reconstituting volume: 0.5–3.0 mL

[^{99m}Tc]Pertechnetate
Concentration: 25.0 mCi/mL
Total volume: 8.0 mL

What volume of [^{99m}Tc]pertechnetate must be added to the kit to prepare the maximum amount of [^{99m}Tc]disofenin from one kit?

a. 8.0 mL
b. 4.0 mL
c. 3.0 mL
d. 2.5 mL

52. One advantage of the in vivo method of ^{99m}Tc red cell tagging is that:

a. all circulating red cells are labeled with tracer
b. no incubation times are required at any step in the process
c. no manipulation of blood samples outside the body is required
d. smaller amounts of stannous chloride are required

53. Boiling a [^{99m}Tc]sulfur colloid preparation for too long will result in colloidal particles that are:

a. too small
b. too large
c. optimal size
d. chemically unstable

54. Which of the following components in a [^{99m}Tc]medronate preparation is a radiochemical impurity?

a. aluminum
b. ^{99}Mo
c. [^{99m}Tc]pertechnetate
d. 0.9% NaCl

55. Which of the following image findings is most consistent with chromatography results of a [^{99m}Tc]oxidronate sample demonstrating 65% radiochemical purity?

a. well-defined bone uptake
b. lung uptake
c. stomach and thyroid uptake
d. gastrointestinal tract activity

56. If 740 kBq of a radiopharmaceutical is to be administered for each kilogram of body weight, approximately how much activity (in megabecquerels) should be administered to a patient who weighs 172 pounds?

a. 9.5 MBq
b. 58 MBq
c. 78 MBq
d. 280 MBq

57. Fifty millicuries of [^{99m}Tc]MAA are available at 0700. How many lung perfusion imaging studies can be performed if the administered dose is 5 mCi and one patient is injected every hour beginning at 0730?

a. 6
b. 7
c. 10
d. 20

58. For cardiac first-pass studies, the prescribed adult dosage of [^{99m}Tc]pentetate is 925 MBq ± 10%. On the basis of the vial label information shown here for [^{99m}Tc]pentetate, what is the maximum volume that should be administered to the patient at 0800 on January 5?

Total activity: 3.7 GBq
Total volume: 2.0 mL
Concentration: 1.85 GBq/mL
Calibration: 0600, January 5

a. 0.57 mL
b. 0.63 mL
c. 0.69 mL
d. 1.0 mL

59. In labeling red blood cells with ^{51}Cr, the final step before reinjecting the labeled red blood cells into the patient is to:

a. add ^{51}Cr to the patient's blood sample
b. wash the labeled red cells to remove excess ^{51}Cr
c. separate the red blood cells from the plasma
d. add ascorbic acid to the tagged blood

60. In what way does the modified in vivo method of labeling red blood cells with [^{99m}Tc]pertechnetate differ from the in vivo method?

a. The modified method mixes [^{99m}Tc]pertechnetate with only a small volume of the patient's blood.
b. The modified method "pretins" only a small volume of the patient's blood.
c. The modified method uses a smaller activity of [^{99m}Tc]pertechnetate.
d. The modified method requires a smaller amount of stannous pyrophosphate.

61. Which of the following statements about the modified in vivo method for labeling red blood cell with [^{99m}Tc]pertechnetate is *true*?

a. Only a sample of the patient's blood is incubated with the reconstituted stannous pyrophosphate.
b. Excess [^{99m}Tc]pertechnetate is removed from the blood sample before the sample is re-injected into the patient.
c. A sample of the patient's "pretinned" blood is incubated with [^{99m}Tc]pertechnetate outside of the patient.
d. Red cell labeling takes place only within the patient's circulatory system.

62. According to NRC regulations, which of the following unit dosages may be administered to the patient?

	Prescribed dosage (mCi)	Measured dosage (mCi)
a.	10	13.5
b.	15	12.5
c.	8–10	10.9
d.	20–25	18.7

63. In the radiochromium labeling process, ascorbic acid is used as which of the following?

a. anticoagulant
b. radiotracer
c. oxidizing agent
d. reducing agent

64. If a vial of ^{99m}Tc-labeled radiopharmaceutical contains 4.65 MBq in 3.5 mL at 0800, what is the concentration at 0930?

a. 1.33 MBq/mL
b. 1.12 MBq/mL
c. 0.90 MBq/mL
d. 0.75 MBq/mL

65. If a unit dosage of [^{99m}Tc]pertechnetate is calibrated to contain 25 mCi in 0.8 mL at 1400, what volume should be removed from the syringe to retain 15 mCi in the syringe at 1200?

a. 0.20 mL
b. 0.32 mL
c. 0.42 mL
d. 0.48 mL

66. If an MAA kit containing 4.5 million particles is prepared by adding 30 mCi in 2.5 mL, how many particles are contained in 3 mCi?

a. 150,000
b. 180,000
c. 216,000
d. 450,000

67. Of the following syringes, which size would be best for withdrawing 1 mL of radiopharmaceutical from a multidose vial?

a. 1 mL
b. 2.5 mL
c. 3 mL
d. 5 mL

68. According to NRC regulations, which of the following signs should be posted in unrestricted areas?

a. No posting is required.
b. "Authorized Personnel Only"
c. "Caution: Radioactive Materials"
d. "Caution: Radiation Area"

69. A package containing radioactive material is monitored and found to produce 12 mR/hr at the surface and 0.9 mR/hr at 1 m from the surface. Which DOT label must be affixed to the outside of the package?

a. "Category I"
b. "Category II"
c. "Category III"
d. No DOT label is required.

70. According to the NRC, decay in storage records must include the date that the radioactive material was:

a. calibrated
b. received
c. disposed of
d. placed in storage

71. All of the following statements about the HVL are true *except*:

a. One HVL reduces the radiation intensity to half its original value.
b. One HVL of lead will absorb the same amount of radiation as one HVL of aluminum.
c. One HVL absorbs 50% of the photons emitted from a radiation source.
d. One HVL of lead is the same thickness as one HVL of aluminum.

72. If a patient receives 20 mCi of [^{131}I]sodium iodide instead of the prescribed dosage of 15 mCi for therapy of hyperthyroidism, which of the following individuals/agencies must be notified?

a. NRC
b. NRC and FDA
c. referring physician
d. NRC and referring physician

73. According to NRC regulations, the annual whole-body occupational dose limit (TEDE) for adults is:

a. 5000 mrem
b. 50 mrem
c. 50 rem
d. 15 rem

74. A "sharps" container reads 50 mR/hr when it is placed in storage. It contains only ^{99m}Tc waste. According to NRC regulations, when can the container be disposed of as nonradioactive biohazardous waste?

a. when the exposure rate drops to 1/10 of the original exposure rate
b. when the exposure rate drops to 1/100 of the original exposure rate
c. when the container gives only a background reading with a survey meter
d. when the container gives only a background reading with a wipe test

75. According to the NRC, areas where therapeutic radiopharmaceuticals are prepared or administered must be surveyed:

a. weekly
b. monthly
c. at the end of each day a therapeutic dosage is prepared or administered
d. after each therapeutic dosage is prepared or administered

76. What is the measured exposure rate shown on the diagram of the G–M meter depicted here?

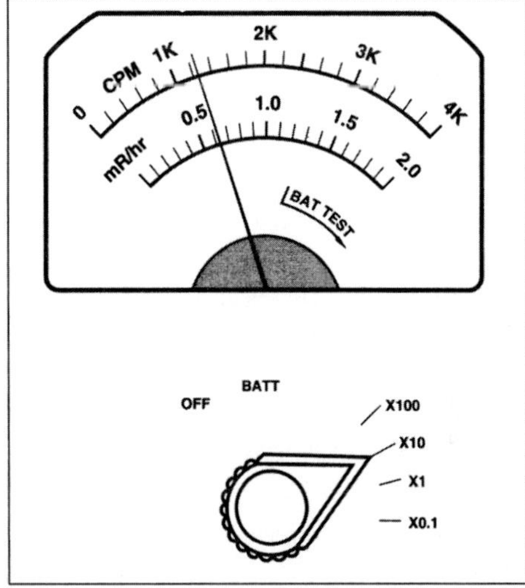

a. 0.06 mR/hr
b. 0.6 mR/hr
c. 6.0 mR/hr
d. 60 mR/hr

77. According to the NRC, the NRC and the final delivery carrier must be notified if the exposure rate at the surface of a package containing radioactive materials exceeds:

a. 100 mR/hr
b. 200 mR/hr
c. 1000 mR/hr
d. 2000 mR/hr

78. Contamination on the surface of the skin is best removed by:

a. flushing the area with hot water
b. cleansing the area with lukewarm water and detergent
c. scrubbing the area with a stiff brush
d. rubbing the area with an abrasive cleanser

79. According to NRC regulations, which of the following concerning restricted areas is *true*?

a. Patient rooms become restricted areas after the patient has received a radiopharmaceutical.
b. Only areas where radiopharmaceuticals are stored must be designated restricted areas.
c. Restricted areas must be locked when authorized personnel are not present.
d. Radiation area monitors are required in restricted areas.

80. According to NRC regulations, radioactive waste can be decayed in storage if:

a. the exposure rate at the time of storage is less than 5 mR/hr at the surface
b. the exposure rate at the time of storage is less than 5 R/hr at the surface
c. it has a physical half-life of less than 120 days
d. it has a physical half-life of less than 1 year

81. If the ambient exposure rate in a hot lab is determined to be 1.2 mrem/hr, what will be the radiation dose to a technologist as a result of 3 hr work in the lab?

a. 0.06 mrem
b. 0.4 mrem
c. 3.6 mrem
d. 40 mrem

82. Which of the following must be performed before a package containing radioactive materials can be returned to a vendor?

a. Confirm that the exposure rate does not exceed background levels.
b. Perform a wipe test to assure there is no surface contamination.
c. Cover each individual vial with a waterproof covering.
d. Notify the NRC that a shipment is being made.

83. Which of the following is a primary source of radiation exposure to the technologist who performs PET imaging?

a. Compton scatter from the patient
b. positrons escaping from the patient
c. γ rays from the long-lived source used for transmission scanning
d. electromagnetic radiation from the PET camera

84. Which of the following personnel monitors would be appropriate for use when monitors are changed at 3-month intervals?

a. film badge
b. TLD
c. OSL
d. TLD or OSL

85. A linearity test was performed on a dose calibrator, and the following data were collected:

Day	Time	Calculated activity (mCi)	Measured activity (mCi)
1	0700	20.0	20.0
	1300	10.0	9.50
	1900	5.0	4.75
2	0700	1.26	1.20
	1300	0.63	0.60
	1900	0.32	0.30
3	0700	0.08	0.076
	1300	0.04	0.038
	1900	0.02	0.019

Based on these results, which of the following statements is *true*?

a. The instrument consistently measures higher than expected.
b. The instrument measures higher activities more accurately than lower activities.
c. The instrument measures lower activities more accurately than higher activities.
d. According to the standard of practice, the instrument is operating within limits.

86. A dose calibrator accuracy test may be performed with which of the following radioactive sources?

a. 100 mCi ^{99m}Tc
b. 60 μCi ^{99m}Tc
c. 75 μCi ^{137}Cs
d. 25 μCi ^{137}Cs

87. On the basis of the spectrometer calibration curve shown here:

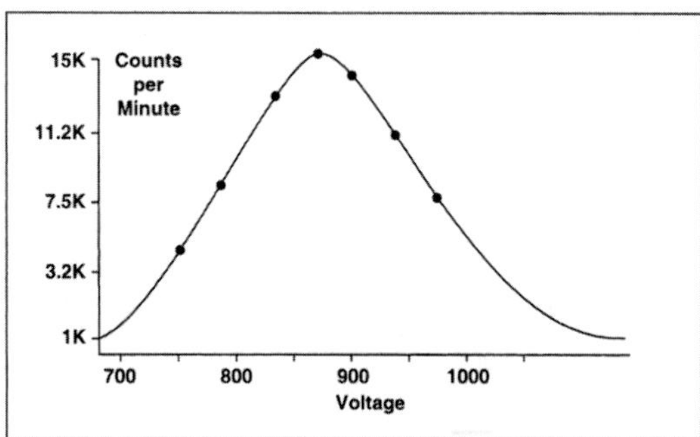

the operating voltage of the instrument is:

a. 800
b. 850
c. 875
d. 885

88. Extrinsic uniformity is performed daily on a scintillation camera with a ^{57}Co sheet source and a low-energy all-purpose parallel-hole collimator. From the data shown here:

Day	Time to collect 2 million counts
June 1	240 sec
June 2	241 sec
June 3	245 sec
June 4	242 sec
June 5	560 sec

all of the following may have caused the decreased sensitivity seen on June 5 *except*:

a. incorrect photopeak/window setting
b. incorrect collimator
c. incorrect acquisition matrix
d. a cracked crystal

89. A technologist performs a uniformity test on a scintillation camera using a ^{99m}Tc point source and obtains the image shown here.

What should the technologist do next?

a. Arrange for camera service.
b. Record the results and proceed with imaging patients.
c. Remove the collimator and repeat the acquisition.
d. Move the point source farther from the face of the detector.

90. According to standards of practice, how often must the accuracy of a dose calibrator be determined?

a. annually
b. quarterly
c. monthly
d. daily

91. The following center of rotation values were obtained on a SPECT camera:

Date	COR value
10/1	32.51
10/8	32.59
10/15	32.48
10/22	32.38
10/29	32.58

On October 29, the most appropriate action for the technologist is to:

a. transfer any SPECT studies to a different computer terminal for processing
b. arrange for camera service
c. acquire SPECT studies using the October 29 value
d. acquire SPECT studies using the October 22 value

92. How frequently should linearity and spatial resolution tests be performed on a scintillation camera?

a. daily
b. weekly
c. monthly
d. quarterly

93. If a ^{67}Ga static image is acquired into a 128 × 128 byte mode matrix using the photopeaks at 93, 185, and 300 keV, how much computer memory is required to store the image?

a. 16 kB
b. 32 kB
c. 64 kB
d. 128 kB

94. Which of the following techniques is used to help eliminate the "star" effect created during tomographic reconstruction?

a. center of rotation offset correction
b. filtered backprojection
c. oversampling
d. uniformity correction

95. A technologist performs a linearity test on a dose calibrator. The expected activity at a given time is 28.2 μCi, and the actual reading is 27.0 μCi. Which of the following statements is correct?

a. The instrument should be repaired or replaced.
b. The instrument can be used to measure activities in the microcurie range.
c. A correction factor of 0.96 should be applied when measuring activities in the microcurie range.
d. A correction factor of 1.04 should be applied when measuring activities in the microcurie range.

96. Which of the following instruments is most appropriate for detecting low-level accidental contamination?

a. thermoluminescent dosimeter
b. Geiger–Mueller counter
c. cutie pie (ionization chamber)
d. pocket dosimeter

97. Image noise can be decreased during dedicated PET imaging by:

a. scanning for a longer time
b. using 2D mode
c. decreasing the dosage activity
d. decreasing the distance between the patient and the detectors

98. What is the standard maximum acceptable % energy resolution measured with ^{137}Cs for a NaI(Tl) scintillation detector?

a. 8%
b. 12%
c. 20%
d. 22%

99. A 10% window for 662 keV is set on a spectrometer with a lower-level discriminator (LLD) and an upper-level discriminator (ULD). If each increment on the discriminator dial equals 1 keV, what should be the settings for the LLD and the ULD?

a. LLD = 596; ULD = 728
b. LLD = 629; ULD = 695
c. LLD = 652; ULD = 672
d. LLD = 657; ULD = 667

100. Which of the following radiation monitoring devices is best suited to survey a patient who has received 150 mCi of ^{131}I for therapy?

a. pocket ionization chamber
b. portable ionization chamber
c. Geiger–Mueller counter
d. dose calibrator

Examination 6

1. If one is receiving 20 mR/hr exposure at a distance of 3 m from a source, at what distance would one receive 500 mR/hr exposure?

a. 0.36 cm
b. 0.36 m
c. 60 cm
d. 0.60 cm

2. If an area survey reveals an ambient radiation level of 7 mR/hr, which of the following radioactive signs would be the best choice to display on the door leading to this area?

a. "Caution: Radioactive Materials"
b. "Caution: Radiation Area"
c. "Caution: High Radiation Area"
d. "Grave Danger: Very High Radiation Area"

3. An ionization chamber is left in integral mode for 10 min and records a total dose of 3 mR. Which of the following area posting signs should be used on the door leading into this area?

a. "Caution: Radioactive Materials"
b. "Caution: Radiation Area"
c. "Caution: High Radiation Area"
d. "Grave Danger: Very High Radiation Area"

4. Which of the following area posting signs would not normally be found in a hospital?

a. "Caution: Radioactive Materials"
b. "Caution: Radiation Area"
c. "Caution: High Radiation Area"
d. "Grave Danger: Very High Radiation Area"

5. Which of the following type of survey instruments would be best to use to survey a spill for removable contamination in a hot lab area where radioisotopes are being stored?

a. G–M detector
b. personal pocket dosimeter
c. dose calibrator with a wipe test
d. well counter with a wipe test

6. Four HVLs reduce the amount of incident radiation exposure to what?

a. 12.5%
b. 6.25%
c. 3.125%
d. none of the above

7. Which of the following is *not* required to be included in the records of a radioactive package receipt check in process?

a. name of patient
b. name of radioisotope
c. amount of activity
d. both external and internal wipe checks

8. A package is reading 2 mR/hr at a distance of 2 m, what is the appropriate DOT label for this package?

a. DOT I
b. DOT II
c. DOT III
d. No labeling is required.

9. The purpose of the transport index is:

a. to list the final destination of the package
b. to indicate the highest activity of the contents at 1 m from the surface
c. not to give emergency personnel information about the contents of the package in an accident
d. not to list the radioisotopes in the package

10. If a patient who is having a bone scan urinates on the floor next to a camera, what would be the best course of action to reduce radiation exposure?

a. Let the radioactive urine decay to background.
b. Move the camera away from the spill.
c. Remove the spill with some absorbent material and cover any residual activity with a lead plate or lead apron.
d. Notify the referring physician of a medical event.

11. Which DOT radioactive labeling is entirely white?

a. DOT I
b. DOT II
c. DOT III
d. DOT IV

12. Which absorber would be the best to use to shield strontium-89?

a. cardboard
b. Plexiglass
c. lead
d. No shielding is required.

13. Which of the following indicates the *amount* of radioactive substance present in a sample or source?

a. activity
b. exposure
c. absorbed dose
d. dose equivalent

14. If the exposure rate is 25 mR/hr and the person being exposed is present for 25 min, what is his/her total exposure?

a. 25 mR
b. 12.5 mR
c. 10.4 mR
d. 5.2 mR

15. What is 120 Sv in millirads (quality factor [QF] = 1)?

a. 8.3×10^{-8} mrad
b. 120,000 mrad
c. 1.2 million mrad
d. 12 million mrad

16. An α particle is similar to what?

a. an electron
b. a proton
c. a helium atom minus its electrons
d. a helium atom minus its neutrons

17. A higher or lower sensitivity is affected by all of the following *except*:

a. thickness of camera crystal
b. collimator design
c. properly set pulse-height analyzer (PHA) and window width
d. instrument deadtime

18. Geometric variation, on a dose calibrator, should be performed:

a. at installation and after repair
b. at installation and yearly
c. quarterly
d. daily

19. Photomultiplier tube drift is associated with which of the following:

a. auto-voltage stabilization
b. auto-gain stabilization
c. energy correction
d. linearity correction

20. A paralyzable counting system will:

a. decrease in count rate after some peak in count rate is obtained
b. never plateau and never obtain a peak count
c. plateau with no decrease in count rate as activity increases, which is the peak count
d. not exhibit any count rate difference

21. Sources of intrinsic nonuniformity include all of the following *except*:

a. "mistuned" PMTs
b. regional variations in Z-pulse amplitude
c. linearity
d. spatial distortion

22. What is added to NaI crystals to allow them to scintillate at room temperature?

a. Tl
b. Xe
c. Ce
d. Ag

23. What is the maximum percentage difference that is acceptable for most regulatory agencies for all four dose calibrator QC checks?

a. ±5%
b. ±7%
c. ±10%
d. ±15%

24. Extrinsic quality control on a camera means quality control is done:

a. with the collimator on
b. without the collimator on
c. inside the camera
d. outside the camera

25. Linearity correction involves:

a. diagonal lines
b. horizontal lines
c. vertical lines
d. horizontal and vertical lines

26. Dose calibrator constancy should be performed:

a. monthly
b. quarterly
c. weekly
d. daily

27. Which of the following quantitative renal techniques require(s) the calculation of kidney depth?

I. Schlegel technique
II. Gates' method
III. Two-compartment effective renal plasma flow (ERPF) determination
IV. Russell's glomerular filtration rate (GFR) method

a. I
b. I and II
c. III and IV
d. II and IV

28. Which of the following functional images represents the magnitude of ventricular contraction?

a. amplitude image
b. paradox image
c. phase image
d. stroke-volume image

29. The background ROI used in determining percentage gastroesophageal (GE) reflux is placed over the:

a. lower left lung
b. small intestine
c. right hepatic lobe
d. upper esophagus

30. Geometric mean is sometimes used in quantization because it corrects for:

a. the size and shape of the organ
b. background activity
c. attenuation and organ depth
d. radioactive decay

31. Given a heart rate of 85 bpm, if a 24-frame gated heart study is acquired, the length of each frame in milliseconds is:

a. 0.06 msec
b. 0.3 msec
c. 29 msec
d. 705 msec

32. Concentric ring artifacts in a reconstructed SPECT image may be caused by:

a. improper collimation
b. large statistical fluctuations in the projection data
c. inadequate uniformity correction
d. too few angles of reconstruction

33. In processing a myocardial perfusion study, a slice from which body axis is used to identify the degree to which the heart points to the left and is used to construct slices in the three opposing cardiac planes?

a. transaxial
b. horizontal long axis
c. vertical long axis
d. short axis

34. The *most* important purpose of center of rotation offset correction is to:

a. eliminate the effects of detector tilt in the reconstructed images
b. minimize count sensitivity variations from one area of the crystal to another
c. ensure that all pixels are uniformly sized over the entire field of view
d. align the center of the computer matrix with the mechanical axis of rotation

35. The *x*- and *y*-axes of a circumferential profile curve are, respectively:

a. *x*-axis: bull's-eye quadrant; *y*-axis: % maximum counts
b. *x*-axis: segment of the myocardium; *y*-axis: maximum counts
c. *x*-axis: time; *y*-axis: activity
d. *x*-axis: rest; *y*-axis: stress

36. Diaphragmatic attenuation may be reduced by:

a. 360° acquisition
b. supine acquisition
c. prone acquisition
d. delayed imaging

37. Which of the following is a definition of sensitivity of a diagnostic test?

a. how good the test is at detecting a true positive
b. how good the test is at detecting a true negative
c. how good the test is at detecting the difference between a true negative and a true positive
d. how good the test is at detecting something

38. In a patient with pulmonary embolism, the perfusion and xenon ventilation lung images will demonstrate the following findings:

	Perfusion	Ventilation
a.	Normal	Normal
b.	Normal	Abnormal tracer retention
c.	Perfusion defects	Normal
d.	Perfusion defects	Abnormal tracer retention

39. Of the following, the biggest disadvantage of ^{133}Xe (xenon gas) for performing lung ventilation studies is its:

a. rapid lung clearance
b. trapping and shielding requirement
c. high cost
d. unavailability

40. Which of the following statements about radiolabeled aerosols used for lung ventilation imaging is *true*?

a. Particle sizes range from 30 to 90 μm in diameter.
b. It is necessary to trap any radiolabeled particles exhaled by the patient.
c. The particles are deposited in ventilated areas of the lungs.
d. Deposition of particles in the central airway is never a problem with lung aerosol studies.

41. An uptake probe is what type of detector?

a. scintillation detector
b. proportional counter
c. ionization chamber
d. Geiger–Mueller counter

42. The purpose of a charcoal filter in a xenon administration unit is to adsorb:

a. bacteria
b. carbon dioxide
c. moisture
d. xenon

43. The concentration of ^{133}Xe gas in the lungs is increasing in which phase of a xenon ventilation study?

a. wash-in
b. equilibrium
c. washout
d. There is no phase of increasing activity.

44. What is the range of particle size, in micrometers, of the majority of particles in [^{99m}Tc]macroaggregated albumin (MAA)?

a. 150–250 μm
b. 100–150 μm
c. 10–90 μm
d. 1–40 μm

45. Following administration of a bone imaging tracer, the patient is instructed to drink fluids to:

a. decrease radiation exposure to the bones
b. clear excess tracer from the blood
c. enhance visualization of the kidneys and bladder
d. remove tracer from normal bone tissue

46. Radioxenon ventilation studies should be performed in rooms whose air pressure is:

a. higher than adjacent areas
b. lower than adjacent areas
c. equal to adjacent areas
d. neither higher or lower than adjacent areas

47. The clinical indication for a diagnostic test is:

a. a list of the patient's symptoms
b. the patient's diagnosis
c. a summary of the patient's clinical history
d. the question the referring physician needs answered

48. In a xenon administration unit, the purpose of soda lime is to absorb:

a. bacteria
b. carbon dioxide
c. moisture
d. xenon

49. If visualized, the gallbladder fossa may be seen on what view(s) of a liver/spleen image?

a. anterior and posterior
b. anterior and right lateral
c. anterior only
d. right lateral only

50. When performing Meckel's diverticulum imaging, which of the following would be visualized in a positive study?

a. malignant thyroid tissue
b. stomach mucosa
c. ectopic stomach mucosa
d. ectopic endometrial tissue

51. Which of the following studies requires radiolabeled red blood cells?

a. infection imaging
b. renal scan
c. MUGA scan
d. liver/spleen scan

52. Twenty-four-hour images are sometimes performed over what area to demonstrate gastroesophageal reflux?

a. lower esophagus
b. lung fields
c. stomach
d. upper small intestine

53. The clinical indication for performing a ^{14}C urea breath test is to:

a. rule out excess urea in the blood
b. determine the cause of gastric reflux
c. detect the presence of *Helicobacter pylori* bacteria
d. diagnose possible causes of abnormal gastric emptying

54. Images acquired during a gastric-emptying study are primarily used for:

a. demonstrating exit of the tracer from the stomach
b. assessing normal biodistribution of the tracer
c. measuring the size of the stomach
d. drawing regions of interest

55. When imaging to determine LeVeen shunt patency, the camera initially is positioned anteriorly over the abdomen, and delayed images can be done:

a. over the brain
b. over the chest or abdomen
c. over the lung or liver fields
d. over the sacroiliac area

56. In a red cell volume determination, it is necessary to add ascorbic acid to the labeled red cells to:

a. prevent additional tagging once the cells are re-injected into the patient
b. remove the ^{51}Cr not tagged to red cells
c. suspend the cells homogeneously
d. prevent coagulation of the whole blood sample

57. Morphine is administered during hepatobiliary imaging to cause the:

a. sphincter of Oddi to contract
b. gallbladder to empty completely
c. cystic duct to open
d. tracer to be diverted to the common bile duct

58. Which of the following is the reason that it is important to have a standardized meal size and composition in a gastric-emptying scan?

a. It can affect the radiation dose to the patient.
b. It can affect the ability to have gastric emptying.
c. It can affect the rate of gastric emptying.
d. It has no effect and is not necessary.

59. Which of the following is/are not indicators of renal function?

a. BUN level
b. peak transit time
c. creatinine clearance
d. CBC

60. If ^{99m}Tc radioactivity in the circulation from a previous nuclear medicine test occurs in a renal scan in the plasma draw:

a. the ERPF will be higher than it should
b. the ERPF will be lower than it should
c. the ERPF will not be affected
d. it is impossible to predict what will happen to the ERPF

61. Static renal parenchyma imaging would be best performed with which of the following radiopharmaceuticals?

a. [^{99m}Tc]mertiatide
b. [^{99m}Tc]pentetate
c. [^{99m}Tc]succimer
d. [^{99m}Tc]gluceptate

62. In a normal kidney, the maximum amount of tracer should be concentrated in the kidney how many minutes after administration of [^{99m}Tc]mertiatide?

a. 1–2 min
b. 3–5 min
c. 8–10 min
d. 30–35 min

63. If the tracer for an ERPF determination using the blood sampling method is administered at 0900, at what time should the blood sample be collected?

a. 0915
b. 0935
c. 0944
d. 1000

64. For a GFR using the camera method one compares the kidney counts to what?

a. dynamic image ROI counts
b. preinjection syringe counts
c. postinjection injection site counts
d. plasma counts

65. Perfusion of the ventricular septum in the heart is provided primarily by which coronary artery?

a. left anterior descending
b. left circumflex
c. right coronary
d. none of the above

66. When performing a left ventricular function examination with ^{99m}Tc-labeled red blood cells, which of the following actions is used to visually separate the ventricles from one another?

a. adjusting the anterior angle
b. adjusting the left lateral angle
c. adjusting the left anterior oblique angle
d. adjusting both the anterior and LAO angle

67. Tachycardia is demonstrated on an ECG strip as:

a. a large P–R interval
b. a normal QRS heart rhythm
c. an increased heart rate
d. a decreased heart rate

68. Adenosine is contraindicated for patients with which of the following conditions?

a. diabetes
b. stress-induced myocardial ischemia
c. chronic obstructive pulmonary disease
d. peripheral vascular disease

69. Consumption of a fatty meal may have the same effect on the hepatobiliary system as which of the following compounds?

a. cimetidine
b. furosemide
c. morphine
d. sincalide

70. Delayed improvement of perfusion following coronary artery revascularization is referred to as:

a. hibernating myocardium
b. infarcted myocardium
c. stunned myocardium
d. necrosed myocardium

71. The percentage ejection fraction calculated from the following data

Diastole: 2,750 cpm

Systole: 1,775 cpm

is:

a. 61
b. 55
c. 35
d. 22

72. Which wave of the ECG is used to trigger the scintillation camera to acquire counts?

a. P wave
b. R wave
c. T wave
d. U wave

73. Which of the following would *not* be a characteristic of an ideal myocardial perfusion agent?

a. high first-pass myocardial extraction proportional to blood flow
b. adequate imaging window
c. ability to complete both rest and stress imaging in 2 days
d. high target-to-nontarget ratio

74. All of the following are advantages of the first-pass method for performing cardiac function imaging *except*:

a. short acquisition time
b. low background activity
c. choice of radiopharmaceuticals
d. multiple views with one tracer dose

75. In the 1-day protocol for myocardial perfusion imaging performed with a ^{99m}Tc-labeled tracer, the larger amount of activity is administered:

a. for the rest study
b. for the stress study
c. for the study performed first
d. for the study performed second

76. Which of the following is most likely to interfere with performing a left ventricular ejection fraction using the gated equilibrium technique?

a. doxorubicin toxicity
b. cardiac arrhythmia
c. cardiomyopathy
d. coronary artery disease

77. An advantage of [^{201}Tl]thallium chloride is that it:

a. has a high photon flux at a high-energy window
b. is a calcium analog
c. has a short half-life
d. redistributes

78. A cardiac shunt would be best demonstrated with which of the following nuclear medicine techniques?

a. equilibrium-gated ventriculogram
b. first-pass radionuclide angiography
c. myocardial infarct imaging
d. myocardial perfusion imaging

79. Functional cardiac studies may be performed to evaluate wall-motion abnormalities caused by all of the following *except*:

a. aneurysm
b. myocardial infarction
c. myocardial ischemia
d. myocardial perfusion patency

80. One advantage of the in vivo method of ^{99m}Tc red cell tagging is that:

a. all the circulating red cells are labeled with tracer
b. no incubation times are required at any step in the process
c. smaller amounts of stannous chloride are required
d. no manipulation of blood samples outside the body is required

81. In preparation for a stress test, patients are instructed to fast to:

a. prevent gastrointestinal upsets during exercise
b. minimize tracer uptake in the GI tract
c. enhance myocardial tracer uptake
d. standardize test conditions among patients

82. Given the decay factor (DF) of a radioisotope is 0.254 for 1 hr and 30 mCi/mL concentration is available at 0700, how much total activity will remain in the vial at 1100 if a total volume of 5 mL was used to make up the kit?

a. 125 μCi
b. 312 μCi
c. 452 μCi
d. 624 μCi

83. Which of the following statements is *true* when transient equilibrium occurs between ^{99}Mo and ^{99m}Tc?

a. The ratio of the ^{99}Mo and ^{99m}Tc activities remains constant.
b. The maximum amount of ^{99m}Tc activity is present.
c. The ^{99}Mo and ^{99m}Tc activities are equal.
d. ^{99m}Tc and ^{99}Mo have the same decay constant.

84. The concentration of [^{99m}Tc]pertechnetate is required to be 60 mCi/mL. If approximately 1,200 mCi [^{99m}Tc]pertechnetate will be eluted from a wet-column generator, which size evacuated vial should be used to collect the eluate?

a. 5 mL
b. 10 mL
c. 15 mL
d. 20 mL

85. The average recommended number of MAA particles to be administered is:

a. 100,000 particles
b. 150,000 particles
c. 350,000 particles
d. 1,000,000 particles

86. What approximate volume of [^{99m}Tc]pertechnetate should be added to the medronate kit to prepare 180 mCi of [^{99m}Tc]medronate?

Medronate Kit
Maximum activity to be added: 300 mCi
Reconstituting volume: 1–8 mL

[^{99m}Tc]Pertechnetate
Concentration: 28.7 mCi/mL
Total volume: 7.5 mL

a. 0.6 mL
b. 6.3 mL
c. 7.5 mL
d. 10.4 mL

87. Bioavailability refers to what concerning pharmacology?

a. fraction of drug that reaches systemic circulation after a particular route of administration
b. fraction of drug that is excreted from the body
c. fraction of drug that is delivered to body on the basis of weight
d. fraction of drug that reaches the heart
e. addresses access to medication across the world

88. Which of the following is *not* a factor in generator yields:

a. time since last elution
b. column cracks
c. air leaks
d. amount of aluminum on the column

89. Radiopharmaceutical kits reconstituted with ^{99m}Tc pertechnetate are prepared in nitrogen- or argon-purged vials to prevent:

a. bacterial growth
b. hydrolysis
c. oxidation
d. radiolysis

90. Which of the following is *not* part of a ^{99m}Tc radiopharmaceutical kit:

a. reducing agent
b. ascorbic acid or stannous ion
c. pyrogenocidal agent
d. lyophilized compound

91. Hydrolysis of reduced ^{99m}Tc during kit preparation is demonstrated on clinical images by radioactivity concentrated in the:

a. kidneys
b. liver
c. lungs
d. thyroid

92. When labeling ^{99m}Tc (VII), in what state is the ^{99m}Tc changed to make it more reactive?

a. ^{99m}Tc (VIII)
b. ^{99m}Tc (VI)
c. ^{99m}Tc (V)
d. ^{99m}Tc (IV)

93. Radiochemical impurities can change:

a. radionuclidic purity
b. generator yields
c. PET blank scans
d. target:nontarget ratios

94. ITLC refers to:

a. instant transverse light chromatography
b. instant tomographic layer chromatography
c. instant thin layer chromatography
d. instant thin light chromatography

95. Possible radiochromatography artifacts include all of the following *except*:

a. using the wrong solvent
b. the strip touches the side of the developing chamber
c. the solvent evaporates before chromatography is completed
d. using tweezers to pick up the chromatography paper

96. An MAA kit has 3,000,000 total particles. If a 5-mCi dose is needed at 1000 and the following information is provided

25 mCi/mL in 5 mL total volume at 0700

what approximate number of particles will be given to the patient?

a. 600,000 particles
b. 120,000 particles
c. 169,635 particles
d. 134,831 particles

97. If a 20-μCi ^{123}I dose is needed on Monday morning 8/15/09, at 0800 CST, what amount of ^{123}I should be sent from Atlanta at 0800 Friday morning, 8/12/09, for the right amount to be available Monday morning?

a. 878 μCi
b. 925 μCi
c. 988 μCi
d. 1088 μCi

98. A 25-mCi dose in a volume of 2 mL is added to 50 mL and a one-sixth serial dilution is performed. What amount of total activity is present in a 5-mL sample of tube no. 33?

a. 3.02×10^{-25} mCi
b. 6.04×10^{-25} mCi
c. 9.08×10^{-25} mCi
d. 12.12×10^{-25} mCi

99. A pharmacokinectic profile of a drug depends on what?

a. time to excretion
b. mode of excretion
c. mode of administration
d. time to administration

100. Which of the following may be used to reduce the allergic effects of contrast media?

a. acetaminophen
b. diphenhydramine
c. air
d. water

Examination 7

1. According to the NRC, survey meters must be calibrated ________ and following any repairs.

a. semiannually (twice a year)
b. biannually (every other year)
c. yearly (once a year)
d. monthly (once a month)

2. The difference between a direct and wipe check radiation survey is that:

a. there is no difference
b. one is qualitative and one is not
c. one is quantitative and one is not
d. one gives an instant reading and one does not

3. An occupational worker has received 14,000 mrem of exposure to the eyes in 1 year on his/her eye dose dosimeter; which following course of action would be appropriate?

a. Recommend eye chelation therapy.
b. Review ALARA standards to reduce exposure because they have exceeded their annual eye dose limit.
c. Review ALARA standards to reduce exposure because they are close to exceeding their annual eye dose limit.
d. Recommend they use leaded eyeglasses to reduce exposure.

4. A nuclear medicine department has an action level of 500 mrem per month whole-body exposure. If you were the NRC inspector, what would your recommendations to this site be?

a. nothing, everything is fine
b. need to reduce their action level to at least 450 mrem per month to be in compliance with annual possible levels of exposure
c. need to increase their action level to 5000 mrem per month
d. need to reduce their action level to at least 410 mrem per month to be compliant with annual possible levels of exposure

5. The allowed dose of ionizing radiation to a declared pregnant women's embryo/fetus is:

a. 10% of the standard occupational workers whole-body dose per year
b. 1% of the standard occupational workers whole-body dose per year
c. 10% of the standard yearly occupational dose for the gestation period
d. 1% of the standard yearly occupational dose for the gestation period

6. In doing a room survey you discover that a therapy patient's room has removable contamination above acceptable levels. What is the acceptable level?

a. $<$200 Bq/100 cm^2
b. $<$200 MBq/100 cm^2
c. $<$12,000 Bq/100 cm^2
d. $<$3.33 Bq/100 cm^2

7. In calibrating your survey meter for your nuclear medicine department, you discover that it has a 12% error. What is your next course of action to remain in compliance with NRC regulations?

a. Use the survey meter as you normally would.
b. Throw it away.
c. Replace the batteries.
d. Recommend that it be serviced.

8. You suspect that a low-level β emitter has been spilled on a countertop. Which of the following survey techniques would be best?

a. pancake probe G–M-type meter
b. scintillation probe-type meter
c. wipe check with a G–M-type meter
d. wipe check with a SCA/MCA-type meter

9. An unrestricted nuclear medicine waiting room is on the other side of the wall from a hot lab. G–M meter readings in the hot lab read 50 mR/hr. Readings on the other side of the wall in the waiting room read 25 mR/hr. What is the minimum number HVLs of Pb that are required in the wall to bring the waiting room reading down into compliance with NRC regulations?

a. 1
b. 2
c. 3
d. 4

10. A G–M meter has a scale of 1–5 mR/hr. If a deflection on the meter reads 4.5 and the meter is set on the ×0.1 setting, what is the reading?

a. 40.5 mR/hr
b. 4.5 mR/hr
c. 0.45 mR/hr
d. 0.045 mR/hr

11. In operating a G–M meter on a daily basis, what is the first thing you should always do?

a. Use a check source to make sure the meter is working correctly.
b. Check the batteries.
c. Insert the batteries.
d. Set it to the most sensitive scale/setting.

12. Form X or NRC Form 3 includes all of the following *except*:

a. the employer is not required to post any notices of violations of the regulations involving radiological working conditions
b. the worker is required to become familiar with the regulations and operating procedures for the work engaged in
c. the worker and employer must abide by the state and federal regulations
d. the employer will make available to the worker a copy of all applicable state and federal regulations, licenses, and operating procedures pertaining to the work

13. The triblade radiation symbol must be which of the following colors on a yellow background?

a. pink
b. purple
c. red
d. brown

14. Which of the following radiation signs would be required if a survey meter reading were 40 mR/hr at 60 cm from a source in the room?

a. "Caution: Radioactive Material"
b. "Caution: Radiation Area"
c. "Caution: High Radiation Area"
d. "Grave Danger: Very High Radiation Area"

15. A DOT II radioactive label is on a package that reads 9 mR/hr at 1 m. What is the appropriate action to take?

a. Log in the package as you normally would.
b. Contact the regional office of the NRC.
c. Inform the vendor that the wrong label was on the container.
d. Notify the DOT that a "shipment event" has occurred.

16. The average energy required to create an ion pair in air is ________.

a. 60 eV
b. 30 keV
c. 5 eV
d. 34 eV

17. The ionization of the *entire* fixed volume of a gas due to secondary ionization is known as the ________.

a. Townsend avalanche
b. Geiger effect
c. proportional effect
d. internal amplification

18. How do the sizes of the pulses produced by the collection of ions in the proportional region compare to those produced by an instrument that operates in the ionization region of the gas curve for radiation detectors?

a. The pulses are larger.
b. The pulses are smaller.
c. The pulses are the same size.
d. The pulses are in resonance.

19. Gas amplification is a phenomenon associated with instruments that operate in the ________ region of the gas curve for radiation detectors.

a. recombination
b. ionization
c. proportional
d. continuous discharge

20. The output pulse-height of a gaseous detector is, in most cases, dependent upon what?

a. the numbers of ions produced in the gas
b. the quantity of radiation that passes through the gas
c. the volume of gas in the detector
d. the pressure of the gas in the tube

21. Which of the following is used for SPECT system performance?

a. high count flood
b. COR offset measurement
c. PLES phantom
d. Jaszczak phantom

22. Which of the following operations would help in improving the image contrast *after* display?

a. use a smoothing filter
b. use an edge enhancement filter
c. use windowing
d. use a formatter

23. Which SPECT cardiac slice is used to generate a polar plot?

a. SA
b. HLA
c. VLA
d. transverse

24. For the majority of studies, "cold" spots are areas on the image display that indicate.

a. increased activity
b. mistuned PMTs
c. necrotic tissue
d. nonlinearity

25. Correction tables are used for:

a. COR correction
b. detector misalignment correction
c. uniformity correction
d. linearity correction

26. Total combined energy of the *two* annihilation photos originating from an annihilation reaction is:

a. 500 keV
b. 511 keV
c. 1 MeV
d. 1.02 MeV

27. The path between the two detectors in PET is referred to as:

a. line of origination
b. line of action
c. line of response
d. line of flight

28. The chance detection of photons from *unrelated* annihilation events within the coincidence timing window is called:

a. true coincidence
b. scatter coincidence
c. random coincidence
d. prompt coincidence

29. A "blank scan" is performed in PET:

a. hourly
b. daily
c. weekly
d. with every patient study

30. Upon performing a blank scan, your final image looks like this (below). What is the likely explanation?

a. perfect blank scan
b. detector malfunction
c. an artifact in the field of view
d. unexplained phenomenon

31. In nuclear medicine, "windowing" (choosing a linear scale with threshold) is used primarily for:

a. background subtraction
b. background normalization
c. image normalization
d. image reconstruction

32. Which of the following is the correct method to calculate gall bladder (GB) ejection fraction?

a. $\dfrac{\text{net min GB counts} - \text{net max GB counts}}{\text{net min GB counts}} \times 100$

b. $\dfrac{\text{net max GB counts} - \text{net min GB counts}}{\text{net min GB counts}} \times 100$

c. $\dfrac{\text{net max GB counts} - \text{net min GB counts}}{\text{net max GB counts}} \times 100$

d. $\dfrac{\text{net max GB counts}}{\text{net max GB counts} - \text{net min GB counts}} \times 100$

33. For SPECT acquisition, a reasonable choice for pixel size would be:

a. 3.12 mm^2
b. 1/3 FWHM of detector resolution or smaller
c. equal to 3 FWHM
d. equal to 2 FWHM

34. The star artifact during SPECT reconstruction can be reduced by ________:

a. increasing the time per projection
b. decreasing the time per projection
c. increasing the number of projections
d. decreasing the number of projections

35. Which one of the following *will not* give information on left ventricular function?

a. gated equilibrium radionuclide angiography
b. gated tomographic myocardial perfusion imaging
c. ungated first-pass study
d. ungated myocardial SPECT

36. When performing a thyroid uptake, the nonthyroidal body background measurement is obtained over the:

a. stomach
b. skull
c. thigh
d. lumbar spine

37. To prepare a patient for a thyroid uptake, the technologist performs a baseline thyroid count and measures radioactivity in the neck that is twice background counts. Which of the actions listed below is the most appropriate for the technologist to follow?

a. Cancel the exam: this is a contraindication for ever performing it in this patient.
b. Administer [^{131}I]sodium iodide instead of [^{123}I]sodium iodide for the uptake.
c. Subtract the baseline counts from the thyroid counts collected at a later time.
d. Calculate a thyroid uptake using only the baseline counts.

38. The therapeutic effectiveness of ^{131}I in treating hyperthyroidism results from the delivery of energy to thyroid tissue from:

a. α particles
b. β particles
c. γ rays
d. X rays

39. Fever, dehydration, and slightly elevated white cell count are all symptoms of:

a. nontoxic goiter
b. hyperthyroidism
c. hypothyroidism
d. benign thyroid goiter

40. In a normally functioning system, an increase in circulating thyroid hormone will cause TSH secretion to:

a. decrease
b. increase
c. remain the same
d. vary unpredictably

41. Which of the following would *not* normally appear as an area of increased activity on the bone image of an adult?

a. anterior iliac crests
b. epiphyseal plates
c. sacroiliac joints
d. nasopharyngeal area

42. For which of the following clinical indications would limited bone imaging ("spot" views) be most appropriate?

a. rule out avascular necrosis of the right femoral head
b. rule out bone metastases
c. determine extent of Paget's disease
d. history of child abuse; rule out occult fractures

43. It is safe to block a portion of the pulmonary circulation with MAA particles in patients with symptoms of pulmonary emboli because:

a. the number of injected particles is very small compared to the number of available precapillary arterioles
b. the particles are made from albumin isolated from human serum
c. the particles are rapidly phagocytized by lung macrophages
d. the albumin is denatured before it is made into particles

44. If tracer concentration is visualized in the stomach, thyroid, and salivary glands on a bone image, the most likely explanation is that:

a. there is pathology in those areas
b. the patient did not drink sufficient fluids
c. the tracer contained unbound [^{99m}Tc]pertechnetate
d. the patient was imaged too soon to allow adequate blood clearance of the tracer

45. Which of the following phrases describes the sensitivity and specificity of bone imaging?

a. sensitive and specific
b. sensitive but not specific
c. not sensitive but specific
d. neither sensitive or specific

46. Ischemia means:

a. necrotic tissue
b. decreased blood flow
c. infarction
d. the superior portion of the pelvis

47. To confirm a referring physician's request for a nuclear medicine theupeutic procedure, the technologist should:

a. confer with the nuclear medicine physician
b. ask the patient why he/she came to nuclear medicine
c. telephone the referring physician for confirmation
d. locate the written directive for the therapy in the patient's medical record

48. All of the following statements about three- or four-phase bone imaging are true *except*:

a. this study includes both dynamic and static imaging
b. the last phase is performed 24 hr post-tracer administration
c. the patient is positioned under the camera prior to tracer administration
d. no special instructions are given to the patient prior to the injection

49. Which of the following structures normally appear as areas of increased activity on the bone images of a child vs. an adult?

a. ribs
b. femur
c. costochondral junctions
d. sternoclavicle joints

50. Nonreactivity toward a particular antigen is called:

a. autoimmunity
b. immunity
c. immunogenicity
d. tolerance

51. The ability of an antibody to react with one and only one antigen is known as its:

a. specificity
b. sensitivity
c. avidity
d. affinity

52. The property whereby an antibody reacts with two or more antigens of similar structure is known as:

a. sensitivity
b. avidity
c. cross-reactivity
d. immunoreactivity

53. The major antibody class found in normal human serum is:

a. IgG
b. IgM
c. IgA
d. IgD

54. All of the following PET radionuclides must be produced very close to the site where they are administered *except*:

a. ^{18}F
b. ^{11}C
c. ^{15}O
d. ^{13}N

55. For what reason is a patient's blood glucose level checked prior to [^{18}F]FDG administration?

a. FDG tends to increase blood glucose levels that may already be elevated.
b. The blood glucose level may need to be increased to ensure good tracer uptake.
c. Hyperglycemia reduces tumor uptake of the tracer.
d. FDG administration is contraindicated in diabetic patients.

56. Preparation of patients undergoing PET imaging for an oncologic clinical indication include all of the following *except*:

a. twelve-lead ECG monitoring
b. installation of IV line
c. hydration
d. fasting

57. Yttrium-90 ibritumomab tiuxetan is used for therapy of which type of cancer?

a. breast
b. prostate
c. non-Hodgkin's lymphoma
d. liver

58. Yttrium-90 ibritumomab tiuxetan is used in conjunction with which chemotherapeutic agent?

a. interferon
b. rituximab
c. cyclosporine
d. methotrexate

59. The size of the spleen can best be determined using what view of a [^{99m}Tc]sulfur colloid image?

a. anterior
b. posterior
c. right lateral
d. left lateral

60. If 4 mCi of [^{99m}Tc]sulfur colloid is administered intravenously, approximately how much activity will be concentrated in the spleen of a normal subject (biodistribution is 80, 15, and 5% to different parts of the body)?

a. 4 mCi
b. 3.2 mCi
c. 0.6 mCi
d. 0.2 mCi

61. Significant visualization of bone marrow uptake on a [^{99m}Tc]sulfur colloid liver/spleen image is most likely due to which of the following?

a. improper colloid particles that are too large
b. insufficient circulation time of the radiopharmaceutical
c. liver dysfunction
d. overactive bone marrow

62. Which of the following diagnostic tests should *not* be performed immediately before liver/spleen imaging with [^{99m}Tc]sulfur colloid?

a. gallbladder examination with ultrasound
b. chest radiograph
c. thyroid uptake with [^{123}I]sodium iodide
d. radiographic upper GI series

63. In a normal hepatobiliary study, excretion of the tracer into the intestine should occur no longer than by how many minutes following tracer administration?

a. 5 min
b. 15 min
c. 30 min
d. 60 min

64. If the gallbladder is not visualized within 60 min during hepatobiliary imaging, which of the following may be administered?

a. cimetidine
b. morphine
c. dobutamine
d. furosemide

65. Very increased serum bilirubin levels will most likely cause which of the following to be visualized on hepatobiliary images?

a. colon
b. kidneys
c. lungs
d. spleen

66. Which of the following framing rates would be most appropriate for a renal function study?

a. 0.1 sec/frame for 260 frames
b. 20 sec/frame for 78 frames
c. 2 min/frame for 13 frames
d. Framing rate is not a relevant consideration for this study.

67. For the detection of liver hemangioma, all of the following imaging is routinely performed *except*:

a. blood flow images
b. immediate blood pool images
c. delayed imaging as late as 3 hr following tracer administration
d. 24-hr delayed imaging

68. Advantages of using [^{99m}Tc]sestamibi for myocardial perfusion imaging include all of the following *except*:

a. acquisition of stress and rest images with one tracer dose
b. acquisition of ventricular function information
c. completion of stress and rest imaging on the same day
d. flexibility in the time of imaging following tracer administration

69. Which of the following agents used for pharmacologic stress testing has the longest plasma half-life?

a. adenosine
b. dipyridamole
c. dobutamine
d. nitroglycerin

70. Which of the following pharmacologic stress agents should *not* be administered to patients with asthma or bronchospastic disease?

a. adenosine
b. dipyridamole
c. dobutamine
d. both adenosine and dipyridamole

71. Dobutamine is contraindicated for stress testing in patients with all of the following conditions *except*

a. severe aortic stenosis
b. unstable angina
c. ejection fraction below 15%
d. blood glucose above 200 mg/dL

72. Which of the following is cited as an advantage of [^{99m}Tc]tetrofosmin over [^{99m}Tc]sestamibi for myocardial imaging?

a. faster tracer clearance from the GI system
b. one-day stress–rest protocol can be used
c. higher activities may be administered
d. stress and rest images can be obtained with one tracer dose

73. Treatment of the adverse effects induced by dipyridamole involves the administration of:

a. adenosine
b. aminophylline
c. antihistamines
d. nitroglycerin

74. When the heart rate is 90 beats/min, how many beats are there per second?

a. 0.011 beat
b. 0.016 beat
c. 0.67 beat
d. 1.5 beats

75. Which agent is preferred for acute myocardial infarction imaging?

a. [^{201}Tl]Cl
b. [^{99m}Tc]pyrophosphate
c. [^{99m}Tc]sestamibi
d. [^{99m}Tc]tetrofosmin

76. Which of the following pharmacologic stress agents indirectly affects adenosine receptor sites on cell membranes?

a. dobutamine
b. adenosine
c. dipyidamole
d. esmolol

77. Which of the following pharmacologic stress agents would be a contraindication for severe aortic stenosis?

a. dobutamine
b. adenosine
c. dipyidamole
d. esmolol

78. ^{89}Sr and ^{153}Sm are used for which of the following indications?

a. cardiac imaging
b. bone palliation therapy
c. bone scan to assess metastasis
d. liver/spleen metastatic disease

79. It is best *not* to administer ^{89}Sr and ^{153}Sm directly via syringe because:

a. the syringe cannot be adequately shielded
b. the radiation dose to the technologist's hands from the β emissions is great
c. there is no means of controlling the rate of radiopharmaceutical administration
d. there is an increased possibility of local irradiation of soft tissue due to infiltration

80. A patient scheduled for PET imaging with [^{18}F]FDG should avoid which of the following foods in the last meal before fasting?

a. steak and mushrooms
b. blackened fish and spinach salad
c. spaghetti and garlic bread
d. eggs and bacon

81. When reporting a medical event to the NRC, which of the following information should *not* be included?

a. identity of the patient
b. licensee's name
c. description of the event
d. remedial action

82. If a physician prescribes a radiopharmaceutical according to the patient's body weight, approximately how much activity should a 185-lb patient receive if 55 μCi/kg is prescribed?

a. 1.6 mCi
b. 4.6 mCi
c. 9.6 mCi
d. 46.0 mCi

83. Which of the following is/are medical event(s) according to the NRC?

a. [^{131}I]Sodium iodide (15 mCi) is prescribed for therapy, but 19 mCi are administered.
b. [^{99m}Tc]DTPA for renal function imaging is requested by the referring physician, but [^{99m}Tc]mertiatide is prescribed by the nuclear medicine physician.
c. A second dose of [^{99m}Tc]MAA is administered after the first is inadvertently infiltrated.
d. A myocardial perfusion dose is given to a therapy patient by mistake.

84. A syringe that contains 50 mCi of a ^{99m}Tc-labeled compound at 0600 will contain how much radioactivity at 1000?

a. 1169 kBq
b. 116.9 MBq
c. 1.17 GBq
d. 11.7 GBq

85. According to the NRC, departmental records of "medical events" must include all of the following pieces of information *except*:

a. identity of the patient
b. referring physician's name
c. nuclear medicine staff involved in the medical event
d. estimated dose to personnel involved

86. Methods to decrease personal radiation exposure when preparing patient doses for injection include all of the following *except*:

a. working as quickly as possible
b. preparing all necessary materials in advance
c. holding the radiopharmaceutical as close to the eye as possible
d. using syringe shields

87. During the IV injection of unit doses, all of the following practices are standard aseptic technique *except*:

a. wearing sterile gloves
b. using disposable equipment before its expiration date
c. aseptically cleaning the venipuncture site prior to injection with an alcohol swab
d. uncapping the needle immediately prior to the injection

88. The prescribed unit dose range for a radiopharmaceutical is 5–8 mCi. The unit dose assayed in a dose calibrator is 19.2 mCi. Which of the following actions is the best for the technologist to pursue?

a. Do not use the dose and call the radiopharmacy for a replacement dose.
b. Administer the unit dose to the patient.
c. Question whether the right radiopharmaceutical has been prepared.
d. Delay the radiopharmaceutical administration until the unit dose has decayed.

89. How many microcuries must be placed in each [^{123}I]sodium iodide capsule to provide approximately 220 μCi at the time of calibration 29 hr following preparation (DF for 1 hr = 0.9488)?

a. 264 μCi
b. 704 μCi
c. 800 μCi
d. 1009 μCi

90. Which of the following is not one of the factors that affect daily planning needs for a nuclear medicine department?

a. types and numbers of each nuclear medicine procedure
b. unit dosages or dosage ranges for each procedure
c. time interval between radiopharmaceutical preparation and administration
d. percentage of "no shows" a department expects

91. The following studies are ordered for the next day: total-body bone image, Meckel's diverticulum localization, and a hepatobiliary study. Which of the following radiopharmaceuticals is *not* needed?

a. [^{99m}Tc]macroaggregated albumin
b. [^{99m}Tc]mebrofenin
c. [^{99m}Tc]medronate
d. [^{99m}Tc]Tco^{4-} (pertechnetate)

92. Bioavailability refers to what, concerning pharmacology?

a. fraction of a drug that reaches systemic circulation after a particular route of administration
b. fraction of a drug that is excreted from the body
c. fraction of a drug that is delivered to body based on weight
d. fraction of a drug that reaches the heart

93. All IV contrast agents have a greater osmolality than plasma. The osmolality of plasma is ________ mOsm/kg.

a. 75
b. 435
c. 285
d. 525

94. Which of the following is not a route of administration of a radiopharmaceutical?

A. inhalation
b. intravenous (IV)
c. intrathecal
d. intraarterial

95. If a concentration equals 25 mCi/mL at 0700 but a dose of 30 mCi needs to drawn at 0200, what volume needs to be drawn if the DF equals1 hr = 0.985?

a. ~1.52 mL
b. ~1.11 mL
c. ~0.77 mL
d. ~0.52 mL

96. Which of the following is most characteristic of a neutron activation product produced from an (n, p) reaction?

a. decay by electron capture
b. can be made nearly carrier free
c. relatively low specific activity
d. more expensive than cyclotron products

97. Which of the following statements about the determination of aluminum contamination in ^{99m}Tc eluate is *true*?

a. The eluate sample is compared to a standard solution with an aluminum concentration of zero.
b. The test for aluminum breakthrough needs to be performed only after the generator has been eluted 10–12 times.
c. The USP states that the aluminum concentration in ^{99m}Tc eluate is not to exceed 10 μg/mL of eluate.
d. An excessively increased aluminum concentration indicates that the elution volume exceeds the capacity of the generator.

98. In practice, carrier-free specific activity means that:

a. the sample contains no chemical contaminants
b. no stable forms of the radioisotope are in the sample
c. all nuclei in the sample will always remain radioactive
d. only stable forms of an isotope are present

99. If no eluate appears in the collection vial during generator elution, the technologist should first:

a. add more elution solvent to the column
b. contact the manufacturer for advice
c. change the generator tubing
d. attempt to eluate the generator with a different (new) collection vial

100. A(n) ________ contrast material may be described as one that does not dissociate or divide into charged particles in solution.

a. ionic
b. nonionic
c. oral
d. osmolar

Answers to Examination 1

1. d Early and Sodee, 1995, p. 345; Christian *et al.*, 2004, pp. 211–213

Explaining the procedure and answering any questions the patient may have are preparations common to any procedure. If the patient is a female of childbearing age, the possibility of pregnancy must also be ruled out before administering the tracer. Pregnancy is a contraindication for procedures involving radiation unless the procedure is being performed for emergency reasons. It is not necessary to have the patient remove any attenuating materials until just before he or she is imaged.

2. c Christian *et al.*, 2004, pp. 506–507

In children, normally increased tracer activity appears in areas of active bone growth. These areas include the epiphyseal plates at the ends of the long bones and the costochondral junctions in the ribs.

3. b Early and Sodee, 1995, pp. 96–103

^{99m}Tc-labeled bone agents are prepared by combining medromite or oxidronate with [^{99m}Tc]pertechnetate. Typically about 3–10% of the pertechnetate does not bind to the medronate or oxidronate, so there is always some unbound or "free" pertechnetate in any bone tracer preparation. However, this percentage is small compared with the amount of [^{99m}Tc]medronate or [^{99m}Tc]oxidronate in the preparation and is not visualized on the bone image. If the radiopharmaceutical was not properly compounded or the ^{99m}Tc-label detached from the chemical compound, the excess [^{99m}Tc]pertechnetate taken up by the thyroid, salivary glands, and stomach is visualized on the bone image.

4. d Early and Sodee, 1995, p. 451

Many of the symptoms of pulmonary emboli are similar to those of rib fracture, myocardial infarction, and pneumonia. A chest radiograph allows the interpreting physician to rule out certain of these conditions, thereby increasing the specificity of the lung image findings.

5. b Early and Sodee, 1995, p. 448

Blood that is withdrawn into the syringe and allowed to mix with the [^{99m}Tc]MAA for a prolonged period may cause the MAA particles to clump together and the blood to clot. If this mixture is then injected into the patient, the clumped particles and "labeled" blood clots are trapped in the lung vasculature and appear as multiple small hot spots on the image.

6. d Christian *et al.*, 2004, p. 395

The NRC sets limits on the airborne concentration of ^{133}Xe. For this reason, ^{133}Xe that the patient exhales must be trapped for decay. Certain xenon-delivery units use activated charcoal for trapping the xenon.

7. d Early and Sodee, 1995, pp. 430–431

The deep venous system of the lower extremities may be imaged with [^{99m}Tc]MAA or ^{99m}Tc-labeled red blood cells. If [^{99m}Tc]MAA is used, the lungs may be imaged after the venogram to rule out pulmonary embolism.

8. d Early and Sodee, 1995, p. 635

Sublingual thyroid tissue occurs when the tissue does not descend from the base of the tongue to the neck during fetal development. It is often associated with hypothyroidism. Mediastinal thyroid tissue is often discovered after investigation of an anterior mediastinal mass visualized on chest X ray.

9. b Early and Sodee, 1995, p. 644

The upper mediastinum between the heart and the thyroid is imaged to visualize ectopic parathyroid tissue.

10. c Early and Sodee, 1995, pp. 384–385

The left anterior oblique view is the projection from which the ejection fraction (EF) is calculated. It is extremely important to separate the two ventricles to obtain an accurate EF value. Typically, 35°–45° of rotation accomplishes the separation. However, the camera should be positioned according to the patient's own anatomy to optimize separation of the two structures.

11. b Early and Sodee, 1995, pp. 409–410

Digestion directs more of the cardiac output toward the gut. Although this probably will not significantly affect myocardial uptake of the tracer, excessive tracer in the upper abdominal viscera interferes with visualization of the myocardial wall, especially when the patient is supine.

12. c Blust *et al.*, 1992, p. 53

Nitroglycerin is not used to induce pharmacologic stress. The plasma half-lives for the agents used in pharmacologic stress testing are:

Agent	Plasma Half-life
Adenosine	<10 sec
Dobutamine	2 min
Regadenoson	1–3 min
Dipyridamole	15–30 min

13. b Christian *et al.*, 2004, p. 462

A 10–15-min time interval is necessary for the colloidal particles to be completely localized within the liver and spleen.

14. b Christian *et al.*, 2004, p. 466

Increased serum bilirubin levels indicate poorly functioning hepatocytes. Therefore, these cells cannot efficiently remove the tracer from the blood, causing the tracer to be excreted through the urinary system.

15. c Christian *et al.*, 2004, pp. 569–570

[^{99m}Tc]pertechnetate is used to visualize a Meckel's diverticulum. Often the Meckel's diverticulum is lined with gastric mucosa that concentrates this tracer.

16. a Early and Sodee, 1995, pp. 526–527

24-hr images are useful in infants for demonstrating aspiration of stomach contents.

17. d Christian *et al.*, 2004, p. 482

ERPF is primarily a measurement of tubular function; therefore, a renal agent that is secreted by the tubules must be used. [^{99m}Tc]mertiatide is secreted by the renal tubules and is used to determine ERPF.

18. c Crawford and Husain, 2011, p. 90

Evaluating the quality of a bolus injection is accomplished by generating a time–activity curve over the superior vena cava and measuring the full width at half maximum (FWHM). If the left ventricular ejection fraction is being determined, an FWHM $\leq$1 sec indicates a technically satisfactory bolus injection. For a right ventricular ejection fraction, an FWHM of 2–3 sec is adequate.

19. a Early and Sodee, 1995, p. 702

In the first 24 hr after administration, the kidneys excrete almost one-third of the ^{67}Ga injected. Hence, renal activity is normally visualized on images up to 48 hr after tracer administration. After 48 hr, renal activity indicates disease.

20. c Adler and Carlton, 2003, pp. 196–197

Transmission-based precautions are applied along with standard precautions when a patient is known to be infected with a communicable disease. They are a second level of precautions that include additional safety measures depending on the method in which the disease in question is transmitted.

21. c SNM Procedure Guidelines Committee, 2011

Pentetreotide is an analog of the hormone somatostatin that is labeled with ^{111}In. It is a peptide rather than an antibody and for this reason does not induce the HAMA effect in patients. The tracer is mostly excreted through the urinary system, but a small amount is also excreted through the gastrointestinal tract.

22. b Park and Duncan, 1994, p. 240

Acetazolamide (Diamox(r)) is used in conjunction with SPECT brain imaging in patients with transient ischemic attacks, carotid artery disease, and cerebrovascular disease, among others. This technique is used to identify ischemic areas in the brain. Acetazolamide induces cerebral vasodilation. After its administration, normal blood vessels dilate, but diseased ones do not.

23. d Steves, 1999, pp. 269–271

Frequently, the radiopharmaceutical for cisternography is administered outside the nuclear medicine department. It is typically the technologist who transports the tracer to the area where the lumbar puncture is being performed and oversees its administration. One of the responsibilities of the technologist is to protect personnel in the work environment by limiting their radiation exposure and confining radioactivity to prevent the spread of contamination. In this instance, the technologist is the onsite expert in handling radioactive materials. Therefore, the technologist should ensure that any contaminated materials used during the lumbar puncture are collected for proper disposal. The administration area and any personnel who handled the radiopharmaceutical should be monitored for contamination before they are permitted to leave the area.

24. b Christian *et al.*, 2004, p. 174

Sodium phosphate ^{32}P is administered intravenously and may be used to treat polycythemia vera.

25. d Seldin, 2002, p. 110

To minimize thyroid uptake of unbound iodine that may be present in the radiopharmaceutical, supersaturated potassium iodide is administered to a patient receiving [^{131}I]tositumomab for treatment of non-Hodgkin's lymphoma. The blocking agent is administered 1 day before and for the next 14 days during therapy.

26. c Adler and Carlton, 2003, p. 243

American Heart Association standards and guidelines indicate that after verification of cardiac arrest has occurred, the rescuer should call for help first and then initiate CPR.

27. a Mallinckrodt, 2004

[^{111}In]pentetreotide should not be administered through an intravenous line containing total parenteral nutrition (TPN) mixtures because the tracer may form a complex with components of the TPN mixture. Because the chemical form of the tracer is now altered, its distribution in the body will be changed.

28. b Christian *et al.*, 2004, p. 458

When liquid and gastric emptying times are to be determined simultaneously, the solid phase is labeled with [^{99m}Tc]sulfur colloid, and the liquid phase is mixed with [^{111}In]pentetate.

29. d Adler and Carlton, 2003, p. 217

For proper drainage, the urine collection bag must always be lower than the urinary bladder. If it is not lower, the urine may reflux back into the bladder, which may result in a urinary tract infection.

30. d Christian *et al.*, 2004, pp. 566–567

Radionuclide cystography is used to assess vesicoureteral reflux. This study may be performed by the indirect or the direct method. In the indirect method, a renal agent is administered intravenously. When the tracer has cleared from the kidneys into the bladder, imaging of the ureters and kidneys is performed during and after the patient voids.

31. b Shackett, 2009, p. 423

There are 2.2 lbs per kg. Therefore,

How many kgs = 175 lbs $\times$ 1 kg/2.2 lbs = 79.54 kgs

How many micrograms of CCK needed = 79.54 kgs $\times$ 0.02 μg/1 kg = 1.59 μg total needed for patient

How many ml needed = 1.59 μg needed $\times$ 1 mL/10 μg = 0.159 mL volume needed for patient

32. d Kowalczyk and Donnett, 1996, p. 170
The term parenteral means "other than through the intestine."

33. d Early and Sodee, 1995, p. 734
The red cell survival test is used to study the lifespan of red blood cells in patients with suspected hemolytic anemia. These patients will have a cell life span shorter than normal.

34. a Christian *et al.*, 2004, p. 212
The referring physician initiates orders for diagnostic testing and enters those orders in the patient's medical record. It is the technologist's responsibility to confirm the order for a nuclear medicine test for each patient.

35. d Christian *et al.*, 2004, p. 528
A probe system equipped with a flat-field collimator should be used to obtain organ counts. This will allow adequate statistics in reasonable time periods and exclude counts coming from areas outside the region of interest.

36. d Early and Sodee, 1995, pp. 726–728, 732
Depending on body weight and gender, the total blood volume normally ranges from about 3 to 6 L. If a plasma volume has been determined to be 15 L, there was most likely some technical error that caused this result. The most plausible explanation is that the tracer was infiltrated. When this occurs, it appears as if the amount of radioactivity thought to be injected has been diluted in a large volume, but what has actually occurred is that not all the tracer was added to the circulation. Then, when a plasma sample is counted, the counts are relatively low compared with a sample in which the tracer has been diluted in a smaller volume. Or, consider the formula used to calculate a plasma volume:

$$\text{PV (mL)} = \frac{\text{volume injected} \times \text{cpm in 1 mL std} \times \text{dilution}}{(\text{cpm in 1 mL plasma})}.$$

The lower the counts in the plasma sample, the smaller the number in the denominator of the plasma volume formula, hence, the larger the calculated plasma volume.

37. d Occupational Safety and Health Administration, 1992, pp. 12–13
Biohazard warning labels are attached to any container of regulated materials. These include refrigerators, freezers, and anything used to store, transfer, or ship blood or infectious materials. Labels are not required on containers of blood that have been released for clinical use, such as blood transfusion.

38. d Early and Sodee, 1995, p. 728
The formula for calculating the total blood volume (TBV) based on the plasma volume uses the corrected plasmacrit in the denominator. Correction is needed to account for trapped plasma and to adjust the venous hematocrit to an average whole-body hematocrit. The formula is:

$$\text{TBV} = \frac{\text{plasma volume}}{1 - (\text{HCT} \times 0.97 \times 0.91)}.$$

39. c Early and Sodee, 1995, p. 728
When residual radioactivity is present in the circulation, it appears as if the amount of radioactivity injected has been diluted in a smaller volume than it actually has. Then when a plasma sample is counted, the counts are relatively high compared with a sample in which the tracer has been diluted in a large volume. Or, consider the formula used to calculate a plasma volume:

$$\text{PV (mL)} = \frac{\text{volume injected} \times \text{cpm in 1 mL std} \times \text{dilution}}{(\text{cpm in 1 mL plasma})}.$$

The higher the counts in the plasma sample, the larger the number in the denominator of the plasma volume formula, hence, the smaller the calculated plasma volume.

40. c Shackett, 2009, p. 423
25–50-mg tablet, usually given orally 1 hr prior to hypertension renal study.

41. d SNM Procedure Guidelines Committee, 2011
Imaging with [^{111}In]pentetreotide routinely includes the head to upper femurs, because detection of both the primary tumor and any metastases is the goal of the examination. If indicated, the extremities may also be included.

42. a Bristol-Myers Squibb Medical Imaging, 2004
If the suspected disease is in the left breast, it would be best to use the contralateral side of the body for injection at a site distant from the breast or lymph nodes, which may also be involved.

43. b Wells, 1999, p. 253

$$\%\ \text{activity in ROI} = \frac{\text{counts in ROI}}{(\text{total counts in all ROIs}))} \times 100$$

$$\%\ \text{activity right lung} = \frac{175{,}362\ \text{counts}}{(175{,}362\ \text{counts} + 325{,}672\ \text{counts})} \times 100$$

$$= \frac{175{,}362\ \text{counts}}{501{,}034\ \text{counts}} \times 100 = 35\%.$$

44. b Chilton and Witcofsi, 1986, pp. 57–60
Elution does not remove all ^{99m}Tc present on the generator column. Elution efficiency is expressed as the percentage of ^{99m}Tc activity on the column that is eluted:

$$\text{elution efficiency} = \frac{^{99m}\text{Tc activity eluted}}{^{99m}\text{Tc activity on column}} \times 100.$$

In this case:

$$\text{elution efficiency} = \frac{342\ \text{mCi}}{375\ \text{mCi}} \times 100 = 91\%.$$

45. b Wells, 1999, pp. 32–33

Conversions between the CGS and SI systems can be accomplished easily if you remember the three following relationships:

$$1 \text{ Ci} = 37 \text{ GBq}$$
$$1 \text{ mCi} = 37 \text{ MBq}$$
$$1 \ \mu\text{Ci} = 37 \text{ kBq}.$$

Then, to convert kilobecquerels to microcuries:

$$250 \text{ kBq} \times \frac{1 \ \mu\text{Ci}}{37 \text{ kBq}} = 6.75 \ \mu\text{Ci}.$$

46. c. Saha, 2004, p. 71

Maximum ^{99m}Tc activity is obtained about 24 hr after the last elution of ^{99m}Tc.

47. d U.S. Nuclear Regulatory Commission, 2003 (10 CFR 35.204)

According to the NRC, ^{99}Mo breakthrough must be measured in the first elution from a ^{99}Mo/^{99m}Tc generator.

48. c U.S. Nuclear Regulatory Commission, 2003 (10 CFR 35.204); Wells, 1999, pp. 224–226

At 0600, the ^{99}Mo contamination in the eluate is below the maximum allowable limit of 0.15 μCi ^{99}Mo per mCi ^{99m}Tc:

$$\frac{10 \ \mu\text{Ci}\ ^{99}\text{Mo}}{416 \text{ mCi}\ ^{99m}\text{Tc}} = 0.024 \ \mu\text{Ci}\ ^{99}\text{Mo/mCi}\ ^{99m}\text{Tc}.$$

To determine the ^{99}Mo concentration in the eluate at 1700, decay correct both the ^{99}Mo and ^{99m}Tc activities obtained at 0600 for 11 hr (0600 to 1700 = 11 hr):

^{99}Mo: 10 μCi × 0.891 = 8.9 μCi
(0.891 is the ^{99}Mo decay factor for 11 hr)

^{99m}Tc: 416 mCi × 0.282 = 117 mCi
(0.282 is the ^{99m}Tc decay factor for 11 hr)

At 1700, then, the ^{99}Mo concentration is equal to:

$$\frac{8.9 \ \mu\text{Ci}\ ^{99}\text{Mo}}{117 \text{ mCi}\ ^{99m}\text{Tc}} = 0.08 \ \mu\text{Ci}\ ^{99}\text{Mo/mCi}\ ^{99m}\text{Tc}.$$

This level is below the maximum allowable limit of ^{99}Mo contamination set by the NRC. Therefore, the eluate may be administered to patients at 1700.

49. b Saha, 2004, p. 75; Eliot, 1990, p. 49

Aluminum is a chemical impurity that is measured using a colorimetric test consisting of a special indicator paper and a reference solution of known aluminum ion concentration. No color change represents an aluminum ion concentration below 10 μg/mL of eluate, the USP limit. Therefore, this eluate may be administered to patients and used to prepare other ^{99m}Tc-labeled radiopharmaceuticals. ^{99m}Tc does contain radionuclidic impurities such as ^{99}Mo, but these impurities are assayed in a different manner.

50. d Saha, 2004, pp. 320–321

Gastric emptying and gastroesophageal relux studies and gastrointestinal bleeding localization all may be performed with [^{99m}Tc]sulfur colloid. [^{99m}Tc]pertechnetate is used to localize a Meckel's diverticulum.

51. c. Early and Sodee, 1995, pp. 627–631, 752

[^{131}I]sodium iodide is the agent used for treatment of hyperthyroidism. [^{123}I]sodium iodide is the agent of choice for thyroid uptake and may be used for thyroid imaging as well. [^{111}In]pentetate is administered for cisternography.

52. b Wells, 1999, pp. 213–214

The volume added to an MAA kit governs the number of particles in each milliliter of radiopharmaceutical and, therefore, the number of particles a patient will receive. For example, if a vial of MAA contains 2 million particles and 2 mL [^{99m}Tc]pertechnetate are added to the vial, there will be approximately 1 million particles in each milliliter. If only 1 mL is added, there will be twice as many particles in each milliliter. Therefore, a patient would receive twice as many particles in a unit dose from the second preparation.

53. d Christian *et al.*, 2004, p. 416

In both the in vivo and modified in vivo techniques, reconstituted "cold" pyrophosphate, containing stannous ions that permit [^{99m}Tc]pertechnetate to permeate red cell membranes, is administered intravenously to the patient. In the in vitro method, the entire labeling process takes place outside the patient. A blood sample is collected, to which stannous ions are added. After an incubation period, [^{99m}Tc]pertechnetate is added to the red cells after they have been isolated from the plasma. After another incubation period, the red cells are washed to remove unbound tracer, reconstituted, and injected back into the patient.

54. c Saha, 2004, p. 123

The contents in the mertiatide reaction vial are light sensitive and must be protected from light.

55. a Saha, 2004, p. 155

The R_f value is the distance traveled by a given radiochemical component compared with the solvent front:

$$R_f = \frac{\text{distance from origin to radiochemical component}}{\text{distance from origin to solvent front}}.$$

In this example, the radiochemical component in question is the radiochemical impurity. Because the impurity remained at the origin, the distance from the origin to the impurity is zero. Thus, the value for the radiochemical impurity is:

$$R_f = \frac{0 \text{ cm}}{8.5 \text{ cm}} = 0.$$

56. c *U.S. Pharmacopeia,* 1990

According to the USP, most ^{99m}Tc-labeled radiopharmacuticals should have a radiochemical purity of at least 90%.

57. d Chilton and Witcofski, 1986, pp. 17–18

The elapsed time between calibration and unit dosage administration is 4 hr (1700–1100). From a decay fact-table from ^{99m}Tc, the decay factor for 4 hr is 0.631. The initial concentration is decay corrected to determine the concentration at 1100:

$$C(t) = C(0) \times \text{DF} = 11.8 \text{ mCi/mL} \times 0.631$$

$$= 7.4 \text{ mCi/mL at 1100.}$$

Then the volume to be administered is calculated based on the prescribed patient dosage and the concentration at the time of administration:

$$\text{volume} = \frac{\text{patient dosage}}{C(t)} = \frac{8 \text{ mCi}}{7.4 \text{ mCi/mL}} = 1.1 \text{ mL.}$$

58. c Wells, 1999, pp. 172–173, 185–186

The elapsed time between calibration and unit dosage administration is 46 hr (1200, February 14 to 1000, February 16). From a decay factor table for ^{201}Tl, the decay factor for 46 hr is approximately 0.646. The initial concentration is decay corrected for 456 hr to determine the concentration at 1000, February 16:

$$C(t) = C(0) \times \text{DF} = 55.5 \text{ MBq/mL} \times 0.646$$

$$= 35.8 \text{ MBq/mL at 1000 on Feb. 16.}$$

Then the volume to be administered is calculated based on the prescribed patient dosage and the concentration at the time of administration:

$$\text{volume} = \frac{\text{patient dosage}}{C(t)} = \frac{37 \text{ MBq}}{35.8 \text{ MBq/mL}} = 1.0 \text{ mL.}$$

59. b Wells, 1999, pp. 172–173, 185–186

The elapsed time between calibration and dosage calculation is 52 hr (0800, June 29 to 1200, July 1). In this example, the radiopharmaceutical is being used before the calibration time. Therefore, the initial concentration on June 29 is the unknown, and the known concentration is divided by the decay factor. The concentration on July 1 is 1.8 mCi/mL (10.0 mCi/5.5mL):

$$C(0) \times 0.609 = 1.8 \text{ mCi/mL}$$

$$C(0) = \frac{1.8 \text{ mCi/mL}}{0.609} = 2.96 \text{ mCi/mL.}$$

Then, determine the required volume:

$$\text{volume} = \frac{\text{activity required}}{C(t)} = \frac{4.0 \text{ mCi}}{2.96 \text{ mCi/mL}} = 1.35 \text{ mL.}$$

60. c Saha, 2004, pp. 116–118

The three methods of labeling red blood cells with ^{99m}Tc all use [^{99m}Tc]pertechnetate. [^{99m}Tc]pertechnetate enters the red blood cell and binds to hemoglobin. Part of the red blood cell labeling process involves administration of a reconstituted "cold" pyrophosphate kit to provide the stannous compound necessary for labeling to occur. [^{99m}Tc]albumin is a blood-pool agent; that is, it remains in the circulation for a period of time after intravenous injection. It does not bind to the red blood cells. [^{99m}Tc]exametazime is used to label white blood cells.

61. b Saha, 2004, pp. 118–121

[^{99m}Tc]exametazime is used to label white blood cells. [^{99m}Tc]pertechnetate is used to label red blood cells. [^{99m}Tc]bicisate is used to demonstrate regional brain perfusion. [^{99m}Tc]sestamibi is used for myocardial imaging as well as other applications.

62. c GE Healthcare, 2006; Christian *et al.*, 2004, p. 169

When [^{99m}Tc]exametazime is used to label white blood cells, methylene blue stabilized is omitted from its preparation.

63. d U.S. Nuclear Regulatory Commission, 2003 (10 CFR 35.63)

The NRC states that the administered dosage must fall within the prescribed dosage range or may not differ from the prescribed dosage by more than 20%. If the prescribed dosage is 4 mCi, the measured dosage must be between 3.2 and 4.8 mCi ($\pm$20% of 4 mCi).

64. a Early and Sodee, 1995, p. 733

Radiochromium should not be added to the ACD solution before the patient's blood because ACD may change the valence of the radiochromium before labeling can take place. Ascorbic acid is added at the end of the labeling procedure to stop the tagging before the blood is returned to the patient.

65. c Wells, 1999, pp. 213–214

The concentration at 1000 is:

$$\frac{148 \text{ MBq}}{0.75 \text{ mL}} = 197 \text{ MBq/mL.}$$

At 1600, after correcting for decay, the concentration is:

$$197 \text{ MBq/mL} \times 0.5 = 98.5 \text{ MBq/mL.}$$

Therefore, the volume of a unit dosage at 1600 is:

$$\frac{148 \text{ MBq}}{98.5 \text{ MBq/mL}} = 1.5 \text{ mL.}$$

The number of particles in 1 mL remains constant over time and is:

$$\frac{325{,}000 \text{ particles}}{0.75 \text{ mL}} = 433{,}333 \text{ particles/mL.}$$

Therefore, the 1600 dosage contains twice as many particles as the 1000 dosage, because the 1600 dosage contains twice the volume to obtain the same unit dosage of 148 MBq:

$$433{,}333 \text{ particles/mL} \times 1.5 \text{ mL} = 650{,}000 \text{ particles.}$$

66. d Wells, 1999, pp. 197–198

Determine the concentration:

$$\text{concentration} = \frac{\text{total activity}}{\text{total volume}} = \frac{4.5\text{ mCi}}{1.2\text{ mL}}$$

$$= 3.75\text{ mCi/mL}.$$

Determine the volume that will contain the required activity:

$$\text{volume} = \frac{\text{activity required}}{\text{concentration}} = \frac{3.5\text{ mCi}}{3.75\text{ mCi/mL}} = 0.93\text{ mL}.$$

Determine the volume that will need to be removed from the syringe:

Total volume − volume required = volume to be removed

$1.2\text{ mL} - 0.93\text{ mL} = 0.27\text{ mL}.$

67. c Wells, 1999, pp. 192–193

Determine the concentration of the eluate:

$$\text{concentration} = \frac{\text{total activity}}{\text{total volume}} = \frac{350\text{ mCi}}{7\text{ mL}}$$

$$= 50\text{ mCi/mL}.$$

Determine the volume of [^{99m}Tc]pertechnetate needed to obtain the required activity:

$$\text{volume} = \frac{\text{activity required}}{\text{concentration}} = \frac{30\text{ mCi}}{50\text{ mCi/mL}} = 0.6\text{ mL}.$$

Because the activity must be contained in a specific volume (5 mL), sterile, preservative-free saline must be added to make up the required volume:

Reconstituting volume = [^{99m}Tc]pertechnetate volume + saline volume

Saline volume = reconstituting volume − [^{99m}Tc]pertechnetate volume

Saline volume = 5 mL − 0.6 mL = 4.4 mL

68. c Wells, 1999, pp. 166–167

In this case, the centrifuge cannot provide the necessary relative centrifugal force (RCF) identified in the protocol. However, by adjusting the time, the same degree of centrifugation may be obtained. The relationship is:

$$T_1G_1 = T_2G_2.$$

where T_1 and G_1 are the minimum time of centrifugation and RCF, respectively, and T_2 and G_2 are the alternative time and RCF, respectively. Solving for the alternative time:

$$T_2 = \frac{T_1G_1}{G_2} = \frac{(5\text{ min})(5000\text{ g})}{2500\text{ g}} = 10\text{ min}.$$

69. b U.S. Nuclear Regulatory Commission, 2003 (10 CFR 20.1902)

The NRC requires that restricted areas, such as imaging rooms, be posted with specific signs depending on the radiation level present. A "Caution: Radioactive Materials" sign should be posted in areas where certain quantities of radioactive materials are used or stored. These quantities are those exceeding 10 times the quantities specified in Appendix C to 10 CFR Part 20. The quantities for commonly used radionuclides that will result in required posting include an excess of 10 mCi of ^{99m}Tc, ^{67}Ga, ^{133}Xe, or ^{201}Tl; an excess of 1 mCi of ^{123}I or ^{111}In; more than 10 μCi of ^{131}I.

70. a U.S. Nuclear Regulatory Commission, 2003 (49 CFR 172.403 and 172.436–440)

The label types and exposure rate limits for packages containing radioactive materials are:

	Exposure Rate (mR/hr)	
Label Category	At Surface	At 1 m
Category I (white)	≤0.5	No detectable radiation
Category II (yellow)	≤50	≤1.0
Category III (yellow)	≤200	≤10

71. b Wells, 1999, pp. 101–102

Use the inverse square law:

$$(I_1)(D_1)^2 = (I_2)(D_2)^2,$$

where I_1 = intensity at original distance (D_1), and I_2 = intensity at new distance (D_2). In this example:

$$(30\text{ mR/hr})(15\text{ cm})^2 = (I_2)(40\text{ cm})^2.$$

Isolate the unknown and solve:

$$I_2 = \frac{(30\text{ mR/hr})(15\text{ cm})^2}{(40\text{ cm})^2}$$

$$I_2 \approx 4.2\text{ mR/hr}.$$

72. c Wells, 1999, p. 107

Each half-value layer (HVL) will decrease the activity to one-half of the previous activity.

No. of HVLs	Exposure Rate (mR/hr)
0	12
1	6
2	3
3	1.5

Thus three HVLs are required to decrease the exposure rate to less than 2 mR/hr. Hence, the thickness of lead required is three times the HVL, or $3 \times 0.3\text{ cm} = 0.9\text{ cm}$.

73. d U.S. Nuclear Regulatory Commission, 2003 (10 CFR 35.3045); Siegel, 2004, pp. 58–59

A licensee must notify the NRC of medical events, which are defined as an administration of a licensed material that results in an effective equivalent dose (EDE) greater than 5 rem, a dose to an organ or tissue that is greater than 50 rem, or shallow dose exposure (SDE) to the skin greater than 50 rem because of any of the following:

- The total dosage delivered differs from the prescribed dosage by 20% or more.
- The total dosage falls outside the prescribed range.
- The wrong radioactive drug was administered.
- The radioactive drug was administered by the wrong route.
- The radioactive dosage was administered to the wrong person.

When a medical event (misadministration) occurs, the NRC requires the licensee to notify the NRC, the referring physician, and the involved individual, unless the referring physician determines, on the basis of medical judgment, that such notification would be harmful to the patient.

74. b U.S. Nuclear Regulatory Commission, 2003 (10 CFR 20.1201); Siegel, 2004, pp. 28–36

According to the NRC, the annual occupational dose limit to the eye is 15 rem or 150 mSv.

75. b. U.S. Nuclear Regulatory Commission, 2003 (10 CFR 35.92); Siegel, 2004, pp. 53–54

According to NRC regulations, decay in storage of radioactive materials requires that the materials remain in storage until the radioactivity is indistinguishable from background radiation using a survey meter on the most sensitive scale and without any shielding in place.

76. a U.S. Nuclear Regulatory Commission, 2003 (10 CFR 35.70 and 10 CFR 20.1501); Siegel, 2004, pp. 43–46

NRC regulations require a survey of areas where radiopharmaceuticals that require a written directive are prepared or administered. This would include therapeutic radiopharmaceuticals and dosages of ^{131}I greater than 30 μCi. As of October 2002, the NRC no longer requires daily surveys and weekly wipe tests. Instead, it allows facilities to establish a survey and wipe test schedule. The schedule must be reasonable, based on the need to determine radiation levels, concentrations or quantities of radioactive materials, and potential radiological hazards.

77. a Thompson *et al.*, 1994, pp. 32–33

The measured exposure rate is the product of the number indicated by the needle on the meter and the scale. In this example, the reading on the meter is 1.7 on a scale of 0.1. Thus, 1.7 mR/hr $\times$ 0.1 = 0.17 mR/hr.

78. b Christian *et al.*, 2004, p. 196

Because it has not been determined that the package is free of contamination, gloves should be put on before the package or its contents are handled.

79. a Christian *et al.*, 2004, p. 202

Decontamination of a radioactive spill should continue until the residual radioactivity is below the action level set by the licensee or until no further contamination can be removed by cleaning the area. If residual radioactivity is present after thorough decontamination, the area should be covered as a reminder for personnel to limit their time in that area.

80. c U.S. Nuclear Regulatory Commission, 2003 (10 CFR 20.1502); Siegel, 2004, pp. 29–36

The NRC requires monitoring of occupationally exposed individuals if they are likely to exceed 10% of the annual allowable limit for external exposure or internal uptake.

81. c U.S. Nuclear Regulatory Commission, 2003 (10 CFR 35.75)

According to the NRC, an individual who has received a therapeutic dosage of radiopharmaceutical can be released if no other individual is likely to receive a total effective dose equivalent (TEDE) exceeding 0.5 rem (5 mSv) as a result of contact with the person who received the radiopharmaceutical.

82. c Christian *et al.*, 2004, pp. 11–13

For each half-life that passes, the activity decreases to half of the previous activity.

No. of Half-lives	Exposure Rate (mR/hr)
0	3
1	1.5
2	0.75
3	0.37
4	0.19
5	0.09
6	0.05

After 6 half-lives, the original activity has decreased to background activity.

83. b U.S. Nuclear Regulatory Commission, 2003 (10 CFR 20.2103); Siegel, 2004, p. 55

According to the NRC, the results of all surveys must be retained for 3 years.

84. c Christian *et al.*, 2004, p. 308

Tungsten is recommended because it will absorb more radiation than the same thickness of lead.

85. d Saha, 2004, p. 221

Only radiation exposure directly related to the practice of nuclear medicine as an occupation is recorded in the individual's dosimetry record. Personal diagnostic and therapeutic exposures are not included.

86. c U.S. Nuclear Regulatory Commission, 2003 (10 CFR 35.60); Siegel, 2004, pp. 50–52; Saha, 2004, pp. 70–71

The NRC requires that dose calibrators be tested for proper functioning according to nationally recognized standards. The standard of practice dictates that the measured activity should be within $\pm 10\%$ of the expected activity when the instrument is tested for linearity. If the instrument exceeds this level of error, a correction factor should be calculated and applied to all measurements in the affected activity range.

87. b Bernier *et al.*, 1994, pp. 80–81

Using a long-lived source, a reading is obtained for each of the commonly used preset buttons on the dose calibrator. Although this does not provide an accurate (true) reading, it shows whether the instrument is performing with precision (reproducibility). The reading should be within $\pm 10\%$ of the expected decay-corrected reading.

88. d Early and Sodee, 1995, pp. 158–162

Voltage may drift slightly from one day to the next, causing the gamma ray spectrum to shift to the right or left, out of the preset window. From the data, it appears that this is what may have happened. Before using the instrument for clinical studies or sending it for repair, the technologist should recalibrate the operating voltage by observing the counting rate at the most recent voltage setting and voltage settings just above and below that setting. If the counting rate increases when counts are obtained off the original operating voltage, the voltage should be adjusted until a maximum counting rate is reached. The voltage at which a maximum counting rate is obtained is the new operating voltage. If there is significant voltage fluctuation from day to day, the instrument should be serviced.

89. b Christian *et al.*, 2004, p. 81

Dose calibrator linearity should be performed quarterly.

90. b Early and Sodee, 1995, p. 262

The round photopenic area corresponds to failure of a single photomultiplier tube. Damage to the crystal would appear more irregular. Because this is an intrinsic flood, the collimator is not in place. However, collimator or damage would also have an irregular appearance. Failure of the x,y localization hardware or software would result in a misshapen flood image.

91. b Early and Sodee, 1995, p. 214

The reference source used for monitoring dose calibrator constancy must be long-lived to permit comparison of measured and predicted activities over an extended period. ^{57}Co (half-life = 270 days) and ^{137}Cs (half-life = 30 years) are sufficiently long-lived to meet this criterion.

92. b Early and Sodee, 1995, p. 247; Powsner and Powsner, 1998, pp. 129–130

The cutoff frequency of a filter determines which frequencies are passed unchanged and which are altered or suppressed. Lowering the cutoff frequency eliminates more of the high-frequency signal that gives the image its sharp detail. As more of the high frequencies are removed, the image becomes smoother or less detailed, eventually decreasing resolution.

93. c Lee, 2005, p. 153

Temporal resolution is the ability to demonstrate changes in radiopharmaceutical distribution over time. Therefore, this is a factor in dynamic and multiple-gated acquisitions, both of which acquire data in sequential frames. The framing rate is the acquisition time per frame (for example, 20 sec/frame). If the framing rate is too long, changes in radiopharmaceutical distribution can be missed. If the framing rate is too short, too few counts will be acquired in each frame, and the resolution of the images may be affected.

94. b Early and Sodee, 1995, p. 235

Temporal smoothing is used in dynamic studies to produce a gradual variation in counts and smoother motion from one frame to the next. Therefore, it is useful in gated studies, but it is not useful in static imaging, such as thyroid or whole-body images or nongated SPECT.

95. b Madsen, 1994, p. 5

Pixel size is determined by the matrix dimensions and the size of the field of view:

$$\text{pixel size (mm)} = \frac{\text{diameter of field of view (mm)}}{\text{number of pixels}}.$$

In this example:

$$\frac{350\ \text{mm}}{128\ \text{pixels}} = 2.73\ \text{mm}.$$

Because pixels are square, the dimensions of each pixel in this 128×128 matrix are 2.73×2.73 mm.

96. c Bernier *et al.* 1994, p. 189

When Geiger counter readings no longer decrease as the cleanup progresses, a wipe test, which is measured in a well counter, is performed. If the wipe test shows activity does not exceed background levels, then all removable contamination has been eliminated. If nonremovable activity remains, shielding of the spill area may be necessary.

97. a Lee, 2005, pp. 8–10, 93–95

A blood-flow study of the feet would be acquired at a framing rate of 2–4 sec/frame, so few counts would be obtained in each frame. Therefore, a small matrix must be used: 64×64. Because there will be few counts per frame, byte mode will be adequate, as it can store up to 255 counts per pixel. In word mode, about 65,000 counts can be acquired for each pixel; however, twice as much computer storage space is needed. Because this level of activity will not be present, it is wasteful—but not harmful—to use word mode.

98. b. Hines *et al.*, 2000, p. 385

For a small-field-of-view camera, 3 million counts should be acquired; for a large field of view, 5 million counts should be obtained. More counts are required as the crystal becomes larger to ensure a minimum of 10,000 counts per pixel. This minimizes the effect of noise and assures an adequate count density so that uniformity can be accurately evaluated.

99. b Christian *et al.*, 2004, p. 67
As a pinhole collimator is moved from a source, the image of the source becomes smaller. As it is moved closer, the image becomes larger.

100. a Wells, 1999, p. 127
When the geometric variation varies from the expected by more than 10%, a correction factor must be calculated and applied whenever that configuration and activity range are measured. To determine the correction factor, the following equation is used:

$$\text{correction factor} = \frac{\text{expected activity}}{\text{actual activity}}.$$

For this example:

$$\frac{212\ \mu\text{Ci}}{253\ \mu\text{Ci}} = 0.84.$$

Answers to Examination 2

1. c Early and Sodee, 1995, p. 345
Static bone imaging performed with a labeled diphosphonate compound is routinely performed 2–3 hr after tracer administration.

2. d Early and Sodee, 1995, p. 348
On bone images of adults, areas of normally increased tracer activity include all those listed as well as the sacroiliac, hip, and acromioclavicular joints and vertebral column.

3. a Christian *et al.*, 2004, p. 64
A photopenic area is one in which a smaller number of photons is visualized—a "cold" spot. A material that absorbs photons may cause an attenuation artifact, an area of falsely decreased tracer concentration. Jewelry, pocket contents, belt buckles, prostheses, and pacemakers are a few examples of objects that commonly cause photopenic areas on bone images. Tracer concentration is increased in the area of dose infiltration, acute myocardial infarction, and osteomyelitis.

4. a Christian *et al.*, 2004, p. 392
Less than 1% of the precapillary arterioles are blocked with the MAA particles; therefore, there is no adverse effect on the patient.

5. c Early and Sodee, 1995, p. 461
A nebulizer is a device that uses ultrasound or pressure to create airborne (aerosol) particles from a liquid. [^{99m}Tc]pentetate (DTPA) is introduced into the nebulizer in liquid form. When the nebulizer is activated, the liquid is converted into small radioactive droplets that are inhaled by the patient through tubing connected to the nebulizer.

6. a Shackett, 2009, p. 94
[^{99m}Tc]MAA is used to image acute deep-vein thrombosis in the lower extremities.

7. c Early and Sodee, 1995, p. 430
The tracer is introduced into the deep venous system of the legs. Therefore, the tracer is administered into the dorsal vein of each foot.

8. b Early and Sodee, 1995, p. 635
The salivary glands and saliva in the mouth, the gastric mucosa and its secretions into the intestine, and the urinary bladder are sites that normally concentrate radioiodine. Concentrations in other sites indicate areas of functioning thyroid metastases.

9. c Early and Sodee, 1995, p. 635
Of the radiopharmaceuticals listed, only [^{99m}Tc]sestamibi concentrates in parathyroid tissue. A computer subtraction technique using [^{99m}Tc]pertechnetate and [^{201}Tl]thallous chloride has been used to image the parathyroids. [^{99m}Tc]pertechnetate concentrates in the thyroid, whereas [^{201}Tl]thallous chloride localizes in both thyroid and parathyroid tissue. In this technique, the [^{99m}Tc]pertechnetate image is subtracted from the ^{201}Tl image. The resulting image demonstrates ^{201}Tl concentration in the parathyroids.

10. b Rowell, 1992, pp. 28–29
The left atrium is partially hidden by the aorta and pulmonary artery. Tilting the detector caudally visually brings the left atrium out from under these structures and separates it from the left ventricle.

11. a Roy *et al.*, 1991, p. 363
[^{99m}Tc]sestamibi is excreted through the hepatobiliary system.

12. c English *et al.*, 1993, pp. 40–42
A cardiac stress test requires a 12-lead ECG tracing, which uses 10 electrodes attached to the patient. For exercise testing, the two arm leads are positioned over the left and right supraclavicular areas, the two leg leads go over the left and right lower quadrants of the abdomen, and six chest leads are placed around the heart.

13. c Early and Sodee, 1995, pp. 489–490
Bone marrow uptake is visualized on liver/spleen images when severe liver dysfunction, such as advanced cirrhosis, is present. In such cases, the spleen has a markedly increased concentration of tracer, and the skeleton (ribs, vertebrae, sternum, etc.) is visualized as a result of increased tracer uptake in the bone marrow.

14. c Christian *et al.*, 2004, pp. 461, 464
If cystic duct obstruction is present, the tracer will be unable to enter the gallbladder. The cystic duct is the passage between the common bile duct and the gallbladder.

15. a Christian *et al.*, 2004, p. 570
For localization of a Meckel's diverticulum, imaging begins immediately after administration of the tracer.

16. a Crawford and Husain, 2011, pp. 89, 92
First-pass cardiac studies to identify or quantify left-to-right shunts are performed with radiopharmaceuticals that can be administered in small volumes of 20–25 mCi. Recommended tracers include [^{99m}Tc]pentetate, [^{99m}Tc]sestamibi, or [^{99m}Tc]tetrofosmin.

17. a Early and Sodee, 1995, p. 590
Determination of the glomerular filtration rate (GFR) requires an agent that is completely filtered by the glomeruli. [^{99m}Tc]pentetate (DTPA) is handled only by glomerular filtration.

18. b Bernier *et al.*, 1994, p. 355
Direct radionuclide cystography is performed by instilling [^{99m}Tc]pentetate, or [^{99m}Tc]sulfur colloid, into the urinary bladder. Imaging is performed as the bladder is filling and emptying.

19. d Dunnwald *et al.*, 1999, p. 110
Although all procedures listed may be performed with [^{99m}Tc]sulfur colloid, only lymphoscintigraphy requires that sulfur colloid be filtered to remove the larger particles. Particle size affects the migration of the tracer through the soft tissue to the lymph system.

20. a Adler and Carlton, 2003, pp. 225–226
Nasogastric tubes are used for gastric decompression. A physician must order the transfer and interruption of suction. The technologist may be required to reestablish suction upon the patient's arrival in the department.

21. d Bernier *et al.*, 1994, pp. 250, 261
In a normal cerebral flow study, the first phase is the arterial phase, indicated by activity in the carotid and anterior cerebral arteries. The capillary phase is followed by the venous phase, indicated by activity in the superior sagittal sinus.

22. c Bernier *et al.*, 1994, p. 217
The injection site should be imaged first to confirm that the tracer has not infiltrated outside the subarachnoid space. Reinjections may be required if infiltration is confirmed and no activity is visualized in the basal cisterns by 2–3 hr after tracer administration.

23. c Early and Sodee, 1995, p. 728
A blood sample collected before the ^{125}I-albumin is injected can provide the background present in the patient's plasma. This will permit counts from the plasma sample containing ^{125}I to be corrected for any residual ^{123}I, and the plasma volume can be performed in a timely fashion without ordering a special tracer.

24. a Early and Sodee, 1995, p. 754
^{89}Sr-chloride is used to relieve bone pain resulting from skeletal metastases.

25. c Christian *et al.*, 2004, p. 365
Although ^{131}I whole-body imaging may be performed as early as 24 hr, optimum images are obtained at 48–72 hr after tracer administration.

26. d Adler and Carlton, 2003, p. 248
Seizure patients may experience a warning that a seizure is about to occur. The technologist should assist the patient to the floor and away from objects that may injure the patient during the seizure. A pillow will cushion the head from the floor.

27. c SNM Procedure Guidelines Committee, 2011
Because the purpose of ^{111}In-penetrotide imaging is to visualize the unknown primary site of the cancer or to demonstrate the extent of the disease, anterior and posterior whole-body images should be performed.

28. c Early and Sodee, 1995, p. 517
Red blood cells labeled with [^{99m}Tc]pertechnetate are used for demonstrating intermittent lower gastrointestinal (GI) bleeding. The area between the xiphoid and symphysis pubis must be included in the field of view to visualize bleeding in the lower GI tract.

29. c Early and Sodee, 1995, p. 378
Any high-flux radiopharmaceutical that is not trapped in the lungs could be used to perform a first-pass cardiac function study. However, if stress and rest examinations are to be performed, it would be best to perform the two studies in as short a time interval as possible. Therefore, a radiopharmaceutical that clears the blood quickly and that does not concentrate in areas that would interfere with the second first-pass study is indicated. Of the tracers listed, only [^{99m}Tc]pentetate meets these criteria.

30. a Peller *et al.*, 1996, pp. 198–203
There is no patient preparation for breast imaging with [^{99m}Tc]sestamibi except explanation of the procedure to the patient.

31. b Christian *et al.*, 2004, pp. 533–534
The Schilling test is used to measure the absorption of vitamin B_{12} in patients with unexplained anemia. The absorption of vitamin B_{12} depends on the secretion of intrinsic factor by the stomach. Pernicious anemia is a vitamin B_{12} deficiency resulting from lack of intrinsic factor.

32. c Crawford and Husain, 2011, p. 92
The arrow indicates tracer prematurely returning to the lungs, an indication of a left-to-right cardiac shunt. Some of the blood on the left side of the heart is being directed back to the right side of the heart, returning to the lungs rather than being ejected out of the left ventricle into the systemic circulation.

33. d Shackett, 2009, p. 166
Subcutaneous injections are needed for a lymphoscintigraphy to determine the sential node.

34. b Christian *et al.*, 2004, p. 521
The hematocrit represents the portion of the blood made up of cellular components, and the plasmacrit represents the fluid portion. Together they comprise the total blood volume. Thus, the sum of the hematocrit and the plasmacrit, each expressed in decimal form, is equal to 1.

35. d Christian *et al.*, 2004, pp. 528–529
Sequestration sites for red blood cells include the liver and spleen. Cardiac counts are used as a standard. Renal areas are not counted.

36. c Early and Sodee, 1995, pp. 727–728
There is leakage of the labeled albumin from the vascular system. The multiple blood samples provide the information needed to estimate the leakage rate and determine the plasma counts before any leakage occurred. The plasma counts as zero-time are extrapolated from the graph.

37. c Klingensmith, 1990–1995, pp. 49–51
Propylthiouracil (PTU) interferes with the organification of iodide by the thyroid gland and is one of the antithyroid drugs available to decrease thyroid hormone production.

38. a Early and Sodee, 1995, p. 728
Injection of about 0.5 mL of heparin is sufficient to maintain the patency of the infusion set tubing used during a red cell mass determination.

39. c Shackett, 2009, p. 110
Gastric emptying studies involve combining [^{99m}Tc]sulfur colloid with eggs.

40. a SNM Procedure Guidelines Committee, 2011
[^{111}In]pentetreotide binds to somatostatin receptors in certain tumors. In the case of suspected insulinoma, there is a potential for inducing severe hypoglycemia. For this reason, an intravenous infusion of glucose should be readily available.

41. b SNM Procedure Guidelines Committee, 2011
Structure normally visualized on an image performed with [^{18}F]FDG include the brain, myocardium, liver, spleen, intestines, kidneys, and urine.

42. b SNM Procedure Guidelines Committee, 2011
The [^{14}C]urea breath test is used to detect the presence of *Helicobacter pylori* bacteria. All patients with duodenal ulcers and 80% of patients with non-drug-induced gastric ulcers are infected with *H. pylori.* The test may be used to initially diagnose the presence of infection as well as for follow-up after treatment.

43. c Wells, 1999, pp. 256–257
In this instance, the capsule that is administered to the patient is first counted as the standard. The counts in the patient's thyroid are compared with the counts in the standard to determine the percent radioiodine uptake. Because the patient's thyroid is not counted until 6 hr after the measurement of the capsule, the capsule counts collected at 0900 must be decay corrected for 6 hr. It will be assumed that room background remains about the same over the 6-hr period. To decay correct the capsule counts, multiply the capsule counts by the 6-hr decay factor for ^{123}I:

$$216{,}789 \text{ cpm} \times 0.73 = 158{,}256 \text{ cpm}.$$

Then, calculate the thyroid uptake using the following formula:

$$\% \text{ thyroid uptake} = \frac{\text{thyroid cpm} - \text{thigh cpm}}{\text{standard cpm} - \text{bkg cpm}} \times 100$$

$$= \frac{94{,}954 \text{ cpm} - 521 \text{ cpm}}{158{,}256 \text{ cpm} - 92 \text{ cpm}} \times 100$$

$$= \frac{94{,}433 \text{ cpm}}{158{,}164 \text{ cpm}} \times 100$$

$$= 60\%.$$

44. b Chilton and Witcofski, 1986, pp. 57–60
Elution efficiency is expressed as the percentage of ^{99m}Tc on the column that is eluted.

$$\text{elution efficiency} = \frac{^{99m}\text{Tc activity eluted}}{^{99m}\text{Tc activity on column}} \times 100.$$

Thus:

$$^{99m}\text{Tc activity eluted} = \text{elution efficiency} \times {}^{99m}\text{Tc activity on column}$$

$$= 0.96 \times 11.7 \text{ MBq}$$

$$= 11.2 \text{ MBq}.$$

45. a Saha, 2004, pp. 69–70
For a dry-column generator, the eluate volume is equal to the saline volume used to elute the generator. In this example:

$$\text{concentration} = \frac{863 \text{ mCi}}{5 \text{ mL}} = 172.6 \text{ mCi/mL}.$$

Using an evacuated vial with a volume larger than the saline volume causes air to be pulled over the column, completely removing any saline. Hence, the name dry-column generator.

46. a Eliot, 1990, p. 50
Loss of vacuum from the elution vial is most likely the cause of this problem and the easiest to rule out. Checking the tubing may cause increased radiation exposure to the technologist because the column shielding meets only U.S. DOT requirements for shipping radioactive materials. Additional shielding is usually required around the generator to decrease radiation exposure to individuals in its vicinity. Also, changing tubing is not practical, because this will compromise the sterility of

the generator components. Adding more saline probably will not force the first saline volume from the column. A vacuum is needed to draw the liquid from the column. Contacting the manufacturer first may delay resolution of an easily solvable problem.

47. b U.S. Nuclear Regulatory Commission, 2003 (10 CFR 35.2204)

The NRC requires that records of ^{99}Mo concentrations in ^{99m}Tc eluates be retained for 3 years.

48. c Saha, 2004, p. 75; U.S. Nuclear Regulatory Commission, 2003 (10 CFR 35.204)

Aluminum is a chemical impurity and not subject to regulation by the NRC. Free pertechnetate is [^{99m}Tc]pertechnetate that is not bound to another compound. ^{99m}Tc is eluted from a generator as [^{99m}Tc]pertechnetate. ^{99}Mo is a radionuclidic impurity, a radionuclide other than the desired one, in ^{99m}Tc eluate. According to NRC regulations, its concentration must be determined in the first elution of a ^{99}Mo/^{99m}Tc generator.

49. a Schwarz *et al.*, 1997, pp. 167–172

The technologist does not need to order or prepare [^{99m}Tc]macroaggregated albumin, the agent used to perform perfusion lung imaging. A renal function study may be performed with [^{99m}Tc]mertiatide, bone imaging with [^{99m}Tc]medronate, Meckel's diverticulum localization with [^{99m}Tc]pertechnetate, and a hepatobiliary study with [^{99m}Tc]mebrofenin.

50. a U.S. Nuclear Regulatory Commission, 2003 (10 CFR 35.2040)

The NRC requires that records of written directives be maintained for 3 years.

51. c Saha, 2004, p. 284

[^{99m}Tc]pentetate is the renal agent used to determine glomerular filtration rate because it is handled by the kidneys solely by glomerular filtration. It is neither bound to protein nor secreted by the renal tubules as are other renal agents.

52. d Wells, 1999, pp. 183, 192–193

The maximum activity that can be prepared from this kit is equal to:

$$\text{maximum reconstituting volume} \times {}^{99m}\text{Tc concentration}$$

$$\text{maximum activity} = 3\text{ mL} \times 75.5\text{ mCi/mL}$$

$$= 226.5\text{ mCi}.$$

To calculate the concentration of the kit, note that the reaction vial contains lyophilized reagents with no appreciable volume. Hence, the total volume in the kit is the sum of the [^{99m}Tc]pertechnetate volume and the volumes in the two syringes:

$$\text{concentration} = \frac{\text{total activity in preparation}}{\text{total vol in preparation}}$$

$$= \frac{\text{maximum activity to be prepared}}{{}^{99m}\text{Tc vol} + \text{vol to be prepared in syringes I} + \text{II}}$$

$$= \frac{226.5\text{ mCi}}{3\text{ mL} + 1.6\text{ mL} + 1.6\text{ mL}} = 36.5\text{ mCi/mL}.$$

53. a Saha, 2004, pp. 114–115, 121–123

Heating is required for the preparation of [^{99m}Tc]mertiatide, [^{99m}Tc]sestamibi, and [^{99m}Tc]sulfur colloid. The preparation of [^{99m}Tc]bicisate requires a 30-min incubation at room temperature.

54. a Chilton and Witcofski, 1986, pp. 54–61

Generator yield, amount of ^{99m}Tc that may be eluted from a ^{99}Mo/^{99m}Tc generator, is calculated by using decay equations that determine the amount of ^{99m}Tc formed from the decay of ^{99}Mo at any given time. The sequence for calculating the generator yield is as follows:

1. Determine the time elapsed between calibration of the ^{99}Mo activity and generator elution.
2. Calculate the amount of ^{99}Mo activity in the generator at the time of elution by decay correcting the initial ^{99}Mo activity.
3. Determine how much ^{99}Tc activity is in the generator by calculating how much has formed from the decay of ^{99}Mo.
4. After elution, measure the amount of ^{99m}Tc activity (with a dose calibrator) collected from the generator.
5. Calculate the generator yield, or elution efficiency, by comparing the measured activity of ^{99m}Tc eluted from the generator to the ^{99m}Tc activity calculated to be in the generator in step 3.

55. b Saha, 2004, p. 155

The R_f value is the distance traveled by a given radiochemical component compared with the solvent front:

$$R_f = \frac{\text{distance from origin to radiochemical component}}{\text{distance from origin to solvent front}}.$$

In this instance, the R_f value for the hydrolyzed-reduced ^{99m}Tc is:

$$R_f = \frac{2.5\text{ cm}}{12.6\text{ cm}} = 0.20.$$

56. b Saha, 2004, p. 59

Specific activity is defined as the amount of radioactivity per unit mass of a radionuclide or labeled compound and is expressed in units of radioactivity per mass. Megabecquerels per mole (MBq/mole), Ci/g, and μCi/mg are units of specific activity. Kilobecquerels per milliliter (kBq/mL) is an expression of concentration, the amount of radioactivity per unit volume.

57. d Wells, 1999, pp. 179–181, 185–186

The elapsed time between calibration and dose calculation is 3 days (May 18–21). In this instance, the radiopharmaceutical is being used before the calibration time. Therefore, the initial concentration on May 18 is the unknown, and the known concentration is divided by the decay factor. The concentration on May 21 is 1.0 mCi/mL (3.0 mCi/3.0 mL):

$$C(0) \times 0.480 = 1.0\text{ mCi/mL}$$

$$C(0) = \frac{1.0\text{ mCi/mL}}{0.480} = 2.1\text{ mCi/mL}.$$

Then, determine the required volume:

$$\text{volume} = \frac{\text{activity required}}{C(t)} = \frac{1.0 \text{ mCi}}{2.1 \text{ mCi/mL}} = 0.48 \text{ mL}.$$

58. b Wells, 1999, pp. 32–33

Calculate the total activity to be administered to the patient based on body weight:

$$15.5 \text{ kg} \times 25 \ \mu\text{Ci/kg} = 387.5 \text{ mCi}.$$

None of the options match this answer unless it is expressed in millicuries. Thus,

$$387.5 \ \mu\text{Ci} \times \frac{\text{mCi}}{1000 \ \mu\text{Ci}} = 0.39 \text{ mCi}.$$

59. d Wells, 1999, pp. 32–33

$$925 \text{ MBq} = 25 \text{ mCi}.$$

The prescribed dosage is expressed as a range, ±10% of 925 MBq or 25 mCi:

$$0.10 \times 25 \text{ mCi} = 2.5 \text{ mCi}.$$

Therefore, the prescribed range is 22.5 mCi (25 mCi − 2.5 mCi) to 27.5 mCi (25 mCi + 2.5 mCi). Any dose calibrator reading between 22.5 mCi and 27.5 mCi verifies that the prescribed activity was withdrawn into the syringe.

60. b Saha, 2004, pp. 116–118

Reconstructed stannous pyrophosphate must be administered first. This step, sometimes referred to as "pretinning," permits [^{99m}Tc]pertechnetate to enter the red blood cells.

61. a Wells, 1999, pp. 192–193

Because the total activity to be prepared is known, it is easiest to calculated the volume of [^{99m}Tc]pertechnetate. The volume of [^{99m}Tc]pertechnetate is equal to

$$\frac{\text{activity desired}}{\text{concentration of } ^{99m}\text{Tc}} = \frac{20 \text{ mCi}}{20 \text{ mCi/mL}} = 1.0 \text{ mCi}.$$

Then, determine the volume of succimer reagent needed. If 1.0 mL = 2 parts, then 1 part must equal half of that, or 0.5 mL.

62. c Adler and Carlton, 2003, p. 202

Materials that have passed their expiration date should not be used with patients. In the case of venipuncture materials, the sterility of the materials may be compromised.

63. d U.S. Nuclear Regulatory Commission, 2003 (10 CFR 35.2204)

Records of ^{99}Mo concentration measurements must contain the ration of ^{99}Mo to ^{99m}Tc, the time and date of the measurement, and the name of the individual making the measurement.

64. b U.S. Nuclear Regulatory Commission, 2003 (10 CFR 35.40)

According to the NRC, a written directive is required for any dosage of [^{131}I]sodium iodide greater than 30 μCi or for any therapy dosage of an unsealed by-product material.

65. b Saha, 2004, p. 182; Chilton and Witcofski, 1986, p. 62

If ^{99m}Tc eluate needs to be diluted to prepare other ^{99m}Tc-labeled products, the correct diluent is preservative-free isotonic saline. Preservatives may act as oxidizing agents that reverse the effect of reducing agents in kits. The reducing agents are necessary to make ^{99m}Tc more chemically active so that it will bind to the compound being labeled.

66. d Wells, 1999, pp. 197–198

Decay correct the total activity for 24 hr (July 9, 0800, to July 10, 0800 = 24 hr):

$$5 \text{ mCi} \times 0.808 = 4 \text{ mCi}.$$

Determine the concentration:

$$\text{concentration} = \frac{\text{total activity}}{\text{total volume}} = \frac{4.0 \text{ mCi}}{2.6 \text{ mL}}$$

$$= 1.54 \text{ mCi/mL}.$$

Determine the volume that will contain the required activity and that will need to be retained in the syringe:

$$\text{volume} = \frac{\text{activity required}}{\text{concentration}} = \frac{3.0 \text{ mCi}}{1.54 \text{ mCi/mL}}$$

$$= 1.54 \text{ mCi/mL}.$$

67. a Wells, 1999, pp. 218–219

The elution efficiency of a generator is expressed as a percentage of the estimated amount of [^{99m}Tc]pertechnetate on the generator column compared to what is actually collected in the elution vial.

$$198 \text{ mCi}/268 \text{ mCi} \times 100\% = \sim 74\%.$$

68. d Lile *et al.*, 2003, p. 273

The volume of a solution in a syringe is measured at the edge of the plunger's stopper where the calibration mark aligns with the edge of the stopper.

69. a U.S. Nuclear Regulatory Commission, 2003 (49 CFR 172 and 173)

The U.S. Department of Transportation (DOT) regulates the packaging and transport of radioactive materials. NRC regulations follow DOT requirements.

70. c U.S. Nuclear Regulatory Commission, 2003 (49 CFR 172.403 and 172.436–440)

The label types and exposure rate limits for packages containing radioactive materials are:

Label category	Exposure rate (mR/hr)	
	At surface	At 1 meter
Category I (white)	≤0.5	No detectable radiation
Category II (yellow)	≤50	≤1.0
Category III (yellow)	≤200	≤10

71. b Wells, 1999, pp. 101–102
Use the inverse square law:

$$(I_1)(D_1)^2 = (I_2)(D_2)^2,$$

where I_1 = intensity at original distance (D_1) and I_2 = intensity at new distance (D_2). In this example:

$$(36 \text{ mR/hr})(0.5 \text{ m})^2 = (18 \text{ mR/hr})(D_2)^2.$$

Isolate the unknown and solve:

$$(D_2)^2 = \frac{(36 \text{ MR/hr})(0.5 \text{ m})^2}{18 \text{ mR/hr}}$$

$$= 0.5 \text{ m}^2.$$

Take the square root of each side:

$$D_2 \approx 0.7 \text{ m}.$$

72. c Bernier *et al.*, 1994, pp. 14–16
If 1.25 cm of lead is one HVL, then twice that thickness (2 × 1.25 cm) is two HVL. Each HVL absorbs 50% of the photons and allows 50% to be transmitted through the shield.

Number of HVLs	0	1	2	3
Photon intensity (%)	100	50	25	12.5
% absorbed	0	50	75	87.5
% transmitted	100	50	25	12.5

73. b U.S. Nuclear Regulatory Commission, 2003 (10 CFR 35.40)
The NRC requires a written directive before administration of ^{131}I in quantities greater than 30 (Ci and any other unsealed by-product material that is used for therapy. [^{32}P]sodium phosphate and [^{89}Sr]chloride are used for therapy, whereas [^{18}F]FDG is used for diagnostic purposes.

74. d U.S. Nuclear Regulatory Commission, 2003 (10 CFR20.1201); Siegel, 2004, p. 28–36
According to the NRC, the annual occupational dose limit to any organ or tissue, other than the eye, is 50 rem or 500 mSv.

75. c U.S. Nuclear Regulatory Commission, 2003 (10 CFR20.2003)
According to NRC regulations, only patient excreta are exempt from any limits when discarded into the sewage system. Disposal limits for other radioactive waste are based on the solubility and rate of waste water discharge from a facility.

76. b Thompson *et al.*, 1994, p. 32
To ensure that the batteries are functional, a battery check should be performed immediately before taking any measurements with a survey meter.

77. b Thompson *et al.*, 1994, pp. 32–33
The needle will register 5 for a full-scale deflection on this meter. The maximum scale is 10. The maximum exposure rate that could be measured is the product of the number at full deflection and the maximum scale. Thus, 5 mR/hr × 10 = 50 mR/hr.

78. a Christian *et al.*, 2004, p. 196
The exposure rate of the packing material is approximately the same as room background, so the carton may be disposed of in the regular trash after any radiation symbols are removed or obliterated.

79. c U.S. Nuclear Regulatory Commission, 2003 (10 CFR 20.1701)
NRC regulations require facilities to use facility design and procedures that will minimize the potential for contamination to the extent practicable. Rooms in which radioxenon is used should be tested to determine the amount of time required for evacuation of gas from the room after a gas spill. A negative air pressure exhaust system would be necessary to draw the xenon out of the room without spreading it to adjacent areas.

80. b U.S. Nuclear Regulatory Commission, 2003 (10 CFR 35.63); Siegel, 2004, pp. 50–51
According to NRC regulations, a unit dosage can be calibrated before administration by one of the following methods: direct calibration using a dose calibrator, or application of a decay factor to the original activity if the dosage has not been manipulated (adjusted) after it was originally prepared and calibrated.

81. c Christian *et al.*, 2004, p. 205
Patients should be given instructions to follow for 3–7 days that will minimize spread of contamination and radiation exposure to others.

82. c Christian *et al.*, 2004, pp. 11–13
For each half-life that passes, the activity decreases to half of the previous activity. In this case, four half-lives are required for the activity to drop to the specified level. If each half-life is 6 hr, the total time required is 24 hr.

83. b U.S. Nuclear Regulatory Commission, 2003 (10 CFR 35.315)
If a person is hospitalized after administration of a therapeutic dosage of ^{131}I, the door of the room must have signage that indicates the length of time a visitor may stay.

84. a U.S. Nuclear Regulatory Commission, 2003 (10 CFR 35.3545)

NRC regulations state that the NRC Operations Center must be notified of a medical event (error) (misadministration) no later than the next calendar day.

85. c U.S. Nuclear Regulatory Commission, 2003 (10 CFR 35.75)

NRC regulations state that written instructions for precautions must be provided to the patient or the patient's parent or guardian if any individual is likely to exceed 0.1 rem (1 mSv) exposure from the therapy patient.

86. a Saha, 2004, p. 71

To ensure that the shields will give accurate results, the decay method must be performed at the same time the shields are first used.

87. b U.S. Nuclear Regulatory Commission, 2003 (10 CFR 35.60); Siegel, 2004, pp. 50–52; Saha, 2004, p. 70

The NRC requires that dose calibrators be tested for proper functioning according to nationally recognized standards. The standard of practice requires the measured value to be within ±10% of the calculated value. In this example, the measured values for ^{57}Co, ^{99m}Tc, and ^{123}I are within that limit. The measured value for ^{201}Tl, however, varies by more than 10% of the calculated value.

$$0.10\ (53.5\ \mu\text{Ci}) = 5.35\ \mu\text{Ci}.$$

The measured value at the ^{201}T1 setting could vary from 48.15 μCi to 58.85 μCi and be within the prescribed limit. However, the measured value is outside this range.

88. a Wells, 1999, pp. 129–130

The full width at half maximum (FWHM) is defined as the width of the photopeak, expressed in keV, at one-half of the maximum or peak counts. This value is used to determine the energy resolution of a scintillation counter. The FWHM is determined by calculating 50% of the highest count obtained. In this example, 50% of 15,000 cpm is 7,500 cpm. Then, a horizontal line is drawn from one side of the photopeak to the other at the 50% point. At the two places on each side of the graph where the horizontal intersects with the graph, a vertical line is dropped to the *x*-axis. The FWHM is calculated by subtracting the larger value from the smaller. In this example, the width of the photopeak is 50 keV (705–655 keV).

89. c Early and Sodee, 1995, p. 214

After the long-lived reference is read on its setting, the same source should be used to obtain a reading on each commonly used radionuclide setting. ^{99m}Tc, ^{201}T1, ^{123}I, and ^{131}I are commonly used radionuclides, whereas ^{125}I is used infrequently. ^{57}Co and ^{137}Cs are reference standards that are counted only on a daily basis.

90. c Bernier *et al.*, 1994, p. 813

The linearity/resolution image was obtained with an orthogonal-hole phantom.

91. c Bernier *et al.*, 1994, p. 80

The standard of practice for performing a dose calibrator accuracy test calls for the use of at least two long-lived reference sources. The measured value should be within ±10% of the calculated value. If the instrument fails to meet this standard, it should be repaired or replaced.

92. d Early and Sodee, 1995, pp. 245–248; Powsner and Powsner, 1998, pp. 126–128

The ramp filter is a high-pass filter; that is, it permits high frequencies to pass through while altering the lower frequencies. This suppresses the star artifact created during filtered backprojection and increases resolution. However, it has little effect on statistical noise, so a low-pass filter, such as Butterworth, Hanning, or Parzen, must be used to eliminate some of this noise, thereby smoothing the image.

93. a Early and Sodee, 1995, pp. 260–261, 267

The UFOV is first determined by measuring the diameter of the largest area that can be inscribed within the collimated field of view. Then, the CFOV is defined as a circle with a diameter that is 75% of the UFOV diameter.

94. b Lee, 2005, pp. 151–152

If the patient's heart rate is 95 beats per minute, then each heart beat or R–R interval is:

$$\frac{60\ \text{sec}}{95\ \text{beats}} = 0.65\ \text{sec/beat}.$$

95. b Wells, 1999, p. 159

The following calculation is utilized when using the point source or line source method for pixel calibration:

$$\text{pixel size} = \frac{\text{distance between sources}}{\text{number of pixels between activity profile peaks}}.$$

In this example:

$$\frac{15\ \text{cm}}{45\ \text{pixels}} = 0.33\ \text{cm}.$$

96. d Early and Sodee, 1995, pp. 197–202

With activities in the millicurie range and sometimes much lower, photons are striking the well-counter crystal at very short intervals. The instrument is in deadtime while many photons are interacting with the crystal. These photons will not be counted and are therefore "lost."

97. a Wells, 1999, pp. 81–82

The 95% confidence level is most commonly used in nuclear medicine. To determine the minimum counts (N) needed to assure a maximum given percent error, the following equation is used:

$$\%\ \text{error} = \frac{(2)(100\%)}{\sqrt{N}}.$$

In this example:

$$2\% = \frac{(2)(100\%)}{\sqrt{N}}.$$

98. d Wells, 1999, p. 173

When the decay factor for a desired time is not available, a combination of decay factors can be used to obtain the correct one. In this case, the 2-year decay factor is multiplied by itself to obtain the 4-year decay factor. The original activity is then multiplied by the decay factor to obtain the expected activity of the source.

$$0.955 \times 0.955 \times 200\ \mu\text{Ci} = 182.4\ \mu\text{Ci}.$$

99. b Wells, 1999, pp. 113–114, 172–173

First, the source activity must be decay corrected for 35 days. When the specific decay factor is not available, a combination of decay factors can be used. To obtain the 35-day decay factor, multiply the 30-days factor by the 5-days factor:

$$0.926 \times 0.987 = 0.914.$$

Determine the decay-corrected source activity by multiplying the original activity by the calculated decay factor:

$$325.8\ \mu\text{Ci} \times 0.914 = 297.8\ \mu\text{Ci}.$$

According to the accepted limits for dose calibrator constancy, the measured activity of the source should be within $\pm 10\%$ of the calculated or expected activity. Determine the $\pm 10\%$ range:

$$297.8\ \mu\text{Ci} \times 0.1 = 29.8\ \mu\text{Ci}$$

$$297.8\ \mu\text{Ci} \pm 29.8 = 268.0 - 327.6\ \mu\text{Ci}.$$

If the dose calibrator reading falls within this range, it meets the standard of practice for dose calibrator constancy.

100. d Wells, 1999, p. 127

When the geometric variation varies from the expected by more than 10%, a correction factor must be calculated and applied whenever that configuration and activity range are measured. To apply a correction factor:

$$\text{true activity} = \text{actual activity reading} \times \text{correction factor}$$

In this example:

$$26.2\ \text{mCi} \times 1.15 = 30.1\ \text{mCi}.$$

Answers to Examination 3

1. b Early and Sodee, 1995, p. 345

Maximum skeletal uptake of [^{99m}Tc]medronate and [^{99m}Tc]oxidronate occurs within 45 min after tracer administration, and imaging is to allow the excess circulating tracer to be cleared from the blood by the kidneys. Such clearance is necessary to increase the target (bone)-to-nontarget (soft tissue) ratio for an optimal image.

2. a Early and Sodee, 1995, pp. 348, 354, 359, 361

Paget's disease, skeletal metastases, and occult fractures resulting from child abuse all have the potential to be widespread throughout the skeleton. For these conditions, then, because their extent is unknown before imaging, total-body bone imaging is indicated. Temporomandibular joint (TMJ) pain is localized; therefore, "spot" view imaging of the skull, face (especially in the area of the TMJs), and cervical spine is indicated.

3. c Christian *et al.*, 2004, pp. 509–510

Early images are important in diagnosing inflammatory conditions such as osteomyelitis. The flow study, the first phase of a multiphase bone image, is important in demonstrating increased blood flow to the affected area. In osteomyelitis, tracer concentration remains increased throughout the other phases.

4. d Christian *et al.*, 2004, p. 394; Early and Sodee, 1995, p. 449

At least six views should be performed in a lung perfusion study: anterior, posterior, right and left laterals, and right and left posterior obliques. Some authors recommend eight standard views; those previously mentioned plus right and left anterior obliques.

5. a Adler and Carlton, 2003, p. 145

Initial feelings of dizziness and faintness when going from a recumbent to an upright position may be the result of a slight drop in blood pressure that occurs when the patient moves too quickly. To help minimize the severity of this orthostatic hypotension, the patient should be encouraged to talk and breathe slowly and deeply. Symptoms should subside within a few minutes. If they do not, the technologist should seek medical help.

6. c Early and Sodee, 1995, pp. 461–462

To perform a ventilation study with [^{99m}Tc]pentetate aerosol, the liquid tracer is placed into the nebulizer, where it is broken up into small airborne particles that are inhaled by the patient. The patient is connected to the nebulizer with tubing and a face mask or mouthpiece. After inhalation of the tracer, the patient is disconnected from the delivery apparatus. Then, the patient is imaged. Because the particles remain where they have been deposited for a period of time, the same views that are acquired for the perfusion images may be acquired for the ventilation images. The nebulizer, tubing, and face mask or mouthpiece all are contaminated with [^{99m}Tc]pentetate and must be handled as radioactive waste.

7. b Bernier *et al.*, 1994, pp. 299–300

The purpose of radionuclide venography is to demonstrate the presence of thrombi in the deep veins of the legs and pelvis (internal iliacs). Therefore, elastic bandages are used to wrap the legs between the ankles and knees to divert blood flow from the superficial circulation to the deep venous system.

8. d Christian *et al.*, 2004, p. 205
It is important to monitor a radioiodine therapy patient daily to determine the earliest possible release from isolation. The measurement should be performed using the same instrument and counting geometry each time the radiation level is monitored to permit comparison of measurements.

9. b Adler and Carlton, 2003, pp. 140–141
The draw sheet is the one on which the patient is lying and is used for transferring the patient from stretcher to imaging table.

10. d Christian *et al.*, 2004, p. 416
An equilibrium ventricular function study requires a radiopharmaceutical that remains in the blood pool. Many departments label the patient's red blood cells with [^{99m}Tc]pertechnetate, but other facilities prefer the immediate availability of [^{99m}Tc]albumin. Currently, [^{99m}Tc]albumin is available only outside the United States.

11. c Crawford and Husain, 2011, p. 40
All of the diagrams are correctly labeled cross-sectional slices of the heart: (1) transaxial, (b) short axis, (c) horizontal long axis, and (d) vertical long axis.

12. a Crawford and Husain, 2011, p. 8
[^{99m}Tc]sestamibi is taken up into the myocardium in proportion to blood flow. It is taken into the myocardial cells, bound, and retained in the myocardium. Therefore, it does not redistribute the way [^{201}T1]thallous chloride does, making it necessary to administer tracer for both the stress and rest portions of the examination.

13. b Early and Sodee, 1995, pp. 505–506
Hepatobiliary agents are cleared from the blood by the hepatocytes in the liver. The tracer is cleared from the hepatocytes into the common bile duct and gallbladder and from there into the small intestine.

14. c Early and Sodee, 1995, p. 504
Ingestion of food may cause the gallbladder to contract, potentially causing a false-positive result; that is, the gallbladder is not visualized. While the gallbladder is contracting, tracer will not be able to flow into it.

15. b Early and Sodee, 1995, pp. 528–529
The physician performs an intraperitoneal injection of the tracer.

16. c Early and Sodee, 1995, p. 587
A transplanted kidney is placed in the iliac fossa. Therefore, a transplanted kidney should be imaged with the patient supine and the camera placed anteriorly over the pelvis.

17. b Rowell, 1992, p. 41
Because an ERPF is a quantitative study, any tracer infiltration will invalidate the calculated ERPF values. Therefore, it is essential to confirm that the entire amount of activity was injected into the circulatory system.

18. c Bernier *et al.*, 1994, p. 355
Direct radionuclide cystography requires that the patient be catheterized and the bladder drained. The tracer is then instilled into the bladder with saline. Although [^{99m}Tc]pentetate, a renal agent, may be used, it is not required. [^{99m}Tc]sulfur colloid or [^{99m}Tc]pertechnetate may be used.

19. c Early and Sodee, 1995, pp. 702–709
Leukocytes accumulate in areas of infection or inflammation. Thus, they would accumulate at ostomy sites, in osteomyelitis, and in dental abscesses.

20. a Adler and Carlton, 2003, p. 240
Pale, cold, clammy skin is characteristic of shock. The patient may also exhibit restlessness and tachycardia.

21. a Early and Sodee, 1995, p. 560
[^{99m}Tc]gluceptate, [^{99m}Tc]pentetate, and [^{99m}Tc]pertechnetate cross the blood–brain barrier only if disease has caused a disruption in the barrier. Therefore, these agents remain in the blood pool unless there is a disruption in the blood–brain barrier. [^{99m}Tc]bicisate and [^{99m}Tc]exametazime normally cross the blood–brain barrier and are taken up in brain tissue in proportion to blood flow.

22. b Mettler and Guiberteau, 1991, p. 74
A ventriculoperitoneal shunt is designed to treat hydrocephalus by directing excess cerebral spinal fluid into the peritoneal cavity, where it is absorbed into the circulation. The patency of the shunt can be ascertained by injecting a tracer, typically [^{99m}Tc]pertechnetate, into the shunt tubing and imaging the movement of the tracer down the tube into the peritoneum. Because of the short duration of this examination, ^{99m}Tc may be used.

23. d Saha, 2004, p. 204
Written consent must be obtained for any radiopharmaceutical that is investigational. These drugs are referred to as investigational new drugs (INDs). All of the radiopharmaceuticals cited have been approved by the FDA for clinical use. That is, their new drug authorization (NDA) has been approved, and they are referred to as NDA drugs.

24. c Elgazzar and Maxon, 1993
Patient preparation for [^{89}Sr]chloride therapy includes total-body bone imaging to demonstrate increased tracer uptake in painful metastatic sites, a complete blood count to confirm adequate platelet and white blood cell counts, and renal function studies because the major route of tracer excretion is through the kidneys.

25. b Steves, 1999, pp. 272–280
In preparation for ^{131}I therapy for thyroid cancer, the patient will need to be instructed about the requirements and limitations associated with being in isolation. If the patient is female, a pregnancy test must be performed immediately before the radioiodine is administered. Pregnancy is an absolute contraindication to ^{131}I therapy. If the woman is breastfeeding, she must discontinue this activity. Oral potassium iodide may be administered to personnel who are exposed to airborne radioiodine as a means of preventing tracer uptake in the thyroid gland.

26. d Adler and Carlton, 2003, p. 266
Verification should be done before injection, and the label should be checked when the radiopharmaceutical is removed from the shelf, when it is dispensed, and when it is returned to the shelf.

27. a Crawford and Husain, 2011, p. 33
The dual-radionuclide myocardial perfusion imaging protocol used [^{99m}Tc]sestamibi for stress imaging and [^{201}Tl]thallous chloride for rest imaging. [^{99m}Tc]tetrofosmin may be used in place of [^{99m}Tc]sestamibi. The dual-radionuclide protocol shortens the time that patients spend in the imaging department and is useful for evaluating myocardial ischemia and viability.

28. a Early and Sodee, 1995, p. 518
[^{99m}Tc]sulfur colloid is cleared from the blood and localized in the liver and spleen within 15 min of administration. Therefore, to demonstrate gastrointestinal bleeding with this tracer, it will have to occur while the tracer is still circulating.

29. a Christian *et al.*, 2004, pp. 413–414
A cardiac first-pass study requires a bolus injection technique to demonstrate each of the cardiac chambers separately. Therefore, a large peripheral vein, such as the median basilic or external jugular, is needed.

30. a Shackett, 2009, p. 319
Patient preparation for ^{131}I therapy includes a low-iodine diet for 1 week prior to therapy to help increase the ability of the thyroid gland or metastatic cancer as a whole to uptake the radioactive ^{131}I versus stable iodine. This will allow for a better uptake of the ^{131}I. Not all salt has iodine added to it.

31. a Shackett, 2009, p. 104
The proper route of administration for ^{67}Ga infection imaging is intravenously.

32. d Early and Sodee, 1995, p. 725
Because radioiodinated serum albumin is "sticky," it has a tendency to adhere to substances, including tissue. Tracer administration and blood sampling should be performed, if possible, in contralateral arms.

33. c Adler and Carlton, 2007, p. 316
An intravenous injection should be done with the needle at about a 15-degree angle to the vein it is being inserted into.

34. c Christian *et al.*, 2004, p. 525
The gamma energy of ^{51}Cr is 320 keV. Therefore, the scintillation detector should be set to accommodate this photopeak.

35. b Crawford and Husain, 2011, p. 40
The short-axis slice displays all walls of the left ventricle.

36. d Early and Sodee, 1995, p. 628
A scintillation probe with a flat-field-of-view collimator is used for a radioiodine uptake test. The flat-field collimator allows for small variations in organ depth without affecting statistical accuracy.

37. b Kowalczyk and Donnett, 1996, p. 234
Cords should be disconnected from the wall by grasping and pulling on the plug, not on the cord.

38. a Crawford and Husain, 2011, p. 40
It is a correctly labeled image of a horizontal long-axis slice of the left ventricle.

39. a Christian and Waterstram-Rich, 2007, p. 371
Ideally, the blood glucose should be less than 120 mg/dL when imaging with [^{18}F]FDG. The [^{18}F]FDG competes for glucose receptors, and a high blood glucose level reduces potential uptake of the [^{18}F]FDG.

40. c Remson and Ackermann, 1977, pp. 77–83
A 1:25 dilution means that the concentration in the diluted solution is 1/25 of the original concentration. Thus:

$$1/25 \times 10\ \mu\text{Ci/mL} = 0.4\ \mu\text{Ci/mL}.$$

41. c Nabi and Zubeldia, 2002, pp. 3–4
In preparation for [^{18}F]fluorodeoxyglucose (FDG) imaging, patients are required to fast to maximize tumor uptake. More [^{18}F]FDG is taken up by cancer cells when the extracellular concentration of glucose is low, which enhances the detection of tumors.

42. c Zevalin® (ibritumomab tiuxetan) [prescribing information]
Before administration of [^{90}Y]ibritumomab tiuxetan therapy, a whole-body image is performed with [^{111}In]ibritumomab tiuxetan to assess the biodistribution of the antibody and to identify areas of normal tissue that may be at risk of exposure to a high radiation dose because of proximity to the tumor.

43. a Saha, 2004, pp. 71–72
The size of a ^{99}Mo/^{99m}Tc generator is expressed as the total ^{99}Mo activity on the column at the time of initial assay (calibration).

44. a Wells, 1999, p. 183
Concentration is expressed as activity per unit volume. It is obtained by dividing the total volume into the total activity. In this case:

$$\frac{1.2\ \text{Ci}}{5.7\ \text{mL}} = 0.210\ \text{Ci/mL}$$

$$0.210\ \text{Ci} \times \frac{1000\ \text{mCi}}{1\ \text{Ci}} = 210\ \text{mCi}.$$

45. d Chilton and Witcofski, 1986, p. 54
The amount of ^{99m}Tc activity eluted from the column will be the same whether 5 or 20 mL of saline are used for elution. For a wet-column generator, however, the eluate concentration is determined by the volume of saline drawn from the supply contained within the generator. The volume of saline is controlled by the volume of the evacuated vial used to remove the eluate. Lower-volume evacuated vials provide eluate with greater con-

centration, and higher-volume vials produce eluate with lower concentration. In this example, the eluate volume is unknown. Thus:

$$\text{concentration} = \frac{\text{total activity}}{\text{eluate volume}}$$

$$\text{eluate volume} = \frac{\text{total activity}}{\text{desired concentration}} = \frac{632\ \text{mCi/mL}}{30\ \text{mCi/mL}}$$

$$= 21\ \text{mL}.$$

A 21-mL evacuated vial is not available, but the 20-mL vial will produce an eluate with a concentration of 31.6 mCi/mL (approximately 30 mCi/mL):

$$\text{concentration} = \frac{632\ \text{mCi/mL}}{20\ \text{mCi/mL}} = 31.6\ \text{mCi/mL}.$$

46. b Saha, 2004, p. 75

Aluminum is a nonradioactive, chemical impurity. The allowable limit is set by the *U.S. Pharmacopeia*.

47. c Wells, 1999, pp. 224–225

^{99}Mo concentration is expressed as a ratio of the number of microcuries of ^{99}Mo to the number of millicuries of ^{99m}Tc. Thus, ^{99}Mo concentration is equal to:

$$\frac{8\ \mu\text{Ci}}{652\ \text{mCi}} = 0.012\ \mu\text{Ci}\ ^{99}\text{Mo/mCi}\ ^{99m}\text{Tc}.$$

48. b Saha, 2004, pp. 75, 114

High levels of aluminum ions in ^{99m}Tc eluate cause the colloidal particles in [^{99m}Tc]sulfur colloid to clump together, forming particles large enough to be trapped in the blood vessels of the lung. Many sulfur colloid kits contain EDTA, an agent that binds the Al^{+3} ions and prevents the aggregation of the colloidal particles into larger ones.

49. d Christian *et al.*, 2004, pp. 175, 511–512

Of the radiopharmaceuticals listed, [^{153}Sm]lexidronam is the agent used for treating bone pain. [^{131}I]sodium iodide is used to treat hyperthyroidism or metastatic thyroid carcinoma. [^{111}In]oxine is used to label white blood cells for infection imaging. [^{32}P]chromic phosphate is used to treat pleural or peritoneal effusions.

50. d U.S. Nuclear Regulatory Commission, 2003 (10 CFR 35.3045)

According to the NRC, reports of medical events made to the NRC should contain the following information: names of all individuals involved in the event, whether the patient or a relative was notified, a description of the incident and why it occurred, the effect on the patient, and remedial actions to prevent recurrence. The patient must not be identified to the NRC.

51. a Saha, 2004, pp. 114–115

Most ^{99m}Tc compounds are prepared with chemically reduced ^{99m}Tc, a more chemically active form of technetium. ^{99m}Tc labeling is accomplished in the presence of a stannous compound that acts as a reducing agent. The stannous ion (Sn^{+2}) reduces the valence state of the technetium in the pertechnetate ion from +7 to +4 or to another reduced valence state. The reduced ^{99m}Tc is a more reactive species, capable of combining with a variety of compounds, such as oxidronate, macroaggregated albumin, and lidofenin. [^{99m}Tc]sulfur colloid incorporates ^{99m}Tc in the unreduced, +7 valence state. Therefore, a reducing agent is not required. The first step in the preparation of [^{99m}Tc]sulfur colloid involves heating together [^{99m}Tc]pertechnetate, an acid, and sodium thiosulfate. During the heating, the elemental sulfur precipitates out of the solution and condenses to form colloidal-sized particles. The ^{99m}Tc is trapped and contained within the particles as they form.

52. a Wells, 1999, pp. 183, 192–193

The concentration of the [^{99m}Tc]sulfur colloid is equal to the amount of radioactivity added to the kit divided by the volume of all the liquid reagents. The volume of ^{99m}Tc required is:

$$\text{volume} = \frac{^{99m}\text{Tc activity required}}{[^{99m}\text{Tc}]\text{pertechnetate concentration}}$$

$$= \frac{125\ \text{mCi}}{26.7\ \text{mCi/mL}} = 4.7\ \text{mL of}\ ^{99m}\text{Tc}.$$

The total kit volume is equal to:

$$^{99m}\text{Tc volume} + \text{acid volume} + \text{syringe A volume}$$

$$= 4.7\ \text{ml} + 0.5\ \text{mL} + 1.1\ \text{mL} + 2.1\ \text{mL}$$

$$= 8.4\ \text{mL}.$$

The final kit concentration is equal to:

$$\frac{^{99m}\text{Tc activity}}{\text{total volume}} = \frac{125\ \text{mCi}}{8.4\ \text{mL}} = 14.9\ \text{mCi/mL}.$$

53. b *U.S. Pharmacopeia*, 1990

According to the USP, 90% of the particles in an MAA preparation should be 10–90 microns in size. No particles should be larger than 150 microns.

54. c U.S. Nuclear Regulatory Commission, 2003 (10 CFR 35.204)

The user must ascertain that ^{99}Mo contamination does not exceed the maximum acceptable limits within the 12-hr period that the eluate may be used. Therefore, decay correct the initial ^{99}Mo concentration for 12 hr to determine its concentration at the end of the time the eluate may be used:

$$^{99}\text{Mo:}\ 0.035\ \mu\text{Ci} \times 0.881 = 0.031$$
$$^{99m}\text{Tc:}\ 1\ \text{mCi} \times 0.251 = 0.251\ \text{mCi}.$$

The ^{99}Mo concentration 12 hr after elution is:

$$\frac{0.035\ \mu\text{Ci}\ ^{99}\text{Mo}}{0.251\ \text{mCi}\ ^{99m}\text{Tc}} = 0.139\ \mu\text{Ci}\ ^{99}\text{Mo/mCi}\ ^{99m}\text{Tc}.$$

This level is below the maximum allowable limit of 0.15 μCi ^{99}Mo/mCi ^{99m}Tc set by the NRC. Therefore, this eluate may be used for 12 hr after elution.

55. d Chilton and Witcofski, 1986, p. 77

Based on the R_f values, the radiopharmaceutical is present on the origin half of the strip, and the radiochemical impurity is present on the solvent front half of the strip. The radiochemical purity is:

$$\frac{\text{counts on origin half of strip}}{\text{total counts (counts on both strips)}} \times 100$$

$$\frac{55{,}632 \text{ cpm}}{55{,}632 \text{ cpm} + 15{,}345 \text{ cpm}} \times 100 = 78.4\%.$$

56. c Saha, 2004, p. 92

Three-phase bone imaging is performed with a bone-seeking agent. According to the label on vial C, the vial contains a bone-imaging agent that has not expired. Vial B contains the previous day's bone agent that has expired. Vials A and D contain radiopharmaceuticals that are not appropriate for performing three-phase bone imaging.

57. b Wells, 1999, pp. 216–217

The elapsed time between calibration and capsule administration is 4 hr. In this example, the radiopharmaceutical is being used before calibration time. Therefore, the activity in a capsule at 0800 is unknown, and the known activity (calibration activity) is divided by the decay factor:

$$A(0) \times 0.810 = 100\ \mu\text{Ci/capsule}$$

$$A(0) = \frac{100\ \mu\text{Ci/capsule}}{0.810} = 123\ \mu\text{Ci/capsule at 0800.}$$

Because the prescribed dose is 400 μCi ± 10% (or 360–440 μCi), the total activity in the number of capsules the patient receives must be within this range. Four capsules contain 492 μCi (4 capsules × 123 μCi/capsule), an activity that exceeds the prescribed dose. Three capsules contain 369 μCi, an amount within the prescribed 360–440 μCi. Two capsules contain 246 μCi, an amount below what is prescribed.

58. c Wells, 1999, pp. 172–173, 185–186

The elapsed time between calibration and dose calculation is 6 days (October 28–November 3; recall that October has 31 days). The concentration on October 28 is 74 MBq/mL (740 MBq/10 mL). Decay correct the initial concentration for 6 days using the appropriate decay factor for ^{131}I:

$$74 \text{ MBq/mL} \times 0.597 = 44.2 \text{ MBq/mL}.$$

Then, determine the required volume:

$$\text{volume} = \frac{\text{activity required}}{C(t)} = \frac{185 \text{ MBq}}{44.2 \text{ MBq/mL}}$$

$$= 4.2 \text{ mL}.$$

59. a Early and Sodee, 1995, p. 726

ACD solution, EDTA, heparin, and sodium fluoride all may be used as anticoagulants. However, for labeling red blood cells with ^{51}Cr, ACD (acid citrate dextrose) solution is the anticoagulant of choice.

60. d Saha, 2004, pp. 116–118

Certain drugs interfere with ^{99m}Tc red blood cell labeling because they inhibit the transport of the stannous ion through the red cell membrane and, hence, entry of [^{99m}Tc]pertechnetate into the red cell.

61. b Wells, 1999, p. 189

The maximum activity that can be made from one pentetate kit is 160 mCi. However, based on the amount of [^{99m}Tc]pertechnetate available, only 125 mCi (25.0 mCi/mL × 5.0 mL) can be prepared; 5.0 mL is also within the reconstituting volume limits (1–8 mL) of the kit.

62. b Christian *et al.*, 2004, pp. 194–196

Disposable gloves serve as a barrier against skin contamination when handling radioactive materials. Syringe shields absorb photon emissions that can dramatically increase radiation exposure to hands and fingers. Keeping radioactive materials at arm's length increases distance between the source and the eyes and torso, thereby decreasing radiation exposure to these areas.

63. a Ceretec® package insert

When [^{99m}Tc]exametazime is used to label white blood cells, methylene blue stabilizer is omitted from its preparation. For this reason, the preparation should be used within 30 min.

64. c Saha, 2004, pp. 151–152

[^{99m}Tc]medronate, a bone agent, should be a clear, colorless solution. Therefore, the technologist should not use the original vial because of its abnormal appearance.

65. a Wells, 1999, pp. 230–231; Saha, 2004, pp. 153–161

The hydrolyzed-reduced ^{99m}Tc impurity is separated using system #1, and the free pertechnetate impurity is separated using system #2. Therefore, the percentage of each impurity in the preparation can be determined directly:

$$\%\ \text{HR-}^{99m}\text{Tc} = \frac{3\ \mu\text{Ci}}{3\ \mu\text{Ci} + 177\ \mu\text{Ci}} \times 100 = 1.7\%$$

$$\%\ \text{free pertechnetate} = \frac{15\ \mu\text{Ci}}{15\ \mu\text{Ci} + 275\ \mu\text{Ci}} \times 100$$

$$= 1.7\%.$$

The radiochemical impurity of the sample is:

$$\%\ \text{HR-}^{99m}\text{Tc} + \%\ \text{free pertechnetate} = 1.7\% + 5.2\%$$

$$= 6.9\%.$$

66. c Wells, 1999, p. 200

Weight-based dose for 95-lb patient:

$$\text{mCi/kg} = 290\ \mu\text{Ci} \times 1 \text{ mCi}/1{,}000\ \mu\text{Ci} = 0.29 \text{ mCi/kg}$$

$$\text{kg} = 95 \text{ lb} \times 1 \text{ kg}/2.2 \text{ lb} = 43.18 \text{ kg}$$

$$0.29 \text{ mCi/kg} \times 43.18 \text{ kg} = \sim 12.5 \text{ mCi}$$

67. d American Pharmaceutical Association, 1999, p. 145

Larger-gauge needles are more likely to damage the rubber closure, especially after multiple withdrawals, causing pieces to fall into the solution in the vial. This is referred to as "coring." Needle gauges of 20–27 are less likely to cause coring with repeated withdrawals.

68. c U.S. Nuclear Regulatory Commission, 2003 (10 CFR 20.1003 and 20.1902)

The NRC requires that restricted areas, such as a radiopharmacy lab, be posted with specifically worded signs depending on the radiation level present. A "Caution: Radiation Area" sign should be posted when an individual could receive more than 5 mrem in an hour.

69. c U.S. Nuclear Regulatory Commission, 2003 (49 CFR 172.403 and 172.436–440)

The U.S. Department of Transportation defines the transportation index of a package containing radioactive materials to be the dose rate measured at 1 meter from the surface of the package.

70. d U.S. Nuclear Regulatory Commission, 2003 (10 CFR 20.2103)

According to the NRC, personnel radiation exposure records must be retained indefinitely.

71. a Wells, 1999, pp.101–102

Use the inverse square law:

$$(I_1)(D_1)^2 = (I_2)(D_2)^2,$$

where I is the intensity at original distance (D_1) and I_2 is the intensity at new distance (D_2). In this example:

$$(50 \text{ mR/hr})(1 \text{ ft})^2 = (2 \text{ mR/hr})(D_2)^2.$$

Isolate the unknown and solve:

$$(D_2)^2 = \frac{(50 \text{ mR/hr})(1 \text{ ft})^2}{2 \text{ mR/hr}}$$

$$(D_2)^2 = 25 \text{ ft}^2.$$

Take the square root of each side:

$$D_2 = 5 \text{ ft}.$$

72. b Saha, 2004, p. 221

An occupationally exposed worker should not wear a personal monitor when undergoing medical procedures that involve radiation. The monitor reading must reflect only the occupational exposure. The monitor should be worn anywhere in the workplace where the technologist may be exposed to radiation, whether within the nuclear medicine department or in other departments or patient rooms. Monitors are worn to determine whether the worker is being exposed to acceptable levels, so removal of the monitor to prevent excessive readings is self-defeating.

73. a U.S. Nuclear Regulatory Commission, 2003 (10 CFR 35.40)

A written directive for administration of [^{131}I]sodium iodide in dosages greater than 30 μCi (1.11 MBq) must include the patient's name and the dosage to be administered. It must be dated and signed by the authorized user before the dosage is administered.

74. b U.S. Nuclear Regulatory Commission, 2003 (10 CFR 20.1301); Siegel, 2004, pp. 36–39

According to NRC regulations, the annual radiation exposure to members of the general public is limited to 100 mrem.

75. b Christian *et al.*, 2004, p. 51

^{32}P is a pure beta-emitting radionuclide. When it is placed in shielding material of a higher atomic number (Z), such as lead or tungsten, bremsstrahlung radiation is produced. This type of x-radiation results from the deceleration of beta particles as they approach the positively charged nuclei of the shielding material. As the beta particles slow down, they lose energy that is emitted as an X ray. Shielding materials of lower atomic number, such as plastic, minimize the production of bremsstrahlung radiation.

76. c Thompson *et al.*, 1994, pp. 32–33

Before any measurements are taken with a survey meter, it should be set on the lowest scale. If the needle of the meter reaches the endpoint at the higher end of the scale, the scale should be adjusted upward until the needle registers a value between zero and the high endpoint of the scale.

77. c Early and Sodee, 1995, p. 329

The trigger level is the exposure rate at which decontamination is performed. This level is set by each licensee with the assistance of the radiation safety officer. A wipe test will determine whether the contamination is removable. If the contamination is removable, decontamination of the site should be carried out until the exposure rate is below the trigger level.

78. c Steves, 1999, p. 270

Medical treatment for life-threatening conditions always takes precedence over any other activity. To prevent the spread of contamination, the victim can be wrapped in a sheet for transport to the treatment area.

79. b Steves, 1999, pp. 276–280

For up to about 1 week after administration of [^{131}I]sodium iodide, iodine that is not bound to thyroid hormone is found in the urine, perspiration, sputum, and saliva. These body fluids are the major sources of contamination from an ^{131}I therapy patient.

80. c U.S. Nuclear Regulatory Commission, 2003 (10 CFR 35.63); Siegel, 2004, pp. 50–51

According to NRC regulations, a dosage cannot be administered if the activity falls outside the range established by the authorized user or differs from the prescribed dosage by 20% or more, unless the authorized user directs the dosage to be administered.

81. c U.S. Nuclear Regulatory Commission, 1998 (NUREG 1556, Vol. 9, Appendix U, Table U.3)

According to the NRC, a woman who is breast-feeding should completely cease breast-feeding that child after she has received [^{131}I]sodium iodide.

82. b U.S. Nuclear Regulatory Commission, 1998 (NUREG 1556)

According to the NRC, wipe test results must be reported in dpm.

83. c Wells, 1999, p. 37

1 mrem = 0.01 mSv, therefore 15 × 0.01 mSv = 0.15 mrem.

84. b U.S. Nuclear Regulatory Commission, 2003 (10 CFR 20.1906)

NRC regulations state that packages containing radioactive material must be monitored no later than 3 hr after delivery during regular working hours or within 3 hr of opening the department for the workday if the package was delivered after hours.

85. d Wells, 1999, p. 93

To determine wipe test readings in dpm:

$$\text{dpm} = \frac{\text{gross cpm} - \text{background cpm}}{\text{efficiency as a decimal}}.$$

In this example:

$$\frac{375\text{ cpm} - 120\text{ cpm}}{0.45} = 567\text{ dpm}.$$

86. c Saha, 2004, pp. 70–71

The results of this linearity test demonstrate that the measured readings are always higher than the calculated activity (the measured readings line is above the calculated activities line). The difference between measured and calculated activities increases in the lower range of activities. To determine if the instrument is operating within limits according to the standard of practice, the technologist next should determine whether the measured values are within ±10% of the calculated values.

87. b Early and Sodee, 1995, pp. 158–162

Calibrating a scintillation spectrometer involves the determination of the operating voltage applied to the dynodes of the photomultiplier tube. A reference standard, such as ^{137}Cs, is counted at various voltage settings, and the counts are recorded. The voltage at which the maximum number of counts is obtained is the operating voltage for the instrument. Calibration results are valid only for the gain setting used during the determination of the operating voltage.

88. b Wells, 1999, pp. 129–130

The percent energy resolution is calculated using the following formula:

$$\%\text{ energy resolution} = \frac{\text{FWHM in keV}}{\text{energy of radionuclide in keV}}.$$

In this example:

$$\frac{53\text{ keV}}{662\text{ keV}} \times 100 = 8\%.$$

89. c Saha, 2004, pp. 70–71

The standard of practice calls for a dose calibrator linearity test to be carried out until the original activity is decayed to 30 μCi or less. If the test begins with 50 mCi, it will take 11 half-lives or 66 hr for the original activity to decay to 30 μCi.

90. b Bernier *et al.*, 1994, pp. 86–87

A PLES phantom contains lead bars that have the same width and spacing. Two images taken 90° to one another can be used to assess linearity over the entire field of view.

91. b U.S. Nuclear Regulatory Commission, 2003 (10 CFR 35.2060); Siegel, 2004, pp. 55–56

All dose calibrator quality control records must be retained for 3 years.

92. b Powsner and Powsner, 1998, pp. 129–130

As the order of a Butterworth filter is increased, more high frequencies are retained in the image. High frequencies add sharpness to the image, so the overall image will be sharper. However, much of the data in the high-frequency range result from noise, so retaining the high frequencies may produce a sharper image that is also less representative of the true distribution of activity. Changing the order of a filter results in more subtle changes in the image than adjusting the cutoff frequency.

93. d Wells, 1999, pp. 154, 156–157

A 64 × 64 matrix is made up of 4,096 pixels. A 256 × 256 matrix is made up of 65,536 pixels. To store data in computer memory, a storage location is needed for each pixel. Because the 256 × 256 matrix has 16 times more pixels than the 64 × 64 matrix, it will require 16 times more storage locations in computer memory.

94. b Lee, 2005, pp. 91–92, 151

When zoom mode is engaged before acquisition, the image is magnified because a small region of interest is represented by a large number of pixels. This increases resolution. Background is actually decreased. Contrast will be determined by the total counts acquired. The amount of memory required remains the same because the same number of pixels (same matrix size) is being used. They are simply covering a smaller anatomical area.

95. c Lee, 2005, pp. 8–10, 93–95

Each image needs to be stored in a separate matrix. Therefore, a set of storage locations in computer memory is needed for each. One 128 × 128 word mode matrix contains 16,384 words or, because there are two bytes per word, 32,768 bytes. Two such matrices require 65,536 bytes. A kilobyte (kB) contains 1,024 bytes. To convert bytes to kB:

$$65{,}536 \text{ bytes} \times \frac{1 \text{ kB}}{1024 \text{ bytes}} = 64 \text{ kB}.$$

96. d Christian *et al.*, 2004, p. 528
A splenic sequestration study requires external counting over the spleen, liver, and precordium. By using the uptake probe with a flat-field collimator, counts from surrounding tissue and background are minimized.

97. a Wells, 1999, p. 156
The total memory required equals matrix height in pixels × matrix width in pixels × number of frames. In this example: 128 × 128 × 30 = 491,520 bytes. The number of pixels in the acquisition matrix corresponds to the number of memory locations or bytes needed for one frame of data.

98. c Wells, 1999, p. 140
Half of the percentage of the window is above and half is below the centerline. The window is expressed as a percentage of the energy of the radionuclide. In this case, the window would be 159 keV ± 12 keV because 7.5% of 159 keV equals 12 keV.

99. b Wells, 1999, pp. 149–150
Calculate the total acquisition time:

$$\text{Acquisition time} = \text{number of projections} \times \text{time per projection}.$$

In this example:

$$60 \text{ projections} \times 0.5 \text{ min/projection} = 30 \text{ min}.$$

Calculate total number of counts based on the acquisition time:

$$\text{total counts} = \text{acquisition time} \times \text{counting rate}.$$

In this example:

$$30 \text{ min} \times 144{,}000 \text{ cpm} = 4{,}320{,}000 \text{ counts}.$$

100. a Wells, 1999, p. 147
Sensitivity is expressed as counts per minute per microcurie. To calculate sensitivity:

$$\text{sensitivity} = \frac{\text{source cpm} - \text{background cpm}}{\text{source activity in } \mu\text{Ci}}.$$

In this example:

$$\frac{30{,}500 \text{ cpm} - 1200 \text{ cpm}}{125\ \mu\text{Ci}} = 234 \text{ com}/\mu\text{Ci}.$$

Answers to Examination 4

1. a. Christian *et al.*, 2004, pp. 497–498
The diagram depicts a posterior view of the lower lumbar spine, the pelvis, and the proximal femurs. The iliac crests would be demonstrated on an anterior view of the pelvis. The distal femurs and the tenth through twelfth thoracic vertebrae are inferior and superior, respectively, to the structures shown in the diagram.

2. c Christian *et al.*, 2004, p. 498
The calcaneus, the heel of the foot, would be best imaged by placing the sole of the patient's foot on the detector. Both feet may be imaged at the same time.

3. b Christian *et al.*, 2004, pp. 509–510
Because the second through fourth phases are performed to determine the presence of increased, persistent tracer uptake in the bone, the study must be performed with a bone agent.

4. c Christian *et al.*, 2004, p. 392
Patients with right-to-left cardiac shunts should be given a reduced number of particles because the particles pass through to the left side of the heart and into the systemic circulation, where they block capillaries and occlude blood flow in the brain, kidneys, heart, and other organs.

5. a Christian *et al.*, 2004, p. 396
In the wash-in/washout method, the patient breathes a mixture of xenon and oxygen for several minutes while a wash-in image is acquired. Air is then added to the system, and the xenon that is exhaled is trapped. Serial images are acquired as the xenon clears from the lungs. This method requires little cooperation from the patient; no breath holding or deep breaths are required. Therefore, the method is well suited for comatose patients as well as for those on ventilators.

6. d McGraw *et al.*, 1992, pp. 228–230; Early and Sodee, 1995, p. 462
There is aerosol leakage at the exhaust of the delivery system. The filter is unable to trap the exhausted aerosol sufficiently to prevent the escape of airborne tracer from the delivery system. The area around the patient's mouth becomes contaminated when a face mask is used. Some of the airborne tracer is not inhaled and is deposited on the patient's face.

7. d Early and Sodee, 1995, pp. 630–631
For routine thyroid imaging, either [^{99m}Tc]pertechnetate or [^{123}I]sodium iodide may be used. [^{99m}Tc]pertechnetate is trapped by the follicular cells of the thyroid. [^{123}I]sodium iodide is trapped and organified (incorporated into the manufacture of thyroid hormones).

8. d SNM Procedure Guidelines Committee, 2011

Nonthyroidal background measurements may be collected over the thigh. The uptake probe should be positioned vertically just above the patient's knee to exclude bladder activity.

9. a Adler and Carlton, 2003, pp. 163–165

In addition to the routine finger method of determining the radial pulse, pulse rates can be determined from the ECG or pulse oximeter. Listening to the heart with a stethoscope will give a pulse rate known as the apical pulse.

10. b Adler and Carlton, 2003, p. 168

Because oxygen is a drug, it must be prescribed by a physician who specifies the amount to be received, the device to be used, and time interval (continuous vs. intermittent). Cessation of oxygen therapy can be done only with the consent or supervision of a physician or attending nurse.

11. b Christian *et al.*, 2004, pp. 429–430

Adverse effects of dipyridamole, a vasodilator, include hypotension, headache, and nausea. These effects may be reversed by administering aminophylline intravenously.

12. d Blust *et al.*, 1992, p. 55

When adenosine or dipyridamole is used for stress testing, the patient should be instructed to discontinue the use of certain substances that interfere with the action of these drugs. Caffeine and medications containing caffeine should not be consumed for at least 12 hr before testing. The use of xanthine derivatives (theophylline, aminophylline) should be discontinued for 24–36 hr before the nuclear medicine procedure. In a normal hepatobiliary study, the duodenum and proximal jejunum are visualized by 30 min after tracer administration.

13. b Christian *et al.*, 2004, p. 465

In a normal hepatobiliary study, the duodenum and proximal jejunum are visualized by 30 min after tracer administration.

14. a Mettler and Guiberteau, 1991, pp. 200–201

A gallbladder ejection fraction is useful in assessing gallbladder dysfunction. In cases of delayed gallbladder visualization, sincalide is administered when the gallbladder is full. Pre- and postcontraction images are used to calculate an ejection fraction.

15. a Early and Sodee, 1995, pp. 517, 524, 526

For the determination of gastric emptying, the patient ingests the radiopharmaceutical. Tracers to detect gastrointestinal bleeding and to image the salivary glands are administered intravenously. Depending on the method used, tracers to detect vesicoureteral reflux are instilled into the urinary bladder via a catheter (direct method) or injected intravenously (indirect method).

16. a Christian *et al.*, 2004, p. 483

Renal function imaging should be performed with the patient in a normal state of hydration. To ensure hydration, the patient should drink 0.5 L of water 30–60 min before the study. False abnormal results may be obtained if the patient is not hydrated.

17. c Early and Sodee, 1995, p. 593

[^{99m}Tc]succimer (DMSA) is used for static renal cortical imaging. Imaging is performed about 2 hr after tracer administration.

18. d SNM Procedure Guidelines Committee, 2011

[^{67}Ga]citrate is excreted in the feces. The activity in the bowel may interfere with the interpretation of the study. Therefore, a bowel preparation may be prescribed at the time the tracer is administered.

19. d Christian *et al.*, 2004, pp. 545–546

At 24 hr after injection, a normal biodistribution of ^{111}In-labeled leukocytes demonstrates tracer uptake only in the spleen, liver, and bone marrow. The greatest uptake is in the spleen, followed by the liver and the bone marrow.

20. d Adler and Carlton, 2003, p. 241

Hypoglycemic patients may exhibit an intense hunger, may be weak, shaky, and sweat excessively. They may become confused and irritable. Most patients will recognize symptoms before they become severe.

21. a Early and Sodee, 1995, p. 574

[^{99m}Tc]gluceptate, [^{99m}Tc]pertechnetate, or [^{99m}Tc]pentetate have been used to demonstrate brain death with a cerebral blood flow study followed by immediate static imaging. [^{99m}Tc]exametazime more recently has been used for this purpose. Because this tracer is normally concentrated in brain tissue in proportion to blood flow, it can visualize the degree of perfusion in the brain.

22. a Early and Sodee, 1995, p. 572

In the case of cerebral spinal fluid leaks through the nose (rhinorrhea) or ears (otorrhea), placing cotton gauze in the patient's nose or ears is helpful in diagnosing such leaks. This technique is particularly useful with small leaks that may not be visualized on images.

23. a Early and Sodee, 1995, p. 755

Colloidal [^{32}P]chromic phosphate is used to treat pleural or peritoneal effusions resulting from a malignancy. The agent is introduced directly into the pleural or peritoneal cavity. It should not be administered intravenously; it will be taken up in the liver, causing localized radiation damage.

24. b Metastron® package insert

It is recommended that incontinent patients receiving [^{89}Sr]chloride be catheterized to minimize the spread of contamination. Because ^{89}Sr is primarily a beta emitter (less than 1% gamma emission), it is not necessary to place patients in isolation or monitor them with a survey meter. Lead shielding should not be used with this beta emitter because bremsstrahlung radiation will be produced in the shielding.

25. a Christian *et al.*, 2004, pp. 330–331
Uptake of SPECT brain agents is primarily in the gray matter of the cerebrum, which has a higher blood flow than white matter. These agents are localized in proportion to blood flow.

26. d Kowalczyk and Donnett, 1996, p. 88
The mask is the most appropriate for airborne respiratory diseases.

27. b Early and Sodee, 1995, pp. 528–529
A LeVeen shunt is used to treat ascites by draining the excess fluid that accumulates in the peritoneal cavity into the superior vena cava. Sometimes the shunt tube becomes blocked. Radionuclide imaging is used to differentiate mechanical blockage of the tube from other reasons for increasing ascitic fluid. Imaging may be performed with either [^{99m}Tc]MAA or [^{99m}Tc]sulfur colloid. After the introduction of one of these tracers into the peritoneal cavity, images of the anterior abdomen (and chest if MAA is used) will demonstrate activity in the liver or lungs, confirming that the shunt is functioning. If the liver or lungs are not visualized, then the tubing is blocked.

28. a Early and Sodee, 1995, pp. 526–528
[^{99m}Tc]sulfur colloid is the radiopharmaceutical used to image gastroesophageal reflux in both adults and children. However, adults are administered a mixture of dilute hydrochloric acid, orange juice, and tracer after fasting from midnight. In infants and toddlers, the procedure is performed at the time of a scheduled feeding, so they may fast as little as 2 hr before receiving the tracer. In adults, an abdominal binder is used to increase external abdominal pressure to demonstrate more subtle instances of reflux. Because the abdominal muscles are important in pediatric respiration, the binder is typically not used with children, particularly infants.

29. a Bernier *et al.*, 1994, pp. 188–190
In general, a quantitative study, any study whose results are a number, should be performed first. In this way, radioactivity from another study will not interfere or need to be accounted for when calculating the results of a quantitative study. An ERPF is performed with [^{99m}Tc]mertiatide. This radiopharmaceutical clears the kidneys quickly. Its 6-hr half-life is short enough to permit bone imaging the next day. [^{111}In]pentetreotide imaging should be performed last. ^{111}In has a 3-day half-life, and the tracer may remain in the body for an extended period.

30. b Christian *et al.*, 2004, pp. 530–531
Intrinsic factor is essential to the absorption of vitamin B_{12}. It binds to the vitamin and facilitates an active transport mechanism for B_{12} absorption in the terminal ileum.

31. b Crawford and Husain, 2011, p. 92
The region(s) of interest for detection of a left-to-right cardiac shunt is (are) drawn around one or both lungs to generate a pulmonary time–activity curve. The curve demonstrates the first pass of tracer through the lungs as well as any tracer that has returned to the lungs and bypassed the systemic circulation.

32. c Adler and Carlton, 2003, p. 161
The normal ranges of vital signs for adults are:

Vital sign	Range
Pulse	60–100 beats per minute
Blood pressure	
Diastolic	60–90 mm Hg
Systolic	95–140 mm Hg
Respirations	12–20 breaths/min
Temperature	97.7–99.5°F (36.5–37.5°C)

33. a Adler and Carlton, 2003, p. 275
A variety of antecubital veins can be used for drug administration, but the two most commonly used are the basilic and cephalic veins.

34. d Christian *et al.*, 2004, p. 529
The red cell sequestration study is performed to determine if the patient's anemia is the result of active splenic sequestration of normal red cells.

35. a Christian *et al.*, 2004, p. 526
Hematocrits vary with vessel size. Smaller vessels yield a lower hematocrit value than larger vessels.

36. c Early and Sodee, 1995, p. 629
The formula for calculating thyroid radioiodine uptake is:

$$\%\text{ uptake} = \frac{\text{net thyroid cpm}}{\text{net standard cpm}} \times 100.$$

Using the data, the percent uptake is:

$$\frac{(2{,}876 - 563 \text{ cpm})}{(10{,}111 - 124 \text{ cpm})} \times 100 = 23\%.$$

37. b Adler and Carlton, 2003, p. 277
An acceptable flow rate for a drip infusion is 10–20 drops per minute. This rate may be adjusted by physician order.

38. c Early and Sodee, 1995, p. 733
The formula for calculating the total blood volume (TBV), based on the red cell volume, uses the corrected hematocrit (HCT) in the denominator. Correction is needed to account for trapped plasma and to adjust the venous hematocrit to an average whole-body hematocrit. The formula is:

$$\text{TBV} = \frac{\text{red cell volume}}{\text{HCT} \times 0.91 \times 0.97}.$$

39. d Christian *et al.*, 2004, p. 526
The formula for calculating plasma volume is:

$$\text{PV} = \frac{(\text{net standard cpm})(\text{dilution factor})}{\text{net plasma cpm/mL}}.$$

From the data supplied:

$$PV = \frac{(839{,}621\ \text{cpm})(15)}{2{,}528} = 4{,}982\ \text{mL}.$$

40. d Remson and Ackermann, 1977, pp. 77–83

A 1:2,000 dilution means that the concentration in the diluted solution is one 2,000th of the original concentration. In this problem, the concentration of the original solution is unknown. Thus:

$$\frac{1}{2{,}000}(?\ \mu\text{Ci/mL}) = 0.05\ \mu\text{Ci/mL}$$

$$\frac{1}{2{,}000} = \frac{0.05\ \mu\text{Ci/mL}}{x}$$

$$x = 2{,}000\ (0.05\ \mu\text{Ci/mL}) = 100\ \mu\text{Ci/mL}.$$

41. d SNM Procedure Guidelines Committee, 2011

In an adult, a normal fasting blood glucose level is 70–115 mg/dL. Because the patient's blood glucose level is within the normal range, the technologist can proceed with the examination.

42. b Wells, 1999, p. 238

% gallbladder ejection fraction:

$$= \frac{\text{max. GB counts} - \text{min. GB counts}}{\text{maximum GB counts}} \times 100$$

$$= \frac{185{,}632\ \text{cts} - 77{,}203\ \text{cts}}{185{,}632\ \text{cts}} \times 100$$

$$= \frac{108{,}429}{185{,}632} \times 100 = 58\%.$$

43. c Saha, 2004, p. 71

Maximum ^{99m}Tc activity is obtained about 24 hr after the last elution of ^{99m}Tc.

44. d Wells, 1999, p. 183

Concentration is expressed as activity per unit volume. In this instance:

$$\frac{2.0\ \text{MBq}}{\text{mL}} = \frac{\text{total activity}}{8\ \text{mL}}$$

$$\text{total activity} = 2.0\ \text{MBq/mL} \times 8\ \text{mL} = 16\ \text{MBq}.$$

45. c Eliot, 1990, pp. 38–42

A wet-column generator is not equipped with a charging port because the saline supply is contained within the generator itself. A dry-column generator, however, uses a charging port to add saline to the column.

46. b Saha, 2004, p. 75

According to the USP, a ^{99m}Tc eluate should contain no more than 10 μg/mL of Al^{+3} in 1 mL of eluate.

47. d Saha, 2004, p. 74

The lead shield method of determining ^{99}Mo contamination is based on the energy differences between ^{99m}Tc photons (140 keV) and ^{99}Mo photons (740, 780 keV). The unshielded vial of eluate is placed into a dose calibrator set to assay ^{99m}Tc, and the ^{99m}Tc measurement is recorded. Then, the vial is placed into a lead shield designed to absorb the lower-energy photons of ^{99m}Tc but to permit transmission of the higher-energy photons of ^{99}Mo. With the dose calibrator set to measure ^{99}Mo, the shielded eluate is assayed for ^{99}Mo, and the ^{99}Mo measurement is recorded. The ^{99}Mo concentration is calculated by making a ratio of the ^{99}Mo and ^{99m}Tc measurements. Thus:

$$\frac{\mu\text{Ci}\ ^{99}\text{Mo}}{\text{mCi}\ ^{99m}\text{Tc}} = \mu\text{Ci}\ ^{99}\text{Mo/mCi}\ ^{99m}\text{Tc}.$$

48. c Saha, 2004, p. 75

The test kit contains an aluminum solution with a concentration of approximately 10 μg/mL, the maximum aluminum ion concentration allowed in ^{99m}Tc eluate as established by the USP.

49. c Saha, 2004, pp. 261–265

[^{99m}Tc]macroaggregated albumin is the tracer used for lung perfusion imaging. Lung ventilation imaging may be performed with ^{133}Xe gas or [^{99m}Tc]pentetate aerosol. [^{99m}Tc]albumin remains in the blood pool and may be used for gated cardiac left ventricular function studies. [^{99m}Tc]sulfur colloid localizes in the reticuloendothelial system and may be used to image the liver, spleen, or bone marrow. [^{99m}Tc]bicisate is used to perform brain perfusion imaging.

50. a U.S. Nuclear Regulatory Commission, 2003 (10 FR 35. 204); Wells, 1999, pp. 224–226

According to the NRC, the maximum allowable ^{99}Mo concentration in a ^{99m}Tc eluate must not exceed 0.15 μCi ^{99}Mo/mCi ^{99m}Tc at the time of administration to the patient. At 0600, the ^{99}Mo contamination in the eluate is below the maximum allowable limit of 0.15 μCi ^{99}Mo per mCi ^{99m}Tc:

$$\frac{15.5\ \mu\text{Ci}\ ^{99}\text{Mo}}{250\ \text{mCi}\ ^{99m}\text{Tc}} = 0.062\ \mu\text{Ci}\ ^{99}\text{Mo/mCi}\ ^{99m}\text{Tc}.$$

A ^{99m}Tc-labeled compound with a shelf life of 8 hr is prepared with this eluate at 1000. If the maximum allowable limit for ^{99}Mo contamination is not exceeded during this 8 hr, the ^{99m}Tc compound may be administered to patients until 1800. However, it must be verified that the radionuclide impurity limit is not exceeded during this period. To determine the ^{99}Mo concentration in the eluate at 1400, decay correct both the ^{99}Mo and ^{99m}Tc activities obtained at 0600 for 8 hr (0600 to 1400 = 8 hr).

^{99}Mo: 15.5 μCi × 0.919 = 14.2 μCi
(0.919 is the ^{99}Mo decay factor for 8 hr.)

^{99m}Tc: 250 mCi × 0.398 = 99.5 mCi
(0.398 is the ^{99m}Tc decay factor for 8 hr.)

At 1400, then, the ^{99}Mo concentration is equal to:

$$\frac{14.2\ \mu\text{Ci}\ ^{99}\text{Mo}}{99.5\ \text{mCi}\ ^{99m}\text{Tc}} = 0.143\ \mu\text{Ci}\ ^{99}\text{Mo/mCi}\ ^{99m}\text{Tc}.$$

This level is below the maximum allowable limit of ^{99}Mo contamination set by the NRC. Therefore, the eluate may be administered to patients at 1400. After decay correcting the ^{99}Mo and ^{99m}Tc activities at 1400 to obtain their activities at 1500:

^{99}Mo: 14.2 × 0:989 = 14.0 μCi

^{99m}Tc: 99.5 × 0.891 = 88.7 mCi

the ^{99}Mo concentration is equal to:

$$\frac{14.0\ \mu\text{Ci}\ ^{99}\text{Mo}}{88.7\ \text{mCi}\ ^{99m}\text{Tc}} = 0.158\ \mu\text{Ci}\ ^{99}\text{Mo/mCi}\ ^{99m}\text{Tc}.$$

This level is above the maximum allowable limit of ^{99}Mo contamination set by the NRC. Therefore, the eluate may not be administered to patients at or after 1500.

51. b Wells, 1999, pp. 192–193

350 mCi of [^{99m}Tc]pertechnetate are available (35.0 mCi/mL × 10 mL = 350 mCi), but this amount exceeds the activity (250 mCi) and volume (5 mL) limits of the kit. Based on the maximum reconstituting volume (5.0 mL) of the kit, 175 mCi can be prepared:

$$35\frac{\text{mCi}}{\text{mL}} \times 5\ \text{mL} = 175\ \text{mCi}.$$

This activity (175 mCi) and volume (5 mL) are within the activity and volume limits for the kit.

52. c Schwarz *et al.*, 1997, pp. 167–168

A sulfur colloid kit contains the following reagents: acid, sodium thiosulfate, the material from which the colloidal particle is formed, and a buffer. To prepare [^{99m}Tc]sulfur colloid, [^{99m}Tc]pertechnetate, the acid, and the sodium thiosulfate mixture are combined in a sterile reaction vial and heated in a boiling water bath. During boiling, sulfur particles are formed and condense, incorporating the ^{99m}Tc. After the boiled mixture is allowed to cool, the buffer is added to adjust the pH of the preparation.

53. c Chilton and Witcofski, 1986, p. 149

[^{32}P]chromic phosphate is a blue-green color. Because this is the radiopharmaceutical's normal appearance, the technologist should continue preparing the unit dose.

54. d Wells, 1999, p. 183

The concentration of the [^{99m}Tc]succimer is equal to the amount of radioactivity, divided by the volume of radioactivity and the volume of succimer reagent. The volume of [^{99m}Tc]pertechnetate required is:

$$\frac{^{99m}\text{Tc activity required}}{[^{99m}\text{Tc}]\text{pertechnetate concentration}} = \frac{30\ \text{mCi}}{18\ \text{mCi/mL}}$$

$$= 1.7\ \text{mL}.$$

The final concentration is equal to:

$$\frac{^{99m}\text{Tc activity}}{^{99m}\text{Tc volume} + \text{sccumer volume}} = \frac{30\ \text{mCi}}{1.7\ \text{mL} + 1.5\ \text{mL}}$$

$$= 9.4\ \text{mCi/mL}.$$

55. b Saha, 2004, pp. 154–160

Based on the R_f values, the free pertechnetate impurity is separated using system #1, and the hydrolyzed-reduced ^{99m}Tc impurity by using system #2. Therefore, the percentage of each impurity in the preparation can be determined directly:

$$\%\ \text{free pertechnetate} = \frac{1716\ \text{cpm}}{1716\ \text{cpm} + 23{,}706\ \text{cpm}} \times 100$$

$$= 6.7\%$$

$$\%\ \text{HR-}^{99m}\text{Tc} = \frac{1200\ \text{cpm}}{1200\ \text{cpm} + 21{,}001\ \text{cpm}} \times 100 = 5.4\%$$

The tagging efficiency, or radiochemical purity, of the sample is:

$$100\% - (\%\ \text{free pertechnetate} + \%\ \text{HR-}^{99m}\text{Tc})$$

$$= 100\% - (6.7\% + 5.4\%)$$

$$= 100\% - 12.1\%$$

$$= 87.9\%.$$

56. a Saha, 2004, pp. 31–32

The technologist did not verify the label information and, therefore, should not withdraw any activity from the vial. According to the label information, the vial should contain a total activity of 555 MBq (10 mL × 55.5 MBq/mL), or 15 mCi:

$$555\ \text{MBq} \times \frac{37\ \text{MBq}}{\text{mCi}} = 15\ \text{mCi}.$$

The technologist should first ascertain that the vial was assayed on the correct radionuclide setting on the dose calibrator. If the radionuclide setting was correctly placed, the technologist should next perform dose calibrator quality control. Only when the technologist has verified that the equipment was used properly and is functioning properly should the manufacturer be contacted.

57. c Wells, 1999, pp. 172–173

The easiest approach is to first equate the calibration time to EST. (Most telephone companies include a map of the time zones in the United States in the front of the telephone directory.) There is a 3-hr time difference between the East and West coasts, with the West Coast being 3 hr earlier than the East Coast. Thus:

0600 PST = 0900 EST.

Once this conversion is performed, the problem is a straightforward decay correction problem. The elapsed time between 0900 EST on March 8 and 1200 EST on March 9 is 27 hr. From a decay factor table for ^{67}Ga, the decay factor for 27 hr is 0.787. The total activity is decay corrected for 27 hr to determine the total activity at 1200 EST on March 9:

$A(t) = A(O) \times D = 5 \text{ mCi} \times 0.787$

$= 3.9 \text{ mCi}.$

58. a Wells, 1999, pp. 179–181, 185–186

The elapsed time between calibration and dosage calculation is 3 days (March 15–18). In this example, the radiopharmaceutical is being used before the calibration time. Therefore, the initial concentration on March 15 is the unknown, and the known concentration is divided by the decay factor. The concentration on March 18 is 0.4 mCi/mL (2.0 mCi/5.0 mL):

$$C(0) \times 0.528 = 0.4 \text{ mCi/mL}$$

$$C(0) = \frac{0.4 \text{ mCi/mL}}{0.528} = 0.76 \text{ mCi/mL}.$$

Then, determine the required volume. Remember that the concentration and activity required must be expressed in the same units. Changing the concentration in microcuries:

$$C(0) = 0.76 \text{ mCi/mL} = \frac{1{,}000\ \mu\text{Ci}}{\text{mCi}} = 760\ \mu\text{Ci/mL}$$

$$\text{volume} = \frac{\text{activity required}}{C(0)} = \frac{50\ \mu\text{Ci}}{760\ \mu\text{Ci/mL}} = 0.07 \text{ mL}$$

59. b Early and Sodee, 1995, p. 733

The patient's blood should be added to the ACD solution before ^{51}Cr is introduced into the vial. Dextrose contained in the ACD solution chemically reduces the hexavalent ^{51}Cr to a trivalent state, which prevents red cell tagging. In a trivalent state, ^{51}Cr cannot penetrate the red cell membrane.

60. d Saha, 2004, p. 117

The in vitro method is recommended when patients are taking certain drugs, such as penicillin or doxorubicin, that have been shown to interfere with red cell labeling. In this method, the red cells can be washed and the interfering substances removed before cell labeling is attempted. The commercially prepared kit eliminates the need for centrifugation with the addition of reagents that oxidize or bind any stannous ion that has not been taken into the red cells, thus localizing the ^{99m}Tc uptake to the red cells. Labeling efficiencies of 95% or greater have been reported for the in vitro method. Labeling efficiencies for the in vivo method are reported to be 80%–90% and for the modified in vivo method to be comparable with those of the in vitro method. Because the red blood cells are removed, labeled, and then reinjected, the risk of hemolysis of the red cells is greater with the in vitro method than with the other methods.

61. d Saha, 2004, p. 113

Particles are viewed with the aid of a microscope. Their size and number can be determined by using the grids on the hemocytometer as a reference.

62. a U.S. Nuclear Regulatory Commission, 2003 (10 CFR 35.2063)

The NRC requires that patient unit dosage records be retained for 3 years.

63. d Saha, 2004, p.131

Ascorbic acid acts as a reducing agent to change the valence of radiochromium from +6 to +3, which stops the labeling process.

64. a Saha, 2004, pp. 151–152

[^{99m}Tc]macroaggregated albumin is made up of aggregated protein particles (albumin). It normally appears as a cloudy, milky solution. Therefore, the technologist should use the vial to prepare unit doses.

65. b Wells, 1999, pp. 230–231; Saha, 2004, pp. 153–161

The free pertechnetate impurity is separated using system #1, and the hydrolyzed-reduced ^{99m}Tc impurity by using system #2. Therefore, the percentage of each impurity in the preparation can be determined directly:

$$\%\text{ free pertechnetate} = \frac{9.2\ \mu\text{Ci}}{107.5\ \mu\text{Ci} + 9.2\ \mu\text{Ci}} \times 100$$

$$= 7.9\%$$

$$\%\text{ HR-}^{99m}\text{Tc} = \frac{8.4\ \mu\text{Ci}}{132.6\ \mu\text{Ci} + 8.4\ \mu\text{Ci}} \times 100 = 6.0\%$$

The radiochemical purity of the sample is:

$$100\% - (\%\text{ free pertechnetate} + \%\text{ HR-}^{99m}\text{Tc})$$

$$= 100\% - (7.9\% + 6.9\%)$$

$$= 100\% - 13.9\%$$

$$= 86.1\%.$$

66. c Wells, 1999, p. 213

A proportion can be used to determine the total volume needed to reconstitute the MAA kit:

$$\frac{\text{particles in kit}}{\text{total volume in kit}} = \frac{\text{particles in patient dosage}}{\text{volume of patient dosage}}$$

$$\frac{6 \text{ million particles}}{x} = \frac{500{,}000 \text{ particles}}{0.4 \text{ mL}}$$

$$x = \frac{0.4 \text{ mL} \times 6 \text{ million particles}}{500{,}000 \text{ particles}} = 4.8 \text{ mL}.$$

67. a Lile *et al.*, 2003, p. 273

The areas of a needle and syringe that must remain sterile are any areas that will come into contact with the sterile solution being withdrawn into the syringe or any part of the needle that will be introduced into the patient.

68. a U.S. Nuclear Regulatory Commission, 2003 (10 CFR 20.1003 and 20.1301)

According to the NRC, an unrestricted area is one in which access is not limited by or under control of a licensee and one in which an individual will receive less than 2 mrem in any hour.

69. a U.S. Nuclear Regulatory Commission, 2003 (49 CFR 172.403 and 172.436–440)

The label types and exposure rate limits for packages containing radioactive materials are:

	Exposure rate (mR/hr)	
Label category	At surface	At 1 m
Category I (white)	≤0.5	No detectable radiation
Category II (yellow)	≤50	≤1.0
Category III (yellow)	≤200	≤10

70. b U.S. Nuclear Regulatory Commission, 2003 (10 CFR 35.2063); Siegel, 2004, p. 56

According to the NRC, dosage measurement records must include the radiopharmaceutical, the patient's name or identification number (if one assigned), the prescribed dosage, the determined dosage (or notation that the dosage is less than 30 μCi or 1.1 MBq), the date and time of the measurement, and the name of the person who measured the dosage.

71. b Early and Sodee, 1995, pp. 72–74

The inverse square law states that by doubling the distance from a point source, the radiation intensity is reduced to one-fourth of the original intensity.

72. d U.S. Nuclear Regulatory Commission, 2003 (10 CFR 35.3045)

A licensee must notify the NRC of medical events, which are defined as an administration of a licensed material that results in an effective dose equivalent (EDE) greater than 5 rem, dose to an organ or tissue greater than 50 rem, or shallow dose equivalent (SDE) to the skin greater than 50 rem because of any of the following:

- The total dosage delivered differs from the prescribed dosage by 20% or more.
- The total dosage falls outside the prescribed range.
- The wrong radioactive drug was administered.
- The radioactive drug was administered by the wrong route.
- The radioactive dosage was administered to the wrong person.

Of the possible answers to this question, only the ^{131}I will result in a radiation exposure meeting the above criteria. In addition, the incorrect radioactive drug was given. Even though options a, b, and c describe errors in the administration of a radiopharmaceutical, the exposure to the patient does not exceed the criteria, and the error does not need to be reported to the NRC.

73. c U.S. Nuclear Regulatory Commission, 2003 (10 CFR 35.40)

A written directive for administration of a therapeutic dosage other than [^{131}I]sodium iodide must include the patient's name, the radioactive drug, the route of administration, and the dosage to be administered. It must be dated and signed by the authorized user before the dosage is administered.

74. d U.S. Nuclear Regulatory Commission, 2003 (10 CFR 20.1208); Siegel, 2004, pp. 29–32

According to NRC regulations, the radiation dose to the fetus of a declared pregnant worker must not exceed 0.5 rem (500 mrem) during the entire pregnancy.

75. a Christian *et al.*, 2004, p. 190

Iodine is taken up into the thyroid gland whether it is ingested, inhaled, or absorbed through the skin. Therefore, using an uptake probe to measure radioiodine uptake the day after handling a radioiodine solution is the method of choice.

76. c Thompson *et al.*, 1994, p. 34

The flat end-window of a G–M meter is the area sensitive to radiation. Therefore, when surveying for surface contamination, the end of the probe should be placed directly over the area being surveyed. To avoid contaminating the probe, the probe should not touch the surface and should be kept approximately 1.5 in. from the surface.

77. d U.S. Nuclear Regulatory Commission, 2003 (CFR 20.1906); Siegel, 2004, pp. 41–43

According to the NRC, all shipments of radioactive materials identified with DOT radioactive labels of White I, Yellow II, or Yellow III must be tested for contamination using a wipe test.

78. a Christian *et al.*, 2004, p. 202

Most contamination may be eliminated by removing personal clothing or protective garb, such as gloves or lab coats. Once contaminated clothing is removed, decontamination of skin surfaces should begin.

79. b U.S. Nuclear Regulatory Commission, 2003 (10 CFR 35.2040)

According to the NRC, written directives must be retained for 3 years.

80. b U.S. Nuclear Regulatory Commission, 2003 (10 CFR 35.63); Siegel, 2004, pp. 55–57

According to the NRC, patient dosage records must be retained for 3 years.

81. a Wells, 1999, p. 98

To determine the total dose, multiply the exposure rate by the time of exposure. In this case, the exposure rate must be converted from mrem/hr to mrem/min by dividing the hourly rate by 60 min:

$$\left(\frac{0.5 \text{ mrem/hr}}{60 \text{ min/hr}}\right) \times 20 \text{ min} = 0.17 \text{ mrem}.$$

82. c Wells, 1999, p. 93

To determine wipe test readings in dpm:

$$\text{dpm} = \frac{\text{gross cpm} - \text{background cpm}}{\text{decimal efficiency}}.$$

In this example:

$$\frac{1{,}240\text{ cpm} - 410\text{ cpm}}{0.35} = 2{,}371\text{ dpm}.$$

83. d Wells, 1999, p. 37

$$1\text{ mSv} = 100\text{ mrem};$$

therefore,

$$10 \times 100\text{ mrem} = 1000\text{ mrem}.$$

84. c Siegel, 2004, p. 35

If an occupationally exposed worker has an exposure reading that approaches the NRC limits, the RSO is required to review the individual's work habits to determine what changes can be made to decrease exposure.

85. d U.S. Nuclear Regulatory Commission, 2003 (10 CFR 35.60); Siegel, 2004, pp. 50–52

The NRC requires that dose calibrators be tested for proper functioning according to nationally recognized standards. The standard of practice includes testing constancy on a daily basis before the instrument is used to measure radiopharmaceuticals.

86. a U.S. Nuclear Regulatory Commission, 2003 (10 CFR 35.2061); Siegel, 2004, pp. 55–56

The NRC requires that survey meter calibration records be retained for 3 years. It does not require records for daily constancy tests.

87. a Early and Sodee, 1995, p. 159

As voltage increases, the gamma ray spectrum moves to the right. Therefore, increasing the voltage will shift the photopeak toward the window and, if the voltage is increased sufficiently, into the window.

88. b Early and Sodee, 1995, pp. 165–167; Wells, 1999, pp. 129–130

As the percent energy resolution increases (the value becomes larger), the energy resolution worsens. This means that the FWHM is becoming larger because the photopeak is broadening and, hence, degrading the energy resolution of the instrument. The energy resolution of any counting system decreases with age as a result of deterioration of both the crystal and the electronics. Sudden changes in energy resolution may indicate a cracked crystal.

89. d U.S. Nuclear Regulatory Commission, 2003 (10 CFR 35.61); Siegel, 2004, pp. 43–45

According to NRC regulations, survey meters must be calibrated before first use, annually, and after each repair.

90. a Bernier *et al.*, 1994, pp. 87–89

This flood demonstrates significant nonuniformity. Therefore, the technologist should first confirm that the image was acquired on the correct radionuclide and window settings. A repeat image should be acquired if the settings were incorrect. If the repeat image also shows the nonuniformity, service should be requested. Patient studies must not be acquired on this instrument until the problem is corrected.

91. b English, 1995, p. 44

It is recommended that the COR offset correction be performed at least weekly.

92. a Bernier *et al.*, 1994, pp. 88–89

The standard of practice calls for acquisition of a uniformity flood every day the camera is used, prior to performing patient studies.

93. c Saha, 2004, pp. 135–138

A static acquisition is performed in studies where the radiopharmaceutical localizes and remains in the area of interest for a period of time long enough for imaging to be completed. The radiopharmaceutical is fixed in the area of interest during the acquisition. For example, the thyroid is imaged after sufficient time has passed for the tracer to be localized in the gland. Data are acquired either for a preset number of counts or for a preset time. Dynamic frame mode acquisitions are used in studies where movement of the tracer is important to document. The blood flow phase (first phase) of a three-phase bone scan and renal function studies are examples of dynamic frame mode acquisitions. A left ventricle ejection fraction (LVEF) determination utilizes a gated technique, which is a variation of a dynamic acquisition.

94. d Early and Sodee, 1995, p. 81; English, 1995, pp. 37–40

The collimator must be in place when uniformity correction acquisitions are performed because collimators have inherent variations that differ from one collimator to another. Because an extrinsic flood is being acquired, a sheet source is required. A point source imaged with a collimator cannot distribute photons evenly over the crystal.

95. b Bernier *et al.*, 1994, pp. 91–92

For uniformity correction maps, it is recommended that high-count flood images be acquired weekly. These flood images should not be confused with daily uniformity flood images that are acquired to check detector response.

96. b Christian *et al.*, 2004, pp. 66–67

The resolution of a parallel-hole collimator is greatest at its surface, so the closer the collimator is to the patient, the better the resolution will be. Increasing the window width will admit more scatter, decreasing the resolution. A high-sensitivity collimator has larger holes that admit photons that are traveling at greater angles. This decreases resolution, because the data are recorded as if the photon traveled on a straight line directly up from its origin to the crystal. If the number of shades of gray in the grayscale is decreased, there will be less detail and, therefore, less resolution.

97. d Christian *et al.*, 2004, pp. 118–119, 258–259

The lower the cutoff frequency, the more high frequencies (which provide image detail) are removed from an image. Therefore, a cutoff frequency of 0.5 cycles/pixel results in an image with the most detail and the most high-frequency noise. At the other extreme, a cutoff frequency of 0.15 cycles/pixel removes many of the high frequencies, resulting in a very smooth image without much detail.

98. b Turkington, 2001, pp. 6–8

As activity increases, so does the number of events. With a large number of events occurring almost simultaneously, there is a greater likelihood that unrelated photons (randoms) will be mistaken as coincident pairs. Deadtime remains the same, but more events occur within that time frame and, therefore, go uncounted. Attenuation is not dependent upon activity; it is present regardless of the amount of activity administered. However, with a higher activity, more "good" events are going to be registered because more of them occur. Noise decreases with an increase in activity because, as the number of events increases, the effect of randomness (noise) decreases.

99. b Wells, 1999, p. 140

The energies accepted within a window centered around a given energy are calculated as follows:

$$\text{energies within window} = \text{centerline energy} \pm \frac{\text{energy (keV)} \times \text{\% window as decimal}}{2}.$$

In this example:

$$364 \text{ keV} \pm \frac{364 \times 0.2}{2} = 364 \text{ keV} \pm 36$$

$$364 \text{ keV} \pm 36 = 328 = 400 \text{ keV}.$$

100. c Yester, 2001

Because the holes are smaller and the septa are often longer in a high-resolution collimator, fewer photons pass through the channels and strike the crystal. This decreases sensitivity. Therefore, it would take more time to acquire the same number of counts using a high-resolution collimator.

Answers to Examination 5

1. d Christian *et al.*, 2004, pp. 497–498

The diagram depicts an anterior view of the rib cage and proximal upper extremities. The acromion processes would be demonstrated on a posterior view of the upper thorax that includes the scapulae.

2. a Cevola, 1993, p. 12

Results of previous bone imaging procedures performed with nuclear medicine or another imaging modality may provide additional information not demonstrated on the current image or indications that the condition has improved or worsened. Healing soft tissue, such as that resulting from recent abdominal surgery, will concentrate bone tracer in an unexpected area. External beam radiation therapy can cause photopenic areas, areas of decreased tracer activity, on the bone image in the area where the therapy was delivered.

3. b Christian *et al.*, 2004, pp. 389–390, 392–394

If the patient is in the upright position, the apices of the lung receive very little blood flow. Consequently, more MAA particles will be distributed in the bases of the lungs than in the apices. In the supine position, although there is a blood flow gradient from anterior to posterior, there is a more homogeneous distribution of particles from apex to base.

4. b Christian *et al.*, 2004, p. 392

For adult patients who have only one lung and, therefore, half the lung vasculature, half the usual dosage is recommended. This reduces the number of particles to approximately half of what is administered in a full dosage.

5. b Adler and Carlton, 2003, p. 137

The footrests should always be moved out of the way. The wheelchair must be properly aligned to the imaging table (depending on patient condition) and locked.

6. d Shackett, 2009, p. 255

No special preparation is really needed for a white blood cell infection imaging other than a possible interference if the patient has had a recent blood transfusion.

7. d Christian *et al.*, 2004, p. 363

A pinhole collimator provides an image with better resolution and offers the ability to obtain oblique views. A parallel-hole collimator used with electronic zoom can provide a magnified image with good resolution.

8. c Early and Sodee, 1995, pp. 207–210

Recall that, as a point source is moved closer to the face of a flat-field collimator, more counts are collected. If the standard represents the total amount of activity administered to the patient, the counts collected from the patient's neck represent a portion of the total amount of activity that concentrated in the thyroid gland. It is important, then, based on the response of the detector at a given distance, to count both the standard and the patient at the same distance. For example, suppose the standard and the patient were both counted at 20 cm, and 20,000 net cpm and 5,000 net cpm were obtained, respectively. The patient's uptake is:

$$\frac{\text{neck counts}}{\text{standard counts}} \times 100 = \frac{5{,}000 \text{ cpm}}{20{,}000 \text{ cpm}} \times 100 = 25\%.$$

If the patient were counted at 5 cm instead of 20 cm, more counts would be collected (i.e., 10,000 cpm). Then, the patient's uptake is falsely increased:

$$\frac{\text{neck counts}}{\text{standard counts}} \times 100 = \frac{10{,}000 \text{ cpm}}{20{,}000 \text{ cpm}} \times 100 = 50\%.$$

9. b Early and Sodee, 1995, p. 392

The counts per minute are obtained from the regions of interest drawn around the end-diastolic and end-systolic images. The counts in each region are then corrected for background. The formula for calculating the left ventricular ejection fraction is:

$$\text{LVEF} = \frac{\text{net end-diastolic counts} - \text{net end-systolic counts}}{\text{net end-diastolic counts}} \times 100$$

$$= \frac{2{,}875 \text{ cpm} - 2{,}162 \text{ cpm}}{2{,}875 \text{ cpm}} \times 100 = 25\%.$$

10. a Adler and Carlton, 2003, pp. 195–197

Standard precautions should be used routinely with all patients. These precautions include activities such as handwashing, wearing gloves, and recapping needles using a safety device. Decontaminating imaging equipment would be performed only if it came in contact with biological fluids from a patient or with a patient known to be infected with a communicable disease.

11. d English *et al.*, 1993, pp. 50–51

The characteristics of normal sinus rhythm as they appear on an ECG tracing are: (1) heart rate of 60–100 beats per minute, (2) R waves at regular intervals (variance of less than 0.12 sec), (3) P waves present and precede QRS complex, (4) PR interval between 0.12 and 0.20 sec long, and (5) QRS complex less than 0.12 sec.

12. b Early and Sodee, 1995, p. 419

Defects visualized on stress images are interpreted as myocardial ischemia if the defects fill in on the resting images. However, the rate of redistribution varies, and ischemic areas may not appear to have reperfused by 4 hr. Administering a second, smaller dose of ^{201}Tl before rest imaging provides additional tracer in the circulation that can be extracted into these areas, improving the image quality and identifying reversible ischemia.

13. b Mettler and Guiberteau, 1991, p. 200

If the gallbladder is not visualized after 1 hr but tracer is seen in the common bile duct and small intestine, morphine may be administered. Morphine acts on the sphincter of Oddi, causing it to contract, thus increasing pressure in the common bile duct and causing tracer to flow into the gallbladder.

14. b Christian *et al.*, 2004, p. 569

Bowel preparations are contraindicated before Meckel's diverticulum imaging because they irritate the intestinal mucosa, possibly causing a false-positive finding. It is recommended that patients fast for at least 2 hr before imaging to reduce stomach secretions that cause migration of [^{99m}Tc]pertechnetate from the stomach into the bowel.

15. c Early and Sodee, 1995, p. 517

Because [^{99m}Tc]sulfur colloid is cleared from the blood within 10–15 min after administration, it is preferred when the patient exhibits active gastrointestinal (GI) bleeding. In cases where the GI bleeding is intermittent and unpredictable, ^{99m}Tc-labeled red blood cells are preferred, because this tracer remains in the blood pool for an extended period that permits imaging up to 24 hr.

16. b Christian *et al.*, 2004, p. 485

Furosemide is a diuretic that increases the production of urine. Activity retained in the collecting system or renal pelvis may indicate an obstruction in that area. Furosemide is used to wash out the activity with an increased production of urine. If the activity clears after the administration of furosemide, there is no obstruction.

17. a Christian *et al.*, 2004, p. 485

Furosemide is a diuretic that increases the production of urine. Activity retained in the collecting system or renal pelvis may indicate an obstruction in that area. Furosemide is used to wash out the activity with an increased production of urine. If the activity clears after the administration of furosemide, there is no obstruction. Clearance of the activity is the normal response.

18. b Early and Sodee, 1995, p. 703

^{67}Ga imaging can be performed from 6 hr to 3 days or longer after tracer administration. When the examination is being performed for evaluation of an inflammatory process, early imaging (6 hr after injection) is indicated.

19. c Adler and Carlton, 2003, p. 194

It is widely accepted that handwashing is considered to be the single most effective way of preventing the spread of infection in a medical care facility.

20. b SNM Procedure Guidelines Committee, 2011

[^{111}In]pentetreotide normally localizes in the pituitary gland, thyroid gland, liver, spleen, bladder, and bowel.

21. c SNM Procedure Guidelines Committee, 2011

For the best image quality, brain imaging with [^{99m}Tc]exametazime should begin no sooner than 90 min after the administration of the tracer.

22. c Christian *et al.*, 2004, p. 342

Normally, cerebral spinal fluid flows out of the lateral ventricles. Reversal of this flow (or reflux) and visualization of tracer in the lateral ventricles is an abnormal finding.

23. b Early and Sodee, 1995, p. 755

Before instilling ^{32}P into the peritoneal space, [^{99m}Tc]sulfur colloid is introduced to demonstrate that the agent will disperse throughout the cavity, thereby uniformly irradiating the peritoneal space.

24. c Christian *et al.*, 2004, pp. 364–365
After a thyroidectomy, the purpose of ^{131}I whole-body imaging is to detect the presence of residual thyroid tissue and/or distant metastases. To enhance the visualization of any metastases, the patient may be instructed to limit dietary iodine. The patient may also discontinue replacement thyroid hormone therapy to permit the metastases to function as thyroid tissue. Exogenous TSH may also be prescribed to stimulate the metastases to concentrate iodine.

25. d Tikofsky *et al.*, 1993, p. 59
It is desirable to image the brain in as close to a "resting" state as possible. Because uptake of [^{99m}Tc]bicisate can be affected by sensory input, distractions (bright lights, noise, pain) should be kept to a minimum.

26. b Christian, 2004, pp. 311–312
Patients who receive [^{18}F]FDG for PET imaging must remain quiet during the interval between tracer administration and imaging. Small changes in tissue metabolism can cause uptake in skeletal muscle that may obscure or be mistaken for disease or can decrease the amount of tracer taken up into the tumor.

27. d Early and Sodee, 1995, p. 524
With the patient upright, imaging should begin immediately after meal consumption for 1 min, then every 15 min for at least 2 hr. Imaging may need to be extended beyond 2 hr if it appears that the stomach is not emptying.

28. b Adler and Carlton, 2003, p. 215
For proper drainage, chest tube apparatus must always remain lower than the patient's chest.

29. b Bernier *et al.*, 1994, pp. 188–190
All of the studies listed are quantitative; their results are a number that reflects some physiologic parameter. In this instance, it is best to perform the study using the least amount of activity first, approximately 0.5 μCi in a ^{57}Co capsule. The thyroid uptake, performed with ^{123}I, which has a half-life of 13 hr, should be performed next. It will be important to count the patient's thyroid before the radioiodine is administered to determine any residual patient background from the Schilling test. After decay of the ^{123}I, the GFR can be performed with several millicuries of [^{99m}Tc]pentetate. At this point, any residual activity from the Schilling test will be negligible, and the activity from the thyroid uptake will have decayed.

30. b Shackett, 2009, p. 67
The sestimibi pharmaceutical for cardiac imaging concentrates in multiple organs and can affect the image. In an effort to clear activity out of the thyroid, liver, and bowel, cold water can be given to the patient prior to imaging to increase the target-to-nontarget ratio for imaging the heart.

31. c Shackett, 2009, p. 67
A nitroglycerin drip will interfere with determining if, at rest, the cardiac arteries are partially occluded. (Patients suffering from angina could be on nitroglycerin therapy.)

32. b Adler and Carlton, 2003, pp. 248–249
The technologist should report the drainage and reinforce the original dressing with additional dressing until appropriate medical personnel are available to address the patient's needs.

33. c Early and Sodee, 1995, p. 728
The red cell and whole blood volumes can be calculated from the measured plasma volume (PV) using the following formulas:

$$\text{total blood volume (TBV)} = \frac{\text{PV (mL)}}{1 - \text{HCT}} \times 100$$

$$\text{TBV} = \frac{3900\text{ mL}}{1 - 0.40} = 6500\text{ mL}$$

$$\begin{aligned}\text{red cell volume} &= \text{TBV} - \text{PV}\\ &= 6500\text{ mL} - 3900\text{ mL}\\ &= 2600\text{ mL}\end{aligned}$$

34. b Christian *et al.*, 2004, p. 527
The time span between injection and blood sampling allows the body to remove cells damaged during the labeling process and allows free chromic ions to be removed from the plasma.

35. a Early and Sodee, 1995, p. 725
Preventing clot formation with the addition of an anticoagulant will result in the fluid portion remaining as plasma. The fluid portion of a blood sample that has been allowed to clot is serum.

36. b Adler and Carlton, 2003, pp. 246–247
CPR should always be administered to a patient in cardiac arrest unless the patient, patient's family, or patient's physician has specifically requested that it not be done. In these cases, DNR (do not resuscitate) should be clearly indicated on the patient's chart.

37. d Shackett, 2009, p. 174
Pentagastrin stimulates ectopic gastric mucosal uptake of pertechnetate by 30%–60% while decreasing emptying time into small bowel and decreasing background.

38. b Christian *et al.*, 2004, p. 527
Red cell survival half-time is obtained from a graph of the net counts per minute of each blood sample plotted on the log scale and time plotted on the linear scale of semilog paper.

39. c Shackett, 2009, p. 42
Place patient in quiet environment before injection.

40. d Remson and Ackermann, 1977, pp. 77–83
When multiple dilutions are performed, the final dilution is the product of the individual dilutions. Thus:

$$\frac{1}{50} \times \frac{1}{200} = \frac{1}{10{,}000}.$$

41. c Williams *et al.*, 1997, pp. 205–207

[^{111}In]capromab pendetide is used in patients who have been newly diagnosed with prostate cancer to more accurately stage the disease before surgery. After surgery or radiation therapy, it is also used to detect recurrence or residual cancer in patients with rising PSA levels but no other evidence of disease.

42. c Wells, 1999, p. 235

Net counts are determined using a background (bkg) region of interest (ROI) drawn near the area of interest. The average counts per pixel in the bkg ROI are subtracted from the cardiac ROI, adjusted for the size of the region.

$$\text{net cardiac ROI counts} = \text{cardiac ROI counts} - \left(\frac{\text{bkg ROI counts}}{\text{bkg ROI pixels}}\right) \times \text{cardiac ROI pixels}$$

$$28{,}503 \text{ cts} - (1859 \text{ cts}/88 \text{ pixels}) \times 417 \text{ pixels}$$

$$28{,}503 \text{ cts} - (21 \text{ cts/pixel}) \times 417 \text{ pixels}$$

$$28{,}503 \text{ cts} - 8809 \text{ cts} = 19{,}694 \text{ cts}.$$

43. a Saha, 2004, pp. 70–72

The yield of ^{99m}Tc is affected by three factors: the amount of ^{99}Mo on the column at the time of elution, the time elapsed since the last elution, and the elution efficiency of the generator. The shorter the time between elutions, the less time the ^{99}Mo has to decay to ^{99m}Tc, resulting in a lower yield of ^{99m}Tc.

44. b Wells, 1999, pp. 32–33

Conversions between the CGS and SI systems can be accomplished easily if you remember the three following relationships:

$$1 \text{ Ci} = 37 \text{ GBq}$$

$$1 \text{ mCi} = 37 \text{ MBq}$$

$$1\ \mu\text{Ci} = 37 \text{ kBq}.$$

Then, to convert millicuries to gigabecquerels:

$$127 \text{ mCi} \times 37 \text{ MBq/mCi} = 4{,}699 \text{ MBq}$$

$$1{,}000 \text{ MBq} = 1 \text{ GBq}$$

$$4699 \text{ MBq} \times 1 \text{ GBq}/1{,}000 \text{ MBq} = 4.7 \text{ GBq}.$$

45. d Chilton and Witcofski, 1986, pp. 54, 57–58

The amount of ^{99m}Tc activity removed will be the same regardless of the saline volume used for elution. However, the amount of ^{99}Mo on the column, the time elapsed since the last elution, and the elution efficiency of the generator all influence the amount of ^{99m}Tc activity eluted.

46. a U.S. Nuclear Regulatory Commission, 2003 (10 CFR 35.204)

According to the NRC, the maximum allowable ^{99}Mo concentration in a ^{99m}Tc eluate must not exceed 0.15 μCi ^{99}Mo/mCi ^{99m}Tc at the time of administration to the patient.

47. d U.S. Nuclear Regulatory Commission, 2003 (10 CFR 35.204); Wells, 1999, pp. 224–225

The ^{99}Mo concentration in this eluate is equal to:

$$45\ \mu\text{Ci}/275 \text{ mCi} = 0.16\ \mu\text{Ci}\ ^{99}\text{Mo/mCi}\ ^{99m}\text{Tc}.$$

This ^{99}Mo concentration exceeds the maximum allowable limit of 0.15 μCi ^{99}Mo/mCi ^{99m}Tc set by the NRC. Therefore, the technologist must not administer the eluate to patients either as [^{99m}Tc]pertechnetate or as some other ^{99m}Tc-labeled compound. Also, remember that radionuclide purity changes with time. Because ^{99}Mo ($T_{1/2}$ = 66 hr) decays more slowly than ^{99m}Tc ($T_{1/2}$ = 6 hr), the ratio of ^{99}Mo to ^{99m}Tc will increase with time, exceeding the maximum allowable limit to a greater extent.

48. c Saha, 2004, p. 75; Ponto *et al.*, 1987, pp. 270, 274

High levels of aluminum ions in ^{99m}Tc eluate can affect the preparation of radiopharmaceuticals and change their biodistribution, including the distribution of [^{99m}Tc]pertechnetate. Therefore, eluate with an aluminum ion concentration exceeding the USP limit should not be administered to patients or be used to prepare other ^{99m}Tc-labeled tracers. High levels of aluminum ions indicate a defect in the preparation of the generator's alumina column, a problem that cannot be corrected onsite in the clinical setting. The manufacturer should be notified, and the generator should be returned for replacement.

49. b Schwarz *et al.*, 1997, pp. 169–172

[^{99m}Tc]apcitide is used to visualize acute deep vein thrombosis in the lower extremities. [^{99m}Tc]succimer is a static renal imaging agent. [^{99m}Tc]exametazime (HMPAO) is a radiopharmaceutical approved for perfusion brain imaging. [^{99m}Tc]tetrofosmin is a myocardial perfusion agent.

50. b Radiopharmaceutical kit package inserts

A review of radiopharmaceutical kit package inserts shows that most prepared ^{99m}Tc agents may be administered for 6–8 hr after preparation. Some exceptions include [^{99m}Tc]succimer, which must be administered within 30 min, and [^{99m}Tc]pentetate, which, when used for glomerular filtration rate determination, must be administered within 1 hr of preparation.

51. c Wells, 1999, pp. 192–193

Based on the activity and volume limits for the kit, up to 100 mCi may be prepared using a volume of 0.5–3.0 mL [^{99m}Tc]pertechnetate. Using the maximum reconstituting volume, 75 mCi of [^{99m}Tc]disofenin can be prepared, an amount within both the volume and activity limits of the kit:

$$3.0 \text{ mL} \times 25.0 \text{ mCi/mL} = 75.0 \text{ mCi}.$$

52. c Christian *et al.*, 2004, p. 416

The major advantage of in vivo red cell labeling is that tagging takes place in the circulatory system. The patient first receives reconstituted "cold" pyrophosphate containing stannous ion that permits [^{99m}Tc]pertechnetate to permeate red cell membranes. After a short incubation period to allow the stannous ion to come into contact with the red cells, the patient is injected with [^{99m}Tc]pertechnetate. After another short incubation period when the tracer becomes incorporated in the red cells, imaging begins.

53. b Ponto *et al.*, 1987, pp. 276–277
The diameter of the colloid particle is increased as a function of heating time. Thus, the longer the ^{99m}Tc preparation is heated, the larger the sulfur colloid particles become. Extended heating times, beyond what is recommended in the package insert, result in particles large enough to become trapped in the lung vasculature.

54. c Saha, 2004, pp. 152–154, 165
Radiochemical purity is defined as the fraction of total radioactivity present in the desired chemical form, in this case, [^{99m}Tc]medronate. [^{99m}Tc]pertechnetate that did not bind to the ligand, medronate, is a radiochemical impurity. Aluminum is a chemical impurity. ^{99}Mo is a radionuclidic impurity. It is a radionuclide other than the desired one, ^{99m}Tc.

55. c Ponto *et al.*, 1987, pp. 268–269
The radiochemical purity of the radiopharmaceutical is only 65%. Tagging efficiencies (radiochemical purities) of 90% or greater contribute to technically satisfactory images. The large amount of impurity (35%), most of which is likely to be free pertechnetate, will be demonstrated as uptake in areas of the body known to concentrate [^{99m}Tc]pertechnetate: the salivary and thyroid glands, and the gastric mucosa of the stomach.

56. b Wells, 1999, p. 195
First convert the patient's body weight into kilograms:

$$172 \text{ lb} \times \frac{\text{kg}}{2.2 \text{ lb}} = 78 \text{ kg}.$$

Next, calculate the total activity to be administered to the patient based on body weight:

$$78 \text{ kg} \times \frac{740 \text{ kBq}}{\text{kg}} = 57{,}720 \text{ kBq}.$$

Then, convert kBq into MBq.

$$57{,}720 \text{ kBq} \times \frac{\text{MBq}}{1000 \text{ kBq}} = 58 \text{ MBq}.$$

57. a Wells, 1999, pp. 189–190
If all patients were being injected at 0700, the maximum number of studies that could be performed is 10 (50 mCi ÷ 5 mCi/patient = 10 patients). However, the injections are beginning at 0730 and on each half hour thereafter. Therefore, the available activity must be decay corrected for 0730 and for each injection thereafter. (See chart below.)

Patient	Time	Decay-Corrected Activity Available (mCi)	Unit Dosage (mCi)	Activity Remaining (mCi)
1	0730	50 mCi ×0.946 = 47.3	5	42.3
2	0830	42.3 mCi × 0.891 = 37.7	5	32.7
3	0930	32.7 mCi × 0.891 = 29.1	5	24.1
4	1030	24.1 mCi × 0.891 = 21.5	5	16.5
5	1130	16.5 mCi × 0.891 = 14.7	5	10.0
6	1230	10.0 mCi × 0.891 = 8.6	5	3.6

58. c Wells, 1999, pp. 29, 172–173, 185–186
The elapsed time between calibration and dosage administration is 2 hr (0600–0800). Decay correct the initial concentration for 2 hr using the appropriate decay factor for ^{99m}Tc:

$$1.85 \text{ GBq/mL} \times 0.794 = 1.47 \text{ GBq/mL}.$$

Then, determine the maximum volume that can be administered to the patient. The maximum prescribed activity, 925 MBq + 92.5 MBq or approximately 1,017 MBq, will make up the maximum volume. Remember that the concentration and the required activity must be expressed in the same units. Changing the required activity to GBq:

$$1017 \text{ MBq} \times \frac{\text{GBq}}{1000 \text{ MBq}} = 1.02 \text{ GBq}$$

$$\text{volume} = \frac{\text{activity required}}{C(t)}$$

$$= \frac{1.02 \text{ GBq}}{1.47 \text{ GBq/mL}}$$

$$= 0.69 \text{ mL}.$$

59. d Early and Sodee, 1995, p. 732
Ascorbic acid is added after red cell tagging has occurred but before the tagged sample is reinjected into the patient. Ascorbic acid reduces any untagged ^{51}Cr in the hexavalent state to a trivalent state, thus preventing red cell tagging in vivo after reinjection.

60. a Saha, 2004, pp. 116–118
In both the in vivo and modified in vivo methods of labeling red blood cells with [^{99m}Tc]pertechnetate, reconstituted stannous pyrophosphate is injected intravenously into the patient. Hence, the same amount of stannous pyrophosphate is administered, and the entire volume of the patient's blood is "pretinned" in either method. Twenty to 30 millicuries of [^{99m}Tc]pertechnetate are used in both methods. The main difference in the modified in vivo method is that only a small volume (~3 mL) of the patient's pretinned blood is mixed with [^{99m}Tc]pertechnetate in a syringe. In the in vivo method, [^{99m}Tc]pertechnetate is injected intravenously 15–30 min after stannous pyrophosphate.

61. c Christian *et al.*, 2004, p. 416
The modified in vivo method for labeling red blood cells involves first administering "cold" stannous pyrophosphate to the patient. Then, a small sample (1–5 mL) of the patient's blood is incubated with [^{99m}Tc]pertechnetate outside the patient. The in vitro method involves collecting a small blood sample that is first incubated with stannous ion, then [^{99m}Tc]pertechnetate outside the patient. The plasma containing unbound [^{99m}Tc]pertechnetate is removed and the red cells washed before reinjecting them. In the in vivo method, all labeling steps occur within the patient.

62. b U.S. Nuclear Regulatory Commission, 2003 (10 CFR 35.63)
The NRC states that the administered dosage must fall within the prescribed dosage range or may not differ from the prescribed dosage by

more than 20%. If the prescribed dosage is 10 mCi, the measured dosage must be between 8 and 12 mCi (±20% of 10 mCi). The measured dosages in choices c and d fall outside the prescribed dosage ranges. Choice b is the correct answer because 12.5 mCi falls within ±20% of 15 mCi.

63. d Christian *et al.*, 2004, p. 525

Ascorbic acid reduces the valence of any remaining free chromium from +6 to +3. The purpose of this step is to stop the red cell tagging process before the labeled blood is reinjected into the patient.

64. b Wells, 1999, pp. 172–173, 183

Decay correct the activity for 1.5 hr (0800–0930) using the 1.5-hr decay factor for ^{99m}Tc:

$$4.65 \text{ MBq} \times 0.84 = 3.91 \text{ MBq}.$$

Determine the concentration at 0930 using the decay corrected activity:

$$\text{concentration} = \frac{\text{total activity}}{\text{total volume}} = \frac{3.91 \text{ MBq}}{3.5 \text{ mL}} = 1.12 \text{ MBq/mL}.$$

65. c Wells, 1999, pp. 197–198

First, determine the total activity in the syringe at 1200 by back decay correcting the activity using the 2-hr decay factor (1200–1400 = 2 hr) for ^{99m}Tc:

$$\frac{25 \text{ mCi}}{0.794} = 31.5 \text{ mCi}.$$

Then, determine the concentration at 1200:

$$\text{concentration} = \frac{\text{total activity}}{\text{total volume}} = \frac{31.5 \text{ mCi}}{0.8 \text{ mL}} = 39.4 \text{ mCi/mL}.$$

Determine the volume that will contain 15 mCi at 1200:

$$\text{volume} = \frac{\text{activity required}}{\text{concentration}} = \frac{15 \text{ mCi}}{39.4 \text{ mCi/mL}} = 0.38 \text{ mL}.$$

Determine the volume that will need to be removed from the syringe:

$$\text{total volume} - \text{volume required} = \text{volume to be removed}$$

$$0.8 \text{ mL} - 0.38 \text{ mL} = 0.42 \text{ mL}.$$

66. d Wells, 1999, p. 213

Based on the volume added to the kit, determine the number of particles in 1 mL:

$$\frac{4.5 \text{ million particles}}{2.5 \text{ mL}} = 1.8 \text{ million particles/mL}.$$

Determine the kit concentration:

$$\text{concentration} = \frac{\text{total activity}}{\text{total volume}} = \frac{30 \text{ mCi}}{2.5 \text{ mL}} = 12 \text{ mCi/mL}.$$

Determine the volume that will contain the required activity:

$$\text{volume} = \frac{\text{activity required}}{\text{concentration}} = \frac{3 \text{ mCi}}{12 \text{ mCi/mL}} = 0.25 \text{ mL}.$$

Determine the number of particles contained in the patient dosage:

$$\text{dosage volume} \times \text{particles/mL} = \text{particles in patient dosage}$$

$$0.25 \text{ mL} \times 1.8 \text{ million particles/mL} = 450{,}000 \text{ particles}.$$

Note that the number of particles in the patient dosage is within the recommended range for adults.

67. b American Pharmaceutical Association, 1999, p. 144

The syringe size is the next size larger than the volume to be withdrawn. If the syringe is filled to its maximum volume, the plunger may easily be pulled out while a volume is being withdrawn or while a patient is being injected with the volume in the syringe.

68. a U.S. Nuclear Regulatory Commission, 2003 (10 CFR 20.1003 and 20.1301)

According to the NRC, an unrestricted area is one in which access is not limited by or under control of a licensee. Unrestricted areas are not posted.

69. b U.S. Nuclear Regulatory Commission, 2003 (49 CFR 172.403 and 172.436–440)

The label types and exposure rate limits for packages containing radioactive material are:

	Exposure rate (mR/hr)	
Label category	At surface	At 1 m
Category I (White)	≤0.5	No detectable radiation
Category II (yellow)	≤50	≤1.0
Category III (yellow)	≤200	≤10

70. c U.S. Nuclear Regulatory Commission, 2003 (10 cfr 35.2092); Siegel, 2004, p. 56

According to the NRC, records of radioactive materials that are allowed to decay in storage must include the date of disposal, the survey instrument used, the background level of radiation, the radiation level at the surface of the waste container, and the name of the individual who performed the survey.

71. d Early and Sodee, 1995, pp. 72–74

The thickness of a half-value layer (HVL) depends on the density of the shielding material and the photon energy of the radionuclide being shielded. The HVL for a radionuclide that emits a higher-energy photon must be thicker than the HVL for a lower-energy photon emitter to absorb 50% if the emitted photons. Thus, the HVL of lead for a low-energy photon emitter, such as ^{125}I (27.5 keV), is 0.04 mm, but the HVL of lead for a higher-energy photon emitter, such as ^{137}Cs (662 keV), is 6.5 mm. Similarly, the HVL for high-density shielding material is less than the HVL for lower-density materials. For example, for ^{131}I, the HVL of a high-density material such as lead is 0.22 cm, but in the case of aluminum, a material with a much lower density than lead, the HVL is 2.6 cm. In this instance, more (a greater thickness) of lower-density material is required to absorb 50% of the emitted protons.

72. d U.S. Nuclear Regulatory Commission, 2003 (10 CFR 35.3045); Siegel, 2004, pp. 58–59

When a medical event (misadministration) occurs, the NRC requires the licensee to notify the NRC, the referring physician, and the involved individual, unless the referring physician determines, on the basis of medical judgment, that such notification would be harmful to the patient.

73. a U.S. Nuclear Regulatory Commission, 2003 (10 CFR 20.1201); Siegel, 2004, pp. 28–36

According to the NRC, the annual whole-body occupational dose limit for adults is 5000 millirem or 5 rem.

74. c U.S. Nuclear Regulatory Commission, 2003 (10 CFR 35.92); Siegel, 2004, pp. 53–54

According to NRC regulations, decay in storage of radioactive materials requires that the materials remain in storage until the radioactivity is indistinguishable from background radiation using a survey meter on the most sensitive scale and without any shielding in place. Before disposal, all radiation labels must be obliterated unless the materials are in a container that will be managed as biomedical waste when released from the licensees.

75. c U.S. Nuclear Regulatory Commission, 2003 (10 CFR 35.70 and 10 CFR 20.1501); Siegel, 2004, pp. 43–46

NCR regulations require a survey of areas where radiopharmaceuticals that require a written directive are prepared or administered. This would include therapeutic radiopharmaceuticals and dosages of ^{131}I greater than 30 μCi. The survey is to be performed at the end of the day. As of October 2002, the NRC no longer requires daily surveys and weekly wipe tests. Instead it allows facilities to establish a survey and wipe test schedule. The schedule must be reasonable, based on the need to determine radiation levels, concentrations or quantities of radioactive materials, and potential radiological hazards.

76. c Thompson *et al.*, 1994, pp. 32–33

The measured exposure rate is the product of the number indicated by the needle on the meter and the scale. In this example, the reading on the meter is 0.6 on a scale of 10. Thus, 0.6 mR/hr $\times$ 10 = 6 mR/hr.

77. b U.S. Nuclear Regulatory Commission, 2003 (10 CFR 20.1906); Siegel, 2004, pp. 41–43

According to the NRC, both the NRC and the final delivery carrier must be notified if the exposure rate of a radioactive package is in excess of 200 mR/hr at the package surface or in excess of 10 mR/hr at 3 feet from the package surface.

78. b Christian *et al.*, 2004, p. 202

Decontamination of the skin should be attempted with a mild detergent and lukewarm water to avoid irritating the skin. Abrasive materials, scrubbing, and hot water all can increase absorption of the radioactivity through the skin.

79. c U.S. Nuclear Regulatory Commission, 2003 (10 CFR 20.1003)

The NRC requires that access to restricted areas must be limited to prevent individuals from being exposed to radiation or radioactive materials that may cause undue risk. To control access, restricted areas must be locked when authorized staff is not present.

80. c U.S. Nuclear Regulatory Commission, 2003 (10 CFR 35.63); Siegel, 2004, pp. 53–54

According to the NRC, radioactive materials must be decayed in storage if the half-life is less than 120 days.

81. c Wells, 1999, p. 98

To determine the total dose, multiply the exposure rate by the time of exposure. In this case:

$$1.2 \text{ mR/hr} \times 3 \text{ hr} = 3.6 \text{ mR}.$$

However, the exposure to people is recorded in mrem. With gamma energies used in diagnostic nuclear medicine, R = rem, so mR can be directly converted to mrem.

82. b U.S. Nuclear Regulatory Commission, 2003 (49 CFR 170–178)

DOT regulations require that a survey of the package be performed to verify that there is no surface contamination before shipping packages containing radioactive materials.

83. a Christian *et al.*, 2004, pp. 307–308

The primary sources of radiation exposure to the technologist who performs PET imaging are from the radiopharmaceutical dosages before and during administration and from the Compton scatter escaping the patient's body. Because they are particles, positrons will be absorbed by body tissue and will not be emitted from the body.

84. d Siegel, 2004, p. 35

Either a TLD or an OSL can be used because the accuracy of the reading is not affected by time. The film in a film badge may begin to fog within this period of time, which may result in inaccurate exposure readings.

85. d U.S. Nuclear Regulatory Commission, 2003 (10 CFR 35.60); Siegel, 2004, pp. 50–52

The NRC requires that dose calibrators be tested for proper functioning according to nationally recognized standards. The standard of practice dictates that the measured activity should be within ±10% of the expected activity when the instrument is tested for linearity. All 9 measured activities are approximately 5% of the calculated values. Therefore, the results of this test are within acceptable linearity limits.

86. c Bernier *et al.*, 1994, p. 80

Various long-lived sources can be used to test accuracy. At least 50 μCi of ^{137}Cs, ^{57}Co, or ^{133}Ba should be used. ^{99m}Tc is not an appropriate choice because it is relatively short-lived.

87. c Early and Sodee, 1995, pp. 158–162

Calibrating a scintillation spectrometer involves the determination of the operating voltage applied to the dynodes of the photomultiplier tube. A reference standard, such as ^{137}Cs, is counted at various voltage settings, and the counts are recorded. Then, the net counts per minute versus the voltage are plotted on linear graph paper. From the graph, the voltage at which the maximum number of counts is obtained is the operating voltage for the instrument. Calibration results are valid only for the gain setting used during the determination of the operating voltage.

88. c Early and Sodee, 1995, pp. 165–167, 272–273

Sensitivity is expressed as counts per minute per microcurie. From the data presented, there is a sudden change in sensitivity from one day to the next. If the window is not set correctly over the photopeak, it will take longer to acquire the specified number of counts. Likewise, using a collimator that has less sensitivity than a low-energy, all-purpose collimator (such as a high-resolution or medium-energy collimator) will require additional time to collect the counts. With a cracked crystal, the photopeak is broadened, thus decreasing the system's energy resolution and causing decreased counts in a given period of time. If an acquisition is set to terminate after a preset number of counts, the matrix size will not affect the length of the acquisition.

89. c Bernier *et al.*, 1994, pp. 88–89; Early and Sodee, 1995, pp. 261–271

Camera uniformity may be performed intrinsically (without the collimator) or extrinsically (with the collimator in place). Intrinsic uniformity images may be acquired with a point source placed at 3–5 UFOV (useful fields of view) from the crystal or with a sheet source placed over the crystal. Extrinsic uniformity must be performed with a sheet source placed on the crystal. The image shown was performed with a collimated point source. Therefore, there is not an even distribution of radioactivity over the face of the crystal. The technologist should either remove the collimator and repeat the image or use a radionuclide sheet source with the collimator in place to obtain the uniformity image.

90. a Bernier *et al.*, 1994, p. 80

According to the standard of practice, the accuracy of a dose calibrator should be tested at installation and annually thereafter.

91. c English, 1995, p. 44

COR values should vary by no more than 1/2 pixel. Deviations greater than 1/2 pixel may degrade resolution in reconstructed images. The values presented are within the 1/2-pixel limit. Therefore, the technologist can use the camera for SPECT studies using the most recent value.

92. b Bernier *et al.*, 1994, p. 89

The standard of practice calls for performance of linearity and spatial resolution testing on a weekly basis.

93. a Lee, 2005, pp. 93–95

Counts from the three photopeaks are collected in one acquisition matrix to form a single ^{67}Ga image. Therefore, one set of storage locations in computer memory is needed. One 128 × 128 byte-mode matrix contains 16,384 bytes. A kilobyte (kB) contains 1,024 bytes. To convert bytes to kilobytes:

$$16{,}384 \text{ bytes} \times \frac{1 \text{ kB}}{1{,}024 \text{ bytes}} = 16 \text{ kB}.$$

94. b Bernier *et al.*, 1994, pp. 254–260

Tomographic images may be reconstructed from the planar projections using a technique called backprojection. This creates a star pattern as the ray sums are projected back along a line in the reconstruction matrix. The use of a ramp filter during the process helps eliminate much of the "star" artifact.

95. b Bernier *et al.*, 1994, p. 81

If the percentage error in the measurement is less than 10%, then the instrument can be used as is. The measured activity falls within ±10% of the expected value. Therefore, no correction factor is needed.

96. b Powsner and Powsner, 1998, pp. 57–58

The Geiger–Mueller (G–M) counter is best suited for detecting low-level contamination because it is sensitive to exposure rates just above background, although the readings are not as accurate as those obtained with an ionization chamber. The G–M has a quicker response time compared with the ionization chamber. Although a pocket dosimeter can give an immediate reading, it cannot be used to localize contamination.

97. a Turkington, 2001, p. 8

The more data, the smaller the effect of the randomness of radioactive decay. Scanning for a longer time increases the number of counts acquired, thereby decreasing noise. Using 2D mode allows for more, because it accepts cross ring interactions. Decreasing the dosage decreases counts and, therefore, increases noise. In a dedicated PET unit, the detectors are stationary on a nonadjustable ring. The distance between the patient and the detectors cannot be adjusted, except to center the imaging pallet in the middle of the ring.

98. b Early and Sodee, 1995, p. 165

The percentage energy resolution should not exceed 12%. If the photopeak has broadened beyond this point, the instrument cannot accurately distinguish one energy from another.

99. b Wells, 1999, p. 142

Half the percentage of the window is above and half is below the designated energy. The window is expressed as a percentage of the energy of the radionuclide. In this case, it will be 662 keV, because 5% of 662 keV = 33 keV. The LLD will be set at the lower limit of the window (629 keV), and the ULD will be set at the upper limit (695 keV).

100. b Early and Sodee, 1995, pp. 131–135

A portable ionization chamber, sometimes referred to as a cutie pie, is used to measure areas of high photon intensity. This instrument gives a direct measurement of the total number of ion pairs produced per unit time and, therefore, is more accurate than a Geiger–Mueller counter when surveying a large amount of radioactivity.

Answers to Examination 6

1. c Christian and Waterstram-Rich, 2007, p. 4

The inverse square law is represented by the equation $I_1(D_1)^2 = I_2(D_2)^2$, with I equaling intensity in mR/hr and D equaling distance. 20 mR/hr represents the I_1 value, while 3 m will be the D_1 value. 500 mR/hr is the D_2 value and the I_2 value can be found by plugging in all the given information to the inverse square law equation and solving for the missing variable.

$$20 \text{ mR/hr } (3 \text{ m})^2 = 500 \text{ mR/hr } (I_2)^2$$

$$(I_2)^2 = 20 \text{ mR/hr } (9 \text{ m}) = 0.36 \text{ m}$$

$$500 \text{ mR/hr.}$$

Take the square root of both sides to get $I_2 = 0.60$ m.

How many cm = 0.60 m × 100 cm/1 m = 60 cm.

2. b Christian and Waterstram-Rich, 2007, p. 207

The "Caution: Radioactive Materials" sign is used in any area where certain quantities of radioactive materials are used or stored. The "Caution: Radiation Area" sign is used in areas where an individual could receive more than 5mrem (0.05mSv) in 1 hr at 30 cm from a radioactive source. The "Caution: High Radiation Area" signs are used where an individual could receive more than 100 mrem/hr (1 mSv) in 1 hr at 30 cm from a radioactive source. Since the ambient radiation exposure is between 5 mrem/hr and 100 mrem/hr, the appropriate caution sign would be "Caution: Radiation Area."

3. b Christian and Waterstram-Rich, 2007, p. 207

The "Caution: Radioactive Materials" sign is used in any area where certain quantities of radioactive materials are used or stored. The "Caution: Radiation Area" sign is used in areas where an individual could receive more than 5mrem (0.05mSv) in 1 hr at 30 cm from a radioactive source. The "Caution: High Radiation Area" signs are used where an individual could receive more than 100 mrem/hr (1 mSv) in 1 hr at 30 cm from a radioactive source. Since the integral dose in 10 min is 3 min, this implies that the total dose for 1 hr is 6 times this amount or 18 mrem/hr. Therefore, the radiation exposure is between 5 mrem/hr and 100 mrem/hr, and the appropriate caution sign would be "Caution: Radiation Area."

4. d Christian and Waterstram-Rich, 2007, p. 207

In areas where personnel would receive life-threatening doses of radiation such as levels over 500 R/hr, the sign "Grave Danger: Very High Radiation Area" would be used. It is unlikely that materials with an activity of lethal dose levels would be stored on the premises of a hospital.

5. d Christian and Waterstram-Rich, 2007, pp. 60, 198–99, 211

G–M detectors are used to survey large areas for contamination that may not always be removable. Pocket dosimeters are used to measure personnel exposure. Dose calibrators are used to measure activity in patient doses. Scintillation probes can be used to detect removable and nonremovable contamination at a higher efficiency than G–M detectors because of its use of a sodium iodide–thallium crystal. Most often, wipe tests with a well counter are used to check for removable contamination.

6. b Christian and Waterstram-Rich, 2007, p. 205

The half-value layer (HVL) is the amount of material needed to reduce radiation intensity by half. Following this logic, 4 HVLs reduce the amount of incident radiation to a transmission factor of 0.0625 or 6.25%.

7. a Christian and Waterstram-Rich, 2007, pp. 203–204

When packages are received, they are inventoried by recording the name of the radioisotope, the amount of activity, and the results of wipe checks as mandated by NRC regulations. Patient name is not relevant at this point because you are just taking inventory.

8. b Christian and Waterstram-Rich, 2007, p. 204

The DOT I transport index or exposure rate at 1 m from the package is mandated to be zero. The DOT II transport index is mandated to be more than 0 but less than 1 mR/hr at 1 m. DOT III is mandated to be more than 1 mR/hr but less than 10 mR/hr at 1 m. This package would fall under the DOT II.

- DOT I (white)
  - At contact not more than 0.5 mR/hr
  - At 3 feet (1 m), no detectable radiation (NDR)
- DOT II (yellow)
  - At contact not more than 50 mR/hr
  - At 3 feet (1 m) not more than 1 mR/hr

- DOT III (yellow)
  - At contact not more than 200 mR/hr
  - At 3 feet (1 m) not more than 10 mR/hr

9. b Christian and Waterstram-Rich, 2007, pp. 203–204

The transport index indicates to all handlers the degree of care that should be taken when handling the package. This index is quantified by an exposure reading taken 1 m from the package or source.

10. c Christian and Waterstram-Rich, 2007, pp. 205–206

When decontaminating a liquid spill, which can include potentially radioactive biologic waste (urine, emesis, etc.) expelled from a patient, the spill can be cleaned up with absorbent material. When contamination cannot be completely removed with thorough cleaning, lead plates or aprons can be used to cover the area of the spill.

11. a Christian and Waterstram-Rich, 2007, p. 204

According to the Department of Transportation, the radioactive label designated as totally white is DOT I. DOT I denotes packages with less than 0.5 mR/hr exposure rate at the surface and with no detectable radiation (NDR) at 1 m.

12. b Christian and Waterstram-Rich, 2007, pp. 15, 587

Strontium-89 is a pure beta emitter. Lead shielding cannot be used to block beta particles because of the production of bremsstrahlung radiation caused by the interaction of beta particles with dense materials such as lead. Cardboard is not dense enough to stop the torturous path of beta particles. Plexiglass is ideal because of its density since bremsstrahlung reactions would be kept to a minimum.

13. a Christian and Waterstram-Rich, 2007, p. 51

Exposure is specifically defined as the amount of charge in the air from interactions with X or gamma radiation, 0 to 3MeV. The unit of exposure is the roentgen: $1\ R = 2.58 \times 10^{-4}$ c/kg. However, activity indicates the amount of radioactive substance in a sample or source. The units are the curie or becquerel.

14. c Christian and Waterstram-Rich, 2007, p. 194

$$25\ \text{mrem/hr}\ (1\ \text{hr}/60\ \text{min}) \times 25\ \text{min} = 10.4\ \text{mrem}.$$

15. d Christian and Waterstram-Rich, 2007, p. 671

$$1\ \text{Sv} = 1\ \text{Gray} = 100\ \text{rad}$$

$$1\ \text{Sv} = 100\ \text{rem}$$

$$120\ \text{Sv} = (100)120\ \text{rad}$$

$$120\ \text{Sv} = 12{,}000\ \text{rad} = 12{,}000{,}000\ \text{mrad}.$$

16. c Christian and Waterstram-Rich, 2007, p. 45

When an alpha particle decays, it loses the two electrons it originally had. Helium nuclei consist of the same number of protons and neutrons.

17. c Prekeges, 2011, p. 96

The thickness of the crystal, collimator design, and instrument deadtime all affect sensitivity and can cause it to be higher or lower from day to day. However, a properly set pulse height analyzer with a proper window around the main peak will not affect the sensitivity and make it higher or lower from day to day.

18. a Christian and Waterstram-Rich, 2007, p. 87

Geometric calibration is performed at installation, whenever a change is made in the type of vial or syringe used in radiopharmaceutical processing, and after the chamber is repaired.

19. b Prekeges, 2011, p. 61

The amplifications of electrons in photomultiplier tubes (PMTs) and, therefore, PMT output are affected by many factors: temperature, PMT age, and earth's magnetic field or unshielded MRIs. Automatic gain stabilization, if not correct, can cause tube drift to occur.

20. a Christian and Waterstram-Rich, 2007, p. 68

In a paralyzable system, as the activity increases, the count rate increases to a maximum valve and then actually starts decreasing at higher activity levels.

21. c Prekeges, 2011, p. 58

The three main sources of nonuniformity are "mistuned" PMTs, regional variations in Z-pulse amplitude (spatial distortion), and edge packing. Linearity is a separate issue and not a part of uniformity assessment itself.

22. a Christian and Waterstram-Rich, 2007, p. 104

NaI (Tl) scintillation camera systems will have an 8% to 12% energy resolution. Thallium acts as an actuator that allows the creation of additional "energy states" within the crystal. Crystals are very sensitive to thermal and mechanical shocks.

23. c Christian and Waterstram-Rich, 2007, pp. 86–87

The limit for percentage difference is $\pm 10\%$ according to the NRC regulations. However, it may be $\pm 5\%$ per manufacturer recommendations, which the NRC says must also be adhered to.

24. a Christian and Waterstram-Rich, 2007, p. 89

Extrinsic testing allows evaluation of the total system as it is used clinically, including the collimator. When a collimator is used during assessment, a source having a uniform radionuclide distribution is placed on the collimator.

25. d Christian *et al.*, 2004, p. 97
Correction involves evaluating the straightness of both horizontal and vertical lines while using a phantom.

26. d Christian *et al.*, 2004, p. 86
Constancy of a dose calibrator is performed every day that it is used. This is usually done using a long-lived radioisotope and comparing daily values to previously measured values.

27. b Chachati *et al.*, 1987, pp. 829–836
Schlegel *et al.*, Brodkey *et al.*, and Gates described noninvasive isotopic methods for the estimation of GFR and ERPF without blood or urine sampling. These methods allow determination of these parameters separately for each kidney and derive values for global renal function.

28. a Lee, 1991, p. 176
The amplitude image is superior to the simple stroke volume image because it shows the actual volume of blood ejected from each region of the heart.

29. a Christian *et al.*, 2004, p. 526
Background subtraction is used to enhance image quality and increase statistical reliability for quantitative studies such as gastroesophageal reflux studies. The lower left lung serves as an appropriate background region of interest close to but not within the field of view of imaging the esophagus and stomach.

30. c Christian *et al.*, 2004, p. 532
The geometric mean calculation and use in quantitative studies allow for a sense of organ depth and where in an organ any possible attenuation is occurring. This could be due to contrast media that could be within a part of the colon but not the entire colon.

31. c Lee, 1991, p. 152
With the patient heart rate at 85 bpm, each beat is 0.7058 sec (60 sec/85 beats = 0.7058 sec). Divide this by 25 frames to get 0.029 sec and then convert to msec by multiplying by 1000 to get 29 msec.

32. c Christian *et al.*, 2004, p. 309
Extrinsic flood field uniformity correction is performed to prevent ring artifacts.

33. a Christian *et al.*, 2004, p. 297
For automatic reorientation of the heart, identify the left ventricle in the transaxial images using a threshold-based approach.

34. d Christian *et al.*, 2004, pp. 302–303
The center of rotation (COR) offset correction makes certain that the COR of the camera matrix corresponds to the COR of the camera heads.

35. b Christian *et al.*, 2004, p. 298
In a circumferential profile curve, segments of the myocardium are listed on the *x*-axis and the maximum counts related to these segments are plotted on the *y*-axis.

36. c Christian *et al.*, 2004, p. 291
Imaging in the prone position minimizes attenuation artifacts in myocardial imaging where the inferior wall of the heart may be shadowed by breast tissue or the diaphragm.

37. a Bolus, 2001, pp. 143–147
Sensitivity is the percentage or fraction of ill patients who have a positive test. Thus, sensitivity is how good a test is at detecting a true positive. Specificity is how good a test is at detecting a true negative.

38. c Shackett, 2009, p. 162
Ventilation study usually presents as normal (uniform and symmetrical uptake and washout in all three phases) in cases of pulmonary embolism (PE). Mismatching areas of activity (usually two or more segmental defects) in the perfusion study are indicators for PE.

39. b Christian *et al.*, 2004, pp. 470–471
Pricing and availability have forced ^{133}Xe into prominence. The more straightforward wash-in, washout method is preferred and can be used even on comatose patients.

40. c Christian *et al.*, 2004, p. 471
Aerosols are deposited in the bronchial tree in relation to particle size, air flow rates, and turbulence. The delivery tubing effectively filters out larger particles 10–15 μm in diameter. Smaller particles are deposited in the larger airways during both inspiration and expiration. Particles less than 2 μm can reach the alveoli and be deposited there, whereas even smaller particles, less than 0.1 μm, probably escape in the expired air.

41. a Christian *et al.*, 2004, p. 65
To count radioactivity in a person, a probe system is often used. The probe consists of a sodium iodide crystal with PMT, electronics, and collimator.

42. d Christian *et al.*, 2004, p. 470
Commercial ventilation units employ xenon traps that utilize activated charcoal to prevent the release of radioactive xenon during the washout phase of a study.

43. a Christian *et al.*, 2004, p. 471
In the wash-in phase, 10–20 mCi of ^{133}Xe diluted in 2 L of oxygen are rebreathed from a simple re-breathing apparatus for approximately 3 min while a static image is taken.

44. c Christian *et al.*, 2004, p. 174
Particles formed have diameters of 10–90 μm, with the majority between 10 and 40 μm.

45. b Christian *et al.*, 2004, p. 577
Unless contraindicated, patients should be hydrated to aid clearance of the radiopharmaceutical from the body. This aids in increasing the target-to-nontarget ratio.

46. b Christian *et al.*, 2004, p. 470
A negative-pressure room is required for xenon ventilation studies to maintain ALARA for staff members and patients in the event of a leak during the study.

47. d Adler and Carlton, 2007, p. 162
The clinical indication is usually associated with the chief complaint and is a question the referring physician needs answered. This involves ruling in or ruling out something that he/she is unable to ascertain just by a patient history.

48. b Christian *et al.*, 2004, p. 470
Carbon dioxide is absorbed in the closed system by soda lime crystals, whereas moisture is removed by calcium sulfate or cobalt chloride crystals.

49. b Christian *et al.*, 2004, p. 541
Views in the anterior are normal while the anterior oblique or right lateral projection may be useful for separating the gallbladder and common bile duct from the duodenum and underlying structures such as the kidneys.

50. c Mettler and Guiberteau, 2006, p. 216
Meckel's diverticulum is based on the visualization of the ectopic mucosa with intravenously administered [^{99m}Tc]pertechnetate.

51. c Shackett, 2009, p. 56
The multigated blood pool acquisition (MUGA) study requires radiolabeled red blood cells that are compartmentalized in the heart to assess ejection fraction and stroke volume.

52. b Christian *et al.*, 2004, p. 526
Delayed images of the thorax can be obtained up to 24 hr to detect reflux leading to pulmonary aspiration.

53. c Christian *et al.*, 2004, p. 546
Helicobacter pylori produces a significant amount of the enzyme urease, which is not present in normal human tissue. When ^{14}C-labeled urea is administered orally to the patient and urease activity is present in the stomach, ^{14}C urea is split into ammonia and $^{14}CO_2$, which is absorbed into the blood and exhaled through the lungs. The ^{14}C activity is trapped in an alkaline solution and measured.

54. d Christian *et al.*, 2004, pp. 526–531
Although conventional gastric emptying is a simple procedure that measures the transit of a standardized radiolabeled test meal through the stomach, the images themselves are not utilized alone. Quantitative information is determined by drawing regions of interest and letting the computer algorithm(s) determine transit times, curves, and graphs,

55. c Shackett, 2009, p. 56
The last part of the procedure is to obtain 2–4-hr delayed images if no lung or liver visualization occurs within 60 min. Under abnormal results, no lung activity after 4-hr delays using [^{99m}Tc]MAA indicates an obstruction. An obstruction is also indicated if no activity in the liver is seen after 4-hr delays using [^{99m}Tc]sodium chloride.

56. a Christian *et al.*, 2004, p. 598
Ascorbic acid is added after incubation to reduce the free chromate to chromic ions, which immediately stops the tagging procedure by keeping the chromic ions from penetrating the red blood cell membrane.

57. a Christian *et al.*, 2004, p. 598
Morphine sulfate contracts the sphincter of Oddi and generates an increase in pressure in the common bile duct and cystic duct.

58. c Christian *et al.*, 2004, p. 598
Gastric emptying is a complex process affected by the physical and chemical composition of the ingested meal. The rate of gastric emptying is determined by many factors including the volume, physical state, caloric content, caloric density, concentration of nutrients, meal distribution, salinity, acidity, and viscosity of the test meal used.

59. d Pagana and Pagana, 2010, pp. 443, 178, 162; Christian *et al.*, 2004, p. 560
BUN is the blood-urea-nitrogen level. Greater than 100 mg/dl indicates serious impairment of renal function. Creatinine is entirely excreted by the kidneys, as is BUN. A level greater than 4 mg/dL indicates serious impairment of renal function. The peak transit time is an indicator of radiopharmaceutical clearance when performing renal scans. CBC is the complete blood count, which is a standard blood test to determine the number of red blood cells, white blood cells, platelets, hemoglobin, and hematocrit.

60. b Shackett, 2009, p. 255
Since the effective renal plasma flow (ERPF) calculation consists of counts of the dose injected divided by counts within a plasma sample taken at approximately 45 min postinjection, a higher amount of counts in the plasma sample would result in an erroneously lower ERPF value.

61. c Kowalsky and Falen, 2004, pp. 299–300
[^{99m}Tc]succimer (DMSA) or succimer injection is indicated for kidney imaging for evaluation of renal parenchymal disorders. [^{99m}Tc]gluceptate is no longer commercially available but is best for renal cortex imaging.

62. b Christian *et al.*, 2004, p. 559
The time–activity curve of a renogram from a normal MAG-3 study shows prompt uptake of tracer 3–5 min postinjection.

63. c Christian *et al.*, 2004, pp. 559–560
In approximately 44–45 min, there will have been a maximum amount of tracer uptake and washing out in the kidneys. The residual plasma level can then be assessed for an ERPF by drawing a blood sample.

64. b Shackett, 2009, p. 255
Right and left kidney counts are compared to the pre- and postinjection syringe counts.

65. a Crawford and Husain, 2011, p. 2
The myocardium receives oxygenated blood from its two major coronary arteries, the left main and right main coronary arteries. They branch and encircle the heart to provide blood to all portions of the myocardium. The left main coronary artery branches into the left anterior descending (LAD) and left circumflex arteries. However, the LAD branch supplies blood to the anterior wall and over 90% of the ventricular septum.

66. d Shackett, 2009, pp. 57–59
Because of the position of the heart and the fact that it turns slightly to the left, positioning the camera anteriorly—typically anterior and left anterior oblique (LAO) (35–60 degrees)—will allow for the best septal wall separation for ejection fraction calculation and processing.

67. c Christian *et al.*, 2004, p. 246
A normal heart rate is 60–90 bpm in an adult. An increased heart rate is greater than 100 bpm, while a decreased heart rate is less than 60 bpm. Tachycardia is a general symptomatic term that does not describe the cause of the rapid rate.

68. c Christian *et al.*, 2004, pp. 493–495
This is a contraindication if the patient has a history of reactive airway disease. The patient must have bronchodilator therapy and resuscitative measures available. A more reasonable pharmaceutical would be Dobutamine or Lexiscan®.

69. d Christian *et al.*, 2004, pp. 541–543
To assess the gallbladder ejection fraction (GBEF) and/or the sphincter of Oddi response to cholecystokinin (CCK), the c-terminal octapetide portion of CCK, sincalide (Kinevac) is given intravenously at a concentration of 0.02 μg/kg in normal saline over a period of 3–30 min.

70. c Mettler and Guiberteau, 2006, p. 135
Areas of stunned myocardium usually present with normal or near-normal perfusion but with absent or diminished contractility. Since the underlying myocardial cells are still viable, once blood flow has been restored, stunning generally spontaneously subsides over several weeks.

71. c Christian *et al.*, 2004, p. 483
Ejection fraction (EF) is the fraction of blood ejected by the left ventricle (LV) during the contraction or ejection phase of the cardiac cycle or systole. Prior to the start of systole, the LV is filled with blood to the capacity known as end-diastolic volume (EDV) during the filling phase or diastole. During systole, the LV contracts and ejects blood until it reaches its minimum capacity known as end-systolic volume (ESV); it does not empty completely. Clearly, the EF is dependent on the ventricular EDV, which may vary with ventricular disease associated with ventricular dilatation.

$$\text{Ejection fraction (EF)} = (\text{EDV} - \text{ESV})/(\text{EDV}) \times 100\%$$

$$\text{EF} = (2750\text{ cpm} - 1775\text{ cpm})/(2750\text{ cpm}) \times 100\%$$

$$\text{EF} = (980\text{ cpm}/2750\text{ cpm}) \times 100\%$$

$$\text{EF} = \sim 35\%.$$

72. b Crawford and Husain, 2011, pp. 110–114
A standard or small FOV camera equipped with a high-resolution parallel-hole collimator is used to perform gated studies. Using the R wave of the ECG to trigger data collection, hundreds of cardiac cycles are collected and stored in a computer. Depending on the computer software, the interval between R waves is divided into frames, most often 16. Typically each frame is acquired in a 64 × 64 matrix; 200–400 thousand counts per frame are obtained for a total of about 3–6 million counts for the entire 16-frame study.

73. c Crawford and Husain, 2011, p. 7
Ideal characteristics of a myocardial perfusion agent include high first-pass myocardial extraction proportional to blood flow, high target-to-nontarget ratio, adequate imaging window, and ability to complete both rest and stress imaging on the same day in as short a time as possible.

74. d Crawford and Husain, 2011, p. 73
The first-pass method for performing cardiac function imaging has a short acquisition time, usually about 30 sec. The first-pass method has a low background activity. Any non-particulate radiopharmaceutical in a volume of 0.3–0.5 mL can be used.

75. d Crawford and Husain, 2011, p. 29
When a 1-day protocol for myocardial perfusion imaging is performed with a ^{99m}Tc-labeled tracer, the smaller dose is administered for the first imaging study, and a higher dose is administered for the second study.

76. b Crawford and Husain, 2011, p. 70
To be valid for systolic and diastolic analysis, MUGA requires a constant regular heart rate and R–R interval. The more arrhythmic the heart rate, the less accurate the representation of diastolic function.

77. d Crawford and Husain, 2011, p. 7
Thallium-201 redistributes, which means rest and stress images can be obtained with one injection. It has a low-energy photopeak and low-photon flux. It is a potassium analog. It has a relatively long half-life of 73.1 hr.

78. b Crawford and Husain, 2011, p. 73
First-pass radionuclide angiography is used to detect and evaluate intracardiac shunts (when blood flow follows any pattern other than going from systemic circulation to the right atrium, right ventricle, the lungs, the left atrium, the left ventricle, and then back to the systemic circulation).

79. d Crawford and Husain, 2011, pp. 67–68
Functional cardiac studies may be performed to evaluate wall motion abnormalities caused by aneurysm (dyskinesia), myocardial infarction, and myocardial ischemia.

80. d Crawford and Husain, 2011, p. 75
The in vivo method of ^{99m}Tc red cell tagging is the easiest for the technologist, with no handling or manipulation of blood products or risk of inadvertent cross-transfusion.

81. b Crawford and Husain, 2011, p. 12
In preparation for a stress test, patients are instructed to fast to reduce tracer uptake in the GI tract.

82. d Shackett, 2009, p. 373
The total amount of activity equals 5 mL × 30 mCi/mL = 150 mCi at 0700. A 4-hr decay factor would be $(0.254)^4 = 0.00416$. A decay factor (DF) of 0.00416 × 150 mCi = 0.624 mCi at 1100 am.

$$? \mu Ci = 0.624 \text{ mCi} \times 1000 \mu Ci/1 \text{ mCi} = 624 \mu Ci.$$

83. a Saha, 2004, p. 23
Transient equilibrium holds true when $(T_{1/2})p$ and $(T_{1/2})d$ differ by a factor of about 10 to 50. The daughter activity grows owing to the decay of the parent radionuclide, reaches a maximum followed by equilibrium, and then decays with a half-life of the parent.

84. d Shackett, 2009, p. 373
Concentration [ ] equals total activity over total volume:

[ ] = total activity/total volume

60 mCi/mL = 1200 mCi/ X

X = 1200 mCi/60 mCi/mL

X = 20 mL.

85. c Christian and Waterstram-Rich, 2007, pp. 467–468; DRAX Image MAA package insert
MAA particles average about 30–40 μm in diameter and, because of this size, become impacted (trapped) in the terminal arterioles and capillaries after they pass through the pulmonary artery. If the recommended dose of particulate material is about 350,000 particles, less than 1 in 1000 pulmonary arterioles are actually blocked. The recommended number of particles per single injection is 200,000 to 700,000, with the suggested number being approximately 350,000.

86. b Shackett, 2009, p. 373

$$\text{volume} = \frac{300 \text{ mCi}}{28.7 \text{ mCi/mL}}$$

volume = 6.3 mL.

87. a Saha, 2004
Bioavailability describes the fraction of an administered dose of unchanged drug that reaches the systemic circulation.

88. d Saha, 2004, pp.67–71
Yield may be reduced by a column defect. Time since last elution is a contributing factor since it will determine how much buildup of ^{99m}Tc is available on the column. Amount of aluminum on the column does not affect generator yield.

89. c Zolle, 2006, pp. 96–97
Introducing nitrogen gas through a sterile filter allows kit contents to be stable for longer periods of time and oxidative processes to no longer affect the labeling yield.

90. c Saha, 2004, p. 106
An ascorbic acid or stannous ion compound, a lyophilized compound, and a reducing agent are all components of the ^{99m}Tc radiopharmaceutical kit. There is no additive that can prevent pyrogens. The presence of pyrogens is tested for as a quality control measure by the manufacturer of the kit.

91. b Kowalsky and Falen, 2004, p. 281
Weak chelates that undergo in vivo hydrolysis are expected to deposit tin in the reticuloendothelial system (RES). The RES is located in the liver, spleen, and bone marrow.

92. d Saha, 2004, p. 98
$^{99m}Tc^{7+}$ is reduced to $^{99m}Tc^{4+}$ in a reaction that occurs during the reduction of technetium by stannous chloride in acidic medium.

93. d Saha, 2004, p. 153
The presence of radiochemical impurities in a radiopharmaceutical can result in poor-quality images due to high background from the surrounding tissues in the blood, which is a result of undesirable radionuclides in the dose. This will affect the target-to-nontarget ratio.

94. c Saha, 2004, p. 106
ITLC stands for instant thin layer chromatography.

95. d Kowalsky and Falen, 2004, p. 412
Grease from fingerprints can alter migration patterns during the development phase of radiochromatography; therefore, using tweezers to pick up the chromatography paper would not cause a radiochromatography artifact.

96. c Shackett, 2009, p. 373

$$\text{activity at } 1000 = 25 \text{ mCi } (0.05)^{0.5}$$

$$\text{activity} = 25 \text{ mCi } (0.05)^{0.5}$$

$$\text{volume needed} = \frac{5 \text{ mL}}{17.68 \text{ mCi/mL}}$$

volume needed = 0.28 mL

$$\frac{3{,}000{,}000 \text{ particles}}{5 \text{ mL}} = 600{,}000 \text{ particles/mL.}$$

$$\text{number of particles} = 0.28 \text{ mL} \times \frac{600{,}000 \text{ particles}}{1 \text{ mL}}$$

number of particles = 169,635.

97. b Shackett, 2009, p. 373

The time difference between Atlanta, which is on Eastern time, and Central time is 1 hr. Factoring this difference into the elapsed time between 0700 CST on 8/12/09 to 0800 CST on 8/15/09 results in 73 hr. The decay factor for ^{123}I for 73 hr is 0.0216279. The precalibration factor is the reciprocal of the decay factor, or 1 divided by 0.0216279, which equals 46.23.

$$46.23 \times 20\ \mu\text{Ci needed} = 924.73\ \mu\text{Ci or} \sim 925\ \mu\text{Ci}.$$

98. a Shackett, 2009, p. 373; UAB NMT Program Course Notes

$$\text{Original dilution} \times (\text{dilution factor})^{\text{no. of tubes} - 1} = \text{dilution factor}$$

$$25\ \text{mCi/52 mL} = 0.48\ \text{mCi/mL}\ (1/6\ \text{dilution})^{33-1}$$

$$= 6.03 \times 10^{-26}\ \text{mCi/mL in tube 33}$$

$$5\ \text{mL} \times 6.03 \times 10^{-26}\ \text{mCi/mL} =$$

$$3.02 \times 10^{-25}\ \text{mCi in tube 33 of serial dilution.}$$

99. c Kowalsky and Falen, 2004, p. 181

The mode of administration will determine the other factors concerning the pharmacokinectic profile of a drug, which include the process by which a drug is absorbed, distributed, metabolized, and eliminated by the body.

100. b Adler and Carlton, 2007, p. 331

Diphenhydramine, which is an antihistamine, can be given to reduce the symptoms if an allergic reaction occurs due to the administration of contrast media.

Answers to Examination 7

1. c Christian and Waterstram-Rich, 2007, pp. 85–86

Survey meters are calibrated annually to make sure that the instrument is performing within the NRC regulation guidelines.

2. d Noz and Maguire, 2007, pp. 114–116

The direct radiation survey will give an instant reading, whereas the wipe check does not give an instant reading.

3. c Siegel, 2004, pp. 29–32

An occupational radiation worker is allowed up to 15,000 mrem/yr dose to the eye. Since this worker is close to but not exceeding the yearly dose, a review of the ALARA concept and a dedicated reduction in eye exposure in the future are recommended.

4. d Noz and Maguire, 2007, pp. 78–79

It is recommended that a radiation occupational worker that is using radiation stay under 410 mrem per month. This limit will keep the worker's radiation levels within the NRC regulations of 5,000 mrem per year whole-body dose.

5. c Forshier, 2002, pp. 113–115, 144–145

It is recommended that women who are pregnant stay within or lower than 10% (500 mrem) of the regular occupational limit of 5000 mrem/yr for the duration of the gestational period.

6. d Siegel, 2004, p. 46

To stay in compliance with NRC regulations, the room radiation levels must be below this level of removable contamination: $<3.33\ \text{Bq}/100\ \text{cm}^2$.

7. a U.S. Nuclear Regulatory Commission, 2003 (10CFR35.61)

A survey is okay to use as long as it does not exceed ±20% of expected readings according to the NRC.

8. d Noz and Maguire, 2007, pp. 158–159

Performing a wipe check with an SCA/MCA would be the best method because it is able to detect the low energies emitted from the beta emitter.

9. d Christian and Waterstram-Rich, 2007, pp. 205–206

For unrestricted areas, it is recommended that the radiation level stay below 2 mrem/hr. Therefore, if the waiting room reads 25 mrem/hr, then 4 HVLs of Pb is needed to decrease the radiation to the acceptable level of 2 mrem/hr.

10. c Prekeges, 2011, p. 9

The reading determined by using the G–M meter was 4.5 mR/hr. However, it was measured on the X0.1 setting. Therefore, the initial reading of 4.5 mR/hr has to be multiplied by X0.1 to correctly get the reading from the meter.

11. b Prekeges, 2011, pp. 11–12

It is always important to verify that the battery in the survey meter is working correctly to ensure proper detector response.

12. a Christian and Waterstram-Rich, 2007, pp. 216–217

According to the NRC, the employer is required to post any notices or violations of the regulations to the employees.

13. b U.S. Nuclear Regulatory Commission, 2003 (10 CFR 20.1901)

Radiation warning signs consist of a purple, magenta, or black tri-blade symbol on a yellow background.

14. c. Christian and Waterstram-Rich, 2007, pp. 4–5, 207

Different radiation caution signs are used depending on the amount of radiation an individual is likely to receive in that area in the course of 1 hr while 30 cm from a radioactive source or surface. Using the inverse square law and the information given, it can be determined that an individual in this circumstance would receive 160 mrem/hr at a distance of 30 cm. For an area where an individual is exposed to radiation levels in excess of 100 mrem/hr, the correct sign to post is the "Caution: High Radiation Area" sign.

15. c Christian and Waterstram-Rich, 2007, p. 205

If a package reads 9 mrem/hr at 1 meter, then it should have a DOT Yellow III shipping label. A DOT Yellow II shipping label is limited to a reading of 1 mrem/hr at 1 m. When a package arrives with the wrong label, the vendor should be contacted.

- DOT I (white)
  - At contact not more than 0.5 mR/hr
  - At 3 feet (1 m), no detectible radiation (NDR)
- DOT II (yellow)
  - At contact not more than 50 mR/hr
  - At 3 feet (1 m) not more than 1 mR/hr
- DOT III (yellow)
  - At contact not more than 200 mR/hr
  - At 3 feet (1 m) not more than 10 mR/hr

16. d Prekeges, 2011, p. 3

The average amount of energy required to cause an ionization depends on the type of gas used in the chamber, but it is generally between 20 and 45 eV per ion pair. 34 eV per ion pair is a commonly accepted value.

17. b Prekeges, 2011, p. 5

Region V of gaseous detectors is the Geiger–Mueller region. Within this region, a charged particle, X ray, or gamma ray will initiate an avalanche of ionization reactions (Townsend avalanche). When one initial ionization event triggers a Townsend avalanche of secondary ions that extends throughout the entire volume of the detector, this is called the Geiger effect.

18. a Prekeges, 2011, p. 5

The sizes of the pulses are determined by the amount of ions created within the gas chamber. More ions are created when there is a greater charge between the cathode and anode. On the characteristic voltage curve for gas detectors, the proportional region operates at a higher current than the ionization region. Because the proportional region operates at a higher current, it produces more ions and has a larger pulse.

19. c Hendee and Ritenour, 2002, p. 132

Within the proportional region of the characteristic voltage curve for gaseous detectors, charged particles collide with gas molecules to produce additional ionization events. This additional ionization results in an amplified current that is proportional to the number of original ion pairs created by the incident radiation. Because ions collide with gas to create an amplified current, this occurrence is called gas amplification.

20. a Prekeges, 2011, p. 5

The pulse height represents the amount of radiation detected in the gas chamber. The amount of radioactivity is based upon the number of ions produced by the interactions between the gas and radiation.

21. d Prekeges, 2011, p. 181

A Jaszczak phantom consists of a 20-cm-diameter Plexiglass cylinder with rod and spheres inserted. The Jaszczak phantom provides excellent information of SPECT performance.

22. c Prekeges, 2011, pp. 135–138

Neither smoothing nor edge enhancement filters will improve image contrast after display. A formatter is no longer widely used in most facilities because it is for a gamma camera using film.

23. a Christian and Waterstram-Rich, 2007, p. 299

Polar plots are circular profiles of the heart created by placing the most apical short-axis slice in the center, surrounded by each successive short-axis slice. The most basal slice becomes the outermost ring of the plot.

24. c Prekeges, 2011, pp. 53, 67; Christian and Waterstram-Rich, 2007, p. 127

Any area that uptakes the radiotracer will display as "hotter" than the background. This means that there is more uptake in these locations. Radiotracer will uptake in active cells and overactive cells. Cold spots are indicative of areas in which the cells are not active, such as dead or necrotic tissue.

25. c Prekeges, 2011, p. 61

Sometimes camera nonuniformity can be attributed to regional variations of insensitivity. Count subtraction/addition would be most appropriate at this point. Most gamma cameras achieve this by using an isotope or collimator specific uniformity correction map to generate an image of final nonuniformity within a ±1–3% range.

26. b Prekeges, 2011, p. 193

A good event in PET is determined by the coincident detection of two 511-keV photons for a total of 1.02 MeV. These two 511-keV annihilation photons originate from the combination of a positron and an electron during the annihilation reaction.

27. c Prekeges, 2011, p. 191

In PET imaging, during coincidence detection, each crystal acts as a separate detector. Each scintillation crystal is allowed to be in coincidence with other scintillation crystals. Each pair of crystals for which coincidence is allowed is designated an individual line of response.

28. c Prekeges, 2011, p. 196

Random coincidence occurs when two photons from two separate annihilations are detected within the coincidence timing window. The system naturally assumes that both photons come from one annihilation event and that the interaction occurred within the line of response for both detectors.

29. b Prekeges, 2011, p. 234

A "blank scan" is a short-timed acquisition that is done at the beginning of each day to verify that the PET's tomography feature is operating correctly for the day.

30. b Prekeges, 2011, p. 235

In PET tomography, since each block has a small number of photomultiplier tubes and uses only one set of electronic devices, a malfunction will oftentimes affect the entire sinogram. Therefore, since blocks typically appear as diagonal lines on the sinogram, a malfunction also appears along a diagonal line.

31. b Lee, 2005, pp. 201–202

The purpose of the window in reconstruction techniques is to limit the reconstruction to data within a range much like a pulse height analyzer on a gamma camera. Thus it is used primarily for background subtraction.

32. c Shackett, 2009, p. 130

This is the only equation given that accurately represents the true total net value of counts from the gallbladder by using the percent difference equation. This equation can also be represented as:

$$\frac{\text{pre-CCK cts} - \text{post-CCK cts}}{\text{pre-CCK cts}} \times 100.$$

33. a Lee, 2005, pp. 223–226

If a test image of two point sources were acquired in a 128 × 128 image matrix, the approximate pixel size would be 3.133 mm in one plane. Both the x and y planes are needed.

34. c Prekeges, 2011, p. 131

Unfiltered backprojection (UBP) is a method of reconstruction used in SPECT imaging. One disadvantage of unfiltered backprojection is that the area of increased count density is greater than the area of increased activity in the object. As more projections are added to the object, the image begins to form a star artifact, and the object's size increases. The more projections are added, the larger and blurrier the star artifact gets. This is why filtered backprojection is commonly used. With regular or filtered backprojection, as it is used clinically, the more projections you have the better the resolution.

35. d Christian *et al.*, 2004, p. 300

The purpose of the first-pass study is to evaluate the ejection fraction of the right and/or left ventricle and to determine the overall functioning capabilities of the heart. When calculating left ventricular ejection fraction, a multiple-gated acquisition is normally used. Gating allows heart motion and contraction to be better resolved by dividing the projections into discrete time intervals throughout an entire cardiac cycle. This gives us more precise and specific information related to a specific portion of the heart. This method includes gated equilibrium radionuclide angiography and gated tomographic myocardial perfusion imaging. A first-pass study occurs too quickly to get any reliable gating, but one does get ventricular function information. Therefore, ungated myocardial SPECT would not provide the information on ventricular function that all the other options here do.

36. c Shackett, 2009, p. 342

The thigh area is used to obtain nonthyroidal body background because it provides a more accurate approximation of the soft tissue uptake throughout the entire body. The camera is positioned over the patient's thigh at the same distance as it is positioned from the thyroid organ.

37. c Shackett, 2009, pp. 343–344

When preparing a patient for thyroid uptake using a thyroid probe, take counts from the thigh and neck (at thyroid level). The thigh counts represent background or baseline counts. Subtract the baseline counts from the actual thyroid counts as part of the calculation for uptake percentage.

38. b Shackett, 2009, p. 332

X-ray alpha particles are not emitted from ^{131}I. ^{131}I is both a gamma and beta emitter; however, the beta particles are what is responsible for the effectiveness of the therapy.

39. b Shackett, 2009, p. 345; Christian *et al.*, 2004, p. 332

Some of the symptoms of hyperthyroidism include fever, sweating, dehydration, palpitations, increased heart rate, and elevated white blood cell counts.

40. a Shackett, 2009, p. 345; Christian *et al.*, 2004, pp. 419–420

An increase in thyroid hormone causes a decrease in the stimulation of TSH. Suppressed TSH is indicative of hyperthyroidism.

41. b Shackett, 2009, p. 31

Iliac crests, sacroiliac joints, and the nasopharyngeal areas are typical "hot spots" in adult bone imaging. Typically there is symmetrical, increased uptake in all joints, junctions, and scapulas. Epiphyseal plates, also known as "growth plates," are bright hot spots in pediatric images. Children are steadily growing, thus causing increased uptake in those areas.

42. a Christian *et al.*, 2004, pp. 578–579

Spot views are individual images of certain areas after the initial whole-body image has been performed. They provide detailed images of areas not clearly visualized on the whole-body images. The right femoral head is a specific area that needs to be imaged, which makes limited imaging the appropriate choice.

43. a Shackett, 2009, p. 152

MAA causes micro emboli in approximately 100,000 capillaries of the 350 million arterioles and 280 billion small capillaries of the lungs. The particles are typically 10–90 μm in size; therefore, the number injected does not compromise the patient. In general, 0.1% of the capillaries are blocked after an injection.

44. c Shackett, 2009, p. 32

Radiotracer tag, like ^{99m}Tc, may break down or be delivered to the body with an insufficient tag. This means that the tracer did not properly attach itself to the pharmaceutical used for the study. It results in unbound pertechnetate or "free Tc" that localizes in the stomach, thyroid, salivary glands, gastrointestinal tract, and some other systems.

45. b Christian *et al.*, 2004, pp. 576–585

Bone imaging is sensitive but not specific. It may be used to determine whether there is an abnormality within the bones. It is also capable of localizing the problem area; however, there is no way to determine the exact location and cause of the problem. Typically other studies are ordered, such as CT or MRI, which are more specific.

46. b Christian *et al.*, 2004, pp. 510–511

Necrotic tissue is that which had undergone premature cell death. An infarction is localized necrosis caused by a lack of blood supply. Ischemia is the term used to describe inadequate or decreased blood flow to an area caused by a blockage.

47. d Shackett, 2009, p. 350

For a therapeutic procedure, there should always be a written directive in the patient's record. It is mandatory that a nuclear medicine technologist have the written directive and that he/she verifies it before administering any therapeutic radiopharmaceuticals. The referring physician or nuclear medicine physicians may not always be readily available for questions. Also, the patient may not always be certain about the procedures he/she is scheduled for.

48. d Shackett, 2009, pp. 28–31

Three- and four-phase bone imaging studies include dynamic images for the flow and blood pool. Static images are also included for images of the extremities and torso. To capture blood pooling and flow as they are occurring, the patient should be positioned under the camera prior to tracer administration. The instructions given to the patient are to drink lots of fluids and to urinate frequently after the injection. 24-hour images are taken by request using the four-phase protocol, thus no special instructions are needed prior to the injection.

49. c Shackett, 2009, p. 31

Normal uptake in children and adults includes the ribs, femur, and joints (sterno-clavicle joints included). However, in children the growth plates show increased activity during bone imaging whereas they do not in adults.

50. d *Taber's Cyclopedic Medical Dictionary*, 2009, p. 2197

Tolerance refers to nonreactivity toward a particular antigen.

51. a *Taber's Cyclopedic Medical Dictionary*, 2009, p. 2033

Specificity refers to the ability of an antibody to react with one and only one antigen.

52. c *Taber's Cyclopedic Medical Dictionary*, 2009, p. 505

The property whereby an antibody reacts with two or more antigens of similar structure is called cross-reactivity.

53. a Christian and Waterstram-Rich, 2007, p. 609

IgG is the major antibody found in normal human serum. It is also the smallest and most common antibody. IgM is the primary antibody against A & B antigen on red blood cells. IgA is primarily an aid in mucosal immunity, and IgD makes up 1% of proteins in plasma membranes of mature B-lymphocytes.

54. a Shackett, 2009, p. 398

^{18}F has the longest half-life of these PET radionuclides. Therefore, it is not necessary for ^{18}F to be produced close to the site where it is administered. ^{18}F has a half-life of 110 min; ^{11}C, of 20 min; ^{15}O, 2 min; and ^{13}N, 10 min.

55. c Shackett, 2009, p. 398

Hyperglycemia reduces tumor uptake of the tracer; therefore, the patient's blood glucose level is checked prior to [^{18}F]FDG administration. FDG does not increase glucose levels and is not a contraindication in diabetic patients. High blood glucose levels do not ensure good tracer uptake; they actually reduce uptake in the tumor.

56. a Shackett, 2009, p. 223

For PET oncologic studies, the patient should hydrate right before the test and fast for at least 6 hr prior to test to reduce insulin levels and uptake in certain organs. An IV should be installed in the patient so the injection can be flushed with saline. A 12-lead ECG monitoring is not required.

57. c Shackett, 2009, p. 313

Yttrium ibritumomab tiuxetan therapy is used for non-Hodgkin's lymphoma. This therapy is not used for breast, prostate, or liver cancers.

58. b Shackett, 2009, p. 314

Yttrium-90 ibritumomab tiuxetan is used in conjunction with rituximab chemotherapeutic agent. Y-90 is not used in conjunction with interferon, cyclosporine, or methotrexate.

59. b Shackett, 2009, p. 144

The spleen is located posterior-laterally in the left upper abdomen, and therefore a right lateral will not show the size of the spleen well. A left lateral view will show the liver and spleen, thereby making it hard to view the size of the spleen. The best view to determine the size of the spleen, therefore, is the posterior view.

60. c Shackett, 2009, p. 142
[^{99m}Tc]sulfur colloid once injected will biodistribute 80% in the liver, 15% in the spleen, and 5% in the bone marrow. If 4 mCi is injected, 0.6 mCi will be concentrated in the spleen.

$4\ \text{mCi} \times 0.15 = 0.6\ \text{mCi}$ of activity.

61. c Shackett, 2009, p. 145
Colloid shifting presents in the bone marrow due to severe liver dysfunction, especially due to cirrhosis, hepatitis, leukemia, infection, or a tumor.

62. d Shackett, 2009, p. 145
A barium study of the colon could cause artifacts or show presumed defects with the liver and spleen.

63. c Christian and Waterstram-Rich, 2007, p. 542
In the normal individual, radioactivity is identified in the gastrointestinal tract by 30 min postinjection.

64. b Christian and Waterstram-Rich, 2007, p. 541
Morphine is usually given to the patient after 60 min because morphine contracts the sphincter of Oddi and increases the pressure in the common bile duct and cystic duct. This causes the gallbladder to fill up with the radiopharmaceutical if the gallbladder is functioning.

65. b Mettler and Guiberteau, 2006, p. 220
Elevated serum bilirubin levels indicating severely jaundiced patients can result in increased renal excretion of the radiopharmaceutical, which can be confused with gallbladder activity.

66. d Shackett, 2009, p. 251
The computer setup for the procedure is usually 20–60 sec/frame for 1800 sec, which is a dynamic study but not a gating study.

67. d Christian and Waterstram-Rich, 2007, p. 540
In liver hemangioma imaging, a blood flow image, an immediate blood pooling image, and a delayed image 2–3 hr after injection are required as a normal imaging protocol. The 24-hr delayed image is not required for a liver hemangioma study.

68. a Christian and Waterstram-Rich, 2007, p. 489
If using [^{99m}Tc]sestamibi, you will have to use more than one tracer dose for the acquisitions of stress and rest images. The sestamibi will have been partially decayed by the time it is ready for both images to be taken.

69. b Christian and Waterstram-Rich, 2007, p. 493
Dipyridamole has a half-life of up to 30 min and can last several hours. Adenosine's half-life is only 10 sec, and dobutamine and nitroglycerin have half-lives of only a couple of min.

70. d Christian and Waterstram-Rich, 2007, p. 493
Adenosine and dipyridamole both have side effects of a feeling of breathlessness and heaviness in the chest. Dobutamine just increases the heart rate and blood pressure by increasing the myocardial work of the heart.

71. d Christian and Waterstram-Rich, 2007, p. 493
A patient that has severe aortic stenosis, unstable angina, or an ejection fraction below 15% is a contraindication for using dobutamine as a stress test. Dobutamine raises the heart rate and blood pressure, hence it could be dangerous for such a patient to undergo this stress test.

72. a Shackett, 2009, p. 68
When given [^{99m}Tc]tetrofosmin, the patient has to wait only 5–30 min for clearance of the GI system. When given [^{99m}Tc]sestamibi, the patient has to wait 45–60 min for clearance of GI system. Therefore, tetrofosmin has a faster GI clearance.

73. b Crawford and Husain, 2011, p. 19
Some physicians administer aminophylline and/or caffeine to all patients as a precautionary measure before releasing them, regardless of symptoms after dipyridamole. Some physicians do this selectively.

74. d Shackett, 2009, p. 373
By using dimensional analysis we know that there are 60 seconds in 1 minute

90 beats/1 min = 1.5 beats

90 beats/60 sec = 1.5 beats/sec.

75. b Shackett, 2009, p. 62
[^{99m}Tc]pyrophosphate is a bone agent that flows with the bloodstream. Pyrophosphate deposition accumulates with calcium in the mitochondria and within the cytoplasm of necrotic myocardial tissue. Thus it is preferred for acute myocardial infarction imaging.

76. c Crawford and Husain, 2011, p. 16
Dipyridamole produces coronary vasodilation and reactive hyperemia by increasing endogenous plasma adenosine levels. Dipyridamole inhibits the clearance pathway of adenosine across the cell membrane; therefore, it indirectly affects adenosine receptor sites.

77. a Crawford and Husain, 2011, p. 20
Dobutamine injection is contraindicated in patients with idiopathic hypertrophic subaortic stenosis (severe aortic stenosis) and in patients who have shown previous manifestations of hypersensitivity to dobutamine.

78. b Shackett, 2009, p. 293
^{89}Sr and ^{153}Sm are used in bone palliation therapy due to their high beta emissions.

79. d Shackett, 2009, p. 294

It is best to administer ^{89}Sr or ^{153}Sm via IV catheter rather than syringe due to possible infiltration and local irradiation of the patient since it is a high beta emitter.

80. c Shackett, 2009, p. 198

There is more emphasis on medications and food surrounding glucose intake (meaning a high-protein and low-carbohydrate diet) and physical activity before PET imaging with [^{18}F]FDG.

81. a U.S. Nuclear Regulatory Commission, 2003 (10 CFR Part 35)

Due to confidentiality rules, the patient identity should not be disclosed in the report to the NRC.

82. b Shackett, 2009, p. 373

2.2 lbs = 1 kg   1 mCi = 1,000 μCi

$$\frac{185\ \text{lb}}{1} \times \frac{1\ \text{kg}}{2.2\ \text{lb}} = 84.09\ \text{kg}$$

$$\frac{55\ \mu\text{Ci}}{1\ \text{kg}} \times \frac{84.09\ \text{kg}}{1} = 4{,}625\ \mu\text{Ci}$$

$$\frac{4{,}625\ \mu\text{Ci}}{1} \times \frac{1\ \text{mCi}}{1{,}000\ \mu\text{Ci}} = 4.6\ \text{mCi}.$$

83. a U.S. Nuclear Regulatory Commission, 2003 (10 CFR Part 35)

Since this is a therapy dose, it must be within ±20% of the prescribed dose. 20% of 15 mCi is 3 mCi, and 3 + 15 = 18 mCi. 18 mCi is thus the maximum that can be given; therefore, 19 mCi would be considered a medical event in this case.

84. c Saha, 2004, pp. 19–21

$A = A_0(0.5)^{n(t/T1/2)}$

$A_0 = 50$ mCi

$T_{1/2} = 6$-hr half-life for ^{99m}Tc

$t = 10{:}00 - 6{:}00 = 4$

3.7 GBq = 100 mCi

$A = 50\ \text{mCi}\ (0.5)^{4/6}$

$A = 31.5$ mCi

$$\frac{31.5\ \text{mCi}}{1} \times \frac{3.7\ \text{GBq}}{100\ \text{mCi}} = 1.17\ \text{GBq}.$$

85. d Siegel, 2004, pp. 102–103, 58

A written report to the appropriate NRC regional office must be submitted within 15 days and must include the licensee's name; prescribing physician; description of event; why event occurred; effect, if any, on the individual(s) who received the dose; actions taken, if any, to prevent recurrence; and certification that licensee notified the individual and, if not, why not. A separate section for occupationally overexposed individuals must also be included in the report and must include employee's name, Social Security number, and date of birth.

86. c Forshier, 2002, pp. 147–148; Christian and Waterstram-Rich, 2007, pp. 204–205

Exposure to ionizing radiation can be reduced by three basic principles: (1) decrease the amount of time spent in the area of the radiation source, (2) increase the amount of distance between the radiation source and the person to be protected, (3) use a shielding material that will attenuate radiation coming from the source. Working as quickly as possible and preparing all necessary materials in advance will decrease the amount of time spent near the radiation source, and using syringe shields will attenuate radiation coming from the source. Holding the radiopharmaceutical as close to the eye as possible does not follow the three basic tenets of radiation safety and will increase radiation exposure. The less time a person is around a radiation source, the lower the exposure; the more distance between a person and a radiation source, the lower the exposure; and the more shielding between a person and a radiation source, the lower the exposure.

87. a Adler and Carlton, 2007, p. 316

Using disposable equipment before its expiration date, aseptically cleaning the venipuncture site prior to injection with an alcohol swab, and uncapping the needle immediately prior to injection are all standard aseptic technique practices. Wearing sterile gloves is not part of standard aseptic technique. Disposable gloves are used during venipuncture.

88. a Siegel, 2004, p. 50

Unless otherwise directed by the authorized user (AU), a licensee may not use a dosage if it does not fall within the prescribed range or if it differs from the prescribed dosage by greater than 20%.

89. d Cherry *et al.*, 2003, p. 35

The decay time is $t = 29$ hr. The decay factor (DF) for 1 hr is 0.9488. Thus, the precalibration factor is 1/DF or $1/0.9488^{29} = 4.59$. The activity that must be placed in each [^{123}I]sodium iodide capsule is 4.59 × 220 microcuries = 1009 microcuries.

90. d Adler and Carlton, 2007, pp. 68–69

Part of planning in a nuclear medicine facility includes the activities and forethought needed to maintain the appropriate amount of supplies and doses to accomplish the type and number of procedures done for the day. The time interval between radiopharmaceutical preparation and administration is also part of the forethought needed. The percentage of no-shows a department expects is not part of the daily planning because all the patients may come, and a facility needs to be prepared.

91. a Shackett, 2009, pp. 28, 125, 148, 173

[^{99m}Tc]medronate is used for total-body bone imaging, [^{99m}Tc]Tco^{4-} (pertechnetate) is used to image Meckel's diverticulum localization, and [^{99m}Tc]mebrofenin is used for a hepatobiliary study. [^{99m}Tc]macroaggregated albumin (MAA) is used for lung perfusion scans and is not needed for the studies that will be performed.

92. a *Taber's Cyclopedic Medical Dictionary*, 2001, p. 247

Bioavailability refers to the rate and extent of the strength to which an active drug or substance enters the general circulation.

93. c *Taber's Cyclopedic Medical Dictionary*, 2001, p. 1538

The osmolality of plasma has a narrow range of 275–295 mOsm/kg.

94. d Shackett, 2009, pp. 28, 79, 125, 148, 160

The route of administration for a lung ventilation study is through inhalation. Many nuclear medicine studies require an intravenous (IV) route of administration. Some examples include bone imaging, HIDA scans, and lung perfusion studies. Cisternography utilizes an intrathecal route of administration. Intraarterial is not a route of administration for a radiopharmaceutical.

95. b Cherry *et al.*, 2003, pp. 34–35

The decay factor for 1 hr is 0.985. The time is $t = 5$ hr. The concentration of activity in the vial is $1/0.985^5 \times 25$ mCi/mL $= 26.962$ mL. The volume required for 30 mCi is 30 mCi divided by 26.962 mCi/mL $= 1.11$ mL.

96. b Christian and Waterstram-Rich, 2007, p. 167

In an (n, p) reaction, the product nuclide is an isotope of a different element, which allows for the production of high specific activity, carrier-free (no stable isotope of the same element) radioisotopes.

97. c Saha, 2004, p. 75

The USP 26 limit states that the limit for aluminum concentration in a ^{99m}Tc eluate is 10 μg/mL for fission-produced ^{99}Mo.

98. b Saha, 2004, pp. 48, 90, 358

Carrier-free specific activity is when no stable forms of the radioisotope are in the sample. This is because no stable form of the radioisotope is expected to be in a sample.

99. d Saha, 2004, pp. 64–77

Attempt to elute the generator with a different (new) collection vial first to see if the evacuated vial was compromised.

100. b Adler and Carlton, 2007, p. 329

A nonionic contrast material may be described as one that does not dissociate or divide into charged particles in solution.

Examination References

Adler AM, Carlton RR, 2003. *Introduction to Radiography and Patient Care.* 3rd ed. St. Louis, MO: WB Saunders Company.

Adler AM, Carlton RR, 2007. *Introduction to Radiography and Patient Care.* 4th ed. St. Louis, MO: WB Saunders Company.

American Pharmaceutical Association, 1999. *The Pharmacy Technician.* Englewood, CO: Morton Publishing Company.

Amersham Healthcare, 2004. Metastron(r). Strontium-89 chloride for injection [package insert]. Arlington Heights, IL. Available at www.amershamhealth-us.com/shared/pdfs/pi/metastron.pdf. Accessed July 2, 2004.

Bernier DR, Christian PE, Langan JK, 1994. *Nuclear Medicine Technology and Techniques.* 3rd ed. St. Louis, MO: Mosby; 298–300.

Blust JS, Boyce TM, Moore WH, 1992. Pharmacologic cardiac intervention: Comparison of adenosine, dipyridamole, and dobutamine. *J Nucl Med Technol.* 20:53–59.

Bolus NE, 2001. Epidemiology for the nuclear medicine technologist. *J Nucl Med Technol.* 29:143–147.

Bristol-Myers Squibb Medical Imaging, 2004. Miraluma kit for the preparation of technetium Tc-99m sestamibi for injection [package insert]. North Billerica, MA. Available at www.miraluma.com. Accessed June 16, 2004.

Brodkey MJ, Schlegel JU, Derouen TA, 1977. Determination of renal plasma flow using the gamma scintillation camera. *Invest Urol.* 14:417–420.

Caretta RF, Vande Streek P, Weiland FL, 1999. Optimizing images of acute deep-vein thrombosis using technetium-99m apcitide. *J Nucl Med Technol.* 27:271–275.

Cevola WE, 1993. *Nuclear Medicine Procedure Specific Clinical History Forms.* Dubuque, IA: Shepherd, Inc.

Chachati A, Meyers A, Godon JP, Rigo P, 1987. Rapid method for the measurement of differential renal function: Validation. *J Nucl Med.* 28:829–836.

Cherry SR, Sorenson JA, Phelps ME, 2003. *Physics in Nuclear Medicine.* 3rd ed. Philiadelphia, PA: Saunders/Elsevier Science.

Chilton HM, Witcofski RL, 1986. *Nuclear Pharmacy: An Introduction to the Clinical Application of Radiopharmaceuticals.* Philadelphia, PA: Lea & Febiger.

Christian PE, Bernier DR, Langan JK, 2004. *Nuclear Medicine and PET Technology and Techniques.* 5th ed. St. Louis, MO: Mosby.

Christian PE, Waterstram-Rich KM, 2007. *Nuclear Medicine and PET/CT.* 6th ed. St. Louis, MO: Mosby/Elsevier.

Crawford ES, Husain SS, 2011. *Nuclear Cardiac Imaging: Terminology and Technical Aspects.* 2nd ed. Reston, VA: Society of Nuclear Medicine.

DraxImage, 2006, MAA kit for the preparation of technetium Tc-99m albumin aggregated injection [package insert].

Dunnwald LK, Mankoff DA, Byrd DR, et al., 1999. Technical aspects of sentinel node lymphoscintigraphy for breast cancer. *J Nucl Med Technol.* 27:106–111.

Early PJ, Sodee DB, 1995. *Principles and Practice of Nuclear Medicine.* 2nd ed. St. Louis, MO: Mosby.

Elgazzar AH, Maxon HR III, 1993. Radioisotope therapy for cancer related bone pain. *Imaging Insights.* 2:1–4, 6.

Eliot AT, 1990. Radionuclide generators. In: Sampson CB, ed. *Textbook of Radiopharmacy: Theory and Practice.* New York, NY: Gordon and Breach Science Publishers; 33–50.

English CA, English RJ, Giering LP, et al., 1993. *Introduction to Nuclear Cardiology.* 3rd ed. North Billerica, MA: Du Pont Pharma.

English RJ, 1995. *Single Photon Emission Computed Tomography: A Primer.* 3rd ed. Reston, VA: Society of Nuclear Medicine.

Forshier S, 2002. *Essentials of Radiation Biology and Protection.* 2nd ed. Clifton Park, NY: Delmar Thomson Learning; 144–145.

Gates GF, 1981. Glomerular filtration rate: Estimation from fractional renal accumulation of ^{99m}Tc DTPA. *Am J Radiol.* 138:565–570.

GE Healthcare, 2006. Ceretec(r) kit for the preparation of technetium Tc-99m exametazime injection [package insert]. Arlington Heights, IL. Available at www http://md.gehealthcare.com/shared/pdfs/pi/ceretec.pdf. Accessed January 26, 2011.

Hendee WR, Ritenour ER, 2002. *Medical Imaging Physics.* 4th ed. Chichester, UK: John Wiley & Sons; 132.

Hines H, Kayayan R, Colsher J, et al., 2000. National Electrical Manufacturers Association recommendations for implementing SPECT instrumentation quality control. *J Nucl Med.* 41:383–389.

IDEC Pharmaceuticals Corporation, 2002. Zevalin (ibritumomab tiuxetan) prescribing information. San Diego, CA.

Klingensmith WC III, ed., 1990–1995. *Nuclear Medicine Procedure Manual.* Englewood, CO: Wick Publishing Company.

Kowalczyk N, Donnett K., 1996. *Integrated Patient Care for the Imaging Professional.* St. Louis, MO: Mosby.

Kowalsky RJ, Falen SW, 2004. *Radiopharmaceuticals in Nuclear Pharmacy and Nuclear Medicine.* 2nd ed. Washington, DC: American Pharmacists Association; 299–300.

Lee K, 1991. *Computers in Nuclear Medicine: A Practical Approach.* Reston, VA: Society of Nuclear Medicine.

Lee K, 2005. *Computers in Nuclear Medicine: A Practical Approach.* 2nd ed. Reston, VA: Society of Nuclear Medicine.

Lile JM, Miller DE, Pakkala JL, eds., 2003. *Pharmacy Certified Technician Training Manual.* 8th ed. Lansing, MI: Michigan Pharmacists Association.

Madsen M, 1994. Computer acquisition of nuclear medicine images. *J Nucl Med Technol.* 22:3–11.

Mallinckrodt, 2004. OctreoScan kit for the preparation of indium In-111 pentetreotide [package insert]. St. Louis, MO. Available at http://imaging.mallinckrodt.com/_Attachments/PackageInserts/Octreoscan%20PI.pdf. Accessed July 2, 2004.

McGraw RS, Culver CM, Juni JE, et al., 1992. Lung ventilation studies: Surface contamination associated with technetium-99m DTPA aerosol. *J Nucl Med Technol.* 20:228–230.

Mettler FA Jr, Guiberteau MJ, 1991. *Essentials of Nuclear Medicine Imaging.* 3rd ed. Philadelphia, PA: WB Saunders.

Mettler FA Jr, Guiberteau MJ, 2006. *Essentials of Nuclear Medicine Imaging.* 5th ed. Philadelphia, PA: WB Saunders.

Nabi HA, Zubeldia JM, 2002. Clinical applications of ^{18}F-FDG in oncology. *J Nucl Med Technol.* 30:3–9.

Noz ME, Maguire GQ Jr, 2007. *Radiation Protection in the Health Sciences.* 2nd ed. Hackensack, NJ: World Scientific.

Occupational Safety and Health Administration, 1992. *Occupational Exposure to Bloodborne Pathogens.* OSHA 3127. Washington, DC: OSHA.

Pagana KD, Pagana TJ, 2010. *Mosby's Manual of Diagnostic and Laboratory Tests.* 4th ed. St. Louis, MO: Mosby/Elsevier.

Park HM, Duncan K, 1994. Nonradioactive pharmaceuticals in nuclear medicine. *J Nucl Med Technol.* 22:240–249.

Peller PJ, Khedkar NY, Martinez CJ, 1996. Breast tumor scintigraphy. *J Nucl Med Technol.* 24:198–203.

Ponto JA, Swanson DP, Freitas JE, 1987. Clinical manifestations of radio-pharmaceutical formulation problems. In: Hlakik WB III, Saha GP, Study KT, eds. *Essentials of Nuclear Medicine Science.* Baltimore, MD: Williams & Wilkins; 268–289.

Powsner RA, Powsner ER, 1998. *Essentials of Nuclear Medicine Physics.* Malden, MA: Blackwell Science; 78–91, 126–131, 144–147.

Prekeges J, 2011. *Nuclear Medicine Instrumentation.* Boston, MA: Jones and Bartlett; 9.

Remson ST, Ackermann PG, 1977. *Calculations for the Medical Laboratory.* Boston, MA: Little, Brown and Company.

Rowell KL, 1992. *Clinical Computers in Nuclear Medicine.* Reston, VA: Society of Nuclear Medicine.

Roy L, van Train K, Bietendorf J, et al., 1991. An optimized protocol for detection of coronary artery disease using technetium-99m sestamibi. *J Nucl Med Technol.* 19:63–67.

Saha GB, 2004. *Fundamentals of Nuclear Pharmacy.* 5th ed. New York, NY: Springer-Verlag.

Schlegel JU, Bakule PT, 1970. A diagnostic approach in detecting renal and urinary tract disease. *J Urol.* 104:2–10.

Schlegel JU, Halikiopoulos HL, Prima R, 1979. Determination of filtration fraction using the gamma scintillation camera. *J Urol.* 122:447–450.

Schlegel JU, Hamway SA, 1976. Individual renal plasma flow determination in two minutes. *J Urol.* 116:282–285.

Schwarz SW, Anderson CJ, Donner JB, 1997. Radiochemistry and radio-pharmacology. In: Bernier DR, Christian PE, Langan JK, eds. *Nuclear Medicine Technology and Techniques.* 4th ed. St. Louis, MO: Mosby; 160–183.

Seldin DW, 2002. Techniques for using Bexxar for the treatment of non-Hodgkin's lymphoma. *J Nucl Med Technol.* 30:109–114.

Shackett P, 2009. *Procedures Quick Reference.* 2nd ed. Philadelphia, PA: Wolters Kluwer Health/Lippincott Williams & Wilkins.

Siegel JA, 2004. *Guide for Diagnostic Nuclear Medicine and Radiopharmaceutical Therapy.* Reston, VA: Society of Nuclear Medicine.

SNM Procedure Guidelines Committee, 2011. Procedure guideline for brain perfusion single photon emission computed tomography (SPECT) using Tc-99m radiopharmaceuticals. *SNM Procedure Guidelines Manual.* Reston, VA: Society of Nuclear Medicine.

SNM Procedure Guidelines Committee, 2011. Procedure guideline for C-14 urea breath test. *SNM Procedure Guidelines Manual.* Reston, VA: Society of Nuclear Medicine.

SNM Procedure Guidelines Committee, 2011. Procedure guideline for gallium scintigraphy in inflammation. *SNM Procedure Guidelines Manual.* Reston, VA: Society of Nuclear Medicine; 105–109.

SNM Procedure Guidelines Committee, 2011. Procedure guideline for somatostatin receptor scintigraphy with In-111 pentetreotide. *SNM Procedure Guidelines Manual.* Reston, VA: Society of Nuclear Medicine.

SNM Procedure Guidelines Committee, 2011. Procedure guideline for thyroid uptake measurement. *SNM Procedure Guidelines Manual.* Reston, VA: Society of Nuclear Medicine.

SNM Procedure Guidelines Committee, 2011. Procedure guideline for tumor imaging using F-18 FDG. *SNM Procedure Guidelines Manual.* Reston, VA: Society of Nuclear Medicine; 171–176.

Steves AM, 1999. Radiation protection in nuclear medicine. In: Dowd SB, Tilson ER, eds. *Practical Radiation Protection and Applied Radiobiology.* 2nd ed. Philadelphia, PA: WB Saunders Company; 263–286.

Taber's Cyclopedic Medical Dictionary, 2001. 19th ed. Philadelphia, PA., F.A. Davis Company.

Taber's Cyclopedic Medical Dictionary, 2009. 21st ed. Philadelphia, PA: F.A. Davis Company.

Thompson MA, Hattaway MP, Hall JD, et al., 1994. *Principles of Imaging Science and Protection.* Philadelphia, PA: WB Saunders Company.

Tikofsky RS, Tremblath L, Voslar AM, 1993. Radiopharmaceuticals for brain imaging: The technologist's perspective. *J Nucl Med Technol.* 21:57–60.

Turkington TG, 2001. Introduction to PET instrumentation. *J Nucl Med Technol.* 29:1–8.

U.S. Nuclear Regulatory Commission, 1998. *Program-Specific Guidance about Medical Use Licenses.* NUREG-1556, Volume 9. Washington, DC: Nuclear Regulatory Commission.

U.S. Nuclear Regulatory Commission, 2003. Federal Regulations, Title 10, Chapter 1, Energy, Parts 19, 20, 35; Title 49 Parts 172, 173. Washington, DC: U.S. Government Printing Office.

U.S. Pharmacopeia, 1990. 22nd ed. Rockville, MD: U.S. Pharmacopeia Convention.

Wells P, 1999. *Practical Mathematics in Nuclear Medicine Technology.* Reston, VA: Society of Nuclear Medicine.

Williams BS, Hinkle GH, Douthit RA, et al., 1999. Lymphoscintigraphy and intraoperative lymphatic mapping of sentinel nodes in melanoma patients. *J Nucl Med Technol.* 27:309–317.

Williams BS, Hinkle GH, Lamatrice RA, et al., 1997. Technical considerations for acquiring and processing indium-111 capromab pendetide images. *J Nucl Med Technol.* 25: 205–216.

Yester M, 2001. Collimators. In: Fahey F, Harkness B, eds. *Basic Science of Nuclear Medicine* [on CD-ROM]. Reston, VA: Society of Nuclear Medicine.

Zolle I, ed., 2006. *Technetium-99 Radiopharmaceuticals: Preparation and Quality Control in Nuclear Medicine.* New York, NY: Springer.

APPENDIX A **Federal Regulations**

Table A.1 U.S. Department of Transportation (DOT), Title 49, Code of Federal Regulations

Topic	*DOT Regulation*
Packaging radioactive materials	§ 173.403 For shipping purposes, radioactive material is defined as any material spontaneously emitting ionizing radiation with specific gravity greater than 0.002 μCi/g uniformly distributed. (Therefore, return of radioactive materials and/or their residues to a radiopharmacy or manufacturer are subject to DOT regulations.) Packaging procedure: 1. Survey package and verify absence of surface contamination with wipe test. 2. Attach appropriate category of "RADIOACTIVE" label and indicate Transport Index. 3. Prepare shipping papers. § 71.0 DOT regulations must be adhered to whenever radioactive materials are shipped, whether or not such shipments are interstate.
Receipt of radioactive materials: removable contamination limits	§ 173.443 Surface levels of removable contamination on packaging must be as low as possible. Levels must not exceed 22 dpm/cm^2 (or 6,600 dpm for wiped surface area of 300 cm^2).

Table A.2 Nuclear Regulatory Commission (NRC), Title 10, Code of Federal Regulations Part 20 (January 1, 2002) and Part 35 (Revisions Effective October 24, 2002)

Topic	*NRC Regulation*
ALARA	§ 20.1003 Acronym for "as low as reasonably achievable." Licensee and occupationally exposed workers must make every reasonable effort to minimize radiation exposure, taking into account state of technology and socioeconomics. NUREG-1556 provides model program that uses 10% of occupational exposure limit as the Investigational Level. RSO would work with any employee exceeding this level to identify methods to bring exposures down. Review of exposures must be at least quarterly.
Radiation protection programs	§ 20.1101 Licensee is required to develop, document, and implement radiation protection program to ensure compliance with NRC regulations. Licensee must develop procedures and engineer work areas to achieve occupational doses and doses to members of the general public that are as low as reasonably achievable (ALARA). § 35.27 All individuals supervised by the licensee must receive instruction in radiation protection procedures and be informed of all applicable regulations and license conditions. Licensee is responsible for assuring that all supervised individuals follow procedures, regulations, and license conditions. § 19.12 All occupationally exposed workers who may receive annual dose of 100 mrem (1 mSv) must be instructed in the following: 1. Storage, transfer, and use of radioactive materials. 2. Radiation protection and applicable NRC regulations. 3. How to report conditions that may violate NRC regulations. 4. How to respond to radiation exposure emergencies. 5. Workers' right to review radiation exposure and bioassay records, if individual requires monitoring.
Dose, occupational, exposure limits	§ 20.1201, § 20.1207, § 20.1208, § 20.1301 (See Table 1.6 for exposure limits.) If dose to embryo/fetus is found to exceed 0.5 rem (5 mSv) at time of declaration, then limit is set to 0.05 rem (0.5 mSv) for remainder of pregnancy.

	§ 20.2104 For occupationally exposed individuals who require monitoring, licensee must determine dose received in current year and, if possible, cumulative occupational radiation dose. Records of exposure from most recent employer must be obtained.
Minimizing contamination	§ 20.1406 Licensees must use facility design and procedures to reasonable extent to minimize contamination and production of radioactive waste.
Personal monitoring requirements	§ 20.1502 Occupationally exposed workers must be supplied with personal radiation monitoring devices if they are likely to receive in excess of 10% of annual limits. § 20.2106 Records of exposures to occupationally exposed individuals who have been monitored should be retained for duration of facility license. § 20.2107 Records showing compliance with dose limits for members of the general public should be retained for duration of facility license. § 20.1301 (See Table 1.6 for exposure limits.)
Restricted and unrestricted areas	§ 20.1003 Unrestricted area is an area not under control of licensee and where access is not limited. Restricted area means access is limited and controlled by licensee in order to minimize radiation exposure to public. § 20.1301 Radiation dose rates in unrestricted areas must not exceed 2 mrem (0.02 mSv) in any hour, exclusive of exposures resulting from presence of patients who have received radiopharmaceuticals. § 20.1802 Radioactive materials cannot be left unattended in unrestricted area.
Surveys	§20.1501 Surveys should be performed as reasonable to determine radiation levels and to evaluate potential radiological hazards. Instruments used for surveys must be properly calibrated. § 35.70 Surveys must be performed at end of each day where by-product materials requiring written directives are used (such as therapeutic dosages of ^{131}I, ^{89}Sr, ^{153}Sm, ^{32}P). Areas where dosage was prepared and administered must be surveyed. § 20.2103, § 35.2070 Survey and calibration records retained for 3 years. Must include date of survey, results, instrument used, and name of individual who performed the survey.
Area posting	§ 20.1003, § 20.1902 Radiation areas should be posted appropriately. 1. GRAVE DANGER: VERY HIGH RADIATION AREA Area in which an individual could receive an absorbed radiation dose in excess of 500 rads (5 grays) in 1 hr at 1 m from source. 2. CAUTION: HIGH RADIATION AREA Area in which radiation levels could result in an individual receiving dose equivalent exceeding 0.1 rem (1 mSv) in 1 hr at 30 cm from the source. 3. CAUTION: RADIATION AREA Area in which radiation levels could result in an individual receiving a dose equivalent exceeding 0.005 rem (0.05 mSv) in 1 hr at 30 cm from the source. 4. CAUTION: RADIOACTIVE MATERIAL Post in areas where radioactive materials are used or stored in amounts exceeding 10 times the quantity of material specified in appendix C to part 20 NRC. (See Table 1.7 for actual activities.) § 20.1903 Caution sign not required if radioactive materials in room for less than 8 hr and person is present at all times who will prevent exposure of individuals in excess of established limits.

Receipt of radioactive materials	§ 20.1906 Wipe tests must be performed on external surfaces of packages labeled with Type I, II, and III radioactive labels. External monitoring (Geiger–Mueller survey) for radiation levels required only for packages containing quantities of radioactive material greater than or equal to Type A quantities. [This exempts essentially all packages received in nuclear medicine departments.] Both wipe tests and G–M surveys required if evidence of leakage or damage to package. Licensee must notify final delivery carrier and NRC if removable surface contamination exceeds 22 dpm/cm^2 (or 6600 dpm for wiped surface area of 300 cm^2) or survey meter reading exceeds 200 mrem/hr from any point on package surface or 10 mrem/hr at 1 m. When packages received during regular working hours, required monitoring must be performed within 3 hr. For packages received outside of regular hours, monitoring must be performed within 3 hr of beginning of workday. § 20.2103, § 30.51 Records of receipt of radioactive shipments retained for as long as material is in possession of the licensee or 3 years after disposal. Package surveys retained for 3 years.
Packaging and transport of radioactive material	§ 71.0 DOT regulations must be adhered to whenever radioactive materials are shipped, whether or not such shipments are interstate. § 71.4, § 71.5 Prior to shipping, packages containing radioactive materials must be wipe tested to verify absence of surface contamination, and an appropriate radioactive label with transport index must be attached to the package.
Disposal of radioactive material	§ 20.1904 Deface or remove radioactive label from containers that no longer contain radioactive materials before disposal. § 20.2001 Dispose of licensed material by transfer to an authorized recipient, by decay in storage, by release in effluents (certain wastes and limits apply). § 20.2003 Patient excreta may be discarded into sanitary sewer (no limits). § 35.315 Materials removed from therapy patient's room must be monitored. If exposure rates from unshielded materials do not exceed natural background readings, can be treated as nonradioactive materials. Materials with readings exceeding background treated as radioactive waste. § 20.2108, § 30.51 Records of disposal retained for 3 years.
Storage area for decay of radioactivity	§ 35.92 Physical half-life must be less than 120 days. Material must be retained until survey meter reading of unshielded waste equals background. Before disposal all radiation labels must be defaced unless they are within container that will be treated as biomedical waste. § 35.2092 Records retained for 3 years for all materials held for decay in storage, then disposed of as nonradioactive waste. Records must include date of disposal, survey instrument used, background reading, survey meter reading at surface of container, name of individual performing survey.
Written directives	§ 35.2, § 35.40 Written directive required before administration of more than 30 μCi (1.1 MBq) [^{131}I]sodium iodide or any other therapeutic dosage of by-product material (Table 1.1). Therapeutic dosage defined as dosage of a by-product material that is intended for palliative or curative treatment. Written directive defined as an authorized user's written order, which must include the following: date, signature of authorized user, patient's name, prescribed dosage, radiopharmaceutical, route of administration. § 35.41 Licensee must develop, implement, and maintain written procedures that verify patient's identity prior to administration of radiopharmaceuticals requiring written directive and that dosage administration is in accordance with written directive.

	§ 35.2040, § 35.2041 Written directives retained for 3 years. Records for procedures for administrations requiring written directive retained for duration of license.
Dose calibrator quality control	§ 35.60 Any dose calibrator used to measure patient dosages prior to administration must be calibrated in accordance with nationally recognized standards or manufacturer's instructions. § 35.2060 Records of the above calibration tests retained for 3 years. Records must include model and serial number of instrument, date of test, results of test, and name of individual performing test.
Calibration of survey meters	§ 35.61 Calibrate survey instruments before first use, annually, and after repair. Calibration date must be conspicuously noted on instrument. A survey meter cannot be used if exposure rate differs from calibrated rate by more than 20%. § 35.61, § 35.2061 Survey meter calibration records retained for 3 years. Records must include model and serial number of instrument, date of calibration, results of calibration, and name of individual performing calibration.
Determination of activity (dosage) administered to patients	§ 35.63, § 35.2 Activity of radiopharmaceutical dosages must be determined and recorded before administration to patient. When unit dosages are used, activity must be measured directly using a dose calibrator, or activity can be determined using decay correction. Unit dosage defined as dosage prepared as single administration to patient without any further manipulation after initial preparation. When bulk kits or solutions are used, dosage activity must be determined directly, or a combination of direct measurement and mathematical calculations may be used. Dosage activity must fall within prescribed range, or must fall within ±20% of prescribed dosage. Variation from range must be approved by authorized user on individual basis. § 35.2063 Dosage records retained for 3 years and must include the following: radiopharmaceutical; patient's name or identification number, if one was assigned; prescribed dosage; actual measured dosage, or notation that activity was less than 30 μCi (1.1 MBq); date and time of dosage determination; name of individual who determined dosage.
Labeling of vials and syringes	§ 35.69 Each vial and syringe containing a radiopharmaceutical must be labeled to identify radiopharmaceutical. Each vial shield and syringe shield must also be labeled with radiopharmaceutical, unless label on vial or syringe is visible.
Release of individuals who have received radiopharmaceuticals	§ 35.75 Individual who has received radiopharmaceutical dosage can be released from control of licensee if no person who is exposed to released individual will receive exposure dose exceeding 0.5 rem (5 mSv). If any person who is exposed to released individual may receive in excess of 0.1 rem (1 mSv), released individual must be given written instructions explaining actions that should be taken to keep exposure to others as low as reasonably possible. If female who receives radiopharmaceutical dosage is breast-feeding and TEDE to nursing infant or child might exceed 0.1 rem (1 mSv), assuming no interruption of breast-feeding, female must be provided with guidance concerning interruption or discontinuation of breast-feeding and an explanation of potential consequences if guidance is not followed. § 35.2075 Records concerning release of patients who have received therapeutic dosages retained for 3 years. Records must be maintained documenting instructions given to patients who are breast-feeding and whose infant/child may receive more than 0.1 rem (1 mSv) assuming no interruption of breast-feeding. These records retained for 3 years.
Mobile service provisions	§ 35.80 Mobile service licensee must have written agreement with each client that permits use of radiopharmaceuticals at client's address and clearly delineates authority and responsibilities of both parties.

	Licensee must check dose calibrators for proper function at each client's address or on each day of use, whichever is more frequent. At a minimum, this must include constancy testing. Licensee must use a dedicated check source to check survey meters for proper operation before use at each client's address. Licensee must perform area surveys as required by Part 20 prior to leaving the client's address. Radiopharmaceuticals can be delivered to client only if client has license allowing possession of by-product materials. § 35.2080 Letters of agreement retained for 3 years after last provision of service to client. Survey records retained for 3 years and must include the following: date of survey, results, instrument used, and name of individual who performed survey.
Generator eluate quality control	§ 35.204 Licensee may not administer to humans a radiopharmaceutical containing more than 0.15 μCi ^{99}Mo/mCi ^{99m}Tc. The first elution from a ^{99}Mo/^{99m}Tc generator must be assayed for ^{99}Mo concentration. § 35.2204 Records of ^{99}Mo assays retained for 3 years. Must include the following: ratio of measured activity expressed as kBq ^{99}Mo per MBq of ^{99m}Tc (or μCi ^{99}Mo per mCi of ^{99m}Tc), time and date of measurement, and name of individual making measurement.
Safety instructions and precautions for patients hospitalized after administration of therapeutic radiopharmaceuticals	§35.310 If patients are hospitalized after administration of therapeutic radiopharmaceuticals, licensee must provide safety instructions for staff caring for such patients. Instruction must include patient and visitor control, contamination control, and waste control. § 35.315 If patient cannot be released after receiving therapeutic radiopharmaceutical because of exposure levels, patient must be given private room with private sanitary facilities or must share facilities with another patient also receiving therapeutic radiopharmaceuticals. Post door of patient's room with "Radioactive Materials" sign. Either a note on the patient's door or in the patient's chart must describe where visitors may sit and how long they can stay in the room.
Medical events involving radiopharmaceuticals (misadministration)	§ 35.3045 Licensee is required to report medical events, which are defined as radiopharmaceutical administrations that: 1. Differ from prescribed dosage by 20% or more or fall outside the prescribed range and will result in a dose that exceeds any of the limits listed below. 2. Are administered to wrong person, by wrong route, or involve wrong radioactive drug and will result in dose that exceeds any of limits listed: Limits: a. 5 rem (0.05 Sv) effective dose equivalent; b. 50 rem (0.5 Sv) to an organ or tissue; or c. 50 rem (0.5 Sv) shallow dose equivalent to skin. Required reports include: 1. Telephone call to NRC no later than next calendar day after discovery. 2. Notify referring physician no later than 24 hr after discovery. 3. Notify patient no later than 24 hr after discovery, unless referring physician chooses to do so or determines, based on medical judgment, that patient would be harmed by being informed. 4. Written report to NRC and referring physician within 15 days after discovery. Report must include brief description of event, why it occurred, effect on patient, actions taken to prevent recurrence. (For staff technologists, the appropriate reporting authority is the chief technologist or nuclear medicine physician. Reports are usually written by the RSO or authorized user.)
Loss or theft of radioactive materials	§ 20.2201 Licensee must notify NRC immediately if specified activities of radioactive by-product are lost or stolen. Activities greater than 1000 times those listed in Appendix C of Part 20 must be reported if an exposure could result to persons in an unrestricted area. See list for actual minimum activities of commonly used nuclear medicine nuclides. The NRC must be notified within 30 days if activities 10 times those in Appendix C are irretrievably lost or stolen.

Table A.3 United States Pharmacopoeia 24 and The National Formulary 19, 2000

Topic	*Standard*
Generator eluate quality	No more than 0.15 μCi ^{99}Mo per mCi ^{99m}Tc.
	No more than 10 mg Al^{+3}/mL of eluate.
Macroaggregated albumin particle size	At least 90% of particles in preparation must have diameter between 10 and 90 microns; none may be greater than 150 microns.

APPENDIX B **Table of Chi Square**

Degrees of freedom* (n − 1)	*There is a probability of*						
	0.99	*0.95*	*0.90*	*0.50*	*0.10*	*0.05*	*0.01*
	that the calculated value of chi square will be equal to or greater than						
2	0.020	0.103	0.211	1.386	4.605	5.991	9.210
3	0.115	0.352	0.584	2.366	6.251	7.815	11.345
4	0.297	0.711	1.064	3.357	7.779	9.488	13.277
5	0.554	1.145	1.610	4.351	9.236	11.070	15.086
6	0.872	1.635	2.204	5.348	10.645	12.592	16.812
7	1.239	2.167	2.833	6.346	12.017	14.067	18.475
8	1.646	2.733	3.490	7.344	13.362	15.507	20.090
9	2.088	3.325	4.168	8.343	14.684	16.919	21.666
10	2.558	3.940	4.865	9.342	15.987	18.307	23.209
11	3.053	4.575	5.578	10.341	17.275	19.675	24.725
12	2.571	5.226	6.304	11.340	18.549	21.026	26.217
13	4.107	5.892	7.042	12.340	19.812	22.362	27.688
14	4.660	6.571	7.790	13.339	21.064	23.685	29.141
15	5.229	7.261	8.547	14.339	22.307	24.996	30.578
16	5.812	7.962	9.312	15.338	23.542	26.296	32.000
17	6.408	8.672	10.085	16.338	24.769	27.587	33.409
18	7.015	9.390	10.865	17.338	25.989	28.869	34.805
19	7.633	10.117	11.651	18.338	27.204	30.144	36.191
20	8.260	10.851	12.443	19.337	28.412	31.410	37.566
21	8.897	11.591	13.240	20.337	29.615	32.671	38.932
22	9.542	12.338	14.041	21.337	30.813	33.924	40.289
23	10.196	13.091	14.848	22.337	32.007	35.172	41.638
24	10.856	13.848	15.659	23.337	33.196	36.415	42.980
25	11.534	14.611	16.473	24.337	34.382	37.382	44.314
26	12.198	15.379	17.292	25.336	35.563	38.885	45.642
27	12.879	16.151	18.114	26.336	36.741	40.113	46.963
28	13.565	16.928	18.939	27.336	37.916	41.337	48.278
29	14.256	17.708	19.768	28.336	39.087	42.557	49.588

*The number of degrees of freedom is usually one less than the total number of observations *n*.
Reprinted, with permission, from Early PJ, Sodee DB, 1985. *Principles and Practice of Nuclear Medicine.* St Louis, MO: Mosby; 348.

APPENDIX C Duel Isotope Counting Spilldown Ratio Data Sheet

High-Energy Radionuclide ____________________ Low-Energy Radionuclide ____________________

Pulse-Height Analyzer Settings:

High-Energy Radionuclide

LLD ____________________

ΔE ____________________

Low-Energy Radionuclide

LLD ____________________

ΔE ____________________

High-Energy Setting

Sample	*Total Counts*	*Time*	*CPM*	*CPM-Bkgrd*
Bkgrd				
(1A) High Energy				
(1B) Mix				

Low-Energy Setting

Sample	*Total Counts*	*Time*	*CPM*	*CPM-Bkgrd*
Bkgrd				
(2A) High Energy				
(2B) Mix				

Data: 1A ____________________ net CPM 1B ____________________ net CPM

2A ____________________ net CPM 2B ____________________ net CPM

Calculation for spilldown ratio (R_{SP}):

R_{SP} = 2A CPM/1A CPM = ______________

1A = net cpm of high-energy sample in high-energy setting

2A = net cpm of high-energy sample in low-energy setting

Calculate net counts of low-energy isotope for spilldown:

Net counts = 2B − (R_{SP} × 1B) = ______________

1B = net cpm of mixed sample in high-energy setting

2B = net cpm of mixed sample in low-energy setting

APPENDIX D **Système International (SI) Unit Conversions**

Quantity	*CGS Units*	*SI (MKS) Units*	*Equivalents*
Length	centimeter (cm)	meter (m)	1 cm = 0.01 m
Mass	gram (g)	kilogram (kg)	1 g = 0.001 kg
Time	second (s)	second (s)	1 s = 1 s
Energy	erg	Joule (J)	1 erg = 10^{-7} J
Radioactivity	Curie (Ci)	Becquerel (Bq)	1 Ci = 3.7×10^{10} Bq
Radiation absorbed dose	rad	gray (Gy)	1 rad = 0.01 Gy
Exposure	Roentgen (R)	Coulomb/kilogram (C/kg)	1 R = 2.58×10^{-4} C/kg
Dose equivalent	rem	Sievert (Sv)	1 rem = 0.01 Sv

Common Prefixes Used in SI

Prefix	*Symbol*	*Numerical equivalent*
giga	G	10^9 = 1,000,000,000
mega	M	10^6 = 1,000,000
kilo	k	10^3 = 1,000
deci	d	10^{-1} = 0.1
centi	c	10^{-2} = 0.01
milli	m	10^{-3} = 0.001
micro	μ	10^{-6} = 0.000001
nano	n	10^{-9} = 0.000000001
pico	p	10^{-12} = 0.000000000001

APPENDIX E **Helpful Web Links**

NMT Certification Board (NMTCB): http://nmtcb.org

American Society of Nuclear Cardiology (ASNC): http://asnc.org

American Society of Radiologic Technologists (ASRT): http://asrt.org

Society of Nuclear Medicine: http://www.snm.org

CDC Just in Time Training Video: http://emergency.cdc.gov/radiation/justintime.asp

Astellas Techtips: http://www.pharmstresstech.com

Mallinckrodt Image Library and Case Studies: http://gamma.wustl.edu/allknown.html

ECG Library: http://www.ecglibrary.com/ecghome.html

US NRC CFR web resource: http://www.nrc.gov/reading-rm/doc-collections/cfr

NUREG site: http://www.nrc.gov/reading-rm/doc-collections/nuregs/staff/sr1556/v9/nureg-1556–9.pdf

Resource for other nuclear medicine websites:
http://www.physics.umd.edu/lecdem/honr228q/specialtopics/nucmed.htm

APPENDIX F Electrocardiogram Interpretation Guide

The guide is a quick review of normal sinus rhythm, rhythms originating in the SA node, rhythms originating in the atria, rhythms originating in the junction, heart blocks, rhythms originating in the ventricles, bundle branch blocks, and pacemakers.

Rhythm	*Rate*	*Rhythm*	*P Wave*	*PR Interval*	*QRS*
Normal Sinus Rhythm Best lead to ck P waves is Lead II 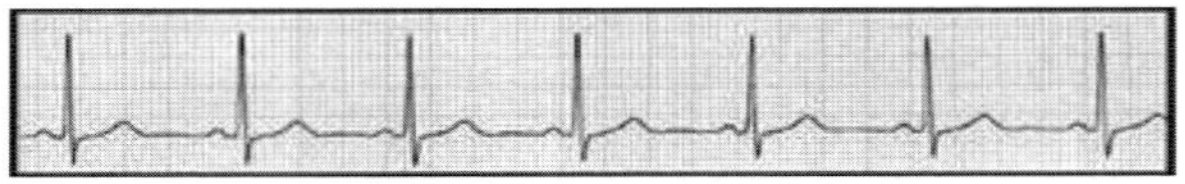	60–100	Regular	Round, upright	12–20	06–12
Rhythms Originating in the SA Node					
Sinus Bradycardia 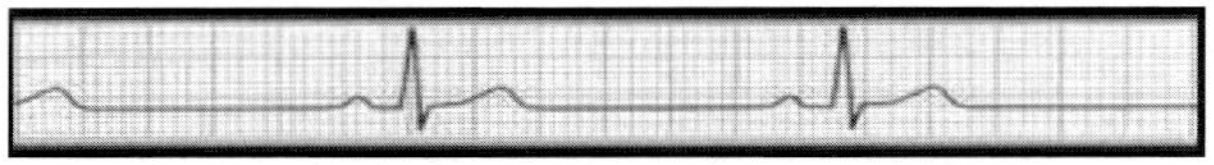	<60	Regular	Round, upright	12–20	06–12
Sinus Tachycardia 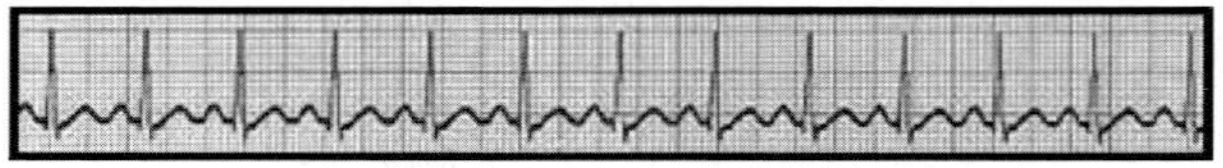	>100, <150	Regular	Round, upright	12–20	06–12
Sinus Dysrhythmia Arrhythmia 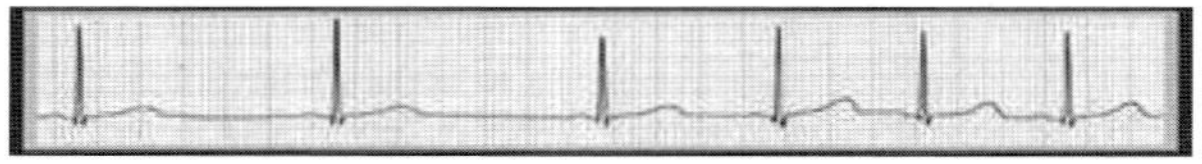	60–100	Irregular	Round, upright	12–20	06–12
Sinoatrial Arrest: (See below) Distance *not* between 3 normal complexes and beat-pause-beat 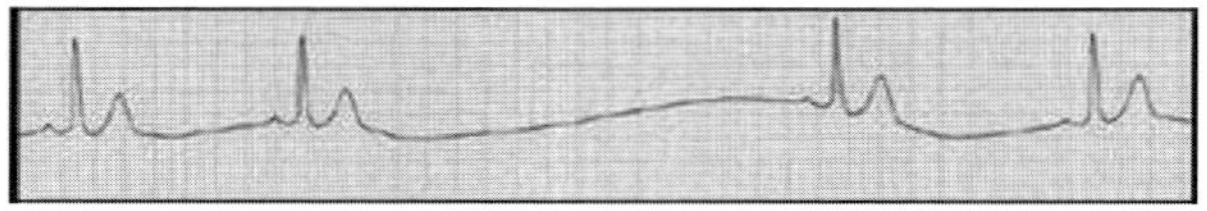	Normal, fast, slow	Irregular with pauses	No P with missed beat	Absent for missed beat	Absent for missed beat
Sinoatrial (SA) Exit Block: Distance between 3 normal complexes equal to distance between beat-pause-beat 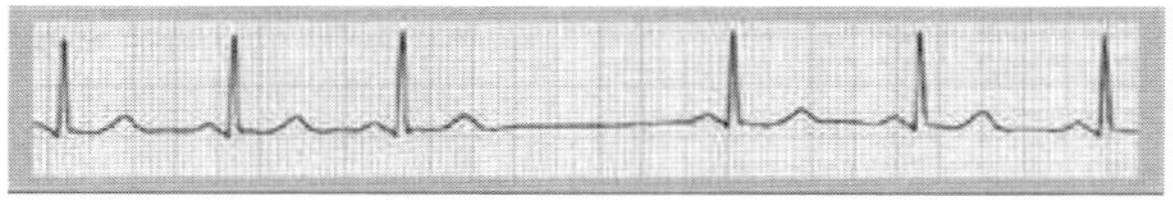	Normal, fast, slow	Irregular with pauses	No P with missed beat	Absent for missed beat	Absent for missed beat

Rhythm	*Rate*	*Rhythm*	*P Wave*	*PR Interval*	*QRS*
Rhythms Originating in the Atria					
Premature Atrial Contraction (PAC) • Can have "blocked" (non-conducted) PAC; may have premature P wave with no QRS	Normal, fast, slow	Irregular	Premature P can look different than sinus P	Usually normal, may be < sinus PR	.06–.12 normal, may be aberrantly conducted
Atrial Tachycardia (can be called SVT)	150–250	Regular	May be hard to ID; may have > P's than QRS	Normal, prolonged, or shortened	.06–.12 normal, may be aberrantly conducted
Paroxysmal Atrial Tachycardia (PAT or PSVT)	150–200	Irregular, with abrupt onset or end	May not be visible P coming into T	Usually unable to measure	.06–.12 normal, may be aberrantly conducted
Atrial Fibrillation	Normal, fast, slow	Irregular R–R	P's not present, wavy or chaotic baseline	None	.06–.12
Atrial Flutter	Normal, fast, slow	Regular or irregular	Sawtooth pattern, picket fence pattern, flutter waves	Not measured	.06–.12

Rhythm	*Rate*	*Rhythm*	*P Wave*	*PR Interval*	*QRS*
Rhythms Originating in the Junction					
Premature Junctional Contractions (PJCs) (Best lead to ck P waves is Lead II)	Normal, fast slow	Irregular	Premature P Inverted before, during (not seen), or after the QRS	Interval associated with the premature beat, usually short	Premature with QRS .06–.12, may be aberrantly conducted
Junctional Rhythm (Best lead to ck P waves is Lead II)	40–60	Regular	Inverted before, during (not seen), or after the QRS	Interval associated with the premature beat, usually short	.06–.12 normal, or may be aberrantly conducted
Accelerated Junctional Rhythm (Best lead to ck P waves is Lead II)	60–100	Regular	Inverted before, during (not seen), or after the QRS	Interval associated with the premature beat, usually short	Premature with QRS .06–.12 normal, or may be aberrantly conducted
Junctional Tachycardia (Best lead to ck P waves is Lead II) Can be called SVT, "paroxysmal" can be PJT	> 100	Regular	Inverted before, during (not seen), or after the QRS	Interval associated with the premature beat, usually short	QRS .06–.12 normal or may be aberrantly conducted

Rhythm	*Rate*	*Rhythm*	*P Wave*	*PR Interval*	*QRS*
Heart Blocks					
First Degree 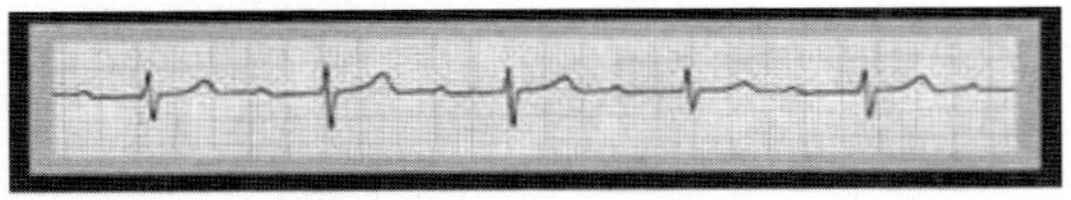	Any rate	Regular	Round, upright	>.20	.06–.12
Second Degree Type I (Wenckebach) 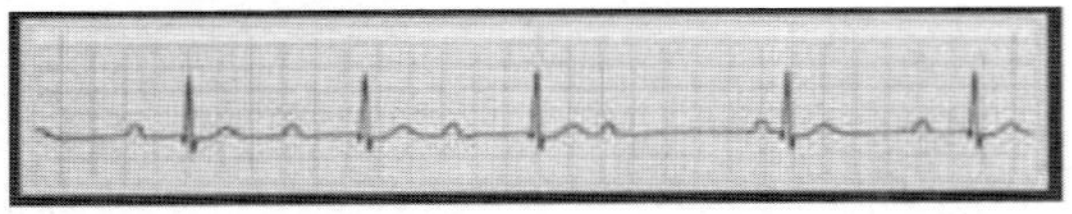	Normal–slow	Irregular	More P's than QRSs	Progressive ↑ of PR, drops QRS	.06–.12 for conducted beats
Second Degree Type II 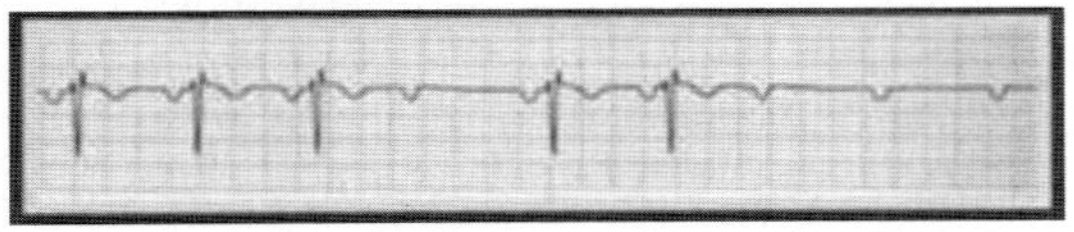	V rate < A	Regular or irregular	More P's than QRSs	PR SAME	Normal or > .12
Third Degree (Complete Heart Block) 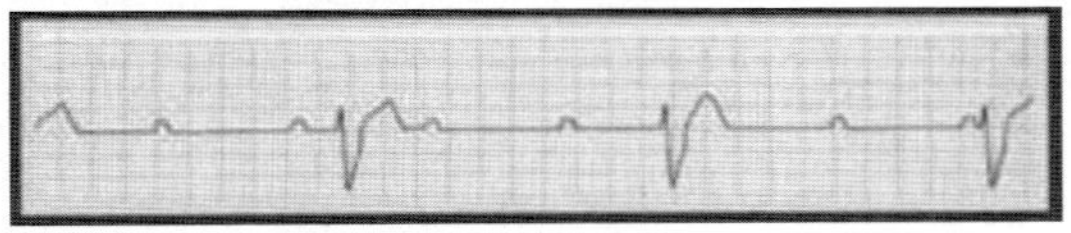	V rate 20–40 A rate < 100	AV dissociation	More P's than QRSs	PR NOT SAME	Normal or wide and bizarre > .12

Quick Way to Remember Heart Blocks!!!

***PR* * Memorize:** * Long (1st) * Long, Longer, Drop (2nd Ty I) * Same (2nd Ty II) * Not the Same (3rd/CHB)

- 1st Degree Φ PR is ***LONG*** (>20)
- 2nd Degree Type I (Wenckebach) Φ PR is ***LONG* < *LONGER* < *DROP*** *QRS*
- 2nd Degree Type II Φ ***Same***, where there is a PR, but drops missing QRSs after some P waves
- 3rd Degree Φ PR is ***NOT the Same***

Rhythm	*Rate*	*Rhythm*	*P Wave*	*PR Interval*	*QRS*
Rhythms Originating in the Ventricles					
Premature Ventricular Contractions (PVCs) Low Risk Patterns: unifocal, occasional, isolated High Risk Patterns: coupled, bigeminal, trigeminal, quadrigeminal, R on T, multifocal	Normal, fast, slow	Irregular	Not usually identified in the premature beat	None associated with the premature beat	Premature, wide QRS > .12 and bizarre, with T wave opposite QRS
Ventricular Rhythm (Idioventricular)	20–40	Regular	Absent	Absent	Wide > .12 and bizarre, with T wave opposite QRS
Accelerated Idioventricular Rhythm	40–100	Regular	Absent	Absent	Wide > .12 and bizarre, with T wave opposite QRS
Ventricular Tachycardia	> 100 often 140–220	Regular	Absent	Absent	Wide > .12 and bizarre, with T wave opposite QRS
Torsades de pointes (Polymorphic Ventricular Tachycardia)	Not measurable	Iregular	Absent	Absent	Wide > .12 and bizarre, QRS direction varies from above baseline to below baseline
Ventricular Fibrillation	Not measurable	Iregular	Absent	Absent	Chaotic waveform, wide and bizarre

Rhythm	*Rate*	*Rhythm*	*P Wave*	*PR Interval*	*QRS*
Bundle Branch Blocks (identified by 12 lead ECG)					
Right BBB RBBB V1	Normal	Regular	Round, upright	.12–.20	• .12 sec • "M" shape / "rabbit ear" QRS in V1, V2
Left BBB LBBB V1	Normal	Regular	Round, upright	.12–.20	• .12 sec • "QS" pattern QRS in V1, V2
Pacemakers (AAI, VVI, DDD) 1st letter of pacer code, chamber paced 2nd letter of pacer code, chamber sensed 3rd letter of pacer code, response to sensing	Normal • May be programmed to any rate desired • VVI usual rate of 70 • DDD usual rate of 60 bpm, upper rate of 120	Regular when paced, may be irregular when instrinsic/own rhythm present	• May be present or not depending on pacer mode • May be upright or inverted after atrial pacing spike • Atrial pacing spike will be before P wave for paced beats	• Normal • Called AV delay • HOCM pts usual AV delay is < 100 msec	• > .12 sec • Ventricular pacing spike will be before QRS for paced beats • Biventricular pacing complexes may be normal and not > .12 sec (CHF pts)

Index